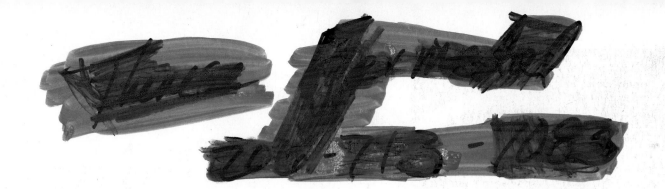

Medical Conditions and Massage Therapy
A *Decision Tree Approach*

Tracy Walton, LMT, MS

Wolters Kluwer | Lippincott Williams & Wilkins
Health

Philadelphia · Baltimore · New York · London
Buenos Aires · Hong Kong · Sydney · Tokyo

Acquisitions Editor: Kelley Squazzo
Product Manager: Linda G. Francis
Design Coordinator: Doug Smock
Illustrations: Dragonfly Media Group
Photography: Stephen Fischer, Eli Kowalski
Manufacturing Coordinator: Margie Orzech-Zeranko
Compositor: SPi Technologies

First Edition

©2011 Lippincott Williams & Wilkins, a Wolters Kluwer business.
351 West Camden Street   **Two Commerce Square, 2001 Market Street**
Baltimore, MD 21201   **Philadelphia, PA 19103**

Printed in China

Library of Congress Cataloging-in-Publication Data
Walton, Tracy.
    Medical conditions and massage therapy : a decision tree approach / Tracy Walton.
        p. ; cm.
    Includes bibliographical references and index.
    ISBN 978-0-7817-6922-8 (alk. paper)
    1. Massage therapy—Decision making.   2. Decision trees.   I. Title.
    [DNLM: 1. Massage—methods.   2. Decision Making.   3. Decision Trees.   4. Treatment Outcome. WB 537 W241m 2010]
    RM721.W23 2010
    615.8'22—dc22

                                                                                                    2010021072

DISCLAIMER

The information in this publication is not intended to be used by massage therapists to diagnose, prevent, or treat disease, and it does not substitute for medical care or constitute medical advice.

Care has been taken to confirm the accuracy of the information presented, and to describe generally accepted practices. However, the author, editors, and publisher are not responsible for errors or omissions or for any consequences from application of the information in this book and make no warranty, expressed or implied, with respect to the currency, completeness, or accuracy of the contents of the publication. Application of this information in a particular situation remains the professional responsibility of the practitioner; the clinical guidelines described and recommended may not be considered absolute and universal recommendations.

The author, editors, and publisher have exerted every effort to ensure that drug selection and dosage set forth in this text are in accordance with the current recommendations and practice at the time of publication. However, in view of ongoing research, changes in government regulations, and the constant flow of information relating to drug therapy and drug reactions, the reader is urged to check the package insert for each drug for any change in indications and dosage and for added warnings and precautions. This is particularly important when the recommended agent is a new or infrequently employed drug.

Some drugs and medical devices presented in this publication have Food and Drug Administration (FDA) clearance for limited use in restricted research settings. It is the responsibility of the health care provider to ascertain the FDA status of each drug or device planned for use in their clinical practice.

The publishers have made every effort to trace the copyright holders for borrowed material. If they have inadvertently overlooked any, they will be pleased to make the necessary arrangements at the first opportunity.

To purchase additional copies of this book, call our customer service department at **(800) 638-3030** or fax orders to **(301) 223-2320.** International customers should call **(301) 223-2300.**

Visit Lippincott Williams & Wilkins on the internet: http://www.lww.com. Lippincott Williams & Wilkins customer service representatives are available from 8:30 am to 6:00 pm EST.

9 8 7 6 5 4 3 2 1

This book is dedicated, as I am, to Sue and Clara.

About the Author

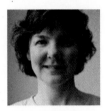

Tracy Walton is a massage therapist, researcher, and educator. She consults to hospitals, schools, and programs in integrative medicine. She has been in private practice since 1990, with a focus on clients with special medical concerns.

As a researcher, she has concentrated her work on massage therapy and cancer, including NIH (National Cancer Institute)-funded clinical trials involving massage by caregivers. Research partners include the Osher Institute at Harvard Medical School, Beth-Israel Deaconess Medical Center, H. Lee Moffitt Cancer Center, and Collinge and Associates. She maintains a bibliography of massage and cancer research on her Web site.

Tracy helped develop the award-winning film, "Touch, Caring, and Cancer," massage instruction for caregivers and partners. She is a frequent contributor to massage therapy publications.

Best known for her leadership and instruction in oncology massage therapy, Tracy also taught physiology and pathology at the Muscular Therapy Institute (now Cortiva Institute) in Cambridge, MA, for 13 years. There, she chaired the science department and served as Academic Dean. As an educator, she integrates the art, heart, and science of massage therapy. In 2003, the AMTA named her the Teacher of the Year.

Tracy holds an MS in biological sciences, with a concentration in biochemistry and cellular physiology. She received her diploma in therapeutic massage from the Muscular Therapy Institute.

Preface

Medical Conditions and Massage Therapy is for massage students, teachers, therapists, employers, standard-bearers, and ultimately for massage clients. At various times in my life, I have been all of these, and hold them in high esteem.

In 20 years of teaching, I have met many seeing, feeling, imaginative learners. Together we have navigated long lists of medical conditions and contraindications that aren't always easy to see, feel, or imagine. Actual clients make these conditions real, but "what ifs?" crowd the classroom: hypothetical clients and unfamiliar diseases with long, intimidating names. Massage therapy contraindications can be overwhelming, especially when there are many different presentations of a single medical condition and there is so much information to know.

I am mindful of the client on the other side of all that information, each condition, and each disease. My own clients have been my truest teachers, and their stories inspired this text. They have taught me about shifts in symptoms, changes in medications, and the deep and difficult experiences of illness. My clients have shown me how differently a single condition can present itself in different people.

This text prepares massage therapists for that range of real and hypothetical clients, and for multiple disease presentations. To that end, easy-to-use tools are presented for managing contraindications in any massage setting. These tools simplify massage planning. With a streamlined way to manage information, a therapist can better attend to the client: that whole, unique person, much greater than the disease, who has come for help, and to be touched.

THE AUDIENCE

This book serves all levels of massage students and therapists. The format makes it usable as a quick reference or as a textbook for deeper clinical thinking:

- As a text, it can be easily used in courses on pathology, massage technique, special populations, medical massage, or student clinic.
- As a reference, it can be consulted quickly in various settings, including the spa, the hospital, the student clinic, or the private massage practice.

No prior medical knowledge is needed to use this book as a text or a reference. Simple vocabulary and clear instruction help students and therapists at any level grasp what is important about a medical condition and how to work safely with it.

Massage teachers are always on my mind as I write. I know what it's like to teach at the edges of massage therapy and medicine. Even with substantial texts in the field, we are still defining how massage affects the body in health and disease. Massage teachers are uniquely responsible for the well-being of their students' future clients. They may feel pressured to

master a huge volume of information—medical conditions, signs, symptoms, and massage contraindications—and to be able to rattle it off on demand.

For those of you who teach, *Medical Conditions and Massage Therapy* can help change your role from an encyclopedia of medical information to a guide in the decision-making process. Liberated from having to have all the answers, you can teach concepts and information-gathering strategies rather than hard-and-fast data, use the general principles, and learn alongside the students as I have. Together, imagine a client scenario and then plot your course and massage plan. Students will then develop the invaluable skill of sorting it out on their own.

ORGANIZATION

The book is divided into three parts. Part I lays a foundation for good decision making, Part II discusses conditions organized by system, and Part III addresses two special topics—cancer and medical treatments—that are brought to bear on many conditions and body systems.

Part I—Foundations

In Part I, a framework for managing massage contraindications is presented. The Decision Tree—the central tool of the book and a roadmap for massage contraindications—is introduced in Chapter 1. In Chapter 2, massage adjustments are described in universal elements, such as pressure, joint movement, speed of stroke, contact, client position, whether a physician should be consulted before a session, and the therapeutic intent of the massage.

General principles for massage contraindications are described in Chapter 3. In Chapter 4, the steps of massage planning are carefully spelled out: questions for the client, information gathering, decision making, explaining the plan to the client, and charting. A sample client health form is introduced, a jumping-off point for conversation.

Chapter 5 presents strategies for involving the client's physician in the massage plan, laying groundwork for productive exchange about massage for the client. Several formats for good physician communication are offered.

Part I concludes with essential information for evaluating massage research (Chapter 6). Clear diagrams and language are used to demystify basic research concepts. This lays the foundation for using the massage research cited throughout the book.

Part II—Conditions by System

Part II (Chapters 7–19) is organized by body system. For each system, sample medical conditions are given full discussion, with complete, "pre-made" Decision Trees. Interview questions are presented for each condition, with massage guidelines based on the client's possible answers. Where available, support for massage is described in the form of research, theory, or clinical observation.

Space limits full discussion of every illness and injury, so each Part II chapter includes a substantial table of additional Conditions in Brief. There, conditions are summarized along with abbreviated interview questions. Massage therapy guidelines are described for common presentations of each condition.

Part III—Special Topics

Part III is devoted to cancer (Chapter 20) and the effects of medical treatments on the body (Chapter 21). Specific types of cancer are presented in Part II chapters by system. Chapter 20 addresses general patterns of cancer spread, cancer treatment, and the effects of treatment. Decision Trees, interview questions, and massage therapy guidelines are presented for typical sites of cancer metastasis and for standard cancer treatments.

Chapter 21 explains common medications and medical procedures in the same format, with Decision Trees and massage guidelines. Both Chapter 20 and Chapter 21 should be used to support specific conditions in Part II.

HOW TO USE THE FEATURES IN THIS BOOK

Several unique, classroom- and clinic-tested tools are presented to help students and therapists work with different conditions. The features presented here can be used in different combinations, all in the service of good decision making and customized massage therapy:

- *The Decision Tree.* This is a simple, visual roadmap for massage contraindications. It divides complex medical issues into small, easier-to-solve parts. It holds a range of client presentations for conditions as diverse as diabetes, hypertension, and prostate cancer. Clear action steps describe concrete massage adjustments for each symptom, complication, and side effect. Consult the pre-made Decision Trees in each chapter for quick highlights of the important massage concerns, or use the Decision Tree as a problem-solving format. The format is easy to learn and quickly becomes automatic, supporting independent thinking in unfamiliar territory. The Decision Tree provides rich detail, picking up where the statement, "Massage is contraindicated," leaves off. It answers the questions, "What is it about the condition that contraindicates massage?" and "What is it about massage that is contraindicated?"
- *The Pressure Scale.* A simple description of five basic massage pressure levels is offered in plain, accessible language. Each pressure level is shown visually and described in down-to-earth terms. Use it to specify the best overall pressure for a certain condition, or the maximum pressure on a specific body area. Many hospital massage programs and clinics are already using it to enhance communication among massage therapists, physicians, nurses, and clients. The pressure scale can be used as a standard in classrooms, clinics, and while working in tandem. It can simplify massage planning and charting.

- *Interview Questions.* Brief, purposeful interview questions are provided for each condition, with follow-up questions throughout the book. Each question is used to identify or explore a possible massage contraindication and is worded at a suitable level for students as well as experienced therapists. Start with the general health questions in Part I (Chapter 4) in a standard intake format. Use the follow-up questions for common health concerns such as pain, medications, injuries, infection, and even diagnostic tests. Questions are sensibly grouped and organized for easy use in fast-paced settings. Adapt the wording to your own personal style, and work these questions into a natural conversation with clients.
- *Massage Contraindications, Linked to Interview Questions.* Clear massage therapy guidelines are presented in specific terms. This text goes beyond one-size-fits-all massage contraindications, because these are often too broad for actual practice. Instead, customize massage contraindications to the client's unique *presentation* of a condition, based on your interview with the client.
- *Principles of Massage Contraindications.* Because a handful of principles are easier to remember than a host of diseases, they are easy to recall and use with a range of client presentations. Use the Vital Organ Principle anytime a major organ is functioning poorly. Use the Sensation Principle whenever sensation is compromised. With these, you can navigate a host of conditions affecting the vital organs (end-stage liver disease, congestive heart failure, or an advanced brain tumor) and a similar range of conditions affecting sensation (diabetic neuropathy, a spinal cord injury, or multiple sclerosis). Some principles have memorable names (The Cardiovascular Conditions Often Run in Packs Principle or The Ask If It's Contagious Principle). Other principles take the guesswork out of hidden conditions (The DVT Risk Principles, The Bone Metastasis Principle, and The Waiting for a Diagnosis Principle).
- *Massage Research.* Check these brief reviews of available massage research to see if there is evidence supporting massage for a condition. Data from clinical trials are summarized modestly, without overstating any claims. Here, research concepts from Chapter 6 are reinforced. To see additional research references, go online at http://thePoint.lww.com/Walton.
- *Possible Massage Benefits.* Even without research, one might make a case for the benefits of massage in certain conditions. Here, look for clinical observations and theories supporting massage for wellness, support, and companionship during illness and injury. There are no sweeping conclusions, just compelling, common sense.
- *Medications and Massage.* Specific drug treatments, side effects, and corresponding massage guidelines are discussed along with each medical condition in this book. But drug treatments change frequently, and massage therapists face a dizzying array of medications, procedures, and massage guidelines. To manage this information, this book supplies several tools: Table 21-1 gathers over 60 common drug side effects into an alphabetized list. Look up each side effect, such as nausea, flu-like symptoms, or bruising, for corresponding massage guidelines. You can also use the Four Medication Questions (Chapter 4) and the Medication Principle (Chapter 3) to decide how to modify the massage plan for a client's medications.

ADDITIONAL FEATURES

- *Therapist's Journals:* Brief, poignant stories of clinical practice, are contributed by massage therapists and written in the first person. These stories reinforce the concepts in each chapter.
- *Selected Clinical Features:* Innovative drawings of human figures show complex conditions such as Parkinson disease, muscular dystrophy, and breast cancer. Areas of the body that are affected by the disease are labeled with key signs, symptoms, and complications, along with factors to consider in the massage plan.
- *Self Test:* A set of study questions is provided at the end of each chapter.

Online Features

The following features are online at http://thePoint.lww.com/Walton:

- The Bibliography lists additional resources for each condition, along with available massage research.
- The Glossary provides definitions for key terms from the book (these terms are shown in blue type throughout the text).
- Detailed discussion and art (including Decision Trees) for four *additional* conditions: *eczema, diverticular disease, thyroid cancer,* and *cerebral palsy.*
- Answers to the Self-Test questions.

Instructor Resources

Online, instructors can find the following:

- Lesson plans with objectives and sample exercises for each chapter, including ideas for building Decision Trees in class.
- An image bank including all Decision Trees and other illustrations.
- The client intake form and physician communication formats, available in printable form.
- Blank Decision Trees.
- Principles of Massage Therapy Contraindications.
- Massage Therapy Guidelines for Common Side Effects of Medications and Procedures (Table 21-1).

CLASSROOM TESTING

I have shared the information in this book during two decades of teaching massage students, practitioners, employers, and teachers. The tools have been used successfully in a variety of settings, including spas, hospitals, massage schools, and private practice settings. The concepts have been taught in various courses: pathology, student clinic, special populations, massage technique, and theory courses.

These tools have been warmly received, often with a sigh of relief. There is no longer a need to memorize impossible volumes of information. The burden lifts, as the method is easy to learn and use. Sorting information in this format is straightforward. Once a clinical problem is laid out in a Decision Tree, the gaps in information need only be filled in with a quick search, a reference, a well-placed question to a client, or a focused communication with the physician. Where information leaves off, principles and good interview questions support the therapist.

A NOTE ABOUT LANGUAGE

Mention of specific massage therapy modalities in this text is minimal, and it's a deliberate omission. For one thing, modality names are not always descriptive, and we don't all agree on their meaning. I have watched therapists argue vehemently over exact pressures and strokes, even when they studied with the same teacher! Although these variances reveal a rich, textured, and dynamic profession, the language for describing it can be confusing.

Instead of modality names, I use more descriptive language and divide massage therapy into its elements: contact, pressure, joint movement, duration, client position, speed, rhythm, and so on. In turn, I steer clear of the debate over terms such as "relaxation massage," "therapeutic massage," and "medical massage." These terms are still being sorted out in the profession.

Throughout this book, massage therapists are referred to as "therapists" or "practitioners." I use "he" and "she" interchangeably to describe therapists, other health care providers, and clients. Health care providers are usually called "physicians" for simplicity, even though a therapist might consult with a client's nurse or nurse practitioner, physician's assistant, or other provider, depending upon the situation.

Under "Massage Research," the benefits of massage for a given condition are supported with research data where available, but a critical analysis of each study is beyond the scope of this book. I tend to use "Research *supports...*" or "Research *suggests,*" rather than "Research *proves...*" to more accurately reflect the available data.

Under "Massage Benefits," any statements about the helpfulness of massage are based on my own observations, others' clinical stories, and common sense. Please take care not to confuse my own opinions with fact or with well-researched outcomes.

COMTA

As of this writing, schools and programs served by the Commission on Massage Therapy Accreditation (COMTA) are required to address six competencies. The concepts in this book support many elements in competencies 1, 2, 5, and 6. There is significant emphasis on the first COMTA competency, planning and organizing a session. Elements of competency 2 (performing massage therapy and bodywork for therapeutic benefit) are addressed in the foundation chapters as well as in specific conditions. Elements of competency 5 (professional referrals and relationships) and competency 6 (research literacy) are reviewed and reinforced throughout this text.

A WORD OF CAUTION

I have made extensive efforts to ensure that the information about each condition in this book is accurate, but medical information changes constantly, and authorities in the massage field have reasonable differences in opinions about the safest, most effective massage approach in each case. As with any textbook, it has not been possible to account for the unique aspects of each client's individual condition. This is particularly true of Conditions in Brief tables that appear in Part II of the book.

As you make your massage plan, I urge you to consult and compare information from multiple sources. If there is any doubt, work conservatively, and direct a focused question to a client's physician, where possible. The more we do this, the more we cultivate productive partnerships with other health care providers.

INTUITION, CONFIDENCE, AND MASSAGE

This book will help therapists get to their destination—the massage table—with purpose and confidence. Good information management and clinical decision making have a powerful place in the daily life of the massage therapist, and acquiring these skills doesn't have to be grinding or difficult. With the right tools, honest work can be pleasurable, even joyful. I've watched therapists, initially intimidated by vast information about a disease, develop mastery over familiar conditions, and soon they are able to extend their skills to unfamiliar conditions with ease. They move almost effortlessly across the Decision Tree.

There is great satisfaction in this process. And best of all is the beauty of the end-product. Once any concerns and contraindications are laid to rest, massage therapists are free to practice with intuition and full presence. With sound clinical thinking, they clear a path for a session with the best of touch, full contact, and heart. Real connections are formed. Therapists provide caring, corrective touch. Clients are healed and inspired. They are fully seen, felt, and heard. This is massage therapy at its best.

Tracy Walton
Cambridge, Massachusetts

Reviewers

Donna Kenny
TESST College of Technology
Towson, Maryland

Thomas Filippi
Morgantown Beauty College
Miami Beach, Florida

Wendy Stone
Muscular Therapy Institute
Cambridge, Massachusetts

Jan Schwartz
Education and Training Solutions, LLC
Tuscon, Arizona

Lisa Mertz
Queensborough Community College
City University of New York
Bayside, New York

Nancy Mezick Cavender
Rising Spirit Institute of Natural Health
Atlanta, Georgia

M.K. Brennan
Charlotte, North Carolina

Acknowledgments

Many people contributed to this text. I am beyond grateful to Linda Francis, my managing editor. Your marvelous sense of humor, endless encouragement, and long view kept me on course, and you are a master at helping make vision into matter. I am also indebted to Betsy Dilernia, my development editor, who mined each chapter for its essence and held the detail and the larger picture at once. Your line editing served me from the first proposal to the very last edit. To the compositor, Ramya Vasudevan, thank you for your sharp eyes, warmth, and professionalism in managing this work to completion. Pete Darcy and John Goucher showed great faith and good sense in this project, as have others at Lippincott Williams & Wilkins: Tanya Martin, Jennifer Clements, Nancy Evans, and Susan Katz. Thank you.

To Sue Mapel, who shared this load with careful edits and perspective, your gifts are remarkable. Your patient cheering edged the manuscript along, and your care and influence are in every line. To Erika Slocum, my research assistant, you kept things running on track, with endless good cheer and organization. You and your enthusiasm arrived at just the right time. Jennifer Green, you filled in patiently and seamlessly, and I'll always be grateful. Stephen Fischer and Eli Kowalski: you provided skilled photography and artful reimaging. Dragonfly Media Group: thank you for your careful, wonderful artwork, and for the humanity you infused into each human form. And to the massage therapists/models—Christine Blake, Stephen Fischer, Algecira Garcia, Devon Leera, and Mica Rie—I appreciate the heart and focus you brought to your work.

I am deeply grateful to Ruth Werner. You all but badgered me to write this text, blazed the trail, and set the example of what was possible. And Gayle MacDonald: thank you for the shared path, vision, care, and purpose. Jean Wible: your textbooks on pharmacology and massage are invaluable, but so is your time; thank you for your many kind eleventh hour consultations.

To the reviewers of this text: you were faithful to the task and forthcoming with great suggestions. Your warm reception meant the world to me. I am grateful, too, to the massage therapists who offered stories about their work, in the form of the Therapist's Journal. When I asked for your help, I received a flood in response. You told your stories with sincerity, style, and deep compassion. There wasn't room for them all in this edition, but each story moved me, and I have held it in my heart.

My students: you inspired and encouraged me along the way. I hope the finished product honors your work as much as you do. To Lee Carpenter: thank you for your all-around kindness and your support for massage therapy and my own efforts.

The community at the Muscular Therapy Institute and Cortiva Institute provided a generous spot to grow up in and a place for warm encouragement. My deepest thank you to those who have shaped my path, including but not limited to Joelle Andre, Erika Baern, Sheila Carroll, Robin Cassel, MaryAnn DiRoberts, Susan Hollister, Barbara Nill, Dianne Polseno, Anne Sheehan, Wendy Stone, Jan Stott, Rick Thompson, Elizabeth Wirth, and Susan White. To Ben Benjamin, the founder of the school: you have been a fabulous teacher, mentor, and friend. And thank you to the many massage instructors I've worked with in the last 20 years. You understand the challenges and joys of teaching and writing in this wonderful and quirky field.

Writing doesn't get done unless the right people are looking after other things. Thanks are due to Anna Geer, MaryAnn Kowalski, and Aren Stone, along with many other neighbors, family, and friends who took wonderful care of my daughter. Adam Frost: thank you for keeping my computer running; I worked it pretty hard.

Moral and physical support also came from Nancy Keyes, K.S. Tsay, Edgar Miller, Maureen Bruno Roy, Rebecca Herrmann, Cathy Thomasen, Christine Moriarty, Marilyn Yohe, Lucille Petringa, Susan Montgomery, Nina Carmel, Yaron Carmel, Stephen Fischer, Will McMillan, Leigh Steel, Joannie Wales, Luata Bray, Lee and Pete Whitridge, Mary Sbuttoni, Mary MacKinnon Boyd, and from my family, which is made up of way too many Waltons and other loved ones to list. Nearby, Bill and Gail Mapel saluted each effort and every milestone. All of you have been close at hand and close to my heart, and for that, I am lucky.

To my clients: your spirits and stories have guided my thoughts on paper and in the classroom. Thank you for your voices, and for walking with me.

A *very* long time ago, three teachers—Darby Giannone, Mary Ellen Henderson, and Bonnita Stahlberg—taught me to love writing things down. As teachers do, you all planted and cultivated without knowing what might come up years later. Your patient instruction still reminds me that teaching is magic, passed along. Thank you.

Contents

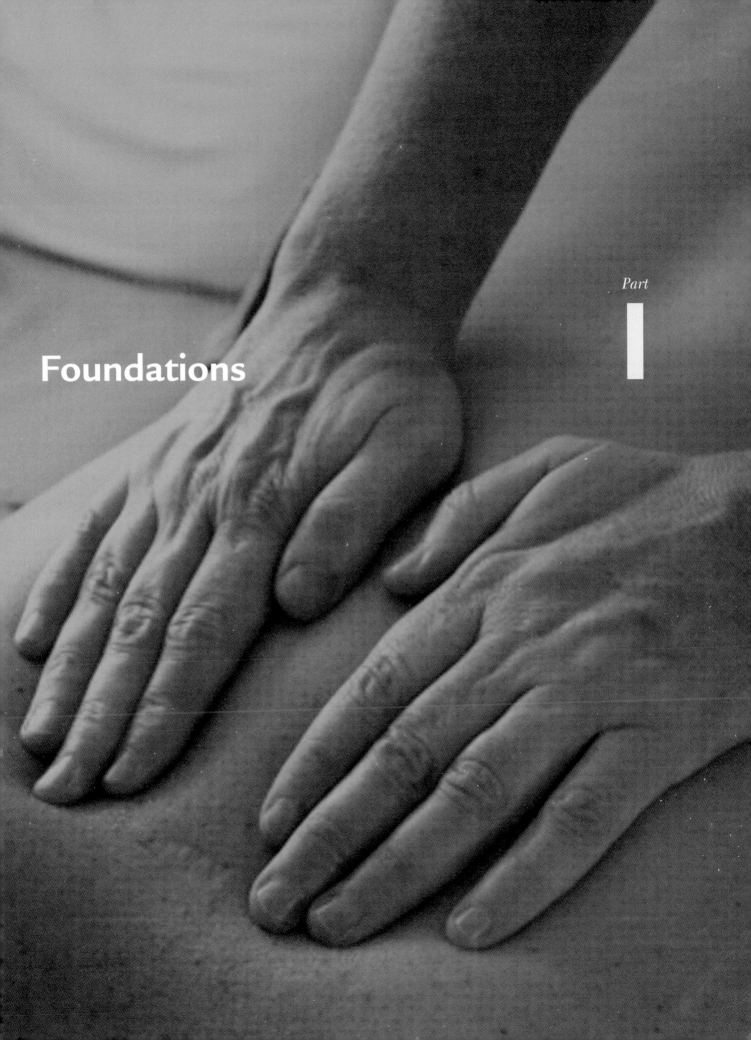

Foundations

The secret of getting ahead is getting started. The secret of getting started is breaking your complex overwhelming tasks into small manageable tasks, and then starting on the first one.
—MARK TWAIN

Massage therapists work with a range of clients, in a variety of settings. The steady growth of interest in massage therapy has moved it firmly into corporate wellness centers and sports venues, airports and hospitals, salons and vacation spots.

This wide range of settings makes massage therapy available to a broad clientele: those in frail health, those who are robust, and everyone in between. At the same time, people are living longer, continuing to function with more illness and injury. Even spa and sports massage therapists see clients with increasingly complex medical conditions.

Across the diversity of massage settings, intake procedures vary: from a single, verbal question about the client's health to a much longer written intake form and interview, combined. Either approach may bring a great deal of medical information to light. Yet no matter how complex a health picture is, there are simple ways to evaluate it, determine any massage contraindications, and arrive at a sensible massage plan.

The Decision Tree presented in this chapter is used throughout the book. It helps the massage therapist simplify an elaborate clinical problem by breaking it into smaller, more manageable pieces. The tree provides a place to arrange relevant information, and follow up on it. Massage therapists can then quickly fill in any gaps in information, identify massage guidelines for an illness or injury, and plan the best session for the client.

The Decision Tree

For some medical conditions, there are just one or two massage adjustments to make. An old back injury might require a slight position change, or a cold with fever could mean rescheduling the session. But more involved conditions require managing more health information, then adjusting several elements of the massage.

One way to do this is to draw a picture of the problem, and organize the information using a **Decision Tree**: a visual display of a medical condition, with guidelines for massaging safely. It shows

the problem and the actions to take. Massage therapists see key information and action steps in one place, and find it easy to use.

Figure 1-1 shows all of the possible information in a Decision Tree. Notice that the medical information is on the left, where the essentials of the condition, any complications, and medical treatments are organized.

Massage therapy guidelines are on the right. Guidelines include elements of massage to avoid or adjust, such as pressure, joint movement, or a client's position. Also on the

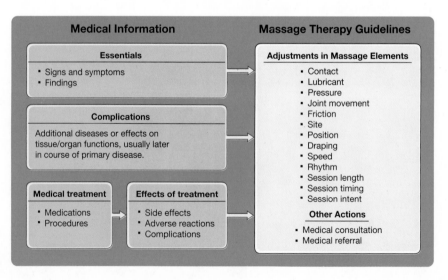

FIGURE 1-1. The basic information in a Decision Tree. Information about the client's medical condition is on the left side of the tree. Massage therapy guidelines for the condition are on the right. Arrows lead from left to right, linking the information and possible actions. This tree shows the thinking process involved in massage therapy contraindications.

right side of the tree are "non-massage" actions the therapist might take, such as consulting a client's physician or making a referral. Placing the medical concerns on the left and the massage precautions on the right draws a firm distinction between the types of information, as the therapist first considers them separately, then together.

The right side of the tree is focused on guidelines for massaging *safely*. It steers clear of indicated or *treatment-oriented* techniques, massage approaches designed to resolve the medical problem.

Together, the two sides of the Decision Tree give more detail to massage contraindications than traditional statements such as "Massage is contraindicated for X." It answers the questions, "What is it about a medical condition that contraindicates massage?" on the left, and, "What is it about massage that is contraindicated?" on the right.

The Left Side of the Tree: Medical Information

To someone with a medical condition—be it poison ivy, a knee injury, AIDS, or a heart condition—there are many layers to the experience. The condition itself is the first concern: the symptoms it causes, the discomfort or disability. Complications, or additional problems created by the condition, can also be a concern. The diagnosis and treatment of the condition are part of the experience, as well. All of these things make up an individual's unique expression of the disease or injury, which is referred to as the client presentation, or *clinical presentation*.

For a given medical condition, client presentations vary considerably. One person with a heart attack history is profoundly disabled by it, left unable to walk; another with a milder history is walking and running 20 miles a week. One person with AIDS is symptom free; someone else is fighting off one infection after another. One person has mild eczema, and another has severe eczema with open, weeping lesions.

The left side of the Decision Tree accommodates these variations and sorts the information into several boxes. Because diseases can present so differently in different clients, there is no single massage plan for a heart attack history, no "one-size-fits-all" approach to AIDS, and no single massage adjustment for eczema. The Decision Tree sets the stage for a customized massage plan for each client.

● ESSENTIALS

The top box holds the basics. It contains any relevant indicators, or factors that are evidence of disease. Signs, or outward indicators of disease (such as redness, a rash, swelling, or a lump), are listed in this box. Symptoms, or subjective experiences of disease (pain, itching, numbness), can also be in this box. This box may include lesions, or abnormalities in a tissue or organ. Lesions can be visible, or they can be things that are not seen or felt, such as a small tumor, a silent blood clot, or a change in a blood cell population that is not yet causing any symptoms. Some lesions might be detected only by a diagnostic test, such as a scan or laboratory analysis. These *medical findings* are also placed in the essentials box.

● COMPLICATIONS

The middle box contains complications. Sometimes a medical condition leads to another health issue that has "a life of its own" and can cause additional problems in the same person, separate from the primary disease. This is called a complication. A complication is also called a *secondary condition*. Examples of complications are:

- Infection from an open sore
- Metastasis (cancer spread) to a tissue, from a primary tumor elsewhere

- Depression during a long-term illness
- Pneumonia developing during a case of influenza
- Heart disease in advanced diabetes

● MEDICAL TREATMENT AND EFFECTS OF TREATMENT

Some medical treatments have strong effects on the body, and these are shown in two boxes at the bottom of the tree. All kinds of medical procedures and medications go in the Medical Treatment box: diagnostic procedures, such as surgeries or scans involving injections; preventive medications and procedures; and treatments, such as surgery or medication. The intention of medical practitioners is to minimize the unwanted effects of a treatment and maximize its effectiveness to resolve the problem. However, unintended negative effects do happen. Effects of Treatment are grouped in the second box; they include side effects, adverse reactions, and complications.

By definition, side effects of treatments are not all negative, but the term is usually used to describe negative effects, such as dry mouth from taking antidepressant medication. An adverse reaction is a strong, often allergic response to a medication such as penicillin. The terms side effect and adverse reaction are often used interchangeably. Side effects can be mild or severe, but adverse reactions and complications tend to be more severe.

A *complication of treatment* is similar to a complication of disease: it is an additional condition or disease that needs treating in its own right, but this time it results from medical treatment rather than another medical condition. If an infection develops after surgery, or osteoporosis develops from prolonged use of steroid medication, it is called a complication of treatment.

In massage therapy, it is more important to get the information on the tree, than to accurately classify it as a side effect, adverse reaction, or complication. However it is labeled, any negative effect of medical treatment goes in the Effects of Treatment box, so it can be considered in the massage design.

● WHICH BOX?

Sometimes it's not clear where to put a certain piece of information on the Decision Tree. Is something a complication, or is it part of the primary disease? Metastasis (cancer spread) is often the first factor in cancer that causes signs and symptoms (which go in the first box), but as a complication, it goes in the second box.

Indeed, some information could go in more than one box. In some cases, it's hard to determine the exact cause. Osteoporosis is one example. An individual could have osteoporosis because she is postmenopausal and there is not enough calcium in her diet. Or she could have osteoporosis as a consequence of long-term steroid medication. The massage therapist could put osteoporosis in the Effects of Treatment box next to the steroid medication that caused it. Or she could give osteoporosis its own Decision Tree.

Deciding which box to put medical information in should not be a source of stress for the therapist. Diagnosing the cause of the osteoporosis is not within massage therapy scope of practice. Instead, it's the therapist's job to adapt the session to the osteoporosis. (See Chapter 9 for a full discussion of osteoporosis and massage guidelines). Again, the important thing is to record the information *some*where and adapt the massage to it.

Ultimately a well-designed massage, customized for the client's condition, matters most. Outlining the condition in a Decision Tree is a reasoning process, not an end result. The Decision Tree process can help break down a large clinical problem into usable bits for following up. It can prompt the therapist to ask good questions in order to complete the tree. When a client mentions a medical condition, an empty Medical Treatment box begs further questions about treatment and any side effects. On the other hand, if a client mentions a medication in the interview, mentally put it in the box, ask what the treatment is for, and start a Decision Tree for that condition. Then fill in any gaps in information—does the condition cause any signs or symptoms, or have there been any complications over the years? A fuller, more accurate health picture emerges, with that client's unique presentation.

The Right Side of the Tree: Massage Therapy Guidelines

The right side of the tree contains guidelines for practice, unique to the territory of massage therapy. Here, appropriate massage therapy responses to each medical condition are described. Together with the left side of the tree, this side shows the flow of thought required to apply massage contraindications.

A **contraindication** is a medical condition or circumstance that makes a certain medical treatment inadvisable. For example, a history of a drug allergy is a contraindication for that drug. In the massage therapy profession, contraindications have described health conditions or circumstances in which massage is thought to cause injury or some other unwanted effect. Historically, lists of massage contraindications have included the common cold, cancer, or treatment with blood thinners. These conditions were said to **contraindicate** massage, to make it inadvisable.

However, in massage therapy literature and education, instruction hasn't always been clear on whether massage is contraindicated altogether, or whether it can be provided with precautions. The resulting confusion has made contraindications difficult to apply. As a consequence, individuals with these and other conditions have been refused massage entirely.

In practice, absolute contraindications to massage and touch are too broad and inflexible for everyday use, and it is seldom necessary to send clients home without massage. Only rarely is massage therapy fully contraindicated, and rarely is an entire massage modality, such as Swedish massage, fully contraindicated.

Instead, with most medical conditions, only fine-tuning is required, with small adjustments in the massage session.

This fine-tuning is reflected in how the term **massage contraindication** is used in this book, to describe a medical condition and the massage adjustments needed to work safely with it. The guidelines on the right side of the Decision Tree describe these specific adjustments. Together with the left side, the right side of the tree refines the picture of what is and isn't advisable for a client's condition.

The terms **massage adjustment** and *massage adaptation* are used interchangeably for common modifications to a session. In addition to hands-on adjustments, massage therapy guidelines can include consulting a client's physician for input, making a good medical referral, or handling an emergency.

For clarity, massage modalities or trade names of techniques are not used on the right side of the tree. Instead, massage and bodywork are broken down into generic elements, such as pressure, contact, joint movement, and the site of massage focus. These massage elements are explained fully in Chapter 2. A few of them are used here, to build a sample Decision Tree. Therapists adjust or adapt these elements according to the client's medical condition. Then, instead of saying flatly, "Massage is contraindicated," only some elements of massage might be contraindicated. These smaller adjustments to the massage reflect typical clinical situations. For example, there are times when *pressure* is contraindicated in a massage, but gentle *contact* would be okay. Sometimes joint movement and pressure should be avoided at a certain *site*, but would be safe anywhere else on the body. In some cases a massage should be shortened, or even rescheduled when a person feels better. For certain conditions, friction should be avoided, or a specific lubricant could aggravate a client's condition.

Building a Tree

Using eczema as a sample condition, we will build a Decision Tree from the beginning. We start with one branch and add on from there.

● ESSENTIALS: THE TOP BRANCH

Figure 1-2, the top branch, shows a massage modification for eczema. Eczema is a common skin condition involving inflammation, irritation, and sometimes open skin. It is described in

detail online at http://thePoint.lww.com/Walton. The Decision Tree for eczema is drawn using a simple "information-action" format.

Suppose a young client named Sam has the common, mild eczema symptoms described in Figure 1-2—dry skin with slight redness, some thickening and swelling, but no open skin. The first element for the massage therapist to consider is the *site* of the condition. Sam's condition appears on both wrists, and the therapist should avoid irritating those areas. The other

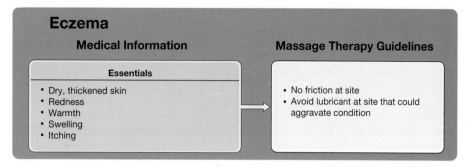

FIGURE 1-2. The top branch of the Decision Tree. Essentials of eczema appear on the left, and corresponding massage therapy guidelines on the right. A full Decision Tree for eczema is shown in Figure 1-6.

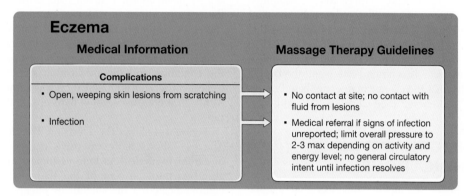

FIGURE 1-3. The middle branch of the Decision Tree. A complication, or secondary condition arising from the primary condition of eczema, is shown on the left. Corresponding massage therapy guidelines for the complication are on the right. A full Decision Tree for eczema is shown in Figure 1-6.

two elements of concern are *friction* and *lubricant*. Friction, which combines pressure and side-to-side movement across the skin, might inflame the area further. Some lubricants could also irritate it. The elements of massage to adjust are friction and lubricant at the site of the condition.

These three elements, combined together, are contraindicated for Sam's presentation of eczema—they are things *not* to do in a session. Decision Trees describe what to avoid or adjust in the massage. Within the limits of these massage adjustments, what is left for the massage therapist to do in the session?

Because the massage adjustments involve only the site of the eczema itself, most types of massage elsewhere on the body would be okay, including any kind of stroke, with any lubricant at any pressure. That's assuming Sam doesn't have other health issues that contraindicate massage elements.

Over the affected area itself, a gentle glide with a nonirritating lubricant might be well tolerated, and not aggravate inflammation. This depends on the individual. Contact with the skin—resting the hands or holding the area—should be fine. Brief stationary pressure, simply pressing in and holding without side-to-side movement, might be tolerated well. On the other hand, repeating this too much or too deeply could irritate the area.

Still, there is a lot left to do with this client: the rest of the body, or modified touch of the affected area. If the eczema is over a small area, the site-lubricant-friction contraindication is not at all restrictive. If the eczema is over a large area, the site constraint might be felt more by the therapist.

As already mentioned, the right side of the tree describes precautions—what is contraindicated or requires adjustment—not what is thought to be beneficial for the condition. Massage

elements outside of those restrictions are likely to be allowable and can be done safely with the given medical condition. Massage benefits for medical conditions are described elsewhere in the chapters ahead.

● COMPLICATIONS: THE MIDDLE BRANCH

Figure 1-3 shows what happens to the Decision Tree when Sam's eczema itches so much that it provokes an "itch-scratch cycle." People with the condition often scratch these areas, worsening the itching, and leading to repeated scratching that breaks the skin in the area. These open, leaking lesions are a complication of eczema, appearing in the middle box. When the skin is broken open, no longer providing an intact barrier between the external and internal environments, the individual is vulnerable to infection. Bacterial and fungal infections are additional complications that may develop when the skin is open, and these are also shown in the Complications box.

This tree now has two branches: a simple Essentials branch, and a Complications branch showing open lesions and infection. A single individual such as Sam could have an uncomplicated case of eczema with closed lesions, a complicated case with open lesions, or a complicated case with infection at those lesions. If he has eczema at more than one site, he could have combinations of those scenarios.

The middle branch of the tree describes these heightened massage concerns, with stricter massage therapy guidelines. In addition to friction and lubricant at the site, contact is contraindicated, to avoid introducing pathogens into the area

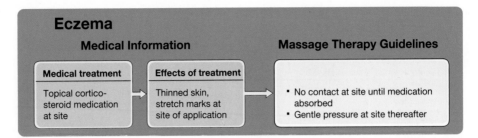

FIGURE 1-4. The bottom branch of the Decision Tree. Side effects on skin from corticosteroid medication are shown at left, with corresponding massage therapy guidelines on the right. A full Decision Tree for eczema is shown in Figure 1-6.

of open skin and causing infection. Direct contact with fluid from the lesions is discouraged, as well, to protect the therapist from infection. In addition, if there are signs of infection that the client hasn't reported to his or her physician, a medical referral is encouraged. If infection is present and being treated, general circulatory massage is contraindicated, and the overall pressure is limited to what the client can tolerate, based on his or her activity level and energy. (See Chapters 2, 3, and 7 for explanations of these guidelines.)

● RESOLVING CONFLICTING CONTRAINDICATIONS

When two contraindications on the same tree don't agree, the most conservative one—in this case, the *contact* contraindication—prevails. Suppose Sam has eczema with open lesions. His therapist doesn't concern herself with the friction precaution, or with finding the right lubricant, she simply avoids contact with the area altogether. Here's another way of explaining this important point: When there are multiple contraindications, the therapist recognizes a built-in hierarchy, and follows the most conservative adjustment or contraindication. Here, the fact that contact is contraindicated encompasses the other prohibitions against friction and lubricant at the site. If there are two distinct sites of eczema, one with open lesions and one without, then Sam's therapist follows the respective contraindication for each site.

In Sam's case, with open lesions, what is left for the therapist to do? As before, contact is permitted elsewhere on the body. If the eczema is only on the wrists and forearms, this leaves a lot of body area to massage, without precautions. If the eczema is distributed widely, the session is a little more limited. Wherever contact is prohibited, the therapist could use off-the-body energy techniques, or reflexive techniques on unaffected areas, such as the feet, hands, or ears.

● MEDICAL TREATMENT AND EFFECTS OF TREATMENT— THE BOTTOM BRANCH

Another component of an individual's health is the medical treatment of a condition. This adds two more boxes to the left side of the tree. The medical treatment itself goes in one box, and the effects of the treatment are in the neighboring box (Figure 1-4).

Suppose Sam has had eczema on both forearms and wrists since early childhood. The skin is thickened from repeated scratching. Because of the severity of a recent flare-up, a physician has prescribed corticosteroid medication (also called

steroid medication) to manage it. Corticosteroid medication for eczema comes in different strengths and has different routes of administration (oral and topical—applied directly to the skin). Treatment with corticosteroid medication is usually of short duration; longer-term treatment depends on the condition and the medication strength. In Sam's case, topical corticosteroid medication was administered over time. Although it controls eczema flare-ups, it also thins the skin at the site.

Figure 1-4 shows the Decision Tree for Sam's treatment. The tree shows more extensive massage adjustments than in earlier examples. As long as topical medication could be absorbed into the skin of the therapist's hands, contact is contraindicated at the site. If the client has thin skin, gentle pressure is required to avoid injury.

Figure 1-5 shows different medical treatments with different effects. Arlene, an older adult with severe, stubborn eczema, uses several treatments to manage it and control complications. In the past, she has taken repeated courses of oral corticosteroid medication, an approach that is in less favor today because of problems arising from prolonged use (see "Corticosteroids," Chapter 21). She takes antihistamines to control itching and uses newer topical drugs called immunomodulators to treat the eczema. In addition, she is completing a course of oral antibiotics to treat a complication of the eczema, a bacterial infection.

Each of Arlene's treatments carries its own massage therapy guidelines. Antihistamines tend to have few side effects, but drowsiness calls for a slow transition at the end of the massage. As with any topical medication, the therapist avoids contact with the topical immunomodulator until it's absorbed, and continues to avoid contact if the preparation causes burning at the site.

Prolonged use of oral corticosteroid medications can leave behind lingering systemic problems: thinned skin and mild osteoporosis. Gentle overall pressure is used in order to avoid injury to tissues. Oral antibiotics can cause gastrointestinal symptoms. Because Arlene experiences mild nausea and diarrhea, the therapist adjusts the massage for these symptoms.

The bottom branch of the tree is more extensive in Arlene's case than in Sam's, requiring multiple massage adjustments on the right side for multiple medical treatments on the left. The right side of the tree in Figure 1-5, Arlene's case, looks different from any of the previous trees for Sam.

Recall that Arlene's case also includes severe and stubborn eczema, and it may affect a sizable area of her skin. In this scenario, one might wonder whether any massage is possible at all. In fact, a massage with gentle pressure overall, with additional care at the site of the eczema itself, could be a wonderful source of stress relief for this client. The portion

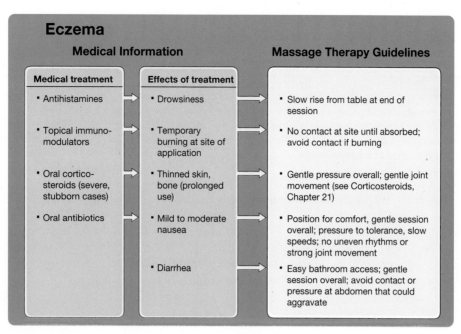

FIGURE 1-5. The bottom branch of the Decision Tree: multiple treatments. Common treatments for eczema, with corresponding side effects, are shown on the left, along with appropriate massage therapy guidelines on the right. Note that multiple treatments require multiple massage adjustments. A full Decision Tree for eczema is shown in Figure 1-6.

of her body affected by eczema seems "off-limits," but as the condition improves or worsens, more or less touch may be possible on these areas. Individual clients respond differently to contact, pressure, drag, or different lubricants. A therapist and client who work together over time will find out which elements of massage are best.

Changing the Medical Elements, Changing the Massage Elements

Notice that the right side of the Decision Tree changes with two very different client presentations. There is no single massage guideline for eczema; instead, there are several depending on the client. These individualized massage approaches allow the therapist to give each client an effective session, with as many elements of massage as possible, instead of following an all-encompassing contraindication to massage or touch. The details shown on the two trees reflect real differences in clinical situations.

When the client's medical condition changes, the massage elements change accordingly. The point of decision making is to gather information about the client's medical condition for the left-hand boxes, and use it to "move to the right side of the tree," where the massage therapy guidelines are shown. Thus, the therapist alters the massage plan according to the client's changing medical condition. Therapist's Journal 1-1 describes another example of different client presentations, with different massage approaches.

Individual Trees Versus Full Trees

So far, the Decision Tree examples have applied to individual clients with eczema, and customized massage guidelines appeared on the right side of the tree. Customized trees can be simple, with one branch, or they can be more involved, with all three branches filled in with information. An individual Decision Tree is unique to a client presentation, as in Sam's and Arlene's cases, above.

Typically, a therapist begins building an individual Decision Tree before the massage, after learning about the client's condition. It can be an informal process, as the therapist mentally sorts through the client's health information, or sketches out a tree on paper. Sometimes this process begins after the client is on the table, when the therapist observes something and asks the client about it, or when new medical information comes to light during conversation. Only that client's unique medical information is used for the tree.

In contrast, a full Decision Tree is more extensive. Instead of one client's clinical picture, it holds a whole spectrum of possibilities for a given condition.

This book contains many "pre-made" full Decision Trees for quick clinical reference. Each tree is devoted to a medical condition, and it includes some of the usual disease indicators and complications, typical treatments, and their effects on the body. Not every possible clinical scenario is captured in the pre-made trees in this book, but the most common scenarios are included, along with those most relevant to massage. A full Decision Tree for Eczema appears in Figure 1-6. It also appears online, along with a complete discussion of each branch.

A full Decision Tree can be a useful tool in massage therapy study as well as in clinical practice. Therapists can use the pre-made full Decision Trees in this book to anticipate client situations, and to jot down interview questions in case they

THERAPIST'S JOURNAL 1-1 *The Medical Treatment Box: Cardiovascular Disease*

I have two clients with cardiovascular disease who are perfect examples of adapting massage to medications. One of them is taking a strong anticoagulant medication, designed to reduce her chances of developing a blood clot, for example, in her leg. The other is taking baby aspirin, also to prevent clot formation. For the first client, the medication is so strong it "overshoots" a little, and instead of being at risk of clotting, she bruises and bleeds easily. Her physician is still adjusting the dosage, but meanwhile she needs gentle pressure in massage, to avoid causing bruising. The second client is only on a weak preventive medication and has no bruising or bleeding, so my usual strong pressures are okay for him except for at a couple of sites.

I had to question both clients carefully about their cardiovascular conditions, history, and treatments, using the interview questions in Chapter 11. There were other issues I had to ask about, too, but the medical treatments stood out. These two medical treatments—one weak, one strong—illustrated for me how useful the Decision Tree can be. Once I had filled in the Medical Treatment box and the Effects of Treatment, it became clear which massage adjustment to use for the woman taking strong medication—gentle pressure overall—and how that adjustment wasn't necessary for the gentleman taking aspirin.

Tracy Walton
Cambridge, MA

come up in practice. Therapists can also generate their own full Decision Trees as exercises, especially if they choose to specialize in certain medical populations. Generating the full Decision Tree in advance of a client's visit, or afterward in order to be better prepared for the next encounter—both approaches work. Therapists can keep copies of pre-made trees on file, then pull one for an individual client, use it in the interview, and highlight or circle key issues that arise from the client's answers.

With so much information, the full Decision Tree might overwhelm some therapists or students. Still, the tree can be a useful, time-saving device. It has most of the medical and massage issues worked out, and a therapist using it during an interview can focus on the information that is true for her or his client, ignoring the rest for the moment. Notice that both Sam's and Arlene's cases are represented on the full Decision Tree for eczema in Figure 1-6.

The Full Decision Tree and the Interview

No matter how much or little time a therapist has for an interview, the full Decision Tree can help it flow smoothly and logically. Looking at Figure 1-6, the therapist can proceed from top to bottom. The first box, Essentials, inspires these questions: "Where is it on your body?" "What are your symptoms?" and "Does it itch?" The Complications box raises the question, "Is there any open skin involved, or any fluid coming from the area?" The Medical Treatment box cues the therapist to ask, "Have you been treated for it in the past, or are you being

treated now?" "Are you taking any oral medications or using any medicated lotions?" "Have you used any of these things over the long term?" "How do the treatments affect you?"

The therapist may not need to ask each one of these questions; answers may come in the natural course of conversation. But the full Decision Tree provides a kind of checklist, so the therapist can be sure that the major areas have been covered. For conditions that are more hidden from view than eczema, this tool is especially useful.

Moving Around the Decision Tree

The Decision Tree provides a flow chart to show how information leads to action. There is a logical progression: It starts with the name of the medical condition, branches into more information about it, and ends with massage guidelines for that condition.

But a Decision Tree is not always built from left to right, or top to bottom. Sometimes the thinking process progresses out of order, and something from the middle of the tree emerges first. For example, during the client interview, a therapist finds out about a medical treatment before learning about the medical condition itself. The therapist fills in the treatment box first, but must backtrack to fill in the medical

condition. This is a common occurrence, because people often forget to report all of their medical problems in an interview. One common scenario occurs when asking about medications; clients may not recall every medical condition, but they will often remember when prompted by the medication.

In this case, the therapist's reasoning process moves backward *and* forward, and the end result is a simple massage adjustment for eczema and its treatment. By "sweeping" around the tree in this way, the therapist covers all the bases. Having laid any concerns to rest, the therapist can then focus on the hands-on work.

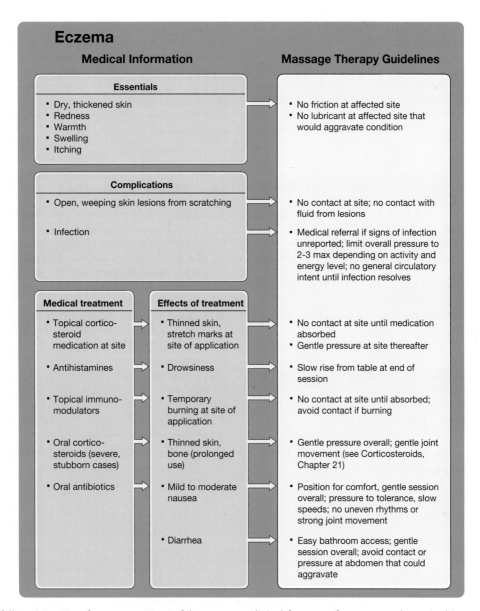

FIGURE 1-6. A full Decision Tree for eczema. Most of the common clinical features of eczema are shown in this tree. Using this tree in the interview, a therapist can highlight relevant areas to customize it to an individual client.

Using Decision Trees in Practice

A client with several health conditions will require several Decision Trees. Suppose a client mentions that he or she has high blood pressure and is taking a certain medication. The therapist will build a tree (and a few interview questions) for the high blood pressure and the medication. The client also has an old back injury that required surgery a few years ago. There might be a second tree (and a few interview questions) for the back injury. He or she has had asthma since childhood. There will be a third tree and interview questions for the asthma.

Constructing multiple trees may seem daunting to some therapists. Even building a single tree may require more time than is available to a therapist on a tight schedule. This is especially true in high-volume massage therapy settings, and in settings where there is only time for a quick verbal interview.

Without the benefit of interview time, written records, or breaks between sessions, a therapist may choose to use the Decision Tree conceptually rather than building each one on paper. From her or his basic questions about medical conditions and treatments, she or he can mentally complete Decision Trees for each condition, being sure to ask follow-up questions about each one (see Chapter 4).

With time constraints, the therapist can also use the pre-made Decision Trees in this book, along with the entries at the end of each chapter in Conditions in Brief. In Parts II and III of this book, there are common clinical features of each condition and massage therapy guidelines to follow. Interview questions are also provided. Although these may serve as quick references, they should *support* the therapist's understanding of each medical condition encountered in practice, rather than *substitute* for understanding.

Is it necessary to build a Decision Tree for every client, every condition, before he or she gets on the table? No. The tree is a tool, a means to an end. It is not the end in itself. For many therapists, the visual Decision Tree becomes automatic, and they think through the possibilities by picturing the diagram in their mind. However it comes to light, it is important to capture key health care information, in order to identify any corresponding precautions. The Decision Tree is a quick way to do so. It tells the story of a client's condition, and how that story should influence massage. The Decision Tree serves as a useful visual guide for directing the therapist's interview, clinical thinking, and, ultimately, the massage therapy session.

SELF TEST

1. List the types of information that go in the Essentials box on the Decision tree.
2. Define a complication of disease. Distinguish between a disease complication and a complication of treatment, using examples.
3. Describe the differences between a full Decision Tree and an Individual Decision Tree.
4. How can a full Decision Tree be used to generate an Individual Decision Tree?
5. When and how is a full Decision Tree typically generated? An Individual Tree?
6. What is a guideline for resolving two conflicting contraindications on the same tree?
7. In which box would you place complications of treatment? Complications of disease?
8. Indicate where you would you place the following on the tree: a headache caused by medication, a concern about strong joint movement, pain from a recent injury, a blood clot following hip surgery, instruction to avoid contact during massage, sensation loss in the leg from multiple sclerosis, a guideline to reduce massage pressure, a side effect of a medication.
9. Can a side effect of high blood pressure medication and a complication of shoulder surgery be placed on the same Decision Tree? Why or why not?
10. Suppose a client has three different health conditions. Can these be collected on one Decision Tree? Why or why not?

 For answers to these questions and to see a bibliography for this chapter, visit http://thePoint. lww.com/Walton.

2 The Elements of Massage Therapy

Creativity is a lot like looking at the world through a kaleidoscope. You look at a set of elements, the same ones everyone else sees, but then reassemble those floating bits and pieces into an enticing new possibility.

—ROSABETH MOSS KANTER

Have you ever had a massage or bodywork session with a massage therapist, then another session of the same modality from a different practitioner? Chances are the sessions were very different, even if one therapist learned it from the other! Each therapist starts with basic ingredients or massage elements, then crafts a session using his or her own creativity and intuition. The beauty of massage therapy is that with each unique combination of elements, the practitioner puts his or her own signature on the massage session.

This individuality can lead to confusion when therapists try to talk about their work and compare techniques. For example, therapists may disagree about the right pressure to use in a certain modality, the right way to position a joint while doing a technique, or other practices, even though they trained together. Most massage therapists employ a variety of modalities, and author their own work in a way that distinguishes it from the work of others and the work they learned in school.

Massage is much more than the sum of its parts, but it is necessary to examine each part individually to determine whether it is safe or contraindicated for a given client condition. Because of the variation in how it's applied, "massage" is not a universally understood term, nor is "bodywork." Even the trade names of some massage modalities are not necessarily descriptive. Different professionals use terms and techniques differently. Massage therapy vocabulary is rich and diverse, but far from consistent across the field. For these reasons, it is rarely accurate to say that an entire massage modality, such as Swedish massage, is contraindicated.

Although the language of touch and movement does not always translate easily into words, with dozens of manual approaches to the human body, a common language becomes necessary. Nowhere is it more necessary than in the realm of contraindications.

Although the phrase "massage is contraindicated" is commonly used, it can mean many different things. The contraindication could refer to stretching, pressure, or even any touch at all, depending on the client's condition and the reasons for the con-

traindication. It could mean that a technique is contraindicated today, but may be safe tomorrow. It could restrict massage of a certain area, but not the rest of the body. The phrase "massage is contraindicated for X" doesn't necessarily capture all the possibilities of touch, nor all the ways the condition X can present in different clients. Recall from Chapter 1 that a single condition, eczema, presented very differently in two clients. The massage guidelines for the two clients differed, as well.

One way to clarify a massage contraindication is to view massage in terms of its elements, or to answer this question: How do the hands travel across the body? It helps to express the elements, or ingredients, of massage in plain, common language. This, in turn, refines massage therapy guidelines. Basic elements of massage are:

- Contact
- Lubricant
- Pressure
- Joint movement
- Friction
- Site
- Position
- Draping
- Speed
- Rhythm
- Session length
- Session timing
- Session intent

Sometimes these elements are modified for a client's medical condition. A massage therapist might lighten the overall pressure, or avoid stretching at a certain joint. He or she might slow down the speed of the strokes, or schedule a session at a time when the client's symptoms have eased.

In addition to these elements of the massage itself, there are two other actions a massage therapist might take. Although they are outside of the hands on session, they can still be central to a client's health and safety. The two actions are:

- Medical consultation
- Medical referral

Each of these elements and actions is explained more fully below, with examples of how they should be modified for certain medical conditions.

Contact

First and foremost, massage therapy includes contact with the client. **Contact** is touch, the meeting of the therapist's hands and the client's skin, clothing, or drape.

Contact of some kind is almost always indicated, regardless of the medical condition.

However, a small number of situations contraindicate contact with skin or even with the client's clothing or linens. Usually contagion is the issue—either the massage therapist or the client has a condition that could be transmitted by contact. Skin conditions such as lice and scabies are examples of this, and even a non-infectious condition such as poison ivy can be spread by contact with the plant oil. A client with a compromised immune system might observe strict contact precautions. Depending on the case, off-the-body techniques may be permitted until a physician or a nurse establishes when it's safe to resume touch as a condition resolves.

Lubricant

Sometimes contact, pressure, and other elements of massage are fine to use, but a certain massage **lubricant** is contraindicated. The ingredients in lotions or oils might irritate an individual's skin, or provoke a genuine allergic response. Some essential oils might be okay for one person but poorly tolerated by another. It may take trial and error to determine which ingredient is poorly tolerated. Once this is identified, another lotion or oil may be substituted, or the session may be performed without lubricant.

Pressure

To apply **pressure**, the force applied to a client's tissues over a given area, the practitioner transfers her body weight or strength through the arms and hands into the tissues. The result is that tissues are compressed or moved aside. Depending on how much pressure is used, the displacement can include skin, fascia, muscle, blood vessels, nerves, joint, and bone.

There are times when heavier pressures are contraindicated, but touch and the other elements of massage or bodywork are not (MacDonald, 2007). Often this is because the tissues are unstable. One example is when a client's blood does not clot properly, and bruising or bleeding can easily occur. In this case, gentler pressure may be safe. The therapist could use pressure that is comparable to applying lotion to the skin, without going any deeper.

Another example of a pressure contraindication is an area of impaired sensation, as in a client with a nervous system condition that affects the ability to feel. The therapist avoids deep pressures over the area, since the usual client feedback mechanism is missing. The client cannot feel how deep the pressure is, nor can he or she warn the therapist away from pressures that are too deep and could cause injury.

Of course, even the term "pressure" is subjective. Light pressure for one therapist or client could feel deep to another, because people have different sensitivities. While there is no universal agreement on the calibration of pressure, there are some ways to describe it that relate to common experiences.

● THE PRESSURE SCALE

For the purpose of discussion, this book uses a consistent scale of five levels of pressure. Each of the five pressure levels is described in terms of the movement of client tissues under the pressure, therapist body use, and common uses of the pressure in clinical practice. For simplicity, client perceptions and preferences do not figure in the descriptions of pressure; instead, the descriptions reflect therapist perceptions and preferences.

The five pressure levels are named and shown in Figure 2-1. They are:

- Pressure level 1: light lotioning
- Pressure level 2: heavy lotioning
- Pressure level 3: medium pressure
- Pressure level 4: strong pressure
- Pressure level 5: deep pressure

The first two pressure levels are commonly referred to by therapists as "light" or "gentle" pressure. The middle pressure level is typically called "medium" or "moderate" pressure. The last two are commonly described in the field as "deep tissue," "vigorous," or "hard."

Although it is not absolute, the scale makes conversation about massage easier. It is used in many facilities where multiple therapists share clients, and common language about pressure allows therapists to provide continuity of care to their clients. They use the pressure levels in charting and in communicating with nurses, physicians, other staff, and clients about massage. Therapist's Journal 2-1 describes the use of the scale in a large medical setting.

● PRESSURE LEVEL 1: LIGHT LOTIONING

In **pressure level 1**, or light lotioning, only the skin is moved by the therapist's hands. It describes the gentlest contact and glide across the skin. This pressure is commonly used by therapists to apply lotion or oil to the skin and spread it around, but not rub it in. For most therapists, it requires little strength in the arms and hands, although therapists inexperienced in light lotioning may feel tension in their arms and hands from the feeling of "holding back." This pressure level is the maximum used with severely medically frail people, such as those with easily damaged or bruised skin. Dawn Nelson and Gayle MacDonald describe this "lotioning" in their teachings with cancer patients and people in later life stages (MacDonald, 2005).

While light lotioning may sound "feathery," almost insubstantial, in fact it can and should be full and firm. Therapists resist the temptation to withdraw energy, presence, and contact from their hands, or the touch becomes partial and unsatisfying. Two consequences of this incomplete touch, "airplaning" fingertips and slightly lifted palms, are shown in Figure 2-2. Instead, a pressure level 1 uses hands resting fully on the skin, taking the shape of the client's tissues. Full, contouring contact, using the whole palm, fingers, and fingertips, provides the most meaningful touch.

Pressure level 1 is unique in that it is so gentle that slow speed is necessary to monitor it. Therapists move through gliding and kneading slowly, to ensure full hand contact without displacing more than the skin. Generally, this watchful approach is not necessary when using higher pressure levels.

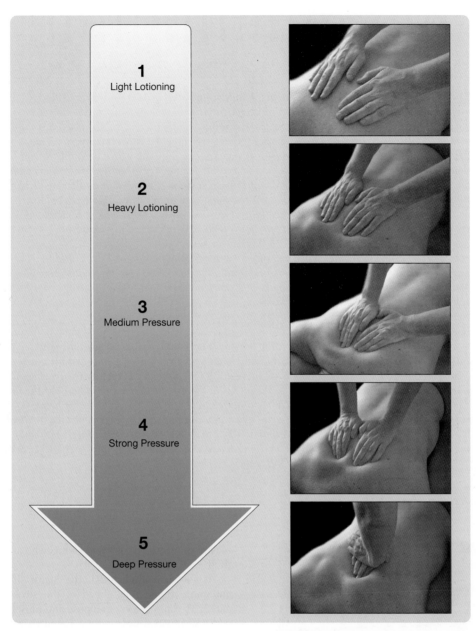

FIGURE 2-1. Massage therapy pressure scale.

● PRESSURE LEVEL 2: HEAVY LOTIONING

Pressure level 2, heavy lotioning, is a shade deeper than light lotioning; it is commonly used to "rub the lotion in" so that no excess lubricant pools or drips. Here, slight displacement of the superficial adipose layer and superficial muscle occurs, as seen in Figure 2-1. Unlike pressure level 1, slow speed is not necessary to monitor this pressure. It is less precise and gentle than level 1, so it can be applied at any speed. Think of rubbing sunscreen or body lotion into a small child's skin—after a bath or in a hurry on the way out the door! Pressure level 2 does not have to be delivered as carefully as level 1, and it involves pressing the lubricant into the skin to rub it in, rather than simply gliding across the skin as in level 1.

Heavy lotioning is commonly used to "introduce" the hands to the client's body at the beginning of a session, and to even out the lubricant. The firm, reassuring introduction is frequently followed by pressure level 3 in a healthy client. For most medically frail clients, it is the deepest pressure used in the session. Wherever it is used, it requires no leaning body mechanics or little strength in the upper extremities. Muscles of the arm are used only for contouring the hands and slight pressing in, gently compressing downward and displacing the skin ahead of the stroke.

Imagine the hands resting heavily on the skin through the drape, often quiet and still, at the beginning and end of many massage sessions. This "hello and goodbye" is often done at a pressure level 2.

● PRESSURE LEVEL 3: MEDIUM PRESSURE

Medium pressure, or pressure level 3, is an everyday pressure used to warm up the muscles in preparation for deeper work. It is commonly used in healthy clients, and may be the

THERAPIST'S JOURNAL 2-1 *Using the Walton Pressure Scale at MD Anderson*

We use the 1–5 pressure scale in our work with patients, families, and staff at MD Anderson Cancer Center. It's been a useful tool for charting—we have the numbers 1–5 on a chart and circle the ones used. Also, it's been a useful tool in communicating with physicians and nurses about our work, eliminating their concern about what we do.

Although we individualize the pressure for each patient, there are some trends in the pressures we use for different patient groups. In palliative care, we generally use just a 1. People come into the world with touch, and they want to leave with it. That level 1 and the simple hold can be just incredible for them. For patients in contact isolation, where we have to gown, glove, and so on, there are a lot of compromised systems. For them and other medically frail patients we will generally stick with 1's and 2's. In the ambulatory treatment center, we'll see inpatients coming in for treatment. Since they're ambulatory they are not as medically frail as some others. We'll look at their blood cell counts and other parameters and adapt our pressure. For them our slow effleurage will usually be at a 2 or 3—sometimes a 1 if they are more compromised.

Outpatients at our integrative medicine center will often receive a combination of 1's, 2's, and 3's. These are cancer survivors, folks who may be pretty robust. Caregivers and family members also visit the center, and they're often as stressed as the patients if not more so. Many of them already receive massage at home. Barring other health problems, they receive a range—usually 3's and 4's, occasionally 5's.

Of course, there are site-specific pressure adaptations, too, and we are gentler near incisions, sites of pain, and over bone metastases.

The pressure scale has been of great use in expanding our work across the center. Physicians who see the five numbers and descriptors, with just 2's circled, can know not only what pressures we are using, but also pressures we are not using. They can see, "the MT's are NOT doing this—a 4—with this patient." Therefore they feel reassured about sending them to us. The pressure scale is really basic. We all knew the pressures we were using but the pressure scale helped us put it all together in five levels of touch. Unlike other aspects of massage—whether it helps, how it helps, the basis of energy work, and other sticking points that arise when you put massage in a conventional medical setting, the pressure scale is really noncontroversial—there's nothing to dispute. It just describes what we've already been doing.

With these simple descriptions, patients, families, and physicians can all see better how we'll take care of people here.

Curtiss Beinhorn
Houston, TX

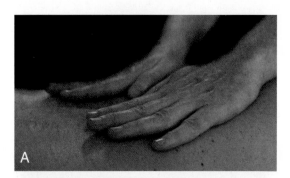
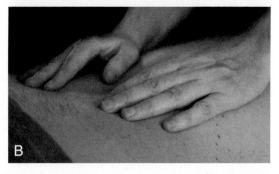

FIGURE 2-2. Incorrect application of pressure levels 1 and 2. (a) slight "airplaning" of the fingertips is evident from the shadows formed at the fingertips. (b) lifting of the palm partially cups the hand, losing the reassuring fullness of good hand contact.

maximum pressure for some clients who are ill, depending on their level of function.

As shown in Figure 2-1, the hands sink in more deeply, and more tissue rolls ahead of the stroke than at levels 1 and 2. Medium layers of adipose and muscle are moved, along with the blood vessels within. Often therapists use level 3 in their warm-up petrissage, as pressure levels 1 and 2 may not provide the grip necessary to squeeze and lift the tissues in the kneading motion.

Several features of pressure level 3 distinguish it from the lower pressure levels. Using a level 3, the therapist observes that massage in one area causes adjacent tissues, including joints, to move or rock slightly with the pressure. For example, massage of the gluteal muscles at this pressure will often passively extend the hip, pressing it into the table or mat. Using medium pressure in lateral movements across the gluteal muscles, the therapist may notice the client's hip joint rotating slightly, rocking the thigh with it.

Another important characteristic of medium pressure is the strength or weight needed to deliver the pressure. In contrast to the easy lotioning of levels 1 and 2, level 3 requires most massage therapists to draw on upper body, arm and hand strength or good body mechanics, with a transfer of the therapist's weight into the tissues.

Depending on how it is used, pressure level 3 may step up the intent of massage. In many Western massage therapy traditions, stroking (effleurage) and kneading (petrissage) at medium and deeper pressures have been believed to increase blood circulation. Because larger blood vessels appear to be compressed, therapists use pressure levels 3 and above with the intention to increase circulation at a single site, or throughout the body. The implications of this are discussed in the massage intent section of this chapter.

● PRESSURE LEVEL 4: STRONG PRESSURE

Pressure level 4, strong pressure, moves deep layers of adipose, muscle, blood vessels, and fascia. Some practitioners use it to focus on areas of muscle tension; others release restrictions in deep layers of connective tissue, including scar tissue. Although there is not yet consensus in the massage profession about the exact meaning of "deep tissue work," most therapists who describe their work as deep tissue are working at pressure level 4 and above. More tissue is compressed and moved aside than at level 3. At lower pressures, most therapists can get by with either upper body strength or good body mechanics; pressure level 4 typically requires both. Therapists may use flats of hands and fingers, or switch to smaller, sharper contact points such as fingertips, knuckles, forearms, or elbows to deliver more focused work.

Most therapists need to lean the body weight into the palms to deliver pressure level 4 in a gliding stroke. However, keeping the fingertips sunk into the tissues can be challenging, requiring finger strength to maintain strong pressure throughout the hands. In some cases, as in Figure 2-1, the palms may lift off slightly to provide the best angle for the fingertips to deliver the pressure. Kneading at this pressure requires substantial hand strength, and most therapists develop this strength after conditioning the muscles during massage training and practice.

Pressure level 4 is commonly used with healthy clients preferring strong overall pressure, and to release restrictions in connective tissue. When it is applied to the soft tissues, the movement of adjacent joints is easily noticeable.

● PRESSURE LEVEL 5: DEEP PRESSURE

Along with pressure level 4, pressure level 5, deep pressure, is used by therapists who describe their work as "deep tissue." This level addresses the deepest layers of muscle and fascia, compressing them against the bone, pushing them aside or ahead of a gliding stroke. Pressure level 5 significantly compresses the tissues; even in the thickest tissues such as in the gluteal area, the bones of the therapist's hands meet the bones of the client's pelvis, and the two move together as a unit. Adjacent tissues often move dramatically with pressure level 5, and the joints will rotate, rocking the limbs or the spine. This pressure is reserved for healthy clients who prefer the

deepest general pressure, or who request focused work on deeper tissues in problem areas.

To work at the deepest level of pressure, a therapist requires excellent body mechanics, and significant strength in the upper torso, arm, and hand. Changes in hand position are often used: Therapists often "stack the hands," bracing one hand with the other as shown in Figure 2-1, or use smaller surfaces such as knuckles, forearms, and elbows. These positions typically make it easier to sustain the deepest pressure over time, and allow the therapist to direct the same amount of body weight and strength into a smaller area.

● A FINAL NOTE ON PRESSURE

The five-level massage therapy pressure scale is not an absolute quantification of massage pressure, or an attempt to impose a rigid standard on therapists. Because pressure is subjective, it is delivered differently by different practitioners. One therapist may have to use effort to deliver medium pressure, while another may easily deliver deep pressure. Moreover, therapists apply pressure to a variety of body types and tissue compositions. In working in an area of high muscle or fat composition, a therapist may use the effort of pressure level 4 to observe a tissue displacement of pressure level 3.

Each of the five levels represents a range, not a narrow measurement, and therapists may find occasional overlap between levels. These variations are to be expected. Rather than an all-encompassing measurement, the five levels express, on a continuum, patterns that are common to many therapists' work. These patterns are derived from observing hundreds of practitioners over years of teaching and practice, and noticing a great deal of agreement in their descriptions of pressure. Many, not all, therapists start using body strength and mechanics when they use pressure level 3. Many, not all, therapists warm up muscles with this pressure. Many, not all, therapists using level 4 or 5 call it deep tissue work.

Standardization in the field may be forthcoming, and may quantify massage pressure in absolute terms, using sensitive equipment. Therapist's Journal 2-2 describes how two therapists, sharing a practice, standardized their pressure in pounds, and then used this system with a variety of client populations.

The 1–5 pressure scale is used throughout this book to describe massage therapy guidelines—when a therapist should stick to a level 1 or 2 over a certain area, or when it seems like the client's condition could tolerate a level 3 overall. These instructions appear on the right side of the Decision Trees and in each Massage Therapy Guideline section. The five levels are useful shorthand in future chapters.

In Table 2-1, each pressure level is described in terms of the depth of the tissues displaced or compressed, the therapist's body use required to deliver that level of pressure, and common uses in massage therapy and everyday life.

Joint Movement

There is a movement aspect to many forms of bodywork, and joint movement is a change in the angle of a joint during massage. The movement can be deliberate or unplanned. Stretching is an example of deliberate movement. So are other

passive movements, such as range of motion or fulcrum techniques. Therapists use these moves to lengthen soft tissues, such as muscle or fascia, but in the process also to move the involved joints.

TABLE 2-1.	FEATURES OF THE FIVE MASSAGE PRESSURE LEVELS

Pressure Level 1: Light Lotioning

Tissues displaced	• Slight skin movement only
Therapist body use	• Little hand strength needed, just for contouring • Use of arms and hands; little upper extremity strength required; no leaning body mechanics required
Common uses	• Applying and spreading massage lubricant • Maximum pressure for clients who are severely medically frail, with highly unstable tissues
Notes	• Slow speed is required to monitor this pressure level • Tendency to go too lightly at this level can result in incomplete hand contact; full, firm contact is important to maintain, taking the shape of the client's tissues

Pressure Level 2: Heavy Lotioning

Tissues displaced	• Slight movement of superficial adipose tissue and muscle
Therapist body use	• Little hand strength needed, just for contouring • Use of arms and hands; little upper extremity strength required; no leaning body mechanics required
Common uses	• Distributing massage lubricant evenly; rubbing in excess • Introducing the therapist's hands to the body at beginning of session • Maximum pressure for most medically frail clients
Notes	• Everyday use of this pressure: rubbing in lotion or sunscreen • Tendency to go too lightly at this level can result in incomplete hand contact; full, firm contact is important to maintain, taking the shape of the client's tissues

Pressure Level 3: Medium Pressure

Tissues displaced	• Some movement of medium layers of adipose tissue, muscle, and blood vessels • Slight movement of adjacent joints may occur with this pressure; for example, neck may rotate a few degrees when pressure is applied in strokes along shoulder
Therapist body use	• Upper body and upper extremity strength or good body mechanics (transfer of therapist's body weight into tissues) necessary to achieve this pressure • Some hand strength is necessary for kneading at this pressure
Common uses	• In healthy populations, used to warm up the tissues and prepare them for deeper pressures or more focused work • Maximum pressure for some clients who are experiencing illness, but are mobile and can participate in some activities of daily living
Notes	• Often used as an "everyday" pressure by practitioners of many modalities, especially in effleurage and petrissage • Effleurage and petrissage at this pressure (and higher) have traditionally been believed and intended to increase circulation

Pressure Level 4: Strong Pressure

Tissues displaced	• Movement of deep layers of adipose tissue, muscle, blood vessels, fascia • Movement of adjacent joints is noticeable with this pressure; for example, hips rotate and thighs roll during hip massage, and significant depression (1–2in.) of the scapula occurs when upper trapezius is pressed inferiorly at this pressure
Therapist body use	• Substantial upper body strength and good body mechanics (transfer of therapist's body weight into tissues) necessary to deliver this pressure with full hand • Substantial hand strength is necessary for kneading • Therapists commonly switch to fingertips, knuckles, forearms, or elbows to apply pressure with less effort
Common uses	• Frequently used in practice with healthy clients to relax tension in medium and deep layers of muscle • Used to release restrictions in connective tissue
Notes	• Often used by therapists describing their work as deep tissue or deep muscle therapy • Along with levels 3 and 5, effleurage and petrissage at level 4 have traditionally been believed and intended to increase circulation

(continued)

TABLE 2-1.	FEATURES OF THE FIVE MASSAGE PRESSURE LEVELS (Continued)

Pressure Level 5: Deep Pressure

Tissues displaced	• Movement of deepest layers of adipose tissue, muscle, blood vessels, fascia • Through compressed soft tissue, therapist engages the bones of the massage site with the bones of therapist's hand (or elbow, forearm, or other massage surface), and the two move as a unit
Therapist body use	• Significant upper body strength and excellent body mechanics (transfer of therapist's body weight into tissues) necessary to deliver this pressure with full hand • Often one hand must be braced with the other hand to deliver this pressure • Therapists commonly switch to knuckles, forearms, or elbows to apply pressure with less effort
Common uses	• Used with healthy, robust clients preferring the deepest pressure • Used to address deep restrictions in soft tissue
Notes	• Often used by therapists describing their work as deep tissue or deep muscle therapy, structural work, deep transverse friction, or mobilization of soft tissue • Along with levels 3 and 4, effleurage and petrissage at this pressure have traditionally been believed and intended to increase circulation

But joint movement is not always a primary purpose of a technique; some happens naturally as a secondary effect. During techniques such as kneading and stroking, the nearby joints flex, extend, or rotate with the other tissues. Even simple stroking techniques at a pressure level 3 on the low back can cause the spine to extend and flex, or the hips to rock gently. A therapist pressing or stroking the shoulder at medium or strong pressure observes rotation and recoil of the neck. For a client lying prone, repeated compressions of the gluteal muscles cause slight hip extension and movement of the lumbar spine. Whether intentional or unintentional, joint movement is usually a positive element of a massage session and can be deeply relaxing.

There are times when joint movement is contraindicated for a certain area. Movement contraindications could include a

THERAPIST'S JOURNAL 2-2 *Quantifying Massage Pressure in Pounds*

Years ago, my business partner, Christopher Deery, and I calibrated the pressure we use on a scale in our office. We established the levels of pressure we use during stationary compression, stroking, and even tapotement, by performing these massage techniques on a scale and noting the pounds used at each level. We even did this with the practitioner blindfolded. For example, I would observe the scale, ask Chris to "give me 5 pounds," then check the scale as he used tapotement, compression, and so on. Then he would apply the same pressure on my arm, then go back to the scale. Then we would switch.

We repeated the process so many times, and have used it for so long in our practices, that our pressure levels are standardized. Standardization makes several things easier: sharing clients, documenting pressure, and educating the physicians, athletic trainers, and physical therapists with whom we work at the hospital and the university. The orthopedic staff was particularly interested in our approach. A physician might be worried about a particularly frail patient if I told him "we used trigger point with that patient," but would relax when said we only used 0.5–3 pounds of pressure.

I have noticed that when Chris, who has larger hands than I do, uses 10 pounds of pressure, it will feel more diffuse than when I apply the same amount. And we have different ranges: Chris uses 0–68 pounds of pressure, I use 0–43 pounds. Usually I work in the 0–20 pound range. He uses 68 pounds of pressure rarely, but most notably on a 500-pound, 7'5" wrestler. Neither of us uses our elbows to work—you can't feel as much through an elbow. We have good body mechanics so we can stick with our hands, and usually anticipate when it's too much. The clients we work with often comment that we seem especially able to "walk the line" of delivering the absolute right amount of pressure without going too deeply. That line is the therapeutic level, where the most releases happen. I believe that our endless practice of pressure quantification—I can describe it in ounces—helps me walk that line more safely and precisely.

It is important to be patient with pressure, and follow the body's response to it before increasing it. Start with just 3 or 4 pounds of pressure and "hang out," or wait for a while. Minutes later you can then go more deeply because the tissues release to let you sink in further. When I used to train massage therapists, I did a "gelatin exercise." I would prepare cubes of gelatin 2.5 inches deep and 3 inches square, one for each student in a dish. Their job was to apply gentle pressure to the top of the cube, eventually touching the bottom of the dish without cracking the gelatin. In order to do so, they had to wait while their fingers warmed it, allowing them in deeper in slow stages. This exercise taught patience, good listening, and the need to gradually increase pressure.

Xerlan Geiser
Tulsa, OK

herniated cervical disk or bone instability, such as in advanced osteoporosis or cancer spread to bone. In some of these cases, massage is still permitted in the region as long as it does not move the area too much. The therapist works in a more contained way, avoiding large movements such as flexion or rotation of the neck in a client with a herniated cervical disk. When massaging a client with advanced osteoporosis, or when cancer has spread to the lumbar spine, it may be more appropriate for the therapist to focus the fingertips in circles on the gluteal or paraspinal muscles, rather than lean the body weight into the area, moving the spine.

Other times, any joint movement may be poorly tolerated, at any site. Joint movement may worsen a client's nausea, or aggravate a headache. In this case, joint movement is generally restricted.

Friction

The common word "friction" calls up an image of rubbing hands together to warm them up. Fires are started with the friction between two sticks. In massage therapy, **friction** is similarly created with back-and-forth or circular motions across tissues. Tissue is compressed, dragged, and stretched as the therapist applies pressure; it is displaced, then restored to its resting place. Wherever it is applied, the pressure used in friction is applied in two directions: vertically into the tissues and transversely across them.

Some motions are directed at superficial tissues such as the skin. Other motions such as *cross-fiber friction* or *transverse friction* are directed at deeper tissues such as tendons, ligaments, and fascia. In deeper friction, the hand catches the skin and upper layers and moves deeper tissues across even deeper ones, generating heat between them.

While friction stands alone as a technique, it is also a component of other massage techniques such as petrissage and effleurage. Both of these strokes generate friction in the skin or deeper tissues, depending on the pressure used.

Friction creates heat, local **vasodilation** (widening of vessels), and **hyperemia** (increased blood flow) in affected tissues. It is often observable as warmth and redness at the skin level. This mild, fleeting inflammation may be a secondary effect of a technique, or an intended effect. At the site of a soft tissue injury, this therapeutic inflammation is thought to loosen scar tissue; reorganize a mass of tissue fibers into stronger, more parallel configurations; and bring blood to the area for restoring the tissues.

Whatever the intent, friction is contraindicated whenever it would worsen inflammation, and friction with pressure is contraindicated wherever that pressure is contraindicated. Experienced therapists may use friction therapeutically for injuries and bypass some contraindications, but therapists using basic massage should respect existing inflammation, not compound it with friction.

Site

As a massage element, **site** refers to a region of the client's body or tissues being considered or addressed in the massage design. If it is an area of concern for the massage therapist, then it may be referred to as a **site restriction** (MacDonald, 2007). The medical condition that specifies the restriction is a *local contraindication* (Werner, 2009). For example, an area of eczema suggests a site restriction, to avoid friction at the site, and eczema is therefore a local contraindication.

An element of massage may be restricted at one or several sites, or it may even be restricted over the whole body, throughout the session. Such an overall adjustment in the session is called a **general restriction**, and the medical condition that calls for it is a *general contraindication*. (Some massage sources describe this as a *systemic contraindication*, but this book uses the term *general* rather than the term *systemic*.)

● SITE RESTRICTIONS/LOCAL CONTRAINDICATIONS

A site restriction cannot stand alone; it must be paired with another massage element to fully specify what to avoid. Massage elements to pair with site restrictions are:

- Contact
- Lubricant
- Pressure
- Joint movement
- Friction

Site restrictions are common in massage, and the massage therapy guidelines in this book are often confined to a single site. One example is a site of open skin, where the therapist avoids making *contact* with the area, and steers clear of any body fluids surrounding it. In another site restriction, massage *lubricant* should not touch some medical devices, such as a nasal cannula worn to deliver oxygen. An easily dislocated shoulder contraindicates *joint movement* at the site, and so on.

These are small, manageable adjustments in the massage session, and they are often obvious from the client's health information. "The Decision Tree" (Chapter 1) links this medical information with these adjustments.

● GENERAL RESTRICTIONS/ GENERAL CONTRAINDICATIONS

A general contraindication, limiting a massage element over the whole body, requires the therapist to be conscious of the restriction throughout the session. Instead of a small massage adjustment, isolated to a single site, the overall session is adjusted. For example, in the client who bruises easily, general pressure is restricted. In a client who is nauseated, the therapist slows the overall speed in the session, and avoids any deliberate or unplanned joint movement that might aggravate the nausea.

Distinctions between site restrictions and general restrictions are provided in this book when needed. It's important to determine when a contraindication limits the work in one area, and when the whole body must be treated with extra care. Table 2-2 provides examples of site restrictions and general restrictions.

TABLE 2-2.	EXAMPLES OF SITE RESTRICTIONS AND GENERAL RESTRICTIONS	
Massage Element	**Site Restriction**	**General Restriction**
Contact	• Open sore on skin • Avoid touching the area, but other areas are usually safe to touch	• Scabies (see Chapter 7) • No contact with client's skin or clothing until condition is resolved or no longer communicable
Joint movement	• Cervical disk herniation • Take care with movement at neck and shoulders, but other joints are safe to move gently	• Advanced osteoporosis (see Chapter 9) • Limit joint movement at all joints
Pressure	• Area of reduced sensation, such as in peripheral neuropathy (see Chapter 10) • Limit pressure at the site, but pressure is safe at unaffected areas	• Tendency to bruise or bleed, as in strong anticoagulant therapy • Limit pressure overall
Friction	• Inflamed area such as acne (see Chapter 7) • Avoid friction at the site, but friction is safe at unaffected areas	• Hives (see Chapter 7) • Avoid friction everywhere

Position

The massage element known as **position** is the placement of the client on the massage table, chair, or other surface. It also includes the use of any additional supports such as bolsters or pillows.

Most massage therapists are familiar with options for positioning the client, and they carry them out instinctively. Usually it's easy to act on a client's position needs by simply asking them about comfort and discomfort. For example, a client with restricted neck rotation could require a face cradle.

Other position adjustments are less obvious, or are good to anticipate and follow up during the interview. Medical devices attached to and inserted in the body, such as an insulin pump or catheter, may require bolsters around them or position changes. A client with a risk of swelling in a limb may need to have it elevated in a neutral position. The therapist needs to know which conditions produce shortness of breath, in order to prepare the table with appropriate bolstering. Options for positions are:

- Supine
- Semi-supine or inclined supine (feet lower than head)
- Prone
- Inclined prone (feet lower than head)
- Seated
- Sidelying

Many options are available to therapists outside of the traditional prone and supine positions. Bolsters can be arranged to achieve some of these modifications, or to support or ease pressure on body areas in any position. The therapist can ask a client how she or he sleeps, in order to get a sense of comfortable positions.

Draping

Therapists have different techniques for **draping**—covering the client—but the goals are similar across disciplines: warmth and discretion for the client, and framing the area of the body to be massaged. Although draping modifications are rare, they may be required around medical devices such as intravenous tubes or catheters. When repositioning a client, the therapist may have to be careful that the drape does not drag across a device and displace it. In addition, the therapist needs to know ahead of time which conditions cause intolerance to cold so that extra drapes are ready before a client becomes chilled.

Speed

Speed, as a massage element, is the rate at which a therapist applies strokes or movements in a session. It can be measured as the number of strokes or movements per minute. Speed also functions in transitions between techniques, and between body regions. Although there is no standard speed for most massage techniques, most therapists agree that slower work is more effective and therapeutic than rapid application of techniques. A long gliding stroke is easier for a client to integrate over several seconds than over 1 or 2 seconds. Therapists observe that slow speeds and gradual transitions enhance general relaxation and make muscles more receptive to deeper work. Clients' breathing deepens and slows during long pauses between techniques. A session at slow speed creates safety and is easier to take in than a rushed session.

Despite this generally accepted notion, many massage therapists feel driven to fit as many strokes into the session as possible. They may feel the pressure of time in a fast-paced, high-volume setting, or the need to address multiple problem areas in an unrealistically short time. Some therapists go on "autopilot" during a session, not realizing how quickly their hands are moving.

Sometimes this faster work is energizing. But many clients, who may not even be aware of their need for slow work, leave feeling jittery, overwhelmed, or even exhausted. The therapist seems hurried or careless. Clearly, some therapists work too quickly as a matter of course.

A client coping with a serious illness, or even a milder condition, typically requires even slower speeds than "normal." A medically compromised client typically benefits from more pauses between strokes, as well as slowing down each stroke.

This speed contraindication is based on common sense: The body, already coping with an illness, doesn't need to cope with too much additional stimulation. This is a time for gentle transitions between techniques and gradual shifts between areas of focus. With enough practice slowing down for medically compromised clients, a therapist may slow down his or her pace for all clients!

Rhythm

In massage therapy, **rhythm** is the pattern or arrangement of massage movements or technique components over time. Rhythm can be influential in a massage session. Even, regular rhythms are predictable to the client and are observed to have a sedative effect. Uneven, syncopated rhythms are surprising and often keep the recipient alert for further changes. Some therapists use uneven rhythms selectively, on the theory that these surprises may slightly increase muscle tension (a "bracing" response) and be followed by deeper relaxation. Whatever the reasons, uneven rhythms may be overwhelming for some clients, similar to their experience of rapid speeds. A client who is medically compromised, anxious, or recovering from a strong medical treatment will appreciate predictable rhythms.

Session Length

The duration of the massage, or **session length**, is typically 50–60 minutes, 30 minutes, or intervals of 30 minutes. Sometimes an entire massage must be shortened in response to a medical condition. A client with a cold, a tension headache, or one who is seriously ill may not be able to tolerate a typical 50-minute session. Even something simple, like 15 minutes of gentle foot massage, can be challenging to very ill clients.

One way to shorten a session for an ill, injured, or especially sensitive client is to do just that: End early. Instead of providing a 50-minute massage, end after 30 minutes when it seems clear the client has had enough. Another way to effectively shorten a session is to reduce the time spent doing more vigorous techniques. Suppose a session was scheduled for 50 minutes, but the client seems too compromised to handle a session for that long. Instead of stopping after 30 minutes of massage at medium pressure (level 3), switch to even gentler techniques such as simple holding, gentle range of motion, off-the-body or on-the-body energy techniques for another 10 or 20 minutes. For some clients even this will be too much, for others not enough, but for some it will be perfect. Less vigorous work for the remaining time may be not only well tolerated but warmly welcomed.

Session Timing

Clients and massage therapists reschedule massage sessions for lots of reasons, and a good one is to ensure a safe, appropriate session. In some medical circumstances, **session timing** is important. Cyclical responses to medication, for example, dictate careful scheduling. Chemotherapy in cancer treatment is one example of this—because patients typically have good weeks and bad weeks. At various times over a chemotherapy cycle, a client may have strong side effects and lower tolerance of touch. The same client might welcome and tolerate a medium pressure massage a week or two later.

Another reason to adjust the session timing is to accommodate good and bad times of day for a seriously ill client. Thoughtful session timing can benefit a client: By scheduling massage before a medical procedure, a therapist might help an individual to manage any pain or anxiety caused by the procedure.

One scheduling contraindication is part of the lore of the massage field: That massaging a person with a cold is contraindicated until the illness has peaked, but massage thereafter is okay and will help the client get better faster. While this approach has little basis in known physiological mechanisms or scientific data, it is widely practiced. Moreover, therapists do observe that clients battling infection seem to feel worse after a vigorous massage. Whatever the reasons behind this observation, it suggests a general mandate: Avoid scheduling massage when it might divert a client's resources from healing. This is an example of an adjustment in session timing.

Session Intent

Therapists use the elements of massage in various combinations to achieve specific therapeutic goals. The session intent is the assumed effect or desired outcome of a massage session.

There are times to pursue the intent, and times to change it to accommodate a client's illness or injury. The aims of a session can vary. Therapists work with many different healing purposes in mind, ranging from the physical to the psychological and spiritual. Physical goals for a session include increasing circulation, readying muscles for a sports event, and releasing restrictions in tissues for better alignment. Therapists may use the other elements of massage, such as joint movement, varying pressures, and positioning, to achieve the goal of the session.

Most massage contraindications currently in use concern the mechanical effects of massage, so the physical (rather than psychological or spiritual) intentions of the session are primarily addressed here. A few principal massage intentions are discussed in detail, below:

- General relaxation
- Muscle relaxation
- Symptom relief
- Increased circulation

● GENERAL RELAXATION

Massage for general relaxation relieves the effects of chronic stress that many people experience. During massage, the breathing and heart rate slow, and the body can rest. Drops in blood pressure and increases in skin temperature are noted—all signs of relaxation. The mechanisms behind these outcomes have not yet been fully determined. A working theory suggests that massage encourages the dominance of the parasympathetic nervous system, the branch of the autonomic system that regulates these measures of relaxation as well as other restorative functions such as digestion and elimination. This "rest-and-digest" state is a needed antidote to chronic stress.

The sympathetic nervous system, responsible for the fight-or-flight responses such as increased cardiac activity, persists in chronic stress (see "Stress," Chapter 17). Certainly chronic stress, by causing the fight-or-flight response to persist for long periods, can compromise a person's health over time.

General relaxation is the intent of most massage therapy sessions, worth preserving as a goal. However, sympathetic nervous system functions are necessary for such activities as getting up off of a massage table, getting dressed, and driving—in addition to responding to danger. The body needs the heart rate to accelerate and the blood pressure to rise and pump blood to the brain upon rising. A gentle re-entry into the functioning world is best for clients who become deeply relaxed. A client with anemia, or another on blood pressure medication, may get dizzy when rising too quickly. Considering these conditions, the therapist can encourage this gentle re-entry by having the client rise slowly from the table. Sitting up for 30 seconds before standing is a good way to do this, and ending with plenty of time for the client to dress and leave on time is also helpful.

Doses of general relaxation are a highly beneficial hallmark of massage therapy. A responsible therapist considers what the client has planned after the massage, advises some "down time" afterward, and aims for the right combination of alertness and relaxation.

● MUSCLE RELAXATION

Massage relaxes muscle: Although it is not the most researched topic in massage therapy, clients and therapists observe muscle relaxation repeatedly. Muscle relaxation is a common goal and outcome of massage, but in some cases this intention is ill-advised: A bit of excess muscle tension can be a good thing. For example, in the case of a recent injury, muscle tension may be needed to help splint the area against movement. The splinting helps prevent re-injury while the tissues heal, and the therapist takes care not to relax the splinting muscles too much.

Specialized practitioners who work more precisely with injuries can assess surrounding muscle tension, but without injury training, it can be difficult to determine how much massage is too much for the involved muscles. The best approach for basic practitioners is to take care not to overtreat the tension, monitor the client's responses over time, and respect the relevant injury and pain principles in Chapter 3. In this way, the intent to relax muscles yields to the need for stability in the area.

Sometimes a client's emotional state or coping mechanisms include tense muscles, and well-intentioned attempts to relax them are ill-advised. Tight muscles may help "hold in" unwanted emotion; they guard against intrusion. They serve as storehouses of emotional tension. This is not an ideal situation over the long term, but it may help someone manage during a hard situation. It's important not to go in and release muscle tension without honoring the reason for its being there in the first place. Relaxing the muscles gradually is best, in a give-and-take process with the client, with clear communication and respect for the whole person.

● SYMPTOM RELIEF

It would be hard to think of a contraindication to symptom relief; indeed, symptoms such as pain, fatigue, anxiety, and nausea indicate massage. Symptom relief is always a worthy goal, and massage may be particularly appropriate for symptoms involving stress and tension: back problems, anxiety, depression, fatigue, and headaches. Even though symptom relief is not contraindicated, it is important to consider *how* to go about it, and use care in combining the other elements of massage to that end. For example, symptom relief of back pain through muscle relaxation is a sensible goal, but methods involving joint movement should be avoided if the client has an unstable back injury. Moreover, if the client comes in complaining of strong, sudden, and unfamiliar back pain, the therapist should refer the client to the physician rather than focus a massage on symptom relief (see Medical Referral, this chapter). Over time with their clients, therapists learn the best approaches to symptom relief.

● INCREASED CIRCULATION

One of the most commonly claimed benefits of massage is an increase in circulation. This statement is at the forefront of many promotional and educational materials. It is mentioned in most massage therapy textbooks, and is a foundation of much of the instruction in Western massage modalities. This increase in circulation is thought to enhance overall health, and to help many conditions, such as swelling, injury, fatigue, and overused muscles.

This belief underlies massage benefits, but it also underlies many contraindications. The logic is that an increase in circulation is inadvisable in some medical conditions such as liver disease, a heart condition, or the common cold. It is argued that such an increase in circulation, beyond what would normally occur physiologically, might overwhelm the tissues and organs, which are already working hard to function in a disease state.

Although the circulatory effect of massage is usually stated as fact, the truth about massage therapy and circulation remains to be determined. There is little evidence in support of this claim, and many research studies in this area are small, poorly designed, decades old, and performed long before sophisticated instruments were devised to measure circulation. In fact, the circulation claim has been sharply questioned in the medical literature and is still an open question (Weerapong, et al., 2005; Tiidus, 1999). Rather than stating, "Massage increases circulation," as certainty, professionals would be more truthful posing it as a belief, an assumption, or, most accurately, a theory.

Without strong data to support this claim, therapists are advised to focus on other massage outcomes that are less open to dispute: observed symptom relief, clients' reports of better sleep, more energy, and fewer headaches, athletes' reports of enhanced sports performance, and so on. Any of these may be seen in a massage practice, without even venturing into the research literature. Yet research support for massage is growing, with well-designed studies on back pain, anxiety, depression, and other conditions.

As tightly as the massage profession clings to its circulatory benefit, research is finding other, more relevant benefits. It is becoming clear to the massage profession that that it's no longer necessary, nor accurate, to claim increased circulation as a primary benefit of massage.

Massage, Circulation, and Contraindications

Even though a circulatory *benefit* of massage is unclear, many massage contraindications are based on the working assumption that increased circulation could cause *harm*. On the contraindication side of massage and circulation, it has been difficult to reason through massage guidelines while its effects are still uncertain. It may be years before the exact role of massage in circulation is well established, as several sizable, rigorous studies are needed to know for sure. If massage *does* increase circulation, research needs to supply the details: In which tissues? Superficially, deeply, or both? Does it affect blood circulation, lymph circulation, or both? Which massage elements, in what measure, cause this effect? What are the physiological mechanisms? Does a circulatory effect extend beyond the area massaged, or is it just a local effect? Can massage increase circulation so that it overwhelms a compromised organ, or does the body's own autoregulation—its ability to control blood flow to organs and tissues—override the effect of massage?

Massage contraindications, however, cannot wait for these evidence-based answers; clinical decisions are being made now. Fortunately, clinical practice provides valuable information for the interim. Therapists report several common, notable observations about massage and circulation:

1. Hyperemia appears at the massage site, as reddening of skin and warming of muscles.
2. Superficial veins, especially at the posterior low leg, appear to empty and refill in response to gliding strokes applied in the direction of the heart.

3. Clients with medical conditions affecting the liver, spleen, heart, and kidney frequently feel unwell after a traditional circulatory massage session.

The first two observations suggest local changes, at or near the site of the massage. The last one suggests general changes in some way. Perhaps the first is a result of friction at the site, and the second, due to the milking action of the strokes. But whether the first two observations actually amount to significant circulatory changes is unclear. Over time, research can sort out that question.

The third observation, about reactions to massage, suggests another open question: Whether circulatory changes are at the root of the clients' unfavorable responses. Perhaps, since the conditions affect blood filters (or, in the case of the heart, the blood pump), massage therapy increases blood circulation enough to overwhelm these structures, causing an adverse reaction. On the other hand, a circulatory effect may not be at fault; instead, ill feeling may be due to heavy pressure, a session that was too long, or other elements that were overwhelming to the client. Until the profession separates and tests each element of massage to determine the offending factor, there is no way to know for sure.

What conclusions can be drawn from these three clinical observations, and how can they inform decision making in the absence of firm data? The first two observations suggest a guiding principle: If a tissue is inflamed, don't aggravate it with circulatory intent at the site (see "The Inflammation Principle," Chapter 3). If massage seems to cause its own transient inflammation, then do not add it to the current level of inflammation.

The third observation is compelling enough to drive another important guiding principle: Avoid general circulatory intent in medical conditions that affect the processing of blood (see "The Filter and Pump Principle," Chapter 3). For good measure, also avoid general circulatory intent when the lymphatic system is strained by infection, generalized edema, and so on.

Until more is known about the precise effects of massage therapy, these working principles can help with many, varied client presentations. The guidelines are also in keeping with the Hippocratic oath: First do no harm. Until it's established that massage therapy is *not* circulatory in effect, it makes sense to assume that it *could be* circulatory. Therefore, many of the contraindications in this book rest on this assumption.

The Massage Plan

How do these guidelines translate into actual hands-on work? There are two kinds of circulatory intent. The first is local circulatory intent. The second is general circulatory intent. Local circulatory intent, or *circulatory intent at a site*, is the aim to raise circulation at a given area such as a low leg, an upper arm, or a low back. Although sources do not agree on how to do this, there seems to be a pattern in the way massage is taught in the Swedish tradition: Effleurage, petrissage, and compressions, applied at medium and deep pressure, are used to increase circulation. This is described in the following components:

1. Effleurage (stroking)
2. Petrissage (kneading)
3. Repeated compressions
4. Medium or deep pressure (pressure level 3 or above)

The first three components are techniques, and the last one is the pressure needed to make those techniques circulatory in intent.

Noncirculatory Alternatives

To avoid local circulatory intent, the therapist stays below a pressure of 3 when kneading, stroking, and applying repeated compressions. Although there may be additional techniques to avoid, such as tapotement and vibration, the most common techniques are emphasized here. A cautious therapist will also avoid any other techniques that are thought to have a circulatory purpose or effect.

When circulatory work is contraindicated at a site, the therapist may draw on many noncirculatory alternatives, such as:

- Kneading and stroking at pressure level 1 or 2
- Joint movement, such as ROM, rocking, stretching (if there is no joint movement contraindication)
- Holding or resting the hands on the area
- A few slow, stationary compressions at pressure levels 1–5 (if there is no pressure contraindication)
- Energy techniques, not designed to raise circulation
- Reflexive techniques, not designed to raise circulation

Using these alternatives, the site may be addressed in a meaningful way without an increase in circulation. Typically, this does not require a major adjustment in the overall session.

A more significant component of massage is **general circulatory intent**. This is the aim to increase overall blood flow or blood flow at multiple sites in the body. This aim is accomplished by using the same four elements—kneading, stroking, and repeated compressions at pressure level 3 or above—on multiple body regions. There is no universal agreement on how many areas to cover and for how long, but many massage instructors emphasize the back and extremities, for a good portion of a 30- or 50-minute massage. Moreover, the circulatory effect is thought to be enhanced in the extremities by **centripetal** placement of strokes—toward the heart, in the direction of venous return of blood.

To avoid general circulatory intent, the therapist avoids these circulatory elements throughout the session. Any other circulatory techniques or modalities are also excluded from the massage plan.

Because a contraindication to general circulatory intent includes so much of the body, it can feel more restrictive than a simple adjustment at a single site. Since kneading, stroking, and compressions at pressure level 3 and above are such staples of massage therapy, therapists may wonder how to fill a session when they are contraindicated, and how to introduce a noncirculatory session to a client who is used to a more traditional one.

The noncirculatory alternatives listed can be utilized fully, in creative combinations. The whole session can be paced slowly, with gradual transitions that enhance general relaxation. And

note that medium, strong, and deep pressure levels are still appropriate as long as they are not paired with kneading and stroking. Unless there are other safety concerns, these pressure levels may still be used in a single stationary compression (or a small number of compressions) in areas requiring more substantial pressure.

For variety, the therapist may also be able to include a few circulatory elements in the session, by strictly limiting them in space and time. For example, a few minutes of kneading at deeper pressure (levels 3–5) on the hands and feet seems unlikely to move much blood since the amount of blood in those areas is small to begin with. And just 1–2 minutes of kneading and stroking on the upper back and shoulders at pressure level 3 is unlikely to influence overall venous return. The therapist uses these elements sparingly, by keeping to a time limit, using them on only one or two sites, and avoiding them on the extremities. Circulatory techniques could be too potent on the extremities, where large, easily compressible veins return sizeable amounts of blood to the heart.

Some therapists feel self-conscious when introducing a noncirculatory session to a client, especially if it seems like a less appealing alternative. A therapist can try this:

"Because of this condition, I'll need to work in a noncirculatory, slightly more conservative way today." Or this: "I can still work deeply if you like, but not with my usual flowing strokes. It might feel a bit different from your usual session, but I can still focus on any trouble areas. Tell me where you'd like me to spend some extra time." Or even this: "We don't know for sure how massage interacts with your condition—but the last thing we want is for you to feel worse! The session I'm describing is for general relaxation, and is likely to help you feel better."

When to Avoid Circulatory Intent

Contraindications to circulatory intent appear throughout this book. Many conditions with localized inflammation of the skin, joint, and muscle are discussed, where circulatory intent should be avoided at the site. This approach is recommended for standard practitioners of massage therapy. (If specialized modalities such as injury and scar tissue treatment or lymph drainage techniques sidestep these limits, it is in the service of other therapeutic goals.)

General circulatory intent is contraindicated in many conditions, as well. Some examples are advanced heart disease, advanced kidney disease, advanced liver disease, and a congested spleen. When infection is present, noncirculatory alternatives are used. Moreover, medication affecting fluid balance, such as steroid medication or diuretics, is also a red flag, and a good time to avoid general circulatory intent. These and other scenarios are discussed in detail in Parts II and III. Until more is known about the effects of massage, noncirculatory alternatives are important to make available.

Other Actions

To respond effectively and safely to some medical conditions, the therapist may take steps that fall outside of the hands-on session. In particularly complex or undiagnosed cases, it is important to involve the client's physician. There are two ways to involve the physician: a medical consultation and a medical referral.

● MEDICAL CONSULTATION

In this book, the term **medical consultation** is used whenever a massage therapist consults with a medical or health care professional (usually the client's physician or the physician's nurse) to determine the advisability of a massage plan.

In some cases, such as a hospital or clinic, physician permission may be necessary in the form of physician orders. In most cases, it is up to the massage therapist to structure the communication. The medical consultation is a dialogue between the massage therapist, the client, and the physician that can be in writing, in person, or by telephone. Chapter 5 addresses when and how to involve the physician in this process.

● MEDICAL REFERRAL

In contrast to a medical consultation, where a medical professional brought into a massage decision, a medical referral is a referral out to a medical professional. The massage therapist refers the client out of the office because she believes the client needs medical attention, and the concern is outside the scope of massage practice.

The immediacy of the referral is specific to the context, and involves a judgment call on the part of the therapist. In most cases, the therapist can urge the client to see his or her physician in the next few days or weeks, for example, if regular massage therapy has failed to address a client's muscular pain. However, in some situations, the therapist urges an *urgent medical referral*, in the next day or two. For example, if a therapist notices a change in the shape of a mole on her client's back, she becomes concerned about a possible aggressive skin cancer. She advises her client to act quickly.

Sometimes more immediate action is needed. In this text, the terms *immediate referral* and *emergency medical referral* are sometimes used interchangeably. *Immediate* typically implies the need to act within a few hours, before a condition could rapidly become more serious, as in compartment syndrome of the lower leg (see Chapter 8). An *emergency medical referral*, involving a call to emergency services, is done when a situation seems life threatening. Although this book occasionally specifies the urgency of the referral as a basic guideline, it is ultimately the therapist's responsibility, with the client, to determine how pressing the need may be in each case. When in doubt, act quickly.

Assembling the Elements: Designing the Massage

Many wonderful elements make up massage therapy. To design the best session for a client, it is important to determine which elements are useful and which are potentially harmful. Instead of assuming all massage is contraindicated, or referring to a technique by its modality name, the therapist can break down the often-used massage terms into their elements for clearer meaning. Then she or he leaves out the elements that could be harmful, and enhances those that could be helpful. Massage therapy elements appear throughout Parts II and III of this book, on the right side of the Decision Trees. Principles governing these elements are in Chapter 3.

The elements are assembled into a massage plan that is safe as well as effective. Once safety concerns are taken care of, the design for the session can be as original and creative as the therapist likes—often when elements are limited by a contraindication, a therapist becomes even *more* creative

with the remaining ones! For example, a therapist who is more comfortable using deeper pressures, suddenly limited to lighter ones by a client situation, may enhance her use of unconventional speeds, rhythms, or attention to certain areas, to great effect in her or his work with clients. A therapist forced to slow down for an ill client may discover that he can relax and slow down much more in his other sessions, or might find his feelings of care for his client flourishing in the generous pauses between strokes. Contraindications to massage elements pose challenges to therapists, but they also can enhance creativity and satisfaction with one's work.

The elements of massage are part of the science of massage. The technical thinking is in the clinical decision making of the Decision Tree. But the right pressure and contact, with caring attention to certain areas, also make up the art of the work, and the right mix of elements is at the heart of it.

SELF TEST

1. What is the drawback of using modality names to describe massage contraindications?
2. Name three massage elements that are common in site restrictions.
3. What is the difference between a site restriction and a general restriction?
4. Which pressure level is typically used to "warm up" the muscles for deeper work?
5. Which pressure level is used to distribute lotion on the skin, but not to rub it in?
6. Compare pressure level 2 with pressure level 3. How are they different?

7. What is the difference between a medical consultation and a medical referral? How are each used?
8. In classical massage, what are the three massage techniques that are thought to raise circulation? What is the minimum level of pressure necessary for these techniques to have a circulatory effect?
9. How does a massage therapist avoid general circulatory intent in a session? Be specific about the elements to avoid. What alternative techniques can the therapist use?
10. What are some possible negative responses to massage strokes that are done too quickly?

 For answers to these questions and to see a bibliography for this chapter, visit http://thePoint. *lww.com/Walton.*

3 Principles of Massage Contraindications

Rules are not necessarily sacred, principles are.

—FRANKLIN DELANO ROOSEVELT

A principle is a guideline for practice or behavior. Different disciplines have their own principles. For example, in health care, an ethical principle of confidentiality guides the policy and practice of protecting the health information of patients. Ethical principles are often expanded to generate a code of ethics for a profession.

In massage therapy, as in any health care practice, principles may be used to guide decision making. Therapists typically use principles every day in practice; the principles are so ingrained that it's often an unconscious process. For example, therapists are taught to begin with gentle pressure to warm up a problem area, then use deeper pressure for more focused work, rather than start with deeper pressure and finish with gentle pressure. This principle might be called The Gentle Warm-up Principle, or a similar name, as it is taught in massage classrooms everywhere.

In this chapter, principles about massage contraindications are gathered in one place. Some are general guidelines for practice, and others are more specific. Many principles introduced here are repeated word for word in later chapters; other times they are stated differently to apply to specific situations.

Using Principles of Contraindications

Therapists can use principles of contraindications in three ways:

1. To get from the left to the right side of the Decision Tree.
2. To generate an appropriate interview question to ask a client.
3. In some cases, after careful reasoning, to override or modify a principle.

Principles make a therapist's job easier. Determining contraindications becomes a simple, straightforward process, without guesswork or memorizing long lists of medical conditions.

● GETTING TO THE RIGHT SIDE OF THE DECISION TREE

Massage principles guide massage practice. On the Decision Tree, medical information is on the left side and massage adjustments are on the right. As shown in Figure 3-1, a principle links the information with the therapist's action. Principles such as the Inflammation Principle ("If an area of tissue is inflamed, don't aggravate it with pressure, friction, or circulatory intent at the site") or the Sensation Principle ("In an area of impaired or absent sensation, use caution with pressure and joint movement") generate appropriate massage guidelines on the right side of the tree.

Principles can be applied more or less broadly to many conditions. For example, no matter what the cause of inflammation is, massage therapists should avoid worsening it. This means that if the inflammation is due to arthritis, acne, chicken pox, or bursitis, the massage therapist practices carefully to avoid aggravating it. Likewise, no matter why sensation is impaired, massage pressure should be gentler than usual because the client cannot give reliable feedback about

pain, and such feedback is necessary to avoid injuring tissue. Sensation could be impaired for various reasons, including multiple sclerosis (MS), a spinal cord injury, advanced diabetes, AIDS, or chemotherapy, but no matter what the reason is, the therapist lightens the pressure.

Principles can be applied to more than one medical condition, so the list of massage principles is much shorter than a list of all the possible medical conditions. Therefore, principles are easier to learn and apply than long lists of specific contraindications. Because they provide a broad basis for practice, principles also tend to be more accurate, as in the following example:

- A principle: If sensation is impaired, massage pressure and joint movement should be gentle.
- A specific contraindication: MS contraindicates pressure.

Both of the statements, above, concern the safe use of massage pressure. The principle is a general one that applies to a host of medical conditions (including some cases of MS). The specific contraindication is only partly true, because there is a range in MS presentations. Only certain clients with MS experience impaired sensation; others have fully intact sensation, stable tissues and robust health, and there is no reason to avoid pressure. Besides sensation impairment, there may be other signs and symptoms of MS that require gentle pressure, but not everyone has these, either.

There is no single, correct massage approach to MS. However, the principle itself is applicable any time sensation is impaired, and is therefore appropriate for many medical conditions which affect sensation. It's often more accurate to use a principle than to try to force a single massage guideline on a given medical condition.

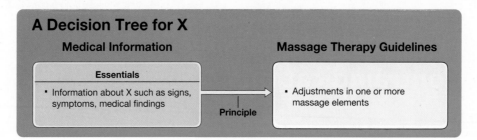

FIGURE 3-1. A massage principle links the left and right sides of the decision tree, directing the practitioner from information to action. Only the top branch of the tree is shown.

● GENERATING INTERVIEW QUESTIONS

Principles can be easily inverted into interview questions. For instance, the Sensation Principle, above, when flipped, becomes this question: "Do you have any health conditions that affect your sensation?" or "Is there any effect of this condition on sensation?" As a therapist, it's good to have a general sense of common diseases that affect sensation, but the list of possibilities is long. By knowing the Sensation Principle and asking the client the relevant question, a therapist can come up with the correct massage adjustment for the whole list of familiar and unfamiliar medical conditions.

Likewise, the Inflammation Principle above can be inverted for a good interview question: "Does this condition involve inflammation?" or "Are any areas inflamed?" A follow-up question expands on it: "Do you have any areas of swelling, redness, pain, or warmth?" Many diseases involve inflammation, and a therapist would be unlikely to encounter them all, even over a long career. Knowing the Inflammation Principle, a therapist can apply it to any possibility, simply by asking a well-placed question about inflammation.

A good intake form (or verbal interview) will include questions drawn from some basic principles, below. For more on the intake and interview process, see Chapter 4.

● CUSTOMIZING A MASSAGE BY MODIFYING OR OVERRULING A PRINCIPLE

In some cases, it's okay to modify or overrule a principle, but only after careful consideration. Continuing with the Sensation

Principle example, it is important for the therapist to use gentler pressure in an area of impaired sensation because the client cannot give dependable feedback about whether the pressure is hurting or not. Not knowing if the pressure hurts, the therapist could damage tissue in the area.

Suppose a client presents with some loss of feeling in his or her feet, perhaps from advanced diabetes. Strictly applying the Sensation Principle, the therapist would work with gentle pressure on the client's feet. But, suppose this client is **ambulatory**, capable of walking regularly. In fact, the client walks a fair amount to public transportation each day to get to work. The tissues of the client's feet look healthy, with no bruises or sores.

Because the activity of walking presses hard on the soles of the feet, it may be appropriate to modify the Sensation Principle. Massage is unlikely to approach the level of pressure applied during walking. Thinking through all of this, a therapist could safely apply broad, medium, or deep strokes (at pressure levels 3 and 4) to the soles of the feet, with slightly lighter pressure (pressure levels 2 and 3) when focusing on small areas of the feet. No hard knuckles or elbows are used, but fairly deep, sweeping pressures from the therapist's fingers and hands would be no more pressure than the feet encounter during the client's daily activities.

In this case, the therapist carefully considers the principle and uses it as a decision-making tool, but then modifies it based on client information. This is different from forgetting to consider it in the first place, or thoughtlessly discarding the pressure contraindication. Instead, the therapist arrives at a thoughtful, defensible approach to this client's feet, with good reasoning behind it. As a result, the client receives a massage session customized to the health of his or her feet.

"First, Do No Harm"

The guiding principle, "First, do no harm" is attributed to the Greek physician Hippocrates and held dear by medical doctors and other health care professionals, including massage therapists. All other principles for the well-being and healing of clients flow from it, and massage contraindications are based on it.

The simplicity of "First, do no harm" makes it easy to remember. The principles presented in this chapter are also simple and broad. These principles are summarized in Table 3-1.

General Principles

The first principles introduced here are all-purpose guidelines for daily massage practice. They are the most broadly applied of massage principles, without any specific medical content.

A therapist who is unsure of how to proceed with a client can often become "unstuck" by drawing on one or more of these general principles.

TABLE 3-1.	PRINCIPLES OF MASSAGE CONTRAINDICATIONS
Name	**Principle**
The Shred of Doubt Principle	If there is a shred of doubt about whether a massage element is safe, it is contraindicated until its safety is established. When in doubt, don't.
The Intuition Isn't Everything Principle	Intuition is one guide in a massage therapist's decision making, but it should not be the only guide.
The Clinical Judgment Improves with Experience Principle	An experienced therapist can more safely and readily predict a therapeutic outcome or modify a principle than a beginning therapist.
The Where You Start Isn't Always Where You End Up Principle	Although a client's condition may call for a conservative initial massage, stronger elements may be appropriate in later sessions, after monitoring the client's response to massage over time.
The Ask the Cause Principle	Consider the cause of a sign or symptom, as well as the sign or symptom itself, when making a massage plan.
The Massage Setting/Continuity of Care Principle	In massage settings favoring single-time rather than repeat clients, lacking continuity of care, or using little or no documentation, therapists should take a cautious approach to medical conditions.
The Activity and Energy Principle	A client who enjoys regular, moderate physical activity or a good overall energy level is better able to tolerate strong massage elements—including circulatory intent—than one whose activity or energy level is low.
The Previous Massage Principle	A client's previous experience of massage therapy, especially massage after the onset, diagnosis, or flare-up of a medical condition, may be used to plan the massage.
The Vital Organ Principle	If a vital organ—heart, lung, kidney, liver, or brain—is compromised in function, use gentle massage elements and adjust them to pose minimal challenge to the client's body.
The Filter and Pump Principle	If a filtering organ (liver, kidney, spleen, or lymph node), or a pumping organ (the heart), is functioning poorly or overworking, do not work it harder with massage that is circulatory in intent.
The Compromised Client Principle	If a client is not feeling well, be gentle; even if you cannot explain the mechanism behind a contraindication, follow it anyway.
The Sensation Principle	In an area of impaired or absent sensation, use caution with pressure and joint movement.
The Sensation Loss, Injury Prone Principle	If a client has lost sensation in an area, inspect the tissues carefully for injury before beginning the massage.
The Physician Referral for Pain Principle	If a client's pain has specific qualities, such as sharp, stabbing, radiating, or shooting pain, or if the pain is accompanied by tingling, numbness, or weakness, refer the client to a physician.
The New, Unfamiliar, or Poorly Managed Pain Principle	Massage for a client with new, unfamiliar, or poorly managed pain should be more conservative than massage for a client with a familiar, well-managed pain pattern.
The Recent Injury Principle	Recent injuries, or injuries that have not been seen by a physician, should not be treated with massage therapy, or massage therapy should be conservative.
The Claim or Litigation Principle	If a client's recent injury involves an insurance claim or litigation, do not complicate the clinical picture with massage that could affect the area.
The Inflammation Principle	If an area of tissue is inflamed, don't aggravate it with pressure, friction, or circulatory intent at the site.
The Unstable Tissue Principle	If a tissue is unstable, do not challenge it with too much pressure or joint movement in the area.
The Stabilization of an Acute Condition Principle	Until an acute medical condition has stabilized, massage should be conservative.
The Emergency Protocol Principle	If a client has a condition with rapid or unpredictable changes in symptoms, ask about any warning signs and appropriate responses in case they occur during a massage.
The Waiting for a Diagnosis Principle	If a client is scheduled for diagnostic tests, or is awaiting results, adapt massage to the possible diagnosis. If more than one condition is being investigated, adapt massage to the worst-case scenario.
The Medication Principle	Adapt massage to the condition for which the medication is taken or prescribed, and to any side effects.
The Procedure Principle	Adapt massage to the condition for which the procedure is advised, and to the effects of the procedure itself.
The Medically Restricted Activity Principle	If there are any medical restrictions on a client's activities, explore and apply any equivalent massage contraindications.

(continued)

TABLE 3-1.	PRINCIPLES OF MASSAGE CONTRAINDICATIONS (Continued)
Name	**Principle**
The Detoxification Principle	If an intent of a spa treatment is to detoxify, avoid using it when the client is significantly challenged by illness or injury, or is taking strong medication.
The Exfoliation Principle	If a client's skin health or overall health is significantly compromised, do not use treatments involving strong exfoliation.
The Core Temperature Principle	Avoid spa treatments that raise the core temperature if a client's cardiovascular system, respiratory system, skin, or other tissue or system might be overly challenged by heat, or if there are comparable medical restrictions.

● THE SHRED OF DOUBT PRINCIPLE

If there is a shred of doubt about whether a massage element is safe, it is contraindicated until its safety is established. When in doubt, don't.

The reasoning behind this principle is that it is better to undertreat than overtreat, minimizing the risk of hurting clients in the goal of helping them. Although the importance of this principle is obvious, at times a massage therapist may be pressured to override it by an insistent client or the therapist's own impulses. In general, a more conservative approach is best when there is doubt about a client's ability to tolerate a given massage element.

● THE INTUITION ISN'T EVERYTHING PRINCIPLE

Intuition is one guide in a massage therapist's decision making, but it should not be the only guide.

The reasoning behind this principle is that, although every health care professional, especially a massage therapist, uses a certain amount of intuition in working with people, intuition is not enough in decisions about contraindications. A therapist also draws on his or her education, experience, and information about each case. Therapists incorporate their own knowledge of anatomy and pathology, the known or suspected effects of massage on the body, information from the client, and in some cases direction from the client's physician.

Additionally, intuition can be compromised from day to day, even in sensitive practitioners with well-developed skills. Factors that can interfere with intuition include stress, fatigue, and poor nutrition. The therapist's own ego, needs, and issues can also cloud his or her judgment. Skilled therapists combine intuition, information, and experience; the best mix of these is true wisdom.

● THE CLINICAL JUDGMENT IMPROVES WITH EXPERIENCE PRINCIPLE

An experienced therapist can more safely and readily predict a therapeutic outcome or modify a principle than a beginning therapist.

The reasoning behind this principle is that, having more experience working with certain conditions or populations, seasoned therapists know better when to follow principles and when to test them or depart from them entirely. A therapist who has seen eight clients with spinal cord injuries has a better sense of the range of client presentations than the therapist who has seen just one. A practitioner with years of experience applying pressure to tissues and feeling responses brings that experience into each clinical decision, often unconsciously. Experienced therapists have a better (although not perfect) ability to predict client responses to the elements of massage than beginning practitioners.

In general, a stricter adherence to massage contraindications and principles is called for in students and beginning practitioners. Later, as skills improve and increase, more experimentation may be possible.

● THE WHERE YOU START ISN'T ALWAYS WHERE YOU END UP PRINCIPLE

Although a client's condition may call for a conservative initial massage, stronger elements may be appropriate in later sessions, after monitoring the client's response to massage over time.

This principle suggests that the client's response to massage elements figures into his or her treatment over time. Without knowing how a client will respond, the therapist works conservatively at the initial session. If the client's symptoms are aggravated or he or she is fatigued by a session, subsequent sessions should be even more conservative. More often, the client's response is favorable, and the strength of the massage elements, such as pressure and joint movement, can be increased over time in small increments.

This principle points to the need for good communication with clients. Here is one way to begin: "Since this is a first-time (or one-time) session and we don't know how massage will affect your condition, I'll begin conservatively. If you receive massage over time, in which case there's a chance to monitor your response, it might be possible to increase the pressure…" This can help a client understand the logic behind the massage plan, to accept it, and to relax fully.

Clients in a new, unfamiliar health crisis or on strong medication may miss their usual, vigorous massage. Still, it's best to start small, and often even a much gentler session can be too much for this "new normal" state of being. The best way to determine the strength of the massage elements is to try them out over a course of massage therapy, inching up in small increments, establishing good communication with the client, and documenting responses (MacDonald, 2005).

● THE ASK THE CAUSE PRINCIPLE

Consider the cause of a sign or symptom, as well as the sign or symptom itself, when making a massage plan.

Different health conditions can cause many of the same signs and symptoms. The causative condition may, by itself, contraindicate one or more massage elements. For example, nausea can be caused by medication or infection. Sensation loss can be caused by a compression injury or chemotherapy. Many of these causes, in and of themselves, require massage adjustments.

Sometimes the cause of a sign or symptom is an even more important massage consideration than the sign or symptom itself. This principle asks the therapist to consider the context of a sign or symptom. For example, edema, a complication of a serious heart condition, infection, or other disease, points the therapist to the primary condition. The primary condition—the diseased heart, or the infection—requires its own Decision Tree and follow-up questions.

● THE MASSAGE SETTING/ CONTINUITY OF CARE PRINCIPLE

In massage settings favoring single-time rather than repeat clients, lacking continuity of care, or using little or no documentation, therapists should take a cautious approach to medical conditions.

The therapist-client relationship and the ability to monitor the client over time are important for providing safe treatment and reducing professional liability. These factors are not equal across massage settings. In high-volume settings with little documentation, fewer repeat clients, and many therapists, a therapist's ability to build a therapeutic relationship and monitor responses to treatment is compromised. This is true of many destination and day spa settings, cruise ships, on-site massage, and massage at special events and large gatherings. Input from the client's physician is not typically possible, and full client schedules and short turnaround times may hinder the therapist's capacity to consider complex health factors. A conservative approach is advisable for a therapist working in these circumstances.

In contrast, a therapist with repeat clients, documentation of each session, time to interview clients, and a higher chance of an enduring therapist-client relationship gains more knowledge about each client. She has time to explore each medical condition with the client, and on her own outside of the session. She monitors the client's responses to massage over time. With this knowledge, she enjoys a more thorough clinical decision-making process. Therefore, she can more safely depart from principles, and step outside of cautious massage guidelines. By documenting the client's feedback, progress, and massage tolerance over a course of treatment, she can try stronger massage elements such as deeper pressure, greater joint movement, and increased circulatory intent over time. By asking, for example, "How did your back injury respond to last week's session," the therapist can gradually increase the massage strength to a desired therapeutic level, or ease off when it becomes too much.

Rapport with a client can ease concerns over safety and liability, but it takes time to develop. In medicine, the role of provider-patient rapport in reducing malpractice litigation is well established. Trust, mutual respect, and good communication reduce the risk of a malpractice claim, even when an actual error results in injury or harm to the patient. A longer-term therapeutic relationship more easily absorbs the occasional mistake than a one-time session. A collaborative relationship with a client fosters client reflection, responsibility, and vital feedback. This is especially important when the client has a medical condition requiring massage adjustments.

Without a strong therapeutic relationship, the therapist is more vulnerable to a client's discontent. Without the ongoing expectation that a client will reflect and report, the burden, by default, falls to the therapist. And without documentation, the therapist has no record of the massage provided or the contraindications she or another therapist followed; she is on shakier ground if a client becomes disgruntled or litigious. Within these constraints, more conservative massage guidelines make sense.

Prediction Principles

It is hard to predict how massage will affect someone with a certain medical condition. A case study might be available, but usually there is no research to consult. In such situations, it can be useful to draw on the client's previous massage experience, or think of an activity that is similar to massage, and ask whether the condition contraindicates that activity. By borrowing a concern from medicine, comparing it to a massage element, then applying it to a client's history, the therapist may be able to predict the effect of a massage. In order to make the best predictions, the therapist asks questions: What are the client's activities of daily living, and how are those similar in some way to massage elements? If the client can tolerate the broad pressure of lying down on a sofa, his back and hips pressing it with his weight, can he tolerate broad massage pressure in the area? If the client walks a mile to work each day, and his energy level is good, can he take a massage with general circulatory intent? If the client stretches and uses a certain joint with his doctor's approval, can he benefit from a massage stretch in that area? These analogies make the work of clinical reasoning about massage easier.

If the effect of a massage element on a given condition is unknown, try to establish an equivalent everyday activity and determine whether it's a well-tolerated part of the client's daily activities, or if it's been medically restricted for the client. Examples are hot showers, saunas, heat applications, cardiovascular activity, body movements, sleeping positions, certain lotions or creams, or the pressure of a seat belt, waistband, or chair against a body part.

The next two principles help a therapist predict, in a limited way, how a client with a given condition might tolerate a massage element.

● THE ACTIVITY AND ENERGY PRINCIPLE

A client who enjoys regular, moderate physical activity or a good overall energy level is better able to tolerate strong massage elements—including circulatory intent—than one whose activity or energy level is low.

Massage is one form of stress on a body—generally a well-received stressor but a stressor, nonetheless. Pressure into the tissues, the stimulation of nervous system receptors, the intention to bring about a change in circulation, joint movement, and the speed of massage are all elements that challenge the body. If a client's body tolerates regular physical activity with a reasonable amount of joint movement, increased circulation, and nervous system stimulation, it's likely that he or she can tolerate and benefit from strong elements of massage therapy. Likewise, if his or her energy level is good overall, it is less likely to be drained by vigorous massage therapy.

This is a useful principle for two decision-making scenarios. First, a client presents with a medical condition about which there is little information in the massage literature. It's hard to predict how massage will interact with the condition, the treatment, or the client coping with both of these. If the client's activity level is good, and he or she is moving through space, then probably the medical condition is not compromising function too much. A strong massage may be welcome and well tolerated.

Second, two people with the same medical condition or treatment can have very different clinical presentations. One person with a heart or nervous system condition might be very active, while another may be unable to tolerate much activity without extreme fatigue. These two clients would probably need very different massage sessions at first. The first could tolerate strong massage elements such as pressure, joint movement, and general circulatory intent; the second would need a massage without these elements, or with much gentler versions of them.

Asking about a client's energy level, activity level, and typical movement patterns is one of the most useful lines of questioning for a massage therapist, especially if the client has a medical condition that seems likely to affect any of these. When asking this question, a therapist might find out some surprising things—a client with a brain tumor is training for a race, or a client with a systemic disease is working out with weights and aerobics four times a week. Such information is helpful when calculating how vigorous a massage to give. On the other hand, a client who has trouble with basic activities of daily living, or who needs to nap twice a day because of fatigue, may need gentle pressure, shorter sessions, careful timing of sessions, and other modifications for a less challenging session.

Asking about activity level is informative in other ways, too: The therapist finds out about injuries, common postural patterns at work, and so on. All of this information can be used to plan an effective massage therapy session.

● THE PREVIOUS MASSAGE PRINCIPLE

A client's previous experience of massage therapy, especially massage after the onset, diagnosis, or flare-up of a medical condition, may be used to plan the massage.

The reasoning behind this principle is twofold. First, any massage experience since the illness or injury began provides a massage history to draw on. The therapist can ask more about what the massage was like, and the client's response to it, to gauge the best level of pressure, speed, and so on for this session.

Second, this information can be used to reset client expectations in some cases. For example, a client who has a history of regular, vigorous massage might not have had it since the onset of a recent health crisis. Although he has no information about how his "new body" might tolerate the familiar, deeper work, he might still want it. The therapist can use this principle to adjust the expectations: "Since this health situation is new for you, I think it's better to start with a more conservative approach than you might be used to. We certainly don't want to make you feel worse. So let's begin with a gentler session. If you feel better, not worse, afterward, then we can experiment with a deeper (or longer, or more vigorous) session next time."

This principle suggests therapists take a strong leadership role in the session. Clients who come with a history of massage might call for deeper pressures, a certain kind of stretching, or a heavy focus in a particular area—a typical "client-centered session." In keeping with the client's medical condition, a therapist may need to define narrower parameters for the session than either the client or therapist would like. This is especially true for a new, unfamiliar medical condition.

Organ Principles

Organs responsible for filtering fluids, pumping blood, and carrying out other functions can be compromised by illness and injury. Therapists adjust several massage elements to accommodate medical conditions affecting organ function. The organ principles help therapists respond to a wide variety of medical conditions that are commonly encountered in practice. These working principles are useful, even though the exact effects of massage on organs and tissues are not yet established.

● THE VITAL ORGAN PRINCIPLE

If a vital organ—heart, lung, kidney, liver, or brain—is compromised in function, use gentle massage elements and adjust them to pose minimal challenge to the client's body.

Someone with an impaired heart, lung, kidney, liver, or brain is typically quite ill, and their tolerance for massage is likely to be limited by the effects of their disease. Examples are congestive heart failure, advanced emphysema, kidney or liver failure,

and severe seizure disorder. These conditions weaken organ function. These organs are vital—the body cannot operate without them—and when they are compromised, overall health is poor. The elements of massage need to be modified so that they are not too challenging to the body, because its resources are primarily needed for managing the disease at hand and for healing. Modified massage elements could include the following:

- Lighter pressure
- Slower speed
- Shorter session length
- Even rhythms
- Sensitive scheduling (at good times of the day so that the client can enjoy the massage with less distraction, or at bad times if it helps the client cope)
- Heightened sensitivity to medical referral needs
- A single position because the client cannot change positions easily
- Greater site restrictions

Also note that not every disease affecting the vital organs significantly affects function. A heart murmur, mild asthma, early cirrhosis of the liver, some kidney diseases, or a mild stroke can affect an organ but not appreciably weaken its function. It is important to ask the client if the *function* of any vital organ is affected by his or her condition. It is also important to list the vital organs on the history form, or ask about each of them at some point.

The Vital Organ Principle should also be considered when there is inflammation in surrounding tissues that puts the organ itself at risk. In these cases, the body is responding to the problem in the neighboring tissues and protecting the vital organ next to it. The person could feel profoundly unwell, and the same gentle elements of massage are in order for this person. One example of this is a urinary tract or bladder infection, with the concern that infection could spread to the kidneys. Other examples are pleuritis, affecting the covering of the lungs; pericarditis, affecting the pericardium (the covering of the heart); and meningitis, affecting the tissues that cover the brain and spinal cord. In these cases, the condition either already impairs the functioning of the neighboring vital organ, or it could spread to affect the organ directly. The Vital Organ Principle is also advised for these conditions because people feel unwell, overall.

● THE FILTER AND PUMP PRINCIPLE

If a filtering organ (liver, kidney, spleen, or lymph node), or a pumping organ (the heart) is functioning poorly or overworking, do not work it harder with massage that is circulatory in intent.

The reasoning behind this principle comes from the belief that massage increases blood circulation, lymph circulation, or both (see Chapter 2). If techniques such as medium or deep (pressure level 3 or above) kneading, stroking, and repeated compressions do indeed increase flow, they might challenge a filtering organ that is already functioning at its capacity. The body's filters are the liver, kidneys, spleen, and lymph nodes. The first three filter blood, and the last filter lymph. The body's pump is the heart, responsible for pumping blood to all tissues.

Strictly practiced, this principle contraindicates massage with general circulatory intent for certain conditions of the liver, kidney, or spleen. This would include any conditions that congest the spleen (such as mononucleosis, other infections, or some blood diseases), or in which the liver or kidneys are compromised in their filtering function (such as liver failure from cirrhosis or kidney failure from advanced diabetes).

If heart pumping is compromised, as in congestive heart failure, then general circulatory intent is contraindicated (see chapter 11). By avoiding the elements that are thought to accelerate venous return of blood, the therapist reduces the risk of overtaxing the heart.

This principle, drawn from the belief that massage can also accelerate lymph circulation, also contraindicates circulatory intent at sites drained by compromised lymph nodes or lymph nodes that are functioning at capacity, such as during infection. Specialized lymphatic techniques might be indicated, instead, and are more likely to honor the natural pace of the filter without overwhelming it.

● THE COMPROMISED CLIENT PRINCIPLE

If a client is not feeling well, be gentle; even if you cannot explain the mechanism behind a contraindication, follow it anyway.

Some principles have logical explanations, based on our understanding of how the body works and established responses to massage. But many do not—there are no physiological explanations for an effect of massage or its contraindication, and no specific risk to an organ is identified. There is little research on massage contraindications or even on the mechanisms of action to aid our reasoning. Instead, principles guiding massage are based on intuition and clinical observation.

For ill clients, it is important for the therapist to modify the session even when there is no established threat to a particular organ. A good example is a client with a cold. Common sense suggests respecting a body during a healing process, and a piece of lore in the massage profession advises against circulatory massage for someone at the beginning of a cold; instead, wait until he or she is past the "peak" and is getting better.

Even though many massage contraindications are based on possible circulatory effects of massage, we are on weak ground when we offer the common explanation for this guideline: that circulatory massage could spread the infection through the body before the immune system can respond, thereby making the client more ill. In reality, whether massage is sufficiently circulatory to cause this to happen is a matter of debate, and the immune response to infection is body-wide as well as local. Instead of trying to explain this guideline, it is better to support it with common sense and clinical observations: for whatever reason, clients in the middle of a cold often feel worse after vigorous massage, not better. Perhaps, in these cases, clients need to conserve their resources for healing.

Although a cold is short term, other chronic or serious medical conditions may call for this principle over the long term. In general, a client whose body is working hard to maintain homeostasis needs support, not more challenge. If it makes sense to bring about change—say, a relaxation in muscle—the massage therapist should coax and invite it rather than force it. This principle is grounded in common sense, rather than clear mechanistic effects of massage.

One challenge for the therapist is knowing when or how to depart from the principle, just a little bit. Can this client withstand a slightly deeper shoulder massage, for a minute or two? Are there other pressure contraindications? Is there time over a series of sessions to test out slightly deeper pressure and monitor the results? Does good record keeping exist? The general principles presented at the beginning of this chapter can help therapists answer these questions.

Principles of Sensation

In some medical conditions affecting nervous system function, sensation loss results. In *impaired sensation*, the loss is partial; in *absent sensation* the loss is complete. Sensations such as pressure, heat, and pain protect the body against injury. Areas of sensation loss are vulnerable to injury, and principles of sensation are designed to protect these areas.

● THE SENSATION PRINCIPLE

In an area of impaired or absent sensation, use caution with pressure and joint movement.

The reasoning behind this principle is threefold: (1) pain is one way the body tells the brain that tissues are being (or are about to be) injured; (2) the perception of pain is necessary for a person to give reliable feedback to a therapist about massage; and (3) in the absence of reliable feedback, massage pressure or movement could injure tissue.

The idea that a massage could cause tissue damage might seem remote to some massage therapists. If the therapist is working sensitively, it is unlikely to happen. However, some therapists using deeper pressures need to be mindful of sensation impairment while working. When the client's feeling of pain isn't there to signal possible injury, the therapist must work more carefully, usually within the range of pressure levels 1–3. Care is given to joint movement, as well; methods such as stretching, positional release, and **range of motion (ROM)** techniques, designed to increase the flexibility of a joint and restore its full spectrum of movement, are cautiously applied. Rather than taking a joint to the very end of its available range, a therapist modifies each movement, staying well within the limits of the joint.

This principle is not just black or white; there are shades of gray. As already mentioned, sensation loss can range from mild impairment to a complete absence of sensation in an area. Likewise, massage pressures and joint movement could range from somewhat gentle to very gentle in response.

While implementing this principle, it is important that the therapist maintain firm, reassuring touch and good contact, avoiding letting the hand contact become too "dribbly" or faint. If the client has partial sensation, a light hand contact can feel ticklish and irritating, and in some nervous system conditions, pressure that is too light can provoke reflexive muscle contraction. It can take time and practice to find the pressure levels that are light enough to protect the tissues, but not so light that they aggravate the condition.

● THE SENSATION LOSS, INJURY PRONE PRINCIPLE

If a client has lost sensation in an area, inspect the tissues carefully for injury before beginning the massage.

This principle is based on the experience of people with conditions that cause profound sensation impairment and loss, such as advanced diabetes and AIDS. In these conditions, loss of feeling in the hands and feet can lead to injury from sharp objects, tight shoes, and other problems. Even small pebbles or other objects, becoming lodged in the tissues, can go unnoticed when no pain is registered.

Because such injuries can break the skin, the therapist looks closely at the tissues before applying lubricant or making contact with the area. By doing so, the therapist avoids making contact with open lesions, and protects herself and her client from infection. Massage therapists, unique in their close contact with the skin, can bring these problems to the client's awareness so that the client can get the proper medical attention.

Pain, Injury, and Inflammation Principles

Clients often seek massage therapy to relieve pain such as back and neck pain and headaches. Massage therapy is ideally suited to address some sources of pain—especially those having to do with stress and tension—but not others. Pain has many causes, and it is often a component of inflammation. Pain can be due to local injury of tissues including muscle, bone, cartilage, ligament, tendon, and fascia. It can also be due to systemic illness. Or it can be of neurologic origin, either trauma to a nerve or systemic illness affecting nerve function. The pain, injury, and inflammation principles help the therapist with basic skills to determine how and when to work with clients in pain. They help identify when it is appropriate to massage, how to massage, and when to refer clients for other services.

● THE PHYSICIAN REFERRAL FOR PAIN PRINCIPLE

If a client's pain has specific qualities, such as sharp, stabbing, radiating, or shooting pain, or if the pain is accompanied by tingling, numbness, or weakness, refer the client to a physician.

In addition, these are specific pain qualities that also signal a physician referral:

- Persistent
- Worsening
- Debilitating
- Not relieved by rest
- Not relieved by movement
- Produced by ordinary movements

The reasoning behind this principle is that any of these specific pain qualities could indicate serious illness or injury, requiring medical attention and diagnostic tests.

● THE NEW, UNFAMILIAR, OR POORLY MANAGED PAIN PRINCIPLE

Massage for a client with new, unfamiliar, or poorly managed pain should be more conservative than massage for a client with a familiar, well-managed pain pattern.

The reasoning behind this is twofold: (1) because unfamiliar and poorly managed pain can be overwhelming, people experiencing it may provide incomplete or conflicting information about it in an interview; (2) without a pain "track record," it is difficult to predict the effect of massage on the pain, or to be sure it won't aggravate the condition.

Although one can argue that all clients with all types of pain should be referred to a physician rather than massaged, this is not usually feasible. There is no hard and fast rule about when, in the course of massage treatment, to make a medical referral. Although many therapists say three or four sessions are enough to determine whether massage can make a difference in the pain, a client with debilitating pain should be seen by a physician well before that.

People often seek massage specifically for pain relief, even when it is severe and debilitating. One client may call in a panic, having reached for something on the floor, then collapsed with severe pain in her lumbar area. She may move with great difficulty, since the pain radiates even with normal movement of the back. These pain qualities suggest that a medical referral is in order, not a massage.

In contrast, another client might come in with a familiar pain pattern that has recurred in five acute episodes following a low back injury 12 years ago. He has been able to manage the pain with rest, ice, heat, and even massage, and has seen his physician a couple of times and was reassured that the injury was not serious. That is a different situation. In this case, the therapist still needs to be careful (especially for a first-time client), but the client's long history with the pain and good client feedback during the massage should contribute to a positive outcome. The massage is less likely to worsen the condition, and more likely to relieve it.

● THE RECENT INJURY PRINCIPLE

Recent injuries, or injuries that have not been seen by a physician, should not be treated with massage therapy, or massage therapy should be conservative.

This principle calls for no treatment, or a conservative approach, for several reasons. First, the body protects a recent injury with **muscle splinting** and swelling. Muscle splinting is an increase in tension in muscles that serves to stabilize the area of injury, preventing it from moving too much and becoming reinjured. Massage should not interfere with this protective effect. Second, the therapist should not use massage pressure or joint movement in the area or adjacent structures if a physician has not examined it, especially if there is any chance of fracture, or severe or widespread ligament injury. Third, the area may include bruising or clotting and therefore should not be manipulated. The client should see his or her physician, and the therapist can gather the physician's input about pressure and joint movement in the area before proceeding with those elements.

This principle overlaps with the Physician Referral for Pain Principle; a medical referral is needed before pressure and joint movement are used. This principle obviously applies more to acute, severe injuries (e.g., recent car accident with neck stiffness) than mild ones (a simple, mild ankle sprain), but even mild bruising and signs of inflammation contraindicate pressure and movement at the site.

● THE CLAIM OR LITIGATION PRINCIPLE

If a client's recent injury involves an insurance claim or litigation, do not complicate the clinical picture with massage that could affect the area.

This principle addresses situations involving medical and legal claims when people are injured. After an injury, a short period of time may pass before a person is evaluated by a physician, undergoes testing, and begins treatment. During this time period, it is important not to complicate the clinical picture with massage. The client's claim of damage during the

injury could be countered by the claim that massage caused the injury, or aggravated it.

If massage therapy clouds the clinical picture of a recent injury, a client's ability to pursue an insurance claim or litigation is jeopardized. In such cases, fair restitution to the client could be put at risk if a company or individual could state that the massage, not an initial injury, caused the symptoms or aggravated the condition, and there is no way to tell how much of the client's discomfort is due to the initial event. This risk is especially high when the therapist does not document the session.

This "hands-off" policy is not indefinite, and it may not apply to all therapists. In fact, advanced therapists, whose work is designed for musculoskeletal injuries, can often intervene effectively very soon after an injury, as long as the physician has done the diagnostic work and it's clear that massage is appropriate. However, therapists with less training and experience may be more likely to make mistakes or overtreat the condition, and should let the claims process take its course for a while, then work conservatively to bring about relief. See Therapist's Journal 3-1 for a story of a client requesting massage right after a car accident.

● THE INFLAMMATION PRINCIPLE

If an area of tissue is inflamed, don't aggravate it with pressure, friction, or circulatory intent at the site.

Inflamed tissue is in the process of healing, and massage could disrupt the process and injure the tissues further. Four signs of inflammation—pain, swelling, heat, and redness—involve complicated physiological processes. Although its ultimate purpose is to heal tissues, inflammation can injure tissues in the process. For example, **edema**, or swelling of the tissue, is one factor in inflammation that, by expanding the space between cells in the area, pushes them farther from their blood supply. This distance leads to **hypoxia**, a shortage of oxygen in the cells farthest from the blood supply, causing cell death. Ultimately, the healing elements of inflammation usually prevail over its damaging ones and resolve the problem. However, in some chronic inflammatory conditions, the injury persists.

In whatever way these processes play out, massage can aggravate them. The pressure and friction of massage causes a kind of brief inflammation, with redness and heat often showing at the surface. Often, clients feel more pain afterward, too. Although more research is needed on the physiological changes in tissues caused by massage, for now the visual signs of inflammation from massage are enough to contraindicate pressure and friction in the area. An exception to this principle can be found in some specialized massage techniques that use inflammation for therapeutic purposes. In such techniques, additional inflammation is deliberate, breaking down scar tissue in ligaments or tendons so that the healing process can build more stable tissue. In this case, friction can be used quite intensely on the tissues, causing direct and obvious aggravation of inflammation. But for the most part, therapists with basic training should be careful not to aggravate inflammation.

Principles for Unstable Conditions

Along the spectrum of health and illness, a client may present with a condition that involves unstable tissue.

This tissue may be vulnerable to massage elements such as joint movement or pressure. Some clients have

THERAPIST'S JOURNAL 3-1 *I Was Rear-Ended on the Way to the Spa*

Believe it or not, I've heard several stories from therapists about their clients getting in minor motor vehicle accidents on the way to their massage appointments. Perhaps they're in a hurry to get there on time! Who knows? I have been asked what to do in that situation.

Massage shouldn't be given to someone who's had a recent accident. A physician needs to examine the person; even if he or she is in no pain right away, he or she could have significant pain in a day or two. There might be insurance claims involved. It is a tricky situation, and massage is one more complication.

One therapist told me she assumed massage was contraindicated on the client's neck in that situation, so she did some passive movement, turning and stretching the neck instead! She thought she was being cautious, but during this tender time, muscles are splinting the area and should not be manipulated by a massage therapist with only basic training.

The most conservative approach would be to avoid massage treatment entirely. At the same time, not all motor vehicle accidents are equal. A gentle tap, 2 days ago, from the car behind at a stoplight, may require a judgment call. In such cases, if therapists work at all they need to work very gently, using no joint movement or pressure on any of the areas that may have been injured, and no joint movement or pressure anywhere on the spine. If the hands and feet were not involved at all, some reflex points or general strokes are probably fine. Documenting the elements of massage used is extremely important here.

Tracy Walton
Cambridge, MA

systemic conditions that may destabilize quickly to become life threatening. Using a few principles, a therapist can be prepared for this range in medical conditions in their practice.

● THE UNSTABLE TISSUE PRINCIPLE

If a tissue is unstable, do not challenge it with too much pressure or joint movement in the area.

The reasoning behind this principle is common sense—to avoid further destabilizing an area that is already unstable. This could apply to skin that is thin and tears easily, or, as in the top branch of a Decision Tree in Figure 3-2, a shoulder that has dislocated recently and is awaiting surgery.

If a joint is unstable, the therapist avoids causing reinjury by avoiding strong stretching or ROM techniques. This tree specifies the elements of massage to adjust pressure and joint movement at a given site. Notice that it does not prohibit stretching muscles across other joints, just the affected area. Depending on the training of the therapist and the level of the client's injury and inflammation, massage of the involved muscles might also be contraindicated so that they can continue to splint the injury and stabilize the shoulder.

If skin, instead of a joint, is the unstable tissue, as in a frail older client or someone with thinned skin as a result of medical treatment, the therapist should consider what the skin is able to tolerate. Pressure level 3 might be fine as long as it is stationary and goes straight into the tissues, without any drag on them. On the other hand, friction or any transverse movement of the skin at pressure level 3 may injure it. The skin issue does not contraindicate joint movement, which would probably be fine as long as the therapist grips the skin gently to move the area.

● THE STABILIZATION OF AN ACUTE CONDITION PRINCIPLE

Until an acute medical condition has stabilized, massage should be conservative.

The reasoning behind this principle is that while the body is struggling with an acute condition, the wrong mix of massage elements might be too much for it. In medicine, the term **acute** is used to describe a symptom or condition of abrupt or recent onset, or rapid progression. In an acute phase of a disease, there may be intense or severe symptoms, requiring urgent medical care. Acute may also describe a disease of short duration, or a flare-up of a chronic disease.

In an acute condition, **homeostasis**, or the body's tendency to return to balance in response to a stressor, may be difficult to achieve. When a client's body is already working hard to maintain homeostasis, it needs supportive massage therapy, rather than any additional challenge. The following conditions, in the acute phase, are examples:

- Heart attack
- Stroke
- Multiple fractures
- Hepatitis
- Traumatic brain or spinal cord injury

Touch may be fine and welcome in these cases, but massage should include conservative elements of pressure, joint movement, and massage intent. Physician input into the massage plan is an important part of this conservative approach.

An acute phase of a disease may be preceded or followed by a subacute or chronic phase, in which the condition is more stable. A **chronic** phase or disease is long or indefinite in duration, and symptoms tend to change slowly. A symptom may also be described as chronic when it has been around for several months, as in chronic pain. In a **subacute** phase, which lies somewhere between acute and chronic, symptoms also tend to be more stable.

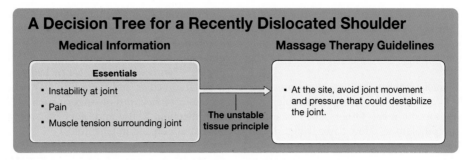

A Decision Tree for a Recently Dislocated Shoulder

Medical Information		Massage Therapy Guidelines

Essentials
- Instability at joint
- Pain
- Muscle tension surrounding joint

The unstable tissue principle

- At the site, avoid joint movement and pressure that could destabilize the joint.

FIGURE 3-2. A Decision Tree for a recently dislocated shoulder, showing the use of the Unstable Tissue Principle. Only the top branch of the tree is shown.

Even if the condition never resolves completely, less conservative massage may be appropriate than in the acute phase.

● THE EMERGENCY PROTOCOL PRINCIPLE

If a client has a condition with rapid or unpredictable changes in symptoms, ask about any warning signs and appropriate responses in case they occur during a massage.

The purpose of this principle is to prepare a massage therapist for acting in an emergency situation. A client with a chronic condition may well receive and benefit from massage therapy, but therapists need more information if the condition can quickly turn acute or life threatening. Examples of chronic conditions that rapidly destabilize are angina pectoris, poorly controlled diabetes, poorly controlled seizure disorders, and very high or poorly controlled blood pressure. It's important for the therapist to ask, "Where do you keep your nitroglycerin in case you have an angina episode?" "What happens to you when your blood sugar drops? What does it look like to others?" "If your blood pressure spikes or drops, what does it feel like, and look like?" For each scenario, also ask "What does your doctor or nurse advise you to do if this happens?" Noting the answers to these questions in the client history and keeping them in mind in advance will make these situations much easier to deal with if they occur during a massage.

Medical Treatment Principles

These principles concern clients in the process of medical diagnosis and treatment. This can be a vulnerable time, and a massage therapist can be an important source of support for a client. As treatment progresses, changes in the client's signs or symptoms, diagnosis, or therapy may require adjustments in the massage plan. These principles help a therapist to adapt to uncertainty and changes in the client's health status.

● THE WAITING FOR A DIAGNOSIS PRINCIPLE

If a client is scheduled for diagnostic tests, or is awaiting results, adapt massage to the possible diagnosis. If more than one condition is being investigated, adapt massage to the worst-case scenario.

The reasoning behind this principle is that if a client's physician is concerned enough to test for a condition, it is best to share the concern and adjust the massage plan for that condition until the test rules it out.

The diagnosis could end up being any of a range of possibilities, but if it is not certain yet, there is an information gap, and the principle "First, do no harm" rules. Applying the physician's concern, the therapist observes massage contraindications for the worst-case possibilities; this is in line with not doing harm.

Finding out the information can take some skill. Asking the client, "Any recent or scheduled diagnostic tests?" and "What are they testing for?" or "What is your doctor concerned about at this point?" may get at the possibilities. This principle may require follow-up research if the client doesn't have the relevant information, and possible consultation with the client's physician. If the information is not available, the most conservative massage or touch session should be offered.

Suppose a client is being tested for hepatitis. Following this principle, the therapist adapts the massage to the worst-case scenario of hepatitis, which would include, among other things, avoiding massage with general circulatory intent (see Chapter 16). If a client is waiting for results of a scan for cancer spread to the spine, the therapist avoids any pressure and joint movement that moves the area (see Bone Metastasis, Chapter 20). If a client's headaches or dizzy spells prompt his physician to run a series of tests for stroke, the therapist treats him as if he is at risk of stroke (see Chapter 10).

Following this principle, the therapist does not have to become an expert on diagnostic tests, she just needs to ask some questions of a client and, at times, investigate further on her own. There are excellent references in the online bibliography for therapists to consult. Therapists can keep a copy of a reference on diagnostics on hand, or do a quick Internet search to find the information quickly.

● THE MEDICATION PRINCIPLE

Adapt massage to the condition for which the medication is taken or prescribed, and to any side effects.

The reasoning behind this principle is twofold: (1) medications are often prescribed for conditions that require massage adjustments and (2) medications can cause side effects that also require massage adjustments.

This is a convenient principle to apply whenever a client is taking a medication. Massage is often adapted to the condition for which the medication is prescribed. This condition may be an issue even though the person is being treated for the problem.

Some medications, such as those for high blood pressure, are not always 100% effective in addressing the problem, or they provide only symptomatic relief. Others, such as antibiotics, often resolve the problem in a few days. If high blood pressure is only partly controlled by medication, the therapist should take that condition into consideration (see "Hypertension," Chapter 11). If medication for migraine headaches is only partially effective at controlling them, massage must be adapted to the headache (see "Headache," Chapter 10).

Massage is also adapted to the unintended effects of the medication, such as side effects, adverse reactions, or complications. Common side effects of medications include nausea, abdominal pain, fatigue, restlessness, hypotension, and headache. A client who is feeling nauseated will need a massage with slow speeds, even rhythms, and minimal joint movement. Abdominal pain might require careful positioning. Medications and procedures are discussed in Chapter 21; see Table 21-1 for an alphabetical list of common side effects and massage guidelines.

● THE PROCEDURE PRINCIPLE

Adapt massage to the condition for which the procedure is advised, and to the effects of the procedure itself.

This principle is nearly identical to the Medication Principle. The reasoning behind the principle is also similar: (1) A procedure is generally ordered to diagnose or treat an existing medical condition, which may require massage adjustments, and (2) procedures, in and of themselves, can cause other problems that could require massage adjustments.

Following this principle, the therapist adjusts the massage plan for procedures such as surgery, radiation therapy, or catheterization. This is because individuals may be left with nausea after anesthesia, fatigue after radiation therapy, and other side effects. Clients who have recently had surgery are common in massage practice, and therapists may need to adapt the massage to complications of surgery, such as blood clots, swelling, and infection. These and other massage guidelines after surgery are discussed in Chapter 21.

● THE MEDICALLY RESTRICTED ACTIVITY PRINCIPLE

If there are any medical restrictions on a client's activities, explore and apply any equivalent massage contraindications.

The therapist needs to share any concerns held by the physician and avoid any massage elements that are discouraged in a medical condition. If the physician prohibits physical exertion or hot whirlpool baths because of a heart condition, the massage therapist should adapt massage so that it doesn't strain the client's heart. In the massage tradition, this has meant that general circulatory intent is contraindicated. If a physician advises a client against sleeping flat on a mattress because of breathing problems, the massage therapist adjusts the positioning accordingly. If a home health nurse recommends a client's leg be elevated to reduce swelling, the massage therapist may need to follow this recommendation during the session.

Therapists can determine the need for this principle by simply asking, "Are there any medical restrictions on your activities?" or "Is your doctor or nurse concerned and advising you to make changes in your day-to-day life?" A general question, "What concerns has your doctor or nurse expressed to you about this condition?" can get at some of this information.

Principles for Spa Treatments

Along with massage, some spa treatments should be adjusted or omitted when medical conditions are present. While little information has been collected on massage contraindications, even less is available about contraindications for spa treatment. However, common sense can fill in the information gap. Therapists can consider the purpose of the spa service, the strength of it, and how it challenges the body in order to determine any contraindications. Many individuals with medical conditions visit spas for health and relaxation, and sometimes turn to other spa services when massage is ill advised.

To decide whether to apply spa principles, it is necessary to ask the client a few questions. The spa health checklist in Chapter 4 has brief massage interview questions for spa guests. In general, asking questions about activity restrictions, activity level, energy level, chronic and degenerative conditions, and the health of skin and vital organs will help bring up contraindications to spa treatments. Therapists can assess each situation and use the following principles.

● THE DETOXIFICATION PRINCIPLE

If an intent of a spa treatment is to detoxify, avoid using it when the client is significantly challenged by illness or injury, or is taking strong medication.

The reasoning behind this principle is that detoxification is inappropriate in some conditions without medical supervision. In most spa settings, where clients are not necessarily monitored over time or followed from one spa service to the next, it is not possible to provide this kind of judgment or supervision. Some spas are the exception, providing customized care through nurse or physician supervision of each client's services. However, many settings do not have the staff with expertise to work with people in complex medical situations.

At times, the Detoxification Principle may seem counterintuitive. Suppose a client comes in between chemotherapy sessions. A therapist might think detoxification is indicated to help remove the toxic medications from the body, and the idea might appeal to the client, as well. But medications have their own clearance rates, and dosages are carefully calculated for individuals. On strong medications, clients are often plagued with side effects as the drugs leave their body over a calculated period of time. If the spa treatment does in fact accelerate this process, the client's symptoms could be aggravated. A spa guest who is on strong medication needs his or her resources for healing, and should not be challenged with a strong spa treatment.

Likewise, systemic illness and significant injury challenge homeostasis, and therapists are discouraged from challenging it even more. Therapists consider the Vital Organ Principle here, and how hard vital organs must work in some conditions to keep the body in balance. If a vital organ is challenged by disease, then a detoxifying spa treatment is contraindicated.

Note that the detoxification principle is based on the *intent* of the spa treatment, rather than the established effect of the spa treatment. As with circulatory intent, there may be little data to verify the effects. But as long as the intent is known, it should be considered in the light of a client's medical condition.

● THE EXFOLIATION PRINCIPLE

If a client's skin health or overall health is significantly compromised, do not use treatments involving strong exfoliation.

This reasoning behind this principle is obvious for skin health—if a skin condition would be aggravated by exfoliation, avoid it. The reasoning is less obvious for overall health. While it's possible that exfoliation could help some conditions, it's also possible that it could aggravate symptoms. If nothing else, The Compromised Client Principle applies here. If used at all with people with complex conditions, exfoliation should be gentle. What is invigorating for a robust person may be fatiguing for someone who is less healthy. The friction, the demand on the cardiovascular system to increase circulation to the skin, possible detoxification intent, and overall nervous system stimulation can be too much for people when they don't feel well. If the client is fatigued, frail, or on strong medications, exfoliation may be too much. At the very least, using gentler exfoliation techniques over less of the body is a good idea, and the client's response should be monitored over a course of treatments to determine whether stronger techniques are appropriate.

● THE CORE TEMPERATURE PRINCIPLE

Avoid spa treatments that raise the core temperature if a client's cardiovascular system, respiratory system, skin, or other tissue or system might be overly challenged by heat, or if there are comparable medical restrictions.

This principle draws parallels between spa treatments and other activities; it is similar to the Medically Restricted Activity Principle. Suppose cardiovascular exercise is contraindicated for a spa guest because of his or her condition; the heart's pumping function is compromised. The guest probably also has medical restrictions on hot tubs, saunas, hot showers, and other activities. The heart cannot provide the increased circulation needed to cool the body, so these treatments are contraindicated.

Another example is a client with lymph nodes missing from the axillary (armpit) area, the inguinal (groin) area, or the neck, after cancer treatment (see "Lymphedema," Chapter 20). With potentially compromised lymph flow, there are often significant restrictions on activities such as saunas and hot tubs. Likewise, wraps involving steam, the application of hot stones to a certain area of the body, or other heat treatments may be contraindicated if they raise core temperature or skin temperature.

A good way to get at this possibility in a short spa interview is to ask the guest if there are any medical restrictions on activities, and ask specifically about heat treatments.

Used with thought and care, the principles in this chapter can help the practitioner manage a variety of medical conditions in massage practice. The principles are especially useful when there are gaps in client information or in the therapist's knowledge. In later chapters, many principles are applied to specific scenarios. Whether general or more specific, massage principles help a massage therapist navigate clinical decision making with confidence.

SELF TEST

1. How are principles used in massage contraindications? List three ways.
2. Suppose you have a first-time client with a chronic neck injury who wants deep neck and shoulder massage. Using the Where You Start Isn't Always Where You End Up Principle, how would you respond to her in the initial session? In subsequent sessions? How would you explain the massage plan to this client?
3. Why should most massage interviews include a question about physical activity?
4. How is the acute phase of a medical condition different from the chronic phase?
5. Name three medically restricted activities that are of particular relevance to a massage therapist in planning a session. How are these activities relevant to massage planning?
6. Suppose your client has a complex medical condition, such as diabetes, and has received regular massage since his or her diagnosis. How might your conversation with

that client differ from a conversation with a client who has had one or two massages, but long before the diagnosis? Which principle are you using?

7. A client informs you of a medical condition that you don't know anything about. While he is getting ready on the table, you ask another therapist what to do. Your colleague advises you "to go with your gut" in order to work safely with him. Which principle or principles can help direct you in this situation?
8. A client presents with a condition ending in "-itis," signifying inflammation. How should you proceed? Which principle most directly applies in this case?
9. If a client reports unstable blood pressure or blood sugar, what questions do you need to ask her before working with her? Which principle applies to this scenario?
10. Your client's advanced AIDS has led to the loss of sensation in his or her feet. What should you do before massaging his or her feet? Which principle are you using in this case?

 For answers to these questions and to see a bibliography for this chapter, visit http://thePoint. lww.com/Walton.

It is the province of knowledge to speak, and it is the privilege of wisdom to listen.

—OLIVER WENDELL HOLMES

Massage therapists listen with their hands and hearts, as well as their ears. They gather information about clients in various ways, for various purposes. They pick up information through their hands as they travel over the client's tissues. As they move the client's joints, they note restrictions. They notice postural habits as the client moves or sits.

This nonverbal information gathering is the classic stuff of massage therapy: human exchanges, beyond words. Through these exchanges, therapists engage the body, and also the mind and spirit, in their hands. For many therapists, this is part of the richness of massage therapy. For clients, the experience of being witnessed in this way may be as healing as the other elements of massage therapy.

Verbal history taking, while different from palpation and observation, can be just as rich as the hands-on experience. Each medical condition, from a broken arm to a life-threatening illness, is part of a client's story, and the interview is a perfect setting to learn about it. Obviously it's not necessary to learn about a client's entire medical history, but buried within it is key, specific information to bring to bear on the session. Interviewing for medical conditions, processing the answers, and charting the massage adjustments are the focus of this chapter. These steps are discussed in the order that they typically occur in practice.

The Purpose of the Interview

Done professionally and well, the client interview builds rapport, the foundation for the therapeutic relationship (Figure 4-1). It gives the client time to get to know the therapist before being touched. In addition, the interview allows the therapist to:

- Gather information on the client's massage experience and preferences.
- Learn about the client's health and establish goals for the session.

- Identify and document the massage contraindications to apply.

Interview styles vary across massage settings and between individual therapists. Some therapists conduct only verbal interviews, others begin with a written form. No matter how it begins, the interview becomes a conversation: an exchange of initial questions, a client's answers, follow-up questions triggered by those answers, more responses, and so on. Throughout, the therapist holds the focus on the client's health, and how that affects the massage plan.

Initial Questions

The primary tool for the interview is the health intake form for massage therapy, also called the *client health form*, shown in Figure 4-2. This form covers the basic information needed to bring common massage contraindications to light.

● BALANCING GENERAL AND SPECIFIC QUESTIONS

Each therapist finds the right balance of general and specific questions. While general questions take less time to ask, they may take more time to answer if they are too open ended. They may also fall flat; for instance, the question, "Is there anything I should know about your health?" is too general. On the other hand, specific questions target some key contraindications, but may miss other important information. And too many specific questions make for a long and tedious interview.

It is not practical or necessary to ask about every disease and injury. Not all medical conditions are equally affected by massage therapy, and the client health form reflects this. For example, cardiovascular conditions, kidney and liver conditions, and skin conditions are mentioned, but immune, lymphatic, and reproductive conditions are left out because of space limitations. The therapist can capture these conditions with other general questions about chronic disease, symptoms, or medical treatment.

Explicit mention of some medical conditions is important, especially common conditions that are most relevant to massage. This prompts clients, jogging their memory about their own health. For example, not everyone would think to write "varicose veins" under "cardiovascular conditions." Yet, depending on how severe they are, varicose veins dictate pressure adjustments at the site. By listing a few other key conditions, the therapist increases the chance of raising important issues before the massage. Initially, a

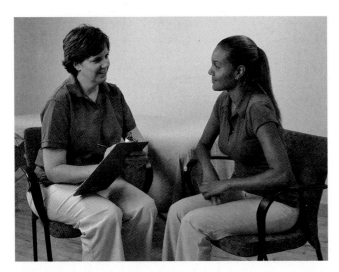

FIGURE 4-1. The client history. The interview is a time for establishing rapport with the client, and for learning about the client's story.

balance between general and specific questions yields useful data without making an interview too superficial, repetitive, or time-consuming.

● LAYERING AND EMPHASIS

It's especially important for massage therapists to consider factors such as skin integrity, bone and joint stability, changes in sensation, and cardiovascular conditions when planning a massage session. Because of the emphasis on these issues, they are queried in different ways in order to prompt the client's memory. This is a layered approach to interviewing. The client health form introduces questions about general health, body systems, and common conditions. There are broad questions about chronic and progressive diseases and injuries. The form concludes with questions about medical treatments.

By organizing questions in this way, the therapist approaches some of the same key information from different angles. For example, a client with a current injury can be prompted by questions about inflammation and swelling, pain, injury history, and activity level. A client with phlebitis might mention the condition when asked about pain, inflammation, cardiovascular conditions, or medical treatment.

Even some follow-up questions, introduced in this chapter, overlap slightly with each other and with initial questions. This built-in redundancy decreases the chance of missing something important in the client's history.

● CUSTOMIZING QUESTIONS

How does a massage therapist decide *how* to ask each question? This may be dictated by the massage setting, a therapist's own focus on a special medical population, or his or her own communication style. Therapists can use the questions in this chapter, purchase stock intake forms, or use one provided in school, but it's best to review each question for relevance and purpose, and then customize a client health form if necessary. In "The History of our History Forms," a therapist describes the pitfalls of using a generic health form without customizing it (see online at http://thePoint.lww.com/Walton).

The questions in this chapter do not need to be read word for word. For the most relaxed, comfortable interview, each therapist can practice asking and following up on questions, in his own words. The best questions are designed or customized by the therapist, who is clear about what he needs to know about, what he doesn't need to know about, and how to use the client's responses. This sense of ownership is important: whatever the setting is, the therapist is in charge of guiding the interview. For each therapist using a set of questions, ease and confidence come from making it his own. The strongest interview is a natural conversation, typically prompted by a written health form.

Accuracy of the Client's Responses

One concern therapists share is the possibility of a client providing incomplete or inaccurate information. This is uncommon, but it does happen, for several reasons: It can be due to "form fatigue"—when a client feels her history is too lengthy to explain on a form, or she leaves out information, not seeing the purpose behind the questions. Inaccurate or incomplete forms also result from language barriers, miscommunication, a client's sense of privacy, or even a client's temptation to withhold information that could jeopardize his or her chances of receiving massage. Sometimes a client is incapable of providing reliable information, due to extreme stress or mental status changes.

Any of these scenarios can result in incomplete or inaccurate information. It's up to the therapist to do his or her best, to be alert for inconsistencies, but not try second guess every answer. Repeating questions verbally, or conducting the entire interview verbally, may remedy the situation. Rewording the questions may help, and a therapist may need to probe a bit more deeply with some clients than with others. Additional information may come forth as the session unfolds. If the information seems incomplete or inaccurate, if a client's answers are circular, vague, or inconsistent, the therapist works conservatively until more information is available.

Follow-Up Questions

A client's response to a question may provide sufficient information, or the therapist may need more details. A thorough interview usually requires at least a few brief follow-up questions focused on possible massage contraindications. Some follow-up questions can be used for a broad range of medical conditions. These gen-

eral questions are introduced in this chapter. Follow-up questions for specific conditions appear in Part II and Part III chapters.

In this chapter, follow-up questions on general topics are grouped by common client presentations such as pain, injury, signs and symptoms, medications, and so on. These all-purpose

**Client Health Form
for Massage Therapy**

**Maria Abutin Massage Therapy
27 Hopedale, Suite 4, Bronxville, NY 10021**

Name _____

Phone _____

Address _____

Date of Birth _____

Massage Therapy

Have you had massage therapy before? _____

Can you describe it? _____

_____

What did you like or dislike about it? _____

_____

Circle areas you would like massage to address:

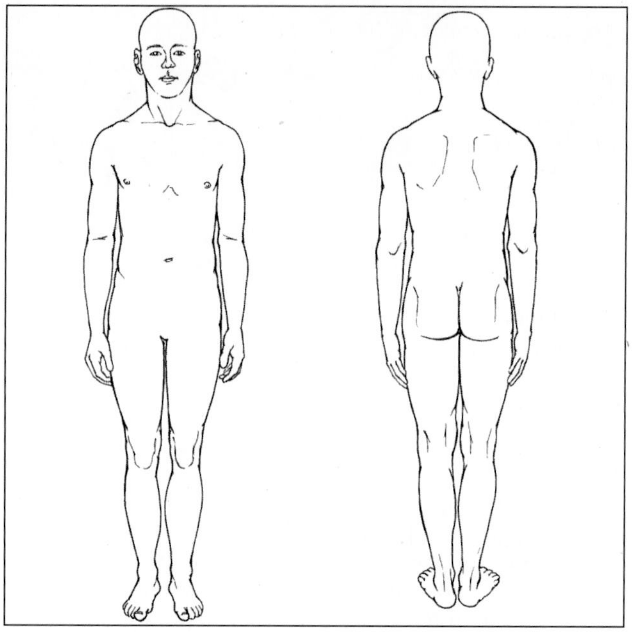

How would you describe your stress level?

0 1 2 3 4 5 6 7 8 9 10

No stress   Worst stress imaginable

How would you describe your pain level?

0 1 2 3 4 5 6 7 8 9 10

No pain   Worst pain imaginable

Activities

Please describe your daily or weekly activities and any exercise or movement you do each week (e.g., work at desk, computer, or telephone; stand at counter; walk to work; heavy lifting; take care of small children; exercise class; swim, etc.)

_____

_____

How would you rate your energy level, on a scale of 0 to 10 (where 0 is no energy and 10 is very high energy)? _____

_____

Health Issues   Past or current, dates, any treatment

General Health

Any areas of pain?	
Any areas of muscle tension?	
Any conditions that seem to be caused or aggravated by stress (e.g., headache, back pain, neck pain, or insomnia)?	
Any inflammation or swelling anywhere in your body?	
Any changes in sensation (numbness, burning, tingling, etc)?	
Any areas of current or recent infection?	
Allergies or sensitivities to certain substances?	

FIGURE 4-2. A client health form for massage therapy.

Health Issues	**Past or current, dates, any treatment**

Skin

Any areas of skin sensitivity, irritation, rash, or open skin?	
Any chronic skin conditions?	
Any tendency to bruise or bleed?	

Muscles, bones, and joints

Any problems with your joints, such as arthritis?	
Any muscle problems, such as pain, stiffness, muscle tension, or tendency to cramp?	
Any bone or spine conditions, such as injuries, osteoporosis, disk problems, or knee problems?	

Nervous system

Any sensation or motor changes?	
Any numbness, tingling, or muscle weakness?	
Any pain?	
Any medical condition that affects your nerves, brain, or spinal cord?	

Cardiovascular system

Have you or a physician ever been concerned about the health of your heart or blood vessels?	
Circle any of the following you have experienced and describe: Varicose veins Phlebitis (inflamed vein) High cholesterol High blood pressure Atherosclerosis or hardened arteries Thrombosis (blood clot) Pulmonary embolism Heart disease Heart attack Heart arrhythmia Angina Stroke or TIA (transient ischemic attack)	
Do you take any medications for blood pressure or other cardiovascular issues?	

Blood conditions

Any conditions that affect your blood or blood cells?	

Respiratory system

Any conditions that affect your lungs, nasal passages, or airway?	

Digestive system

Any conditions that affect digestion or elimination?	

Liver

Any conditions that affect your liver function, such as hepatitis, cirrhosis, or other liver disease?	

FIGURE 4-2. (*Continued*)

Health Issues	Past or current, dates, any treatment
Glands and hormones	
Any conditions that affect the function of glands, such as the pancreas or thyroid, or hormones?	
Kidney and urinary	
Any conditions that affect your kidneys, bladder, or urinary tract?	
Headache	
Any history of headache—migraine, tension, or other kinds of headaches?	
Injuries or accidents	
Have you ever had a serious injury—car accident, fall, fracture, or sprain?	
Cancer	
Any history of cancer or suspected cancer?	
Diabetes	
Any history of diabetes or blood sugar problems?	
Pregnancy	
Is there any chance that you are pregnant?	
Chronic conditions	
Have you had any chronic, recurrent, or ongoing conditions?	
Progressive or degenerative conditions	
Have you had any degenerative or progressive (worsening) conditions?	
Other	
Any other condition or concern not mentioned here?	

Medical Treatments	Please describe
Are you currently or were you recently in a doctor's care for any condition?	
Are you taking any medications?	
Have you taken any strong medications in the recent past?	
Have you ever had surgery?	
Any hospitalization in the past 5 years?	
Any recent, scheduled, or significant diagnostic tests?	
Are there any activities suggested or restricted by your doctor or other health care professional?	

FIGURE 4-2. (*Continued*)

questions often help in a pinch, when the therapist encounters an unfamiliar medical condition in practice. With answers to these general questions, the therapist can devise a massage plan for that session.

Of the questions introduced here, the questions about pain, activity, and medications are the most commonly used. These appear in Boxes 4-1 to 4-3.

More specific follow-up questions, aimed at particular conditions, are provided in Parts II and III of this book.

● FOLLOW-UP QUESTIONS ABOUT ANY CONDITION

For any condition, familiar or unfamiliar, the therapist can ask these questions to complete the Decision Tree:

1. What are the signs and symptoms of the condition? If it was a long time ago, does it still affect you in some way?
2. Are there any complications of the condition? Does it have an effect on any other organs or tissues in your body?" (Questions 1 and 2 might also be combined as: How does the condition affect you?)
3. How is it treated? How does the treatment affect you?

Use the client's answers to complete the left side of a Decision Tree. Compare it to a corresponding pre-made Decision Tree in this textbook, or to the Conditions in Brief tables at the end of each chapter in Part II. If there is no full discussion of this condition in this book, then see Gathering Additional Information, this chapter.

● FOLLOW-UP QUESTIONS ABOUT SIGNS AND SYMPTOMS

For any sign or symptom, such as rash, swelling, pain, or discomfort, the therapist can ask:

1. Do you know what the cause is?
2. Have you seen a doctor for this condition?

Use the first question to apply the Ask the Cause Principle from Chapter 3. Complete a Decision Tree for the causative condition. If the condition is the result of a medication, complete the Medical Treatment and Effects of Treatment boxes and apply the Medication Principle.

It may be that the cause itself is a massage contraindication, or calls for more follow-up to fill out the tree. Suppose the client answers "yes" to a question on the health form about swelling because he or she has swollen glands. Swollen glands under the jaw contraindicate pressure and circulatory intent at the site. But the cause is usually infection, which contraindicates general circulatory intent as well.

> **The Ask the Cause Principle. Consider the cause of sign or symptom, as well as the sign or symptom itself, when making a massage plan.**

The question about whether the client has seen a physician can be used for two purposes: The first is to find out the causative condition and adapt to it. For many reasons, including lack of access to health care, people self-diagnose and self-treat their own conditions. For conditions that could be serious, a therapist needs a physician's diagnosis; otherwise, it

is left to the therapist to determine whether a medical referral, a massage adjustment, both, or some other action is in order. In the example of swollen glands, a therapist's concern increases if the client reports that the condition appeared suddenly, persists, is severe, or has no identified cause. Each of these factors calls for a medical referral.

On the other hand, a clear, identified cause can diminish the concern, as in slight premenstrual puffiness that has persisted for years, or minor swelling on the hand from banging it against something. These require a good judgment call on the part of the therapist, but it is probably safe to massage the premenstrual puffiness directly, while the swelling on the hand contraindicates pressure levels 3–5 and friction at the site if it is acute.

● FOLLOW-UP QUESTIONS ABOUT PAIN

A common reason to seek massage therapy is pain, but pain can stem from a variety of causes. How should the therapist determine whether a client's pain is caused by something within the therapist's scope of practice? Or whether it's a symptom that massage might help relieve?

If a client reports pain, either on the client health form or in the interview, several follow-up questions help the therapist learn more about the pain, determine whether to work with it at the site, adjust massage appropriately, or suggest a medical referral. The Pain Questions provide a way to navigate many different client presentations, and they are used repeatedly in practice (Box 4-1).

● FOLLOW-UP QUESTIONS ABOUT INJURIES

The role of massage therapy in treating injuries may vary according to state and provincial regulations, and be subject to different levels of training. These questions are generally helpful, no matter what the context is:

1. Where is your injury?
Have the client point to it and establish the site. It is advisable to document the site in the client record.
2. When did it happen? Has it happened before?
Work conservatively with a recent injury, and provide a medical referral where necessary. With a recurrent injury, the client already knows how to get better, knows the injury will probably heal and how long it will take, and may even have experience with how massage helps. With this information, it's easier for you to provide massage that will help, rather than aggravate the injury. In general, it's easier to predict a massage outcome for a familiar condition than a new one.
3. Have you seen a doctor about it? (This especially applies to a recent injury.) If so, what was the diagnosis?
If the client has seen his or her physician and has a diagnosis, determine if there are any massage contraindications. If the client has not seen his or her physician, then apply the Recent Injury Principle.

> **The Recent Injury Principle. Recent injuries, or injuries that have not been seen by a physician, should not be treated with massage therapy, or massage therapy should be conservative.**

BOX 4-1 THE PAIN QUESTIONS

1. Where is the pain?
   Have the client point to it, so the site is clear. It's advisable to document the area in a client record.
2. Describe the pain; what does it feel like? (Dull, achy, sharp, stabbing, radiating, shooting, burning, tingling, and so on.) Does it appear suddenly? On a scale of 0–10, with 0 being no pain and 10 being the worst possible pain, how would you rate your pain?
   Pain with "nervy" qualities—sharp, stabbing, radiating, shooting, burning, or tingling—requires a medical referral. But a dull, achy pain may be muscular in origin and amenable to massage. However, if dull, achy pain is chronic or persistent, a medical referral is advised. Review the Physician Referral for Pain Principle in Chapter 3.
   Use the client's answers to the verbal analogue (0–10) scale for before and after assessments, to determine whether massage is helping. Also, pain that is above a level 2, or is very disturbing to the client, is cause for a medical referral.
3. Is there any numbness or tingling, or weakness with the pain?
   If yes, refer the client to his or her physician, as these symptoms need urgent or immediate attention.

   The Physician Referral for Pain Principle. If a client's pain has specific qualities, such as sharp, stabbing, radiating, or shooting pain, or if the pain is accompanied by tingling, numbness, or weakness, refer the client to a physician.

4. Would you describe the pain as stable or unstable? Unstable means that slight movements or position changes bring on sudden or strong pain.
   If the pain is unstable, the client should see a physician. If you must provide massage in the moment, minimize disturbance to the area: limit pressure and joint movement, and use careful positioning. Review the follow-up questions about injury in this chapter as well as the Pain, Injury, and Inflammation Principles in Chapter 3.

   The Unstable Tissue Principle. If a tissue is unstable, do not challenge it with too much pressure or joint movement in the area.

5. How long have you had it? Has it happened before?
   You can get a sense of how familiar, recurrent, and well managed the pain is, and whether the client has her own methods and a track record of relieving the pain herself. With unfamiliar pain of recent onset, be more cautious; people often feel anxiety that can aggravate pain, and if strong massage temporarily worsens the condition, it could be more problematic than for someone who can manage the pain. If the client has prior experience of the pain and has treated it successfully, she is likely to be less anxious about it.

   The New, Unfamiliar, or Poorly Managed Pain Principle. Massage for a client with new, unfamiliar, or poorly managed pain should be more conservative than massage for a client with a familiar, well-managed pain pattern.

6. Does it interfere with your usual level of function? Does it restrict any positions or activity?
   A medical referral is necessary if the pain is disabling. In milder cases, massage is usually okay, but monitor massage outcomes over time. If several sessions of massage fail to provide relief, the client should see his or her physician.
7. Does gentle stretching or movement provide relief, or does it aggravate the pain?
   If it relieves pain, massage is also likely to help. If it aggravates pain, be much more cautious.
8. Do you know what causes or caused the pain?
   Working backward on the tree, investigate the cause for any needed massage adjustments.
9. Have you brought it to the attention of your doctor?
   This information is always useful, but is especially pertinent to Questions 2, 3, 4, and 6, above. Without a diagnosis, proceed cautiously.
10. In general, how do you manage the pain? What aggravates it? What relieves it?
    Use this information to try to avoid aggravating factors such as certain positions in the session, and to optimize relieving factors such as positions and pressure from the client's daily life. You can get a sense of which muscles are involved. Advanced massage therapists can use this information to evaluate an injury.
11. Does it limit your activities? If so, because it's stiff, or because sudden, strong pain occurs with movement?

(continued)

(Continued)

If the pain limits movement by coming on suddenly and strongly, make an urgent medical referral (see Question 2, above.) If it is just stiff, monitor the massage results over time, as massage may help.

12. Have you used massage for the pain? If so, has massaged helped or aggravated the pain? If you can, describe what it is about massage that has helped or worsened the pain—certain strokes or movements, pressures, positions, or focus on some areas?

If the client has not used massage for the condition, approach conservatively for the first session, and monitor the results since there is no massage track record for this condition. If the client has used massage, draw on the history of aggravating and relieving factors to design the current session. This is in keeping with the Previous Massage Principle.

> *The Previous Massage Principle. A client's previous experience of massage therapy, especially massage after the onset, diagnosis, or flare-up of a medical condition, may be used to plan the massage.*

4. Were any tests performed, such as an X-ray?

It's important to know there's no fracture or other unstable tissue before applying pressure or moving joints in the area.

5. How was it treated?

Refer to the "four medication questions" in Box 4-3, this chapter.

6. Are there any medical restrictions on activities, or recommended activities?

Compare these activities to the elements of massage. If there are activity restrictions, apply the Medically Restricted Activity Principle. If there are recommended activities, comparable massage pressure and joint movements are probably permissible and may be helpful.

7. Is there any pending insurance or worker's compensation claim, or possible litigation arising from this injury?

Consider your own skill level in injury work, the timing, and the client's ongoing assessments by a physician in doing massage in this case. Avoid doing anything—usually joint movement and pressure levels 3 and above—that could be perceived as causing or aggravating the injury. On the other hand, if the client's injury has been documented by a physician, you have injury treatment skills, and your work is part of an approved or integrated treatment plan, then massage does not have to be so cautious.

> *The Claim or Litigation Principle. If a client's recent injury involves an insurance claim or litigation, do not complicate the clinical picture with massage that could affect the area.*

After completing injury questions, the therapist continues with the questions about pain (this chapter). If a client has impaired or absent sensation and the pain questions don't apply, it is important to consult the physician to learn which structures are injured and how to safely apply massage.

● FOLLOW-UP QUESTIONS ABOUT SENSATION CHANGES

1. Where is the sensation change?
2. Describe the feeling.
3. Do you know the cause?
4. Have you brought it to the attention of your doctor?
5. Is this accompanied by any weakness in your muscles, or other nervous system symptoms?

If the answer to question 2 is numbness or loss of sensation, follow the Sensation Principle.

> *The Sensation Principle. In an area of impaired or absent sensation, use caution with pressure and joint movement.*

If the answer is any other sensation, such as burning, or something unfamiliar, gentle massage in the area may be okay, but go to questions 3 and 4 first. If the client knows the cause, complete the Decision Tree for the cause and investigate any massage contraindications. If the client has not told his or her physician about the problem, strongly encourage him or her to do so. Be extremely gentle in the area until she has further information from his or her physician. If the sensation change is accompanied by muscle weakness, other nervous system symptoms, or other unfamiliar symptoms, then an urgent or immediate medical referral is the best action.

● FOLLOW-UP QUESTIONS ABOUT INFECTION

1. What is the nature of the infection? What is affected?
2. Has it been diagnosed?
3. Is it something you need to take precautions for, to avoid infecting others?
4. Are you having any fever or chills? Do you continue to feel worse, or are you feeling better?

Use these follow-up questions to get at several issues: where the infection is, whether you are at risk of contracting it, whether it's acute, and how to work with the client if it is advisable.

If your client is fighting an infection, for example, a cold or flu, he or she is not a good candidate for massage with general circulatory intent. This is especially true if it's acute, and he or she is experiencing fever or chills. Follow the Compromised Client Principle.

> *The Compromised Client Principle. If a client is not feeling well, be gentle; even if you cannot explain the mechanism behind a contraindication, follow it anyway.*

On the other hand, if your client is past the peak of infection and has been feeling better for a few days, he or she is probably better able to tolerate general circulatory intent.

Suppose the infection seems minor, such as a very slight swelling around a hangnail, minimal discomfort, and no other symptoms. Avoid contact at the site, and circulatory intent on that limb, but if there are no chills or fever, general circulatory intent elsewhere is probably not contraindicated. However, if the swelling is uncomfortable, or there are other signs of acute infection, see "Lymphangitis," Chapter 13.

With the name of the infection and the area affected, you *can* establish whether you are at risk of contracting it during a massage. Some fungal, bacterial, or viral infections of the skin, such as ringworm, impetigo, and herpes, are transmissible by contact. Other conditions, such as athlete's foot, are also transmitted by contact, but infecting others is not easy unless they are immunocompromised or particularly susceptible. Other parasitic infestations, such as lice or scabies, are highly communicable, regardless of everyone's immune status. And some respiratory infections, such as the common cold, are transmissible by contact with skin or fluids from mucous membranes. Learn about the client's infection, determine where it is, then check in this book or other resources for the level of risk to ensure that contact and massage are safe for you. If in doubt, contact the health department in your area; a nurse can provide useful information about touch and communicable disease.

● FOLLOW-UP QUESTIONS ABOUT ALLERGIES AND SENSITIVITIES

1. Are you sensitive to any of the following ingredients in the lotion/oil I use?
List the ingredients. Nut oils and preservatives are common offenders. If the client has a history of reaction to any known ingredient, avoid using it.
2. What happens when you have an allergic reaction or sensitivity?
Use this question to identify signs of a reaction if they arise during the session and discontinue using the lotion or oil if so.
3. Do you have a favorite lotion or oil you'd like me to use for massage?
Within limits, you might be able to use a lotion or oil the client brings in, one with a known track record. This is advisable if the client is especially sensitive, or is sensitive to multiple factors.

● FOLLOW-UP QUESTIONS ABOUT ACTIVITY AND ENERGY

In determining contraindications, the therapist can draw on elements that are common to both exercise and massage therapy. Questions about activity level, activity tolerance, and activity restrictions are some of the most useful in predicting the client's response to massage. Together with a client's energy level, this information can help the therapist plan a massage session of appropriate strength (Box 4-2).

● FOLLOW-UP QUESTIONS ABOUT DIAGNOSTIC TESTS

One valuable question—Have you had any recent, scheduled, or significant diagnostic tests?—helps establish how the physician is monitoring the client's health, and what their concerns are. This question may be asked of all clients, or of any client who reports a symptom or medical condition.

The questions about diagnostic tests help the therapist identify massage contraindications. There might be information from X-rays about a fracture, or from blood tests about a client's vulnerability to infection. Massage modifications such as pressure, or infection control precautions, flow from these.

If the client reports a recent, scheduled, or significant test, the follow-up questions are:

1. What were (or are) they testing for?
If the client is scheduled for an important test, or has had it, but is still waiting for test results, then his or her doctor could be investigating a worst-case or best-case possibility. Apply the Waiting for a Diagnosis Principle until the actual results come back.

> *The Waiting For A Diagnosis Principle.* **If a client is scheduled for diagnostic tests, or is awaiting results, adapt massage to the possible diagnosis. If more than one condition is being investigated, adapt massage to the worst-case scenario.**

2. What were the findings?
Adapt the massage to the new diagnosis or any change in health status. If the client has a life-limiting condition such as cancer or advanced heart disease, ask this question gently, with a warm and matter-of-fact tone. It's possible that everyone in the client's life is asking the same question, and that the client feels burdened by keeping them up to date, or by not always being able to provide good news.
3. What was the procedure (or anticipating the procedure) like for you?
Use this last question judiciously; it might not be appropriate to ask of all clients, or for minor procedures. But by asking, you can learn useful information: Did he or she have to hold still for the procedure? Was his or her body in a certain position? Did it cause him or her pain or discomfort, something that massage might address? Is it stressful to anticipate the test, or to wait for the results?

By asking these questions, you offer the client an opportunity to say how the experience affected him. Some diagnostic tests are painful and stressful, cause concern to the client's loved ones, and are part of life-changing experiences of injury or illness. Along with physical side effects, procedures can be surrounded by stress—the hope of good news to report, and the need to take care of others when the news is bad.

Important client experiences lie within this line of questions about diagnostics. Essential information for massage planning may emerge, as well.

● FOLLOW-UP QUESTIONS ABOUT MEDICATIONS

Many massage clients are taking prescription or over-the-counter medications, and some are taking several. The dizzying array of brand names, generic names, chemical actions, and side effects can be intimidating. The information expands as new drugs are added to the market. Complete command of this information would be difficult, but therapists practicing at the basic level can use thoughtful questions and several resources to determine the massage implications of a client's medications. There are excellent textbooks on this topic (Wible, 2009; Persad, 2001), listed in the bibliography.

Much of the time, the massage and medication issues can be captured with four medication questions. In many cases, a client's

1. What is your activity level? Can you describe your average movements and activities each day? Each week?
   This question gives you a sense of how the client's medical condition or medical treatment affects his or her movement habits and activity, and how well he or she might tolerate massage. Apply the Activity and Energy Principle (see Chapter 3).

   If you are evaluating the client closely for muscle tension patterns and restrictions, this information is also useful to determine any activities or movements that contribute to the muscle tension.

   Note that sometimes this question can make an individual feel uncomfortable and guilty about not exercising, and tempted to report exercise above his or her true levels. Ask this question in a neutral tone, without judgment. "Can you tell me what kinds of things you were able to do yesterday and today?" Probe gently for the information.

2. How is your tolerance of activities? Do you stay pretty strong or do you feel fatigued from your schedule and activities?
   Use the client's responses to gauge the best strength of the massage. A high activity level might reflect necessity (such as working full-time, or taking care of children) rather than true energy reserves. Even if your client keeps an impressive schedule, if he or she is overwhelmed by fatigue from his or her health, work, or family responsibilities, massage should be gentle.

3. Are there any medical restrictions on your activities?
   If your client's physician has restricted his activities because of a condition or medical treatment, then adjust the massage, in kind: usually joint movement or general circulatory intent should be limited.

   The Medically Restricted Activity Principle. If there are any medical restrictions on a client's activities, explore and apply any equivalent massage contraindications.

   If spa services such as hot wraps are being considered, ask specifically whether cardiovascular exercise, heat applications, or raising core temperature is restricted, and see "Principles for Spa Treatments," Chapter 3.

4. Can you describe your overall energy level? If it is low, are there good or bad times of the day or week?
   If the client's energy level is compromised by illness or medical treatment, apply the Activity and Energy Principle. Establish whether there are cyclical symptoms to work around or address. You might try timing massage sessions during low points if massage seems to energize the client. Or provide massage at end of day when the client's energy is no longer needed for daily activities, and massage can help his or her sleep. If the client prefers vigorous massage, you might schedule the session for expected higher energy times, when he or she might be able to tolerate slightly stronger work.

answers to these standard questions provide enough information to proceed with the massage session in the moment.

These four medication questions (Box 4-3) have an additional use: Once the word "procedure" is substituted for "medication," they become "the four medical procedure questions." These address other kinds of treatments such as surgery, laser or radiation therapy, and physical therapy protocols.

Many medications and procedures appear in the Full Decision Trees in Parts II and III. Each tree is devoted to a medical condition, and shows some of the most common therapies for that condition. Often, there are too many side effects to list them all, but the side effects that are most relevant to massage planning are listed. Treatments and their effects point to massage therapy guidelines on the right side of the tree.

Qualities of a Good Interview

No matter how long an interview is, the dialogue at the start of a massage can be pivotal for the session. The conversation allows the therapist and client to get to know one another, exchange important information, and plan the massage. These are qualities of a good interview:

- Thorough
- Short duration
- Focused
- Sets clear expectations
- Unhurried
- Establishes rapport

Some of these qualities seem to conflict: How does a therapist establish rapport, collect thorough health information, and maintain an unhurried pace in a short amount of time? This may take practice: by conveying interest, using a relaxed, friendly tone, and gently steering the interview in the direction of the necessary information.

Limiting the interview length can be challenging when the client health form seems long, but in reality, most interviews can be accomplished in 10–15 minutes. More time may be necessary in student clinics or in settings specializing in medically complex client populations. With practice, most therapists can move quickly through the information, because they

BOX 4-3 THE FOUR MEDICATION QUESTIONS

1. How do you spell it?
   Having the correct spelling helps you look it up. Even if your client doesn't know the correct spelling, a close approximation will enable you to look up the drug in a book, on the Internet, or in a product information reference. Be careful of similar-sounding brand names, though, such as Celebrex and Celexa, two very different drugs with different properties.
2. What is it for?
   By itself, the condition being treated may contraindicate one or more massage elements. Investigate whether this is so.
3. Is it effective?
   Establish whether the condition has resolved, or if there are still problems such as signs, symptoms, or effects on tissue function. Many medications control symptoms but do not address the underlying cause. Adapt massage to any remaining problems.
4. How does it affect you? Are there any side effects or complications of this medication?
   Common side effects of medications, such as nausea, fatigue, hypotension, and digestive disturbances, require their own massage adjustments. Find out how the drugs are affecting your client, and adapt the massage plan accordingly.

Used well, these four questions satisfy the Medication Principle (see Chapter 3). When the format is used to ask about a medical procedure such as surgery or laser treatment, it satisfies a similar principle, the Procedure Principle (see Chapter 3).

The Medication Principle. Adapt massage to the condition for which the medication is taken or prescribed, and to any side effects.

recognize areas that require more focus, and areas that are less important.

Because most clients prefer to spend the time actually receiving massage than talking about it, therapists should set an approximate time frame for the interview, and let the client know the purpose behind the questions. This helps the client to relax, knowing that the massage treatment is forthcoming:

Thank you for filling out this form. The information you gave me is very helpful. I'll be focusing with you for a few minutes on the things that help me plan your massage session. We'll talk for about 15 minutes, plan your session together, and make sure we have you ready on the massage table around 5:15 so we don't interfere with any of your hands on time.

Some clients, when prompted by health questions, may talk at length, prolonging the interview. It is up to the therapist to manage the interview, and there are gracious ways to guide the discussion when it goes on too long:

Since we just have a couple of minutes left, tell me how these two medications affect you, and what they are for. Then we can get started on the massage.

Or

I wonder if I can jump in for just a moment. How about if we continue this conversation after you've gotten on

the massage table? Right now I need to know some quick information about something else you mentioned so we can plan the session without cutting into your massage time—I'm aware that it's already 5:20.

Or even give the client a choice:

It seems like you have more to say about this condition. I'm aware of the time, and the need to begin the massage in order to finish by 6:30. If you want, we can keep talking and shorten the massage by a few minutes. Or, I can gather the other information I need right now, and we can continue this conversation after you've gotten on the table. Which would you like?

In the last example, the client may choose to continue talking, but the therapist can relax, having defined the overall time limits, and knowing that the client probably needs more conversation in order to be comfortable. This can contribute to rapport. When delivered in a relaxed manner, the therapist conveys interest in the client, without sacrificing the point of the interview: a safe, effective massage session.

That said, therapists who set their own schedules may opt for a longer interview, preferring the time to ask open-ended questions and get to know the client before beginning the massage. Therapist's Journal 4-1 describes a less structured interview, focused on the client's experience as well as the therapist's need for information.

Processing and Decision Making

How does the therapist use the information that emerges from the client interview? A health history can contain an overwhelming amount of information, especially from an older adult with multiple conditions, yet not all of the information is relevant to massage. Even after thorough

questioning, and an excess of information, there may be gaps in information. Swiftly and thoughtfully, the therapist needs to come up with a massage plan, using the right massage guidelines. There are three steps in this decision-making process:

THERAPIST'S JOURNAL 4-1 *A Client-Centered Health History*

I'm not a big fan of generic history forms. In the beginning of massage therapy study or practice, I think they are necessary in order to provide a framework and make sure everything is covered. But after 20 years of interviewing people in nursing and massage therapy, I have honed the process enough so that I do a more narrative, open-ended history taking.

In my practice, I begin by asking clients what brought them to massage, and asking more about their reasons for coming. What comes out can take you in a very different direction than a generic form. If they're comfortable, clients may tell you about the stressors in their life. Sometimes asking about stress outright, to rank their stress level on a 1–5 scale, can prompt this process.

I've provided massage to a lot of different populations who may feel alienated by a form, whose tolerance of bureaucracy may be limited. I've worked with homeless people, folks with mental health problems, people with substance-abuse problems, and so on. I also work with many people for whom English is not their first language, and some of them feel lost and confused in bureaucratic systems that insist on more forms to fill out. Often with people who might feel marginalized by a written form, I'll start with getting them to move, looking and touching the area of their complaint, and pointing at diagrams of the body to indicate what is going on. We move quickly to the reason they want massage therapy, making it relevant. I find out the other things on a history form along the way, but without necessarily ticking through a checklist. The stressors they talk about might be a five-hour wait in a welfare line, a methadone clinic that is closed, or a new symptom of HIV infection.

There's a good argument for forms that are gender-specific and age-specific. Adolescents and young adults may have more body image issues for me to consider; for women who have given birth, I'll ask about postpartum issues that can linger long after the last baby was born. With middle-aged and older adults, I make sure I attend to chronic, degenerative, and age-related disease so that I don't miss anything important.

As a massage therapist, I feel responsibility: for some people, massage therapy is a point of entry into the health care system. We need to be vigilant, looking for common diseases and red flags, so that we can refer the client appropriately to other health care professionals when necessary.

The most important thing is for therapists to listen carefully and come to the interview without judgment. They need to show unconditional positive regard in every exchange with clients. They need to demonstrate that they have listened by asking good follow-up questions in the interview, and then acting on the client's major concerns during the massage session.

An intake interview needs to be client centered, not just therapist centered. Whichever method the therapist uses to gather data, the client should feel comfortable.

Isobel McDonald
Van couver, BC, Canada

1. Sort and prioritize the information.
2. Apply appropriate principles and Decision Trees to the scenario.
3. Gather additional information if necessary.

● SORTING AND PRIORITIZING CLIENT INFORMATION

When a great deal of history emerges in the health history, how does a therapist wade through it? Sorting and prioritizing are necessary during the interview, to guide it to the relevant topics, and afterward, to generate massage guidelines.

A Decision Tree provides one way to sort information, and Chapter 1 provides guidance for the interview using a pre-made Full Decision Tree, or generating an individualized one in the moment.

Prioritizing is a skill that comes with practice, and becomes second nature, even on a tight schedule. It can help the therapist to ask himself a few key questions: Does this information cue me to any massage principles from Chapter 3? Is it possible that there is impaired *function* or stability of an organ or tissue? Is something inflamed, or injured? Is it something I've never heard of? Is it something sudden, new, recent, unfamiliar, poorly understood, or pending a diagnosis? If the answer to each of these common-sense questions is no, then it may not require follow-up. If the answer is yes, the therapist consults

this book—either a chapter, section, or Conditions in Brief—for follow-up questions and massage contraindications.

Let's consider the question about surgery on the client health form. Having asked three clients about their history of surgery, the therapist might find out the following:

1. A 57-year-old client had surgery to remove his tonsils at age 5.
2. A 36-year-old client had a procedure 2 years ago to unblock her fallopian tubes.
3. A 43-year-old client had back surgery 14 months ago.

Does this reflect impaired function or stability of an organ or tissue? This is a good test question for each of these scenarios. In the first scenario, a tonsillectomy 52 years ago would not have appreciably affected the function or stability of any organ or tissue, and would have no effect on the massage plan.

In the second scenario, a procedure to unblock fallopian tubes has little bearing on the massage itself, as there is no specific principle or contraindication to apply. Nothing within reach is likely to be inflamed or injured. However, a follow-up—Have you had any related procedures or medications more recently?—might begin a conversation about a current struggle with fertility treatment, the related stress, or an upcoming procedure that could have massage contraindications (see "Female Infertility," Chapter 19). The client might even state a therapeutic goal—reduced stress—to help her cope with the treatments. During these conversations, the therapist can use the opportunity to build trust and rapport with warmth, lack of judgment, and careful listening.

In the third scenario, a conversation about the surgery could alert the therapist to tension patterns to guide the massage, any stabilizing metal in the back on which to avoid pressure, old and recurring injuries to bear in mind, and current pain levels or restricted mobility. The therapist might draw on one or more principles from Chapter 3, such as the Previous Massage Principle, to develop a plan for the session.

● USING THE INTERVIEW, PRINCIPLES, AND DECISION TREES

How does a therapist use the interview along with the Decision Tree, and the principles from Chapter 3? These tools reinforce each other, and can be used in different sequences. Figure 4-3 shows different ways to use these decision-making tools. As shown in Figure 4-3A, the Full Decision Tree suggests questions to ask about a client's condition, and a therapist can go quickly down the left side of the tree, asking about each aspect of it. Or, checking principles, such as those about inflammation, pain, injury, and medical treatment, the therapist questions the client about each of these topics.

In another sequence in Figure 4-3B, the interview brings out health information that can be sorted into boxes on the left side of an Individual Decision Tree, then checked against a pre-made tree. Key health information often emerges in a more or less random fashion, so the therapist might start anywhere on the tree, then move backward, forward, and upward. Here is an example of this: during the conversation, a piece of information pops up, such as a drug the client is taking. The therapist uses the four medication questions to learn more about the drug, discovering that it controls blood sugar, and that the client has diabetes. Questioning the client further, he or she sketches out an individual Decision Tree, then checks it against a full, pre-made tree for diabetes (see Chapter 17) in this book to complete the right side.

Often, the information that comes out in the interview injects a healthy dose of reality into the clinical thinking process, as shown in Figure 4-3C. Suppose a client mentions that he or she had a heart attack 3 years previously. According to the full Decision Tree for heart disease, one complication is heart failure—an impaired ability to pump blood (see Chapter 11). This serious impairment, on the middle branch of the Decision Tree, contraindicates general circulatory intent. This follows the Filter and Pump Principle.

> *The Filter and Pump Principle. If a filtering organ (liver, kidney, spleen, or lymph node), or a pumping organ (the heart) is functioning poorly or overworking, do not work it harder with massage that is circulatory in intent.*

Yet, as the interview continues, the therapist learns about the client's heart function, activity level, and activity tolerance. After the heart attack, the client gradually returned to a very high level of activity; running several miles a week; doing heavy, supervised workouts at the gym, taking aerobics classes. In this case, the Activity and Energy Principle prevails, effectively overriding the Filter and Pump Principle.

Thanks to the activity and energy questions (see Box 4-2) and the four medication questions the therapist learns of no significant complications, and few medications. The therapist crosses out the middle branch of the tree for this client, and part of the bottom branch. A moderate to vigorous massage session is appropriate, with general circulatory intent. This session is ideal for the client's actual health picture and activity level.

> *The Activity and Energy Principle. A client who enjoys regular, moderate physical activity or a good overall energy level is better able to tolerate strong massage elements—including general circulatory intent—than one whose activity or energy level is low.*

A therapist working under time constraints might not be able to complete a tree for each condition, but may rely on a principle or two to determine what to do. Either way, good questions for the client supplement the other decision-making tools in this book. By using the massage principles, the Decision Tree, and the interview in just the right balance, a therapist is able to customize massage for each client's health and needs.

● GATHERING ADDITIONAL INFORMATION

Most clients are able to provide reliable, complete information about their own medical conditions, but even after a thorough interview, the therapist may need to look something up to determine the best massage plan. This may occur after an initial phone conversation with the client, after the interview, or even between sessions. Often a therapist has only a few minutes to hurriedly gather information while the client gets on the massage table. Three places to turn to for more information are Massage therapy literature, patient education literature, and, in some cases, the client's physician or nurse.

Massage Therapy Literature

The chapters in Part II and III of this text provide Decision Trees, Interview Questions, Massage Therapy Guidelines, and Conditions in Brief. All are designed for quick consultation.

Several massage therapy textbooks are useful sources of medical and massage information. Therapists can draw on books on pathology, medications, concerns in special settings, and special client populations. The bibliography (online at http://thePoint.lww.com/Walton) lists many of these sources (Werner, 2009; Wible, 2009).

Patient Education in Print and Online

When a patient is diagnosed with a medical condition, he or she often receives literature about it from his or her nurse as part of patient teaching. Booklets, pamphlets, and Web sites that inform patients and families about health conditions offer accessible and helpful information for therapists, *even if there is no explicit mention of massage contraindications*. Without mentioning massage therapy directly, these resources often have practical guidance for the massage setting. Here are some examples:

1. A Web site on stroke describes common areas of impaired sensation. Applying the Sensation Principle, the therapist

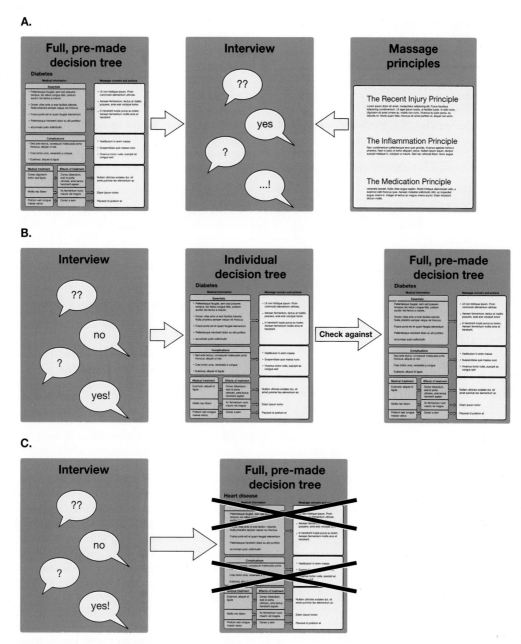

FIGURE 4-3. Decision-making tools for massage therapists. The interview, Decision Tree, and principles can be used in various ways. (A) A Full Decision Tree and one or more massage principles guide the interview. (B) The therapist uses the interview to create an Individual Decision Tree, then checks it against a Full Decision Tree for completeness and accuracy. (C) A client's answers to interview questions are used to cross out irrelevant information on the Full Decision Tree.

asks the client about these areas, in case he or she needs to use less pressure there.

2. A booklet on respiratory disease describes positions that can aggravate breathing problems. The therapist can apply the information to positioning and bolstering the client on the massage table.

3. A brochure on a medication mentions that skin reactions can occur. A therapist, using the brochure, asks the client whether side effects include skin problems and avoids friction, lubricant, and possibly contact on affected areas.

A simple Internet search for a medical condition or its treatment can yield additional information for patients. For example:

1. Typing "emphysema" and "treatment" provides links to Web sites with common treatments for emphysema.

2. Typing the brand name of a drug or treatment and the words "side effect" provides links to Web sites that list common side effects of the drug.

3. Typing the brand name of a drug followed by ".com"—such as "Wellbutrin.com" or "Arimidex.com"—brings up the manufacturer's Web site with information about why the drug is prescribed, and common side effects.

4. Typing in a health condition and ".org"—such as "stroke. org"—often generates a nonprofit association or foundation devoted to research on the condition, patient advocacy, and education.

A word of caution: Not everything on the Internet is accurate. However, government Web sites (such as nih.gov), sites run by hospitals for their patients (such as clevelandclinic.org), and large nonprofit associations are often reliable sources of information. As of this writing, excellent, carefully reviewed information about medications is available from the University of Maryland Medical Center site (umm.edu), at drugs.com, and safemedication.com. Even though advertising is a primary function of a pharmaceutical Web site, such sources are also educational. Drug companies share data about their products in a standard format, useful for health professionals and patients, alike. It is always a good idea to consult several Web sites to look for consistency, especially about key information. Recommended web resources appear in each chapter bibliography online.

The Client's Physician or Nurse

After using the resources listed above, a therapist can usually design a massage plan, but may still need to fill in gaps in information by consulting with the client's physician. Chapter 5 discusses the steps of physician communication in detail.

Presenting the Massage Plan to the Client

Once the therapist has arrived at a massage plan for the client's presentation, it's time to tell the client about it and explain the rationale. Some therapists also choose to put it in writing, in an informed consent process.

● EXPLAINING MASSAGE CONTRAINDICATIONS

Typically, therapists and clients plan out other elements of the session together, including areas of focus, preferred pressure and modalities, and so on. Massage adjustments for the client's medical conditions are a natural part of this conversation (Figure 4-4).

When talking to the client about massage contraindications, a therapist may feel self-conscious, as though he or she were offering something less to the client. This is most often the case when deeper pressure is contraindicated, or it's necessary to avoid a certain area of the body. The therapist may feel the weight of a client's expectations, or pressure from an employer to please a customer. Yet, most clients are receptive to massage changes, especially when they understand the reasons for them, and feel included in the decision. Here is one way to explain a contraindication to a new client:

> I understand you prefer very deep pressure, and that's what you've liked about massage in the past. Today I'm learning toward gentler pressure on your back, because of your osteoporosis. In massage therapy, we don't work too vigorously on areas that may be unstable. On the other hand, there are places I can use a bit more pressure on, such as your feet and shoulders. Are those areas that would like attention during the massage? How does this approach sound to you?

This explanation has several useful components:

1. A clear description of the massage adjustment, and why there is a need for it.
2. Acknowledgement of the client's past and preferences, and how this session might be different.
3. Alluding to general practices in the massage profession—"*we* don't work too vigorously"—as a foundation for the decision, rather than the therapist's personal preference or whim.

Occasionally, a therapist encounters a client who resists or dismisses the need for the massage adjustment. He or she might feel that the therapist is too cautious, or that his or her medical condition shouldn't make a difference in the massage. Perhaps he or she feels singled out, or misses the "normal" massage he or she received before becoming ill or injured. This is more likely to occur in a new therapist-client relationship than in an established one.

When a client balks at a massage plan, the therapist may need to assume more of a leadership role, explaining that he or she needs to abide by the limits for the client's well-being. This is a different paradigm than "the customer is always right," and it can be challenging to implement in settings that emphasize client-centered care and customer satisfaction. It is easier to navigate a client's resistance when remembering the purpose of the contraindication: to do no harm. It can be helpful to tell the client, "I think we should be gentle—the last thing we want is for you to feel worse after the massage. We'd much rather have you feel better!" And it may be that future sessions can be more vigorous, once the client's massage tolerance is established. (See "the Where You Start Isn't Always Where You End Up Principle," Chapter 3.)

● INFORMED CONSENT

Some therapists describe the massage plan in a process called informed consent. **Informed consent** is an educational process, in which a patient reviews his or her medical treatment plan in writing. It includes the purpose, possible benefits and risks, and the details of the treatment. In medicine, informed consent is vital when invasive procedures are performed, with possible side effects and complications that range from bothersome to life threatening.

In the process of informed consent, the patient has a chance to ask questions of the health care provider administering the informed consent form. The patient signs a statement saying

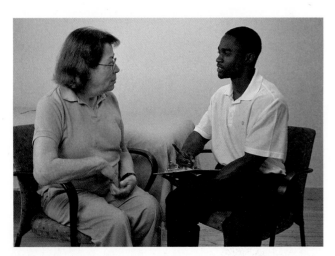

FIGURE 4-4. Explaining the massage plan.

that these steps took place, and that he or she understands and accepts the treatment.

In massage therapy, informed consent is used to set expectations for the session or course of treatment. Some therapists use written informed consent, and others use a less formal verbal exchange. Informed consent can be multipurpose: parameters such as session length, draping practice, clothing to be removed, and the areas to be massaged are often included. The therapist describes the need for communication during the session, and the client's responsibility to disclose any medical conditions and treatments to the therapist. Informed consent is a chance for the therapist to welcome the client's input on areas and pressures, and to underscore the client's choice of how to be touched. The therapist may describe his or her scope of practice: that he or she does not diagnose or treat disease, for example. He or she may include general office practices such as the office cancellation policy.

Informed consent provides one framework for presenting massage contraindications to the client. This is also an ideal time to educate a client about possible side effects of massage, such as mild, temporary soreness. These are small risks of massage, common to massage practice. But larger risks, such as bruising, infection, or fracture, have no place in massage therapy, not even if a client consents to them in writing. Unlike informed consent before surgery, informed consent before massage should never be used to justify massage that could cause strong side effects, more serious complications, or lasting damage to tissue.

A common question for massage therapists arises from the following scenario: Suppose a client insists on deep pressure or a strong stretch, even against the therapist's advice. Perhaps the client's tissues are unstable, or another medical factor is a concern for the therapist. Is it appropriate for the therapist to offer informed consent, releasing the therapist from liability if he or she complies with the client's request? The answer is no. Informed consent is not designed to dismiss a massage contraindication.

Here is another way to state this important point: Even if a client is open to the risk, and willing to state that in writing, the therapist is ethically bound to do no harm. Informed consent does not release the therapist from liability if injury or illness occurs, and few practitioners would be comfortable working unsafely, even with informed consent. Informed consent is for education and communication, not overriding professional judgment. Any document intended for legal purposes should be reviewed by an attorney before use.

Charting Massage Contraindications

There is a range of record keeping in massage therapy, from extensive records, to no written notes at all. Factors that influence a therapist's charting include the amount of training in documentation, his or her own personal style, and the facility in which he or she works. Some therapists take formal SOAP notes with standard abbreviations. Others keep informal notes on the client's medical information, his or her progress over time, and their own observations during a session.

No matter how the therapist documents the session, the chart should include massage contraindications that were followed, with this information:

- The conditions—illness or injury—requiring the adjustments (from the left side of the Decision Tree).
- The elements of massage that were adjusted in the session, such as site, joint movement, pressure, intent of the session, and so on (from right side of the Decision Tree—see Chapter 2).

Any conversations or correspondence with a client's physician or nurse should also be noted, and dated.

A Decision Tree is one format for documenting the massage contraindications that were followed; written notes are another. A pre-made diagram of the human body can supplement these methods, providing an efficient recording format. Therapists mark directly on the diagram with a few notes, a format that allows simple retrieval of the information. Here are examples of written notes (in longhand, without standard medical abbreviations) and supporting diagrams:

Client has mild eczema and both forearms, extensor surfaces. Avoided friction and oil on affected areas

Figure 4-5A is a visual record of these adjustments for eczema.

Client has end-stage liver disease with swelling in the abdomen, osteoporosis. Avoided prone position because of swelling (used left sidelying). Overall pressure 2 maximum. Avoided general circulatory intent (followed Filter and Pump Principle).

Figure 4-5B is a visual record of some adjustments for liver failure (see "Liver Failure," Chapter 16; "Osteoporosis," Chapter 9).

The chart should be kept up to date for a subsequent session or course of treatment. Each time, the therapist records the client's response to the previous session, and any changes in health status. Asking, "Have there been any changes in your symptoms, diagnostic tests, or treatment since I saw you last?" and "Have any other health changes occurred since the last session, anything new?" can be an effective way to monitor the client over time.

With a session clearly recorded in the chart, the therapist can return to it at subsequent sessions, or reference it when seeing another client with a similar clinical picture. A clear record of massage adjustments also provides a form of legal protection for the therapist if his or her liability for injury to a client is ever questioned.

Special Populations and Settings

In the rapidly growing field of massage therapy, interviewing and documentation methods are still being developed. Even though there are excellent texts on these subjects (see Bibliography), there is no universal agreement on what the therapist should ask a client, or on how to document and apply the answers. Therapists interview differently for different populations of clients, or when working in certain massage settings.

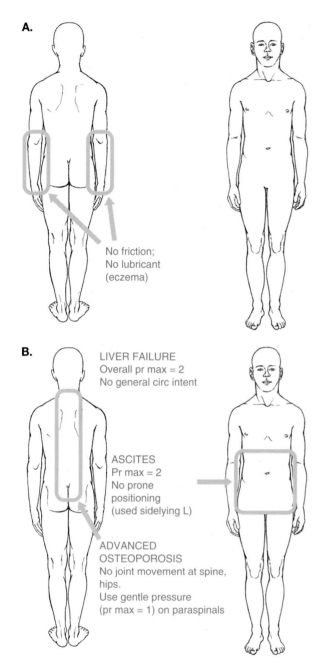

FIGURE 4-5. A diagram of the contraindications followed in a massage session is used to supplement handwritten notes. Two examples are shown. In (A), the therapist recorded his or her massage adjustments at sites of eczema on the client's forearms. This corresponds to the top branch of the Decision Tree for eczema. (B) The therapist recorded several massage adjustments for a client with advanced liver failure.

FORMS FOR SPECIAL POPULATIONS

Many therapists specialize in certain kinds of work, such as prenatal massage, geriatric massage, or massage with athletes. One way to streamline the interview process is to include commonly used follow-up questions on a single form, perhaps aimed at specific medical populations. For instance, working with several people with fibromyalgia, a therapist discovers a simple way to ask some common questions. He or she develops a quick fibromyalgia checklist for any client with this

condition, and a diagram of characteristic fibromyalgia tender points to mark, using the client's self-report of pain or tenderness. Another therapist designs a form for pregnant and postpartum women; another has a form for people with cancer.

A therapist specializing in injury work might include questions about certain injuries for clients. The follow-up questions on pain can be an excellent checklist to send out to a client ahead of time, asking him or her to reflect on his or her pain and describe it fully. Therapists who accept third-party reimbursement for massage therapy, especially as part of injury treatment, have many resources available to them for interviewing and documentation, listed in the bibliography. No matter what the therapist's purpose for it is, a specialized form usually saves time. Therapists who develop them may be better prepared to serve that population.

CHALLENGES IN DIFFERENT MASSAGE SETTINGS

The massage setting influences interviewing and charting, and there is variation in these practices across the profession. An interview in a hospital inpatient setting might be brief: the patient is fatigued, the massage therapist has already reviewed the patient's medical chart in detail and checked with the nurse for key information. The massage session may be recorded in detail in the patient's chart. An interview in another clinical setting might be more extensive, including a thorough history and goals for a course of massage treatment, also recorded in a patient's chart. Standard medical vocabulary and abbreviations may be necessary in both of these settings, for insurance reimbursement, or for multiple practitioners seeing the same client.

An interview in private practice may reflect a therapist's specialty, or be broad based, and the therapist's notes may be highly individualized. In high volume massage settings, such as spas, resorts, and cruise ships, the interview may be constrained by a short turnaround time between clients. In these cases, the interview might be extremely brief, amounting to a question or two, or a more fully developed checklist of medical conditions.

In on-site or "chair massage" settings, located in shopping malls, airports, and special events, there is usually no charting. Contraindications may be managed by a quick sign-in or release form, asking the client to review a quick checklist of conditions or symptoms and verify, by signature, that he or she is not experiencing any of them. While interviewing and charting would offer some protection against liability in such settings, it would also lengthen each exchange and diminish the possible volume. Conventional practice in these and other massage settings is likely to evolve as the field of massage therapy continues to develop.

INTERVIEWING FOR CONTRAINDICATIONS IN THE SPA

Although many therapists are employed by spas, the spa setting can provide challenges in the areas of interviewing, documentation, and massage contraindications. In some spas, a full medical intake is performed by a nurse or another professional, upon entrance to the spa, who designs the guest's spa services with his or her health history in mind. However, in most spas, little or no health information is solicited, and no records are kept.

BOX 4-4 THE SPA HEALTH CHECKLIST

1. Do you have any medical conditions? Have you been recently or currently treated for any medical condition?
   Ask the follow-up questions for any condition.
2. Any recent or scheduled medical procedures?
   Follow the Procedure Principle, and ask the follow-up questions about diagnostic tests (this chapter) to determine whether there is a medical condition to consider.

   The Procedure Principle. Adapt massage to the condition for which the procedure is advised, and to the effects of the procedure itself.

3. Are you taking any prescription or over-the-counter medications?
   Ask the four medication questions.
4. Do you have any condition that affects your bones, joints, or muscles?
   Keep the Unstable Tissue Principle in mind, as well as the pain, injury, and inflammation principles. The Previous Massage Principle can be extremely useful here.
5. Any conditions that affect your skin?
   If there are, some of the follow-up questions about infection should be asked to determine communicability. Be familiar with the skin principles in Chapter 7. For most skin conditions, the Exfoliation Principle (see Chapter 3) should be applied, at least at the site.
6. Any conditions affecting your nervous system, heart, lungs, liver, or kidney?
   Ask about whether the condition affects the function of the organ. If it does, apply the Vital Organ Principle; also apply the principles concerning spa treatments—the Detoxification Principle, the Exfoliation Principle, and the Core Temperature Principle.
7. Is there any cancer or cancer treatment in your health history? Any removal or irradiation of lymph nodes, if so?
   Even if the cancer was a long time ago, some treatments have lingering effects. Depending on the case, the Quadrant Principle for Lymphedema Risk could be important to apply, and additional follow-up questions about cancer history are essential for working safely (see Chapter 20).
8. Are there any surgeries in your health history?
   Use the Procedure Principle. If the surgery was recent, follow the Unstable Tissue Principle or the Stabilization of An Acute Condition Principle, as needed. Review "Surgery," Chapter 21.
9. Any pain or discomfort anywhere? Where and from what?
   Principles concerning pain, injury and inflammation should be considered here.

Yet massage therapists in these settings encounter a broad range of client presentations: serious illness and injury, chronic and progressive conditions. Therapists seeing clients in these high-volume settings, with many first-time clients, may be scheduled so tightly that there's no time for an extensive interview. In such settings, therapists are often confined to the single question: Is there anything that I should know about your health?

There is a problem with this approach, putting the burden on the client to know and understand which health information is relevant to massage. Only the therapist can determine whether a client can safely receive massage and spa services, and it is up to the therapist to ask the right questions. A brief spa health checklist, condensed from the longer client health form, can get therapists started at obtaining the essential information from their clients (Box 4-4).

To make quick decisions with one-time clients, without the time to explore each condition fully, complete a Decision Tree, or look up specific information, a therapist may rely more heavily on broad massage principles. Principles introduced in Chapter 3, and additional principles in Parts II and III, are easy to use quickly, and can be invaluable to spa staff. Therapists in such settings should *always* be mindful of the Massage Setting/Continuity of Care Principle.

The Massage Setting/Continuity of Care Principle. In massage settings favoring single-time rather than repeat clients, lacking continuity of care, or using little or no documentation, therapists should take a cautious approach to medical conditions.

A therapist who grows comfortable with interviewing, decision making, and charting is richly rewarded in his or her work. Able to work confidently with a range of ages, illnesses, injuries, and levels of health, a skilled therapist draws clients with complex presentations to his or her practice. Through exchanges with some of the most challenging experiences of the human condition—those that affect the human body—the therapist may deepen her experience of her clients and the work of skilled touch.

Each person's body tells its own unique story of health and healing, illness and injury, tension and movement. Questions start the conversation between a therapist and client, and during a massage session, that client's story continues to be told through touch. Depending on many factors, the conversation could last for the next hour or for a decade. However long it lasts, the therapist's notes chronicle the ongoing exchange of information, the client's response to massage, and the massage provided. Listening with his or her ears, hands, and heart, the therapist attends to the client's story as it continues to unfold.

SELF TEST

1. How could you find out, online, the common side effects of a medication a client is taking?
2. Why is it important to use a layered approach to interviewing, asking for some of the same information in several ways?
3. What are three follow-up questions to ask about a medical condition, in order to complete a Decision Tree for that condition?
4. If you discover in the interview that a client's pain or injury is accompanied by muscle weakness, what do you advise?
5. Regarding a client scheduled for a diagnostic procedure, what questions do you ask, and which principle do you apply to design the massage plan? State the principle in your answer.
6. There are four questions to ask about each of a client's medications. State the four questions and their purpose.
7. If a client has an illness or injury, then what questions should you ask about his or her activity and energy level? How the client's answers influence the specifics of the massage plan?
8. List three guidelines for locating reliable medical information on the Internet.
9. List three things a therapist can do when he or she suspects that a client is giving incomplete or inaccurate health information during an interview.
10. Why is it essential to ask a recently injured client about any insurance claim or litigation involving the injury?

 For answers to these questions and to see a bibliography for this chapter, visit http://thePoint. lww.com/Walton.

Communicating with the Client's Physician

A dialogue is more than two monologues.

—MAX KAMPELMAN

In some cases, the client's health status requires outside advice on massage contraindications, and the massage therapist needs input from the client's physician or other health care providers. On the Decision Tree, the shorthand for this action is medical consultation. A physician may be consulted, but depending on the context, the provider might be one of the physician's representatives, such as a nurse practitioner (NP), nurse, or physician assistant (PA). For simplicity, this book uses "physician consultation" and "medical consultation" as collective terms that mean communicating with any of these providers about a client's massage plan. Several communication samples are introduced in this chapter. For some client presentations, a physician consultation can play an important role in massage therapy.

In many countries, there is no defined relationship between massage therapy and medicine. Although this is changing, the lack of an organized connection to conventional health care has made it challenging, at times, for therapists and physicians to join in partnership in patient care. Many massage therapists, unaccustomed to medical language and practices, are uneasy about approaching conventional health care professionals for dialogue about the interactions of medical conditions and treatments with massage therapy. When an opportunity for conversation does occur, it may be complicated by ambiguity about the benefits and contraindications of massage.

Without a formal infrastructure for dialogue, therapists have been advised to simply request a permission note from a client's physician, approving massage therapy for the patient with a medical condition. In this chapter, the limitations of this approach are discussed, along with alternative methods of communication. Guidelines for consulting with a physician collaboratively are introduced, together with a clear picture of what is needed from the physician in order for the massage plan to go forward.

The Pitfalls of the Simple "Doctor's Note"

In the massage field, lists of massage contraindications have often included the need for a physician's permission for massage, and many therapists are trained to ask for such a note when there is any question about the safety of massage. Often this note is requested of the client, who, in turn, requests it from his or her physician. Unfortunately, this form of communication is usually too brief and one-dimensional to be meaningful. Its usefulness is limited, for several reasons:

1. In asking for permission for *any* massage rather than input on specific massage elements, the therapist's request is too general.
2. The physician may not be well informed about massage therapy, or about the specific therapist's work.
3. With little information available in the literature about the effects of massage, the physician may not have considered how massage elements interact with the patient's medical condition and cannot effectively address the therapist's question.
4. Deference to the client's physician in these decisions sidesteps the therapist's professional responsibility for investigating massage contraindications on his or her own.

In medicine, there is no established line of thinking to approve a patient for massage therapy. Compare this to other, more familiar activities: A physician gives permission for a patient to drive 6 weeks after surgery or to begin to operate machinery after successful treatment for a seizure disorder. A physician may prescribe supervised exercise at a certain point after a heart attack or give permission for a patient to participate in school sports. These are familiar activities with predictable effects on the body. The interplay of massage therapy and medical conditions is less clear, without established guidelines or practices.

In the absence of such guidelines, the massage therapist takes on more of a leadership role in physician communication, encouraging the flow of information in both directions. The therapist asks questions about the client's condition and the advisability of certain massage elements and raises the physician's awareness about massage contraindications. The physician offers needed medical information and a medical perspective on the massage plan. The physician and the massage therapist put their heads together for the welfare of the client.

Roles and Responsibilities

Clear roles and responsibilities can pave the way for good communication. If the therapist is clear about what he or she needs, the steps to take, and what he or she expects of the physician, it increases the likelihood of a productive exchange.

● THE MASSAGE THERAPIST'S RESPONSIBILITIES

A physician consultation involves planning and preparation. Before initiating communication with the physician, the therapist does the following:

1. Gathers as much information as possible about the client's health in the client interview;
2. Educates herself or himself about the client's condition, using medical literature and patient education resources;
3. Searches the massage literature, including this text, for massage therapy guidelines for the condition;
4. Answers as many questions as possible for herself or himself, perhaps by sketching one or more Decision Trees, reviewing massage principles, or asking the client a few more questions (see Chapters 1–4);
5. Identifies any unanswered questions, focusing them on specific medical information that has bearing on the massage plan;
6. Prepares questions for the physician.

The therapist is not expected to have a vast store of medical knowledge about the client's condition. However, by carrying out the first four tasks mentioned above, the therapist might answer his or her own questions, making physician communication unnecessary. This is especially true as the therapist grows in experience.

> *The Clinical Judgment Improves with Experience Principle. An experienced therapist can more safely and readily predict a therapeutic outcome or anticipate a problem than a beginning therapist.*

If the therapist does identify unanswered questions, she makes them as clear as possible and is then ready to consult the physician. At this point, her responsibility is to facilitate the consultation, guiding it as well as possible to a productive exchange.

● COMMUNICATION STEPS

A consultation with a client's physician involves four steps:

1. *Communication*: Establishing a method of communication between the therapist and the physician.
2. *Education*: Informing the physician of the practice of adapting massage therapy to medical conditions, the specific concerns about the client's condition, and the proposed massage adjustments for the client.
3. *Input*: Requesting information from the physician about the client's medical condition and potential interactions with massage.
4. *Approval*: Obtaining the physician's permission to proceed with the massage plan (in certain cases).

By initiating contact and establishing lines of communication with the client's physician, the therapist can then raise the physician's awareness about massage contraindications and the adjustments that might be in force for a particular client. This paves the way for the physician's acknowledgment of the massage plan, input into it, or permission for it to go forward.

In steps 3 and 4 mentioned above, the distinction between *information* from the physician and physician *permission or approval* is an important one. If permission is necessary, it usually satisfies requirements of a facility serving a medically vulnerable population, or even a licensing law. Asking for information is another thing altogether—it is a request for dialogue.

● THE PHYSICIAN'S RESPONSIBILITIES

By engaging the physician in a discussion about a client, the therapist is asking the physician to:

- Consider the therapist's questions about the patient's medical condition;
- Give weight to the therapist's concerns about the interactions of massage and the condition;
- Answer the therapist's questions with any information, insights, and medical perspective that are needed for the massage plan.

It is not part of the physician's role to teach the therapist all about the client's medical condition. Nor should the physician be expected to substitute for a good intake interview—it is not the physician's responsibility to supply information that the therapist could reliably get from the client. Finally, it is not up to the physician to shoulder the responsibility for the safety of the massage; that responsibility is the therapist's.

Consulting a Physician

One of the therapist's primary responsibilities in consulting a physician is to define specific questions. Having phrased these questions as clearly as possible, the therapist determines the best health care provider to approach. But before the therapist communicates directly with that person, he or she obtains the client's written authorization for the communication.

● THE CLIENT'S AUTHORIZATION

A client's authorization to release medical information is required for any direct correspondence between his massage therapist and his physician's office. By its nature, any correspondence between the therapist and the physician involves

Shawn MacKinnon Massage Therapy
1745 Vista Drive   West Orange, CA 93631   714 555 6162

Authorization to Release Medical Information

Client Name:

Date of Birth:

Address:

City, State/Province:

Telephone Number

Contact Person (if other than client): _____   Phone: _____

I:_____ authorize Shawn MacKinnon to disclose my health care information to the following health care provider:

Name:

Address:

The following information may be disclosed (check all that apply):

☐ All health care information in my medical chart.

☐ Only health care information relating to the following injury, illness, or treatment:

_____

☐ Only health care information for the following dates or time periods:

_____

☐ Including information regarding HIV, sexually transmitted disease, mental health, drug or alcohol abuse.

I give my authorization to release health care information for the following purposes (check all that apply):

☐ To share information with my health care team in an attempt to coordinate care
☐ To obtain payment of care expenses I have incurred for my treatments
☐ To take part in research
☐ Other:

_____

This authorization expires on:

Date: _____ (no longer than 90 days from the date signed)

Event: _____

I understand that I may refuse to sign this authorization.
I may also revoke this authorization at any time by writing a letter to Shawn McKinnon Massage Therapy.
I understand that once my health care information is disclosed there is the potential for unauthorized re-disclosure and it may no longer be protected by HIPAA or state privacy laws. Shawn MacKinnon Massage Therapy will continue to maintain the confidentiality of patients' medical records mandated by the Federal HIPAA Privacy Rule.

I also understand my obtaining care cannot be conditioned on my signing this release.

Signature _____   Date _____

FIGURE 5-1. Sample authorization to release medical information. (Adapted from Thompson D. *Hands Heal,* 2nd ed. Philadelphia: Lippincott Williams & Wilkins, 2006.)

exchanging private information about the client's health. In the United States, this is called **protected health information (PHI)**. PHI includes information documented in the client's medical records and massage records. Even the fact that he or she is receiving massage therapy is PHI, and other data—the client's date of birth, address, other identifying information, and any medical conditions—are likewise private and protected. A client's written, signed, and dated authorization, on file in both the massage therapist's office and the physician's office, is necessary in order for a therapist and a physician to discuss this information. A sample client authorization to release medical information is in Figure 5-1.

Different countries have different laws about confidential health information, and even different states or provincial laws complicate matters. But no matter where the massage therapist practices, client confidentiality is one tenet of professional ethics and the therapist-client relationship. This confidence can be broken only by written permission from the client. In the United States, regulations governing the protection and handling of PHI are contained in the **Health Insurance Portability and Accountability Act (HIPAA) Privacy Rules** of 1996. HIPAA resources for massage therapists are listed in the bibliography at http://thePoint.lww.com/Walton.

● QUESTIONS TO ASK

The questions in a medical consultation should be thoughtful and focused—the question, "Is it okay for this person

TABLE 5-1.	SAMPLE PHRASING OF QUESTIONS FOR A CLIENT'S PHYSICIAN	
Medical Condition	**Possible Massage Adjustment**	**Question to Physician**
Scabies	General contact	I need to know if this patient's skin condition, scabies, has resolved and is no longer communicable before I can provide any touch therapy. Can I offer her massage and touch on my table, without any risk to myself or other clients?
Osteoporosis	Joint movement, pressure	I am aware of this client's osteoporosis. She prefers deep massage pressure, but it is unclear, from my interview with her, how stable her spine is, so I have not provided deep pressure. In my practice, I use stretching, range of motion, and five levels of massage pressure (attach pressure scale). In my opinion, medium pressure—a maximum pressure of 3 on her paraspinal muscles—and only gentle movement at her hip and shoulder joints are appropriate, but we need your input on the safety of this. Are you concerned about this pressure or about any other activities for this patient? What is her risk of pathologic fracture from this kind of intervention?
Spinal Cord Injury	Overall pressure, varying positions, joint movements	This client recently sustained a spinal cord injury. Since it has been only a few weeks since the accident, I want to ask you about autonomic dysreflexia (see "Spinal Cord Injury," Chapter 10). Is his blood pressure stable enough for him to receive massage of his upper body, with various pressures, positions, and joint movements? Is there anything I need to be concerned about or certain signs of dysreflexia that I should be alert for?

to receive massage?" is too general. Instead, the therapist includes specific elements of massage in the question. Perhaps the client has a sign or symptom that seems to contraindicate deeper pressure levels or the movement of joints in a certain area. Or maybe the therapist needs to know whether contact is safe, if an infection has resolved. These are reasonable questions to ask of a client's physician or physician's representative. Examples of questions and phrasing are in Table 5-1.

● APPROACHING VARIOUS PRACTITIONERS

A therapist seeking a medical consultation may also need to determine which practitioner to consult. Some people see several different physicians for a single condition, or for multiple conditions. This could include a primary care practitioner (PCP), an orthopedist, a cardiologist, or an oncologist. Many physicians' offices also include a PA or NP, both of whom are licensed to diagnose, treat, and manage disease. With the authority to prescribe medications and order tests, these providers can also be consulted for advice, acknowledgment, or approval of a massage plan.

For a question about a condition or treatment, consult the treating physician or physician's representative. If a client has multiple conditions or treatments, the best person to contact is usually the physician or representative who sees the client regularly, often the client's PCP. Although the PCP might not be treating the condition in question, he or she still has an understanding of how multiple treatments can affect the different body systems. The client usually has the easiest access to that person and has established rapport and an ongoing relationship.

Consulting the Nurse

In most situations, the massage therapist ends up communicating with the physician through the physician's nurse, which is ideal. Often, the nurse is the front line of communication from the physician's office, fielding questions and requests from the client and client's family, and is "the way in" to communicating with the physician. The physician's nurse may be more available by phone and often communicates with other practitioners. She or he may help process paperwork, such as a care plan or form sent by the therapist, and is a natural intermediary. Communication with the nurse has several advantages:

1. *Training in massage.* Massage as a comfort measure has traditionally been part of nursing training; nurses tend to understand the dynamics of massage and appreciate its benefits and contraindications.
2. *The benefits of touch.* Nurses have often championed massage therapy for patients, and much of the research on massage therapy appears in nursing journals. Many nurses go on to study touch and energy modalities in an effort to bring touch and massage back into nursing care.
3. *Handling the body.* In normal nursing care, nurses handle the body more often, and for longer periods than most physicians—applying lotion, supporting and repositioning patients, and checking for vital signs. They can readily consider equivalent modifications in contact, lubricant, pressure, movement, and positioning in massage therapy.

Formal physician approval for massage must come from the client's physician, physician's assistant, or NP, and each time a medical consultation appears on a Decision Tree, it signals communication with one of these providers. But input from nurses is vital to most massage conversations. The nurse is a valuable resource, not just as an intermediary, but because she or he can provide useful insights and direction for massage therapy.

More and more physicians and other health care providers are becoming familiar with massage and touch therapies and welcoming these for their patients.

Communication Methods

There are several ways to initiate communication with a physician whom the therapist has not worked with or met:

1. Direct communication, using a personal letter
2. Direct communication, using a pre-made format, such as a massage therapy care plan
3. Indirect communication through the client, by asking the client to bring a question to his or her physician

Direct contact with a physician is usually most effective when it is in writing, giving him or her a chance to read and respond on his or her own schedule. By writing, the therapist has time to formulate questions and collect thoughts and to make it as professional as possible. Written correspondence documents the communication between the massage therapist and the physician. Where necessary, a telephone call can follow the written contact.

● THE PERSONAL LETTER

In a personal letter, the therapist draws on information in Chapter 2 to describe massage therapy in plain, universal terms, using the elements of massage and avoiding trade names and modality names. The therapist includes relevant factors in the client's condition and specific concerns for the physician to address. It is not necessary to restate massage principles, include Decision Trees, or attach the completed client health form, as these are tools for clinical decision making rather than finished correspondence. Instead, the therapist introduces a provisional massage plan and asks the physician for one or more of the following:

- Health information to fill in any gaps
- Input on massage contraindications
- Approval for the patient to receive massage

A written inquiry to the physician should be brief—no more than one or two pages. The note should be well organized and contain clear information. The questions should be as specific as possible. Figure 5-2 is a sample of a personal letter to the physician with specific questions about a massage plan.

In the letter, outline exactly what is needed from the physician and a clear, easy, and useful way for the physician to respond. Most physicians' offices have a staggering volume of paperwork. A request from a massage therapist can be a daunting additional task to complete. One way to smooth the feedback process is for the therapist to ask the physician to complete a form enclosed with the letter, or even within it, then sign it and return it to the therapist (see Figure 5-2).

Presumably the physician's office will copy or record these communications for their patient record, but even if they do not make a copy, the therapist has a convenient, complete record of the correspondence on one or two pages.

● STREAMLINING COMMUNICATION: THE MASSAGE THERAPY CARE PLAN

Generating a personalized letter to every client's physician, for every question that comes up, can become tedious. A therapist can save time by developing *massage protocols* for common situations or for a population of the therapist's specialty. Among other things, a protocol describes the massage approach, expected outcomes or benefits, and massage contraindications. A protocol can be set down in a format called a massage therapy care plan. The term *massage plan* is an informal term used throughout this book, usually to describe massage contraindications for an individual session. The term *care plan* has a broader meaning in the context of medical care. In medicine and nursing, a care plan is not only for contraindications; it also describes a course of treatment, expected treatment outcomes, ways to measure them, and a timeline for the course of treatment. A massage therapy care plan includes all of these elements adapted to massage therapy.

Typically, care plans in medicine are informed by clinical research about which therapies are effective. In massage therapy, there is not yet a sufficient body of research to support one massage approach over another for a certain client presentation (see Chapter 6). Until research is available, care plans in massage therapy are based on therapists' clinical observations, case reports in professional literature, and the advice of instructors and colleagues.

Figure 5-3 is a basic massage therapy care plan for a client in cancer treatment and a request for the physician to review the plan, acknowledge it, and comment on the plan if he or she feels it is necessary. The care plan is somewhat generic, in that it includes common massage issues for this population (see Chapter 20). The therapist left some of the general information in the plan but customized much of it to his or her individual client before sending it to the physician, along with a short note. Similar forms are used by many oncology massage therapists in the United States (MacDonald, 2007).

In this example, the care plan is not designed to start a lengthy dialogue about a specific question; instead, the therapist asks for acknowledgment of the care plan and invites comment. However, depending on the

(*text continues on page 64*)

Joanne Lightfoot Massage Therapy
1463 Pearl Street
Prospect Valley, PA 19320
Telephone: 484 555 0000

Date

Dr. Frances Lin
Valley Medical Associates
123 Pleasant Street
Prospect Valley, PA 19320

Dear Dr. Lin:
Your patient, Mr. Gene Werner, DOB 5/12/58, has given me permission to contact you. Mr. Werner would like to receive regular massage therapy in this office. I am writing to ask your input on massage therapy and movement for him, and approval for going forward with our massage plan. Because this patient sustained whiplash injuries in a motor vehicle accident 10 weeks ago, I would be grateful for your input.

Provisional Massage Therapy Plan

Overall, the massage session would include kneading, stroking, and stationary pressure, using gentle to medium, "warming up" pressure on the muscles of the back, shoulders, hips, arms and hands. No deep pressure would be used at the occiput, neck, or shoulders. I am asking for your recommendations, for or against the following:

- Massage of the neck muscles, lateral and posterior, with gentle to medium pressure, engaging the medium layers of muscles, pressure slightly more than that needed to "rub in" lotion or sunscreen.

- Medium, focused fingertip pressure to the attachments at the occiput, including the SCM attachments at the mastoid.

- Gentle movement of the neck, perhaps passive rotation up to 30 degrees right and left, and passive side flexion to 40 degrees right and left, to patient's tolerance.

In your best estimation, can these techniques be done safely at this point, without aggravating the patient's discomfort or injury, or interfering with medical treatment? Is this plan appropriate? Please comment below on this provisional plan and return it to my office at the above address. Also, please feel free to call with questions or concerns.

Thank you for your consideration.

Kind regards,

Joanne Lightfoot

Joanne Lightfoot

Physician Recommendations for Massage Therapy Plan

I have reviewed the above massage plan for my patient, Mr. Gene Werner, and circled yes, below, next to techniques I recommend, and no, below, next to techniques I do not advise:
(Please circle yes or no in each case)

Yes No   Direct massage of neck muscles, lateral and posterior, with gentle to moderate pressure.

Yes No   Focused fingertip pressure at moderate pressure to attachments at the occiput, including the
           mastoid process.

Yes No   Gentle passive rotation of neck to 30 degrees, right and left

Yes No   Gentle passive lateral flexion of neck to 40 degrees, right and left

I have noted any additional exclusions or recommendations below:

_____

_____

_____   _____
Physician's Signature   Date

_____
Print Physician's Name

FIGURE 5-2. Sample personal letter for physician consultation.

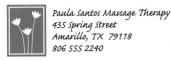

Paula Santos Massage Therapy
435 Spring Street
Amarillo, TX 79118
806 555 2240

Deval Montgomery, MD
Oncology Associates of Amarillo
24 Curtis Ave.
Amarillo, TX 79118

Dear Dr. Montgomery:

Your patient, Earlene Sikes, DOB 1/19/49, would like to receive massage therapy during the course of her cancer treatment. I'm enclosing the massage therapy care plan for your review, and welcome your input. The care plan lists common massage adaptations for patients in cancer treatment, and I have circled those that are relevant for this patient.

Please return a signed copy of the care plan in the enclosed envelope, and feel free to call me at the number above if you have questions or concerns. Thank you for your time and consideration.

Warm regards,

Paula Santos
Paula Santos, LMT

Paula Santos Massage Therapy
435 Spring Street
Amarillo, TX 79118
806 555 2240

Massage Therapy Care Plan

Client is in treatment for breast cancer: Left lumpectomy and axillary lymph node dissection December 2009, chemotherapy planned through March 2010, to be followed by a six week course of radiation therapy.

Client complains of nausea, fatigue, muscle pain in neck and shoulders, and sleep disruption.

Goals of Massage Therapy Treatment (Outcomes Assessed at Each Treatment)
- Improvement in client self reports of overall relaxation
- Improvement in self reports of sleep quality and duration
- Muscle relaxation, as measured by palpation, observation of posture, client self reports of pain and stiffness
- Reduction of complaints of nausea, as reported through verbal analogue scale (0-10)

Course of Massage Therapy Treatment

One-hour relaxation massage sessions, 1X/week, until completion of cancer treatment

Course of Massage Therapy Treatment

General relaxation massage with focus on areas of muscle pain
Kneading, stroking, and compressions to the tissues
Gentle passive stretching and range of motion
Range of massage pressures, from movement of the skin (as in applying lotion, or "lotioning") to compression of medium layers of muscle.

Common Massage Therapy Adaptations for Clients in Cancer Treatment (Relevant conditions are circled):

Sites affected by surgery, radiation therapy, skin conditions, pain, edema, or bone involvement
Avoid deep pressure and in some cases medium pressure and even contact on affected areas.

Areas at risk of lymphedema
If there is any removal or radiation of lymph nodes with lymphedema risk, use only "lotioning" pressure on the extremity and on the associated trunk quadrant. If needed, the limb is elevated during the massage.

Unstable tissues due to malignancy, easy bruising, bone metastasis
Gentle overall pressure or gentler pressure at specific sites, as needed.

Side-effects of cancer treatments
Limit pressure depending on symptoms and massage tolerance (begin with ("lotioning"), use slow speeds, even rhythms, and limited joint movement, to avoid aggravating symptoms (nausea, pain, fatigue, poor sleep):

Possible increased risk of DVT, secondary to malignancy, cancer treatment, or other factors
Limit joint movement, avoid use of medium or deep pressure on lower extremities if risk of thrombosis exists.

Physician Acknowledgement of Massage Therapy Care Plan

I have reviewed the above massage therapy care plan for my patient, Ms. Earlene Sikes, and noted the massage adjustments circled.

If I suggest any additional massage adjustments, have any other information, or have any concerns about the appropriateness of the above plan for this patient, these are described below:

_____

_____

_____   _____
Physician's Signature   Date

_____
Print Physician's Name

FIGURE 5-3. Sample massage therapy care plan.

therapist's intent, she can word her correspondence differently. She may:

- Request the physician's formal approval of the care plan by adding a statement of permission or approval for the physician to sign.
- Request specific information by adding a question to the correspondence and a means for the physician to answer it easily.

Because care plans collect the typical massage therapy issues and approaches in one place, they are worth developing for common, medically complex conditions such as heart disease, diabetes, cancer, or HIV/AIDS. A prepared massage therapy care plan has four obvious benefits:

1. In the process of preparing the care plan, the therapist familiarizes himself or herself with the common massage adjustments for a particular medical condition. This is a valuable learning experience.
2. By targeting specific outcomes of a session or a course of treatment, the therapist attends to massage benefits as well as contraindications.
3. By using the care plan format, the therapist enhances the professionalism of his or her work.
4. The care plan serves as a template, ready to modify for a client presenting with that condition. This saves time later, smoothing the way for good communication with the next client's physician.

By requesting the physician's signature, the therapist links the education of the physician to an acknowledgment, input, or approval mechanism. If the therapist needs a certain question answered, he or she can put it in the accompanying note or put the care plan into a yes/no format, similar to the personal letter in Figure 5-2.

The care plan eases the communication process for both the physician and the therapist. It may introduce a pause into the blizzard of the physician's paperwork, a moment to consider the therapeutic benefit of massage and the importance of contraindications. Although the primary purpose of such a form is communication, it can also draw attention to the therapist's work. In "Raising Awareness with Paperwork," a massage therapist describes several examples of this (see online at http://thePoint.lww.com/Walton).

● COMMUNICATING THROUGH THE CLIENT

Although direct, written communication is advised for a medical consultation, some therapists find occasion to communicate with the physician through the client. This method can be simpler, although sometimes it is more complicated than direct communication. The therapist may ask the client, for instance, "Please ask your doctor about this skin rash you told me about, and find out if she's sure it's not communicable before we schedule an appointment." Or, "Ask your doctor if it's okay for you to stretch at that joint, and for me to give you what we call 'a passive stretch.' Or does she think we should wait?" If needed, the therapist

jots down his or her questions for the physician to help the client remember them.

This through-the-client method of communication has advantages. It is generally quicker and takes less effort than working up a written communication to the physician. Because the client controls the flow of information, it does not require an additional written release of medical information. It also empowers clients in the dialogue about their health and the potential for it to interact with massage therapy. The approach may work well in high-volume massage settings with little or no record keeping, where the client sees the same therapist regularly and there is no infrastructure for written communication, but questions arise over a course of treatment.

This communication method has disadvantages, too. For it to be meaningful, the therapist has to trust the client to clearly convey the concern to the physician and then to accurately return the physician's response. The information might be too complicated for the client to describe to the physician, and he or she might not be able to answer the physician's follow-up questions. Therefore, to use this method, the therapist needs to be confident that the client understands the concern, shares it, and can be a reliable intermediary. In "Reliable Communication Is Key," a therapist describes a scenario in which it would be unwise to go through the client to communicate with the physician (see online).

Another disadvantage of communicating through the client is the lack of a formal paper trail. Without a written record of the exchange, the therapist cannot reference it over time but must rely on his or her own memory and the client's memory of what the physician said. The lack of documentation also leaves the therapist professionally vulnerable if something goes wrong, and a complaint is made against the therapist.

If the information can be reliably conveyed through a client intermediary, it may be the fastest, most meaningful way to communicate. But occasional communication through a client is not appropriate for a complicated question or for a serious condition, where real injury could result. Typically, a written exchange provides a more thorough route, one that is safer for everyone.

● FOLLOWING UP

As the client's health changes, the documentation should likewise be kept up to date. Whether this requires periodic physician consultation is another question. There is no set rule for how often to contact the physician about an ongoing health issue; it is an individual decision, based on massage issues that arise. If changes in a client's health status lead the therapist to specific questions or concerns, an updated medical consultation is probably necessary.

Advantages of regular correspondence with a physician include the opportunity to remind him or her of the benefit that the client is receiving from massage and continued prompting about the role that massage therapy plays in the client's life. These reminders may strengthen the professional relationship and build bridges between massage therapy and medicine.

Problem Solving

Consulting with a client's physician often goes smoothly, including all the desired steps. However, problems sometimes occur, such as the following:

- There is no response from the physician to the therapist's inquiry.
- The physician's response seems incomplete—he or she seems to have approved the massage plan without considering all of the issues.
- Conflicting opinions arise between the physician and the therapist or between two other health care providers regarding massage therapy and the client's condition.

These scenarios are discussed below, along with some possible strategies. Whatever exchange ends up occurring between the therapist, physician, and client, the therapist should ask himself or herself afterward: Do I have the answer to my question? Am I convinced that the massage plan is safe? If the answer is yes, the massage plan can proceed. If not, there is more work to do.

● HANDLING NONRESPONSE

Even after a therapist sends a well-written form, or the most personalized letter, some physicians' offices may not respond. Reasons for nonresponse vary. The office might be backed up on processing paperwork. A key person involved in processing paperwork could be out of the office due to illness. The physician may have seen the form but set it aside, wanting to give it more attention later. Because a variety of factors can interfere with the timely processing of a therapist's correspondence, it is important not to take it personally if there are delays.

Unless a facility or regulation requires physician approval for massage, a communication delay does not typically hold up massage therapy entirely; more likely, it postpones a specific massage plan. The therapist leaves out the massage elements in question but can begin cautious work with a new client or continue with a current client, until the physician consultation is complete.

If delays are prolonged, it is primarily the client's responsibility, rather than the massage therapist's, to engage the physician (or, if a client is unable to advocate for herself or himself, it is her or his family's or health care proxy's responsibility). If the physician does not respond to the therapist's request for communication, the client is in the best position to facilitate an exchange.

One reason for nonresponse might be the physician's concern about being liable if something goes wrong during massage, or a concern that massage will harm the client. In these situations, more communication is needed, not judgment or snap decisions. Perhaps another way to communicate can be worked out; a physician who is reluctant to sign a form might prefer phone conversation. Ideally, the correspondence should be in writing, but if the physician's input comes over the phone, there is still a chance for dialogue.

Any verbal exchange must be documented: The therapist records the name and position of the physician or nurse, the date and time of the conversation, and all relevant and specific information exchanged.

● INCOMPLETE RESPONSES

Sometimes it might appear that the physician responded to a massage question too hastily, signing a form without considering all the issues. In this case, the physician's acknowledgment, input, or approval of the plan was obtained, but it is not clear whether communication and education took place. The physician's response may be empty without these steps. There are a couple of ways to address incomplete responses. One is to persist, in writing, by phone, or through the client. Another is to follow it up with a yes/no format described below.

If the therapist decides to pursue an expanded response from the physician, by phone or letter, it is important to be polite, understanding, and specific. For example:

> Thank you for responding to the massage therapy care plan I sent you. On the form, I noticed that you approved general pressure, but I don't see any mention of pressure on this specific area, given the patient's vascular condition. Because of the condition, I need to know your thoughts about pressure there. I hope we can talk more about that, since the client is asking for specific pressure on that area. We'll be able to proceed with the massage once you give us your opinion. Thank you for making time to respond.

Occasionally, the therapist may need to be even more direct and focused in an inquiry, especially in questions about massage pressure and unstable tissue. Being explicit about pressure may help, as in the following example:

> If appropriate, I could lean in and use a fair amount of pressure in this area. Generally at my medium and deep pressure levels, joints move. At the deepest pressures, the deep muscles and vessels are compressed and I engage the underlying bone. I am concerned about the stability of the tissues in the area. Would you recommend this level of pressure, or should I hold back? Can you tell me which factors you consider in your recommendation?

Depending on the therapist's tone, these statements could sound terse or challenging. Maintaining a friendly, receptive tone, while remaining professional, is the key to getting the best possible response.

The Yes/No Format

When a form for the physician is returned with no detail on it, it is hard to know whether the physician was able to take a good look at it before signing. Another way for the therapist to get specific questions addressed is to use a yes/no format. The physician simply circles the answer and signs the form. See Figure 5-2 for a yes/no format, in this case, as part of a personal letter to the physician.

An inquiry to the physician in a yes/no format can be in a letter, a care plan, or any other checklist. The questions need to be focused, and the therapist should avoid asking the physician to recreate the client health form by asking questions that are better directed to the client. For instance, asking the physician about each symptom or sign of a client's condition, such as nausea or headache, can be a waste of time, and symptoms can change frequently. Yes/no questions can be presented to the physician in the form of statements, such as:

- Because of this patient's medications, he is susceptible to bruising and bleeding.
- This patient's blood pressure is well controlled and stable and is unlikely to spike unexpectedly.
- This patient's spine is stable enough to withstand a level 4 massage pressure, as in the attached pressure scale (see Chapter 2).
- This patient is at elevated risk of deep vein thrombosis, and massage pressure in the lower extremities should be limited to level 1 or 2.
- This patient's hip is stable enough to withstand strong stretching or range of motion.

This yes/no format can serve as a follow-up measure to an incomplete response. Some therapists may also choose the yes/no format for an initial exchange (see Figure 5-2) to lower the chances of the form being "waved through" without close consideration of the therapist's concerns. Whenever it is used, the yes/no format can be very useful to the massage session. However, in most cases, it should not substitute for gathering information from the client himself.

● MANAGING CONFLICTING OPINIONS

In opening communication with a client's physician, a massage therapist opens himself or herself to possible disagreement on the right course of action for the client's massage sessions. This is not necessarily a bad thing. Dialogue between massage therapists and physicians is necessary for coordinated care, and disagreement can be a positive sign, that the physician is engaged in the issue and is seriously considering the therapist's concerns.

Disagreement can take different forms and, in some cases, can include the client. For example, a client might feel that massage is "no big deal" and that the consultation process is unnecessary, even if the massage therapist is in favor of it. A physician may join a client in the view that the therapist is excessively conservative in his or her decisions. Or, a massage therapist and client could favor a certain care plan, but the physician is concerned and will not approve the plan.

The Shred of Doubt Principle can help massage therapists navigate this terrain. If any one of the three parties involved—client, massage therapist, or physician—disagrees with the others, a shred of doubt still exists about the massage approach. In this climate, the mostconservative

course is advised. The client, of course, has the right to refuse a technique or massage element, no matter how much benefit or how little harm it might hold. The physician has the right to withhold approval, if concerned about the plan. And the massage therapist has the right to omit massage elements that he or she thinks are potentially harmful, even if the other parties are in favor of it.

> *The Shred of Doubt Principle.* **If there is a shred of doubt about whether a massage element is safe, it is contraindicated until its safety is established. When in doubt, don't.**

In the client-therapist-physician triad, if conflicting opinions result in strong disagreement or dispute, the best response is more communication and education. Become curious about the opposing view, and be inquisitive. Try more communication, written or verbal. Consult resources in the literature. Work with, rather than against, the other to reach agreement. If appropriate, involve the client in the exchanges. If disagreement persists, then the Shred of Doubt Principle prevails and the most conservative approach is best.

● OVERRIDING A PHYSICIAN'S INPUT

If opinions conflict, when is it appropriate for the massage therapist to override the physician's input or approval? It depends on the circumstances. Several scenarios are possible, and two of them are discussed here: In one, the physician is more conservative, and in the other, the massage therapist is more conservative.

If a physician supports a conservative massage plan, or no massage at all, in conflict with the therapist and client, then it is unwise for the therapist to override the physician's input. Even if the physician is not well informed about massage, or unresponsive to the client's and the therapist's efforts to educate her, the therapist should stick with the physician's position. This might rankle some therapists, but let us consider the possibilities. Suppose a physician refuses to approve a massage plan for the client. Perhaps she advises against it because her own experience of massage is that it is very deep and feels strongly that massage would therefore be harmful to the client. Perhaps she persists in her view, despite the massage therapist's carefully outlined, gentle, conservative massage therapy care plan. This scenario is unusual, but it does happen.

The massage therapist is in an awkward position. He believes that he can provide a perfectly safe, effective session with modifications. The client and possibly even the client's family or friends are eager for the work, but the physician disagrees or will not approve it. The therapist is caught in the middle. Many therapists would be tempted to go ahead and provide massage in this situation, but they should think twice. If anything goes wrong, such as an adverse response to massage, or the client's condition worsens, the massage therapist who overruled the physician's advice would be professionally vulnerable. The massage therapist is accountable to not only the client and the physician but also the client's family. The answer to this kind of dispute is more education and dialogue, not rebellion.

Now, let us consider the other scenario: Suppose a physician supports massage, but the therapist has doubts about some elements. An example is a massage therapist who does not feel comfortable applying strong pressure or circulatory massage, even after the physician has given the go-ahead and the client wants it. The therapist's hands and judgment are on the line, not the physician's. The massage therapist *does* have the right to refuse to provide work that he thinks might be harmful, even if the physician and the client are in favor of it. In this case, the therapist's concerns override the other perspectives. However, if the therapist intended at the outset to stick to a cautious massage plan, he might not have needed to seek the physician's input in the first place. In "The Nurse's Advice," a therapist tells a story of working more conservatively than a physician's recommendation (see online).

At first, it is important to use caution and follow up on any information that suggests a contraindication. With more dialogue and information, or a track record of positive client responses to the pressure, a less conservative massage plan may develop over time.

The Where You Start Isn't Always Where You End Up Principle. Although a client's condition may call for a conservative initial massage, stronger elements may be appropriate in later sessions, after monitoring the client's response to massage over time.

● MAINTAINING ALLIANCES

On rare occasions, consulting with a client's physician can be difficult, if not exasperating. This is usually due to the heavy demands placed on medical personnel, leaving little time for correspondence. If a therapist has difficulty carrying out communication with a client's physician, the therapist must not complain to the client. The patient-physician relationship is vital to the client's care and is distinct from the relationship the therapist has with either the client or the physician. The alliance between a physician and a patient is essential, as is the alliance between the massage therapist and a client.

If, during a breakdown in communication between the therapist and a client's physician, the client wants to know the progress of the exchange, the therapist shares the information in a neutral, professional way: "I haven't heard back yet, perhaps it's because of the long weekend." "I called the office a couple of times yesterday, but didn't receive a return call." "Your physician did not seem in favor of massage, so I'm trying to find out more about his concerns so we can respond to them."

If a client complains about the physician's nonresponse, or, for that matter, if she complains at all about the care she is receiving, the therapist does not join in and gang up on the physician, adding ammunition from her own experience. Instead, she stays neutral and global in her response and sticks with reflective listening. "It sounds like you've tried hard to get through to the office to get the form processed. I'm sorry you've had to keep trying."

Sometimes clients bring their complaints about their health care to massage therapists. Within long massage sessions, there is ample time to express themselves. Again, reflective listening and neutral responses, not judgment, are the most supportive. The most important point is not to compromise the client's care, or her alliance with her physician. Asking questions like "Do you need to talk with someone about the care you're receiving?" might be helpful. A therapist must remember her own role as a health care professional—she would not want a client and his physician to complain about her, either.

Record Keeping

In keeping with the therapist's code of ethics, all correspondence with a client's physician should be kept confidential, with the client health record in a secure location. Electronic records must be stored in accordance with the HIPAA privacy rules or other regulations. A record should be updated as needed, most often when new questions for the physician arise, or when the client's health status worsens significantly. With an ongoing client, the therapist asks for a health update at each session and records the client's response. If changes occur in the client's report over time, it may be time to revise the massage therapy care plan and check it with the physician.

The therapist should also document how the physician's input was used in the session, for example, if he or she made adjustments to the massage based on the physician's advice. If the exchange was purely verbal, over the phone or through the client, a written summary of the exchange should be included in the notes, along with the date and the physician's or nurse's name. Even if communication with the client's physician was unsuccessful or incomplete, the details should be documented. If disagreement occurred between the therapist, client, and physician, specific points of disagreement should be charted along with the therapist's massage plan.

Physician Communication and Professional Liability

Whether written or verbal, a physician consultation does not automatically transfer liability from the massage therapist to the physician. While it may be tempting for a therapist to seek safe haven under the umbrella of the physician's license in these decisions, it is not a true refuge. In the end, it is the therapist, not the physician, who worked with the client, making the final decision about how and where to move his or her hands. It is the therapist who is considered responsible for any real or perceived harm, just as the therapist is responsible for any therapeutic benefit.

A physician consultation does widen the sphere of decision making to include the physician, and this good faith effort may, in some instances, be viewed favorably in the unlikely event of litigation. If weighed in court, written evidence of physician communication is much more reliable than verbal recall, and a therapist with a paper trail of completed forms and careful charting can show that he or she offered the massage plan to the client's physician for comment and advice before proceeding.

The sample communications in this chapter are not designed to be legal documents; instead, they are tools for meaningful discourse between a massage therapist and a physician. The true purpose of physician communication is the well-being of the client. Any document planned for formal legal purposes should be reviewed by an attorney before it is used.

The Benefits of Physician Communication

The benefits of a physician consultation are broad and deep. By involving the client's physician in massage decisions, the therapist models care and professionalism. By preparing thoughtfully and methodically for the exchange, the therapist enhances his or her own knowledge base about massage and the client's condition. The communication is an opportunity for the therapist to work responsibly and collegially with other health care professionals.

Everyone learns from such an exchange. Therapists broaden their knowledge of various medical conditions. Physicians broaden their understanding of massage therapy. Clients may be empowered in the decisions that affect their health and massage treatment. And finally, responsible massage adjustments, made after necessary research and consultation, safeguard the health and well-being of the client.

Ongoing communication with other health care professionals, especially when it is repeated, can lead to name recognition for the massage therapist. This, in turn, can lead to referrals from medical offices. Therapist's Journal 5-1 describes examples of professional alliances forged from this process.

The massage therapy profession is developing rapidly, and some therapists have less training in medical conditions and massage contraindications than others. Determining contraindications can be challenging. A temptation in the profession to lean on the simple "note from the doctor" might offer some comfort, but no real information. On

---

THERAPIST'S JOURNAL 5-1 *A Paper Handshake: Forms as Marketing Tools*

Usually following a conversation about my work, I hand the person my business card, with my name and contact information. In my practice, connection with my clients and the other practitioners in their circle of health care is valued. I prefer face-to-face communications, but initial community connections in business are often not in person. In these cases, I reach out with a paper handshake: a personalized mailing.

At a massage course focusing on massage for people with cancer, I was introduced to a physician consultation form designed to assist communication between oncologists and massage therapists in regard to clients receiving massage therapy during treatment. After careful consideration of my audience (there was a palpable curiosity among physicians about the safe delivery of massage to cancer clients) and my own practice beliefs, I adapted this form to meet various needs. I renamed it a Cooperative Care Plan, signifying that each chosen health care provider involved is an invited guest in this client's circle of care. Knowing that I am competently trained to deliver safe massage therapy for cancer patients, I utilized collaborative, nonhierarchical language in these revised forms. The result was a form that fostered cooperation and directly empowered the client's voice in the process of healing.

I sent a direct mailing of 200(+) to all health care providers listed by my clients on their intake forms and to all local oncologists. I personalized a warm letter, introduced my practice, and included my brochure and a blank copy of the Cooperative Care Plan. I did a combination of calls preceding the mailing and follow-up phone calls. This mailing planted the seed for future professional relationships. There were immediate return calls and referrals, and 100% of those contacted had positive feedback. But more importantly, the groundwork for trusted, competent delivery of services was initiated. I required a Cooperative Care Plan to be completed for all clients with cancer. Naturally, my reputation as a quality therapist and personality factored into the success of this marketing effort. But the forms we devise for our practices often are our signatures. This mailing was a significant tool in maintaining a thriving oncology massage practice of 6 years.

Sarah Moore Sturges
Le Mars, IA

the other hand, a little research and preparation arms the therapist with tools and reduces his or her anxiety about the unknown, and it sets the stage for a meaningful exchange with a client's physician.

Over the course of a career, a massage therapist may weather an occasional unpleasant or hurried exchange with another health care provider, but therapists tell many stories of productive communication and mutual respect. Focused on clear questions, bearing the goals of communication in mind, the therapist can guide a successful exchange that benefits the physician, the therapist, and, ultimately, the client who deserves the care.

SELF TEST

1. Suppose a client has a medical condition that raises possible massage contraindications. Why is a simple note from the doctor, approving massage, insufficient for the massage therapist?
2. A massage therapist plans to correspond directly with a client's physician about the client's medical history. Describe what the therapist needs from the client in order to contact the physician.
3. What are the four steps of a physician consultation?
4. List three advantages of involving a physician's nurse in a medical consultation about the advisability of massage therapy.
5. What are the components of a massage therapy care plan? List the advantages of having a standard massage therapy care plan prepared for a certain client population.

6. Describe the responsibilities that a massage therapist should carry out before initiating contact with a client's physician.
7. What are the disadvantages of communicating with a client's physician through the client, without a written record?
8. In correspondence with a client's physician, how should the therapist describe the massage modalities that he or she uses?
9. If a therapist causes a real or perceived injury to a client with a medical condition, does written consultation with a physician transfer liability for the injury to the physician? Why or why not?
10. In the event of a physician consultation, what should the therapist record in his or her client records about it?

 For answers to these questions and to see a bibliography for this chapter, visit http://thePoint. lww.com/Walton.

If we knew what it was we were doing, it would not be called research, would it?

—ALBERT EINSTEIN

As massage therapy becomes more visible to consumers and in health care, the call for massage therapy research is growing stronger. Massage therapy is gaining ground as a health care modality, and there is reason to look beyond individual client stories and chart some collective wisdom.

Research can influence the profession of massage in many ways. Four of the principal contributions are:

1. Solid research in support of massage helps to promote massage therapy to the public, to other health care professionals, and to health care policy makers.
2. If research establishes health care cost savings with massage therapy, it offers convincing evidence to policy makers for the support of massage.
3. Any documented adverse effects of massage can be used to establish safety guidelines for massage therapy.
4. By documenting approaches that are most effective for certain clinical presentations, research can direct the best practices in the profession.

The first two research contributions address the basic question of *whether* to massage. The last two suggest *how* to massage. Knowledge of any adverse effects of massage is as important as knowledge of its benefits, since both can guide the practice of massage. Ongoing sophisticated research will yield even more precise data about the "best practice" of massage, refining therapists' approaches to various clients. Best practice research compares different massage protocols, the massage dose, the best muscle groups to focus on, and other factors in clinical success. When research shows a consensus about the best massage protocols to use for various clinical problems, these protocols will become part of accepted massage therapy care plans for various clinical problems.

Many of the best practice guidelines in medicine are available in the National Guideline Clearinghouse (NGC), available on the Internet. At the time of this writing, the Massage Therapy Foundation has published a report outlining the need for best practice guidelines and plans for submitting massage therapy guidelines to the NGC (Grant et al., 2008).

A few massage studies at the frontier of massage research have begun to look at best practice (Aourell et al., 2005; Cambron et al., 2006). From these and other efforts, the rich knowledge in the profession will become easier to transfer: from therapist to therapist, and from teacher to student. With this growing attention to massage, it is an exciting time for the profession.

A Collection of Stories

Although research methods, language, and statistics can be intimidating to many therapists, a research study is simply one way to collect stories from people about massage. Each time a client leaves a massage session claiming, "My headache is better!" or "The pain in my leg is gone," he or she tells a story about massage therapy. Each time a pregnant or laboring woman tells her massage therapist, "Thank goodness you are here—it's helping me through this," it is a massage therapy story. In research, these stories are systematically collected and analyzed, to determine whether they show clear cause and effect, and whether the same kind of massage can be helpful on a larger scale in the general population. In Therapist's Journal 6-1, a massage therapist tells a story of a patient in a massage study.

As such, collections of individual stories, archived by researchers and told through research, can be as inspiring and useful as individual testimonials from clients. They can build a collective, shared understanding of the role and influence of massage therapy.

Massage therapy wisdom has been passed along primarily by oral tradition. Therapists tell their stories to other therapists, to massage students, and to their clients. While it's important to relay these, it is also important to write them down. An experience of an individual client, handful of clients, or groups of clients in a massage research study reaches a wider audience if it's recorded in the literature. Once such experiences are published, others can evaluate it, agree or disagree with it, and echo it from their own experiences.

The stories people tell about skilled touch and its impact on pain, sleep, anxiety and experiences of labor are compelling, and worth telling. Research is one forum for these stories, and is a good way to see if these individual experiences are shared by others—that is, if they are **generalizable** to a larger group of people. Clinical research attempts to answer this question: Could the intervention help a significant number of people, to a significant enough degree, to justify recommending its use for a given population?

THERAPIST'S JOURNAL 6-1 *The Night Before the Procedure*

One night at the hospital, after the dinner trays were cleared, I went to see an inpatient who was part of our massage study. She was scheduled for the active treatment, in a study looking at massage for people with advanced cancer. I knocked on her door and she invited me in. I introduced myself, and we chatted for a few minutes. I prepared my things, added pillows to support her, and we began the massage.

I remember this patient well. She was quiet for much of the session, but as I massaged her feet, she began to talk. She told me about an extremely painful procedure that was scheduled for the next morning. She was dreading it. She told me she was even more afraid of how advanced her cancer was, that she was, in fact, dying. But her biggest fear was for her family. She feared for her husband and children. She had held their household together for years, and she worried about whether they could get along without her.

She talked for a while, listing her fears, then rested again, more deeply as the session went on. I finished some data collection, then slipped out, quietly, so she could continue to rest. She gave me a sleepy wave. Clinical research is often seen as dry, cold, and analytical. My experience in this study, and on that particular evening, was otherwise; it was a deeply human exchange.

The next day, the patient told the research assistant that she was astonished that she had slept better than she could have imagined that night. She was so grateful for the massage. Over the course of the study, we heard many stories like hers. In this population, improved sleep is a theme. So is easing painful procedures. As research on massage continues to grow in the coming years, I am eager to see how these experiences are affected by massage.

Tracy Walton
Cambridge, MA

Determining Clear Cause and Effect

Conventional Western medicine is a world of **evidence-based practice**, in which clinical decisions are often based on results of systematic research. Researchers ask one or more questions: Did the massage cause the desired effect, or was it due to something else? If massage has an effect, what quality or feature produced that effect? How do we design further research to learn about cause and effect?

Researchers are interested in *variables*, or things that change in a study. For example, if we vary the length of massage, will the client's back pain vary, as well? This question is expressed in independent variables and dependent variables, or cause and effect. In clinical research, an **independent variable** is a therapy or intervention that is manipulated by a researcher to see if it affects another factor, the dependent variable. In a massage study, massage therapy—say, the presence or absence of it, or the dose or frequency of it—is the independent variable. A **dependent variable** is an outcome of an experiment, measured to see if it does, in fact, depend on the independent variable. Dependent variables are usually signs or symptoms, such as back pain, sleep quality, blood pressure, or relaxation.

The Current State of Massage Research

The massage therapy profession has benefited from small studies of massage over the last few decades, much more in the past 20 years. After so much time without recognized research, the profession has welcomed this development, and in some cases, has embraced the available research without questioning it. However, in many cases, too much has been made out of the small body of research. The profession is just beginning to incorporate the high standards of research use and design that are characteristic of medicine. Instead, the credibility of massage therapy still suffers from the ways research has been used:

- Citing massage research of uneven quality
- Overstating results from small studies
- Making too much out of a single study, rather than quoting a body of literature on a research topic

While the body of massage research is growing, it is still small, and in many cases, it is too early to draw strong conclusions from it. Some studies have been poorly designed and poorly reported, without explicit mention of important data or design steps when published. Sometimes the researchers' own bias in favor of massage influences the study results or the tone of the report. Often published studies report a cause and effect relationship between massage and patient improvement, but the investigators haven't accounted for other possible explanations for the improvement.

The available research is frequently given too much weight in massage-marketing materials, trade journals, and texts. Many of the claims made about massage have little or no research behind them, or the research is not conclusive. The profession is on stronger ground when massage therapists carry out the following responsibilities:

1. *Make accurate claims about massage.* Look closely at the statements that are commonly made about the effects of massage, and whether they are supported by research or by thoughtful clinical observations.
2. *Use research accurately.* Avoid overstating available research, and recognize strengths and limitations in published research.

Distinguish between stronger and weaker levels of evidence in massage research.

3. *Track massage research*. Follow the development of research in a topic of interest, such as massage and back pain, massage after surgery, or massage and cancer symptoms.

4. *Treat clinical work as a form of research inquiry*. Focus on therapeutic outcomes, and use measurement tools from research to determine what is effective for different client presentations. Document and share successes and failures.

Massage therapists do not have to become research experts, and not all therapists are drawn to it. But research is more accessible and interesting than it often appears, and everyone benefits from good research. The Internet makes it easy to find, appreciate, and use.

From the list above, the first two areas of focus are ethical and professional responsibilities, expected of all health care providers. The last two may interest some therapists more than others. Each area is discussed in this chapter, with suggestions and resources for implementing it.

Making Accurate Claims about Massage

There are many building blocks of evidence-based medicine, and the massage profession is beginning to adopt them. Several key concepts in medical research are explained below, with applications to massage therapy:

- Research reviews
- Randomized, controlled trials (RCTs)
- Sufficient sample sizes
- Levels of evidence

Even as the profession moves toward an evidence-based approach, many unsubstantiated claims are being made about massage therapy. In fact, some of the most often-repeated claims about massage have the least research support. Table 6-1 lists three of the most common claims about massage, along with the status of research at the time of this writing. The claim about massage and circulation is the most deeply rooted of the three, but, in fact, the evidence to support it has not yet arrived.

Unfortunately, these claims about circulation, endorphins, and the immune system have been made for so long that they are deeply ingrained in massage promotion, practice, and instruction. Therapists have repeated them innocently enough, without knowing the gaps in the evidence. But it's better for the profession to recognize its lore, and drop it from the many lists of massage benefits. If solid, convincing research emerges one day in support of these claims, they may be reinstated. Until then, they verge on false claims about massage therapy. More humble and accurate claims, based on clinical observations and the intent of massage, also appear in Table 6-1.

Using Research Accurately

Massage trade journals, promotional materials, and massage training curricula have made strong statements of weak research, using it to "prove" the claim of massage benefits. Yet, undeniable proof is not a common thing, even in medical science. Even when research makes a statement, it is not always definitive; a single study does not prove a point. Instead, a study needs to be around for a while, reviewed by other experts in the field, and considered alongside other evidence from other investigators in order for firm conclusions to be drawn. In medicine, a number of studies from different researchers are typically necessary in order to say that there is clear cause and effect between a therapy and a therapeutic outcome.

By simply avoiding the word proof, and using more moderate language, such as "research suggests," or "research supports," a therapist is already in more honest territory. In more clear-cut cases, discussed below, a therapist might even be able to say "Strong evidence for massage benefit is shown in the following research review: ___." In general, a dose of humility when making massage claims, or any claim, is well received in an evidence-based medical world.

● USE A BODY OF RESEARCH VERSUS A SINGLE STUDY

In fact, even the most well-designed study does not stand alone as convincing evidence of a therapeutic effect. Any one study, no matter how large or well constructed, could be vulnerable to the bias of the research group, or a mistake along the way that wasn't caught. It is better to look at the whole body of

work on a topic than a single study, and assess the pool of evidence. To review the evidence adequately is a daunting task, however, and one might have to look through many studies to determine which ones are strong enough to include in the assessment. Limitations on time, resources, and expertise make this impossible for most health professionals. Instead, they rely on research reviews by experts. There are two types of research reviews: the narrative review and the systematic review. Think of a review as "a study of the studies" on a topic.

The Narrative Review of Research

In a **narrative review**, researchers focus on a topic of interest and search the medical literature for relevant studies. They might decide to look at general massage effects, or the effects of massage on a given problem or population. They report on their findings: the number and strength of the studies, and the direction that the evidence seems to lean. They do not subject the studies to any statistical tests, as is done in the systematic review, but give their impressions of the available data. Done well, a narrative review is given more weight than any single study.

Although a narrative review is a broad synthesis of other studies, it is still subject to the bias of the reviewers, especially in the selection process. The reviewers' own preferences and relationships with other researchers may influence the studies that they select to include in the review. Still, narrative reviews can be valuable compilations of data on a topic, even though there is no formal statistical processing. On topics of

TABLE 6-1.	COMMON CLAIMS ABOUT MASSAGE
"Massage increases circulation."	
Status of the Evidence	As of this writing, only a handful of studies exist on massage and circulation, all are small, and the results are mixed. Older studies with less sophisticated measurements suggest that massage increases blood and lymph circulation. The information from more recent studies, using ultrasonography and other measurement techniques to measure circulation, is inconclusive.
References	Weerapong et al. (2005); Mori et al. (2004); Hinds et al. (2004); Taniwaki et al. (2004); Morhenn (2000); Agarwal et al. (2000); Shoemaker et al. (1997); Tiidus and Shoemaker (1995)
More Accurate Claim	It's too early to say whether massage increases circulation at the site of massage, or increases systemic circulation—the evidence is unclear. In clinical practice, we observe temperature and color changes at the site of massage that may be attributable to a change in circulation.
Massage Intent	When appropriate, we work with the intent to increase circulation.
"Massage releases endorphins."	
Status of the Evidence	As of this writing, only two small studies, published 20 years ago, have looked closely at massage and endorphins. One found no change in endorphins using Swedish techniques. The other suggested some change associated with a specialized form of connective tissue massage, not with common techniques.
References	Kaada and Torsteinbo (1989); Day et al. (1987)
More Accurate Claim	There is insufficient evidence to answer this question—we don't know whether massage acts directly on endorphins. In clinical practice, our clients commonly report pain relief during and after massage. Whether endorphins are responsible for this has yet to be seen. The body of research on massage for pain, stress, and quality of life is growing, though, and it will be interesting to see what is found.
Massage Intent	We practice with the intent to relieve pain and increase well-being.
"Massage boosts the immune system."	
Status of the Evidence	As of this writing, only a handful of small studies report this claim, and the body of evidence does not conclude that massage enhances the immune response.
References	Hiller et al. (2010); Billhult et al. (2008); Hernandez-Reif (2005); Hernandez-Reif (2004); Shor-Posner et al. (2004); Diego et al. (2001); Goodfellow (2003); Field et al. (2001)
More Accurate Claim	We don't have enough research to know how massage affects immunity. In clinical practice, our clients report stress relief and increased well-being. It is possible that these factors influence immunity.
Massage Intent	We practice with the intent of reducing our clients' stress and supporting their well-being.

great interest, there may even be multiple reviews by multiple authors. One example of this is massage for people with cancer, with reviews by Corbin (2005), Myers et al. (2008), and Weiger et al. (2002) (see online bibliography at http://thePoint. lww.com/Walton). Narrative reviews provide important compilations of data on a topic, even though there is no statistical processing.

The Systematic (Quantitative) Review of Research

In evidenced-based practice, a systematic review is given the highest ranking (see "Levels of Evidence," this chapter). It is given more weight than a narrative review, because it includes statistical processing of available studies. It pools the data from multiple studies that meet specific standards.

In a **systematic review**, the gold standard in research, reviewers use quantitative methods to determine whether a therapy is effective. They begin by searching the literature

on a topic, mining it for suitable studies that meet explicit, rigorous selection criteria. As part of the process, the reviewers make note of the studies that are most vulnerable to bias. Their selection methods are transparent and open to scrutiny because they are published in the review. If the studies generated by a systematic review are comparable enough, the reviewers can use established statistical methods known as **meta-analysis**, or *meta-analytic methods* to treat the collection of different studies as one large study and determine whether an intervention convincingly produces a given outcome. Assuming this is done according to protocol, with a minimum of bias, the information it generates is extremely useful. Using meta-analytic methods, the systematic review has the advantage of assembling larger numbers than is possible with small studies.

The systematic review is a powerful tool for answering research questions, and in establishing results that can be generalized to large numbers of people. After going through the review process, authors typically return one of three conclusions:

1. That the therapy appears to be effective enough to warrant current practice or wider use.
2. That the therapy does not appear to be effective enough to warrant current practice or wider use.
3. That the number or strength of the available studies is too small to determine the effectiveness of the therapy, and it is too early to say for sure, in either direction.

Systematic reviews often include suggested directions for further research, which can help guide researchers in the area.

In health and medicine, the most widely recognized source of systematic reviews is the Cochrane Collaboration, which maintains a searchable database on the Internet. A **Cochrane Review** is a systematic review on a topic in medicine, including massage therapy and other CAM therapies. The reviews performed by the Cochrane Collaboration fit well-established protocols, and are therefore a reliable source of information for this level of evidence. Cochrane reviews are updated periodically, and it is possible to simply view the abstract and a plain language summary or the full text of the review. Cochrane reviews have been performed on topics such as:

- Massage and HIV/AIDS (Hiller et al., 2010)
- Massage and touch for people with dementia (Hansen et al., 2006)
- Effect of massage on preterm infants (Vickers et al., 2004)
- Deep transverse friction massage for tendinitis treatment (Brosseau et al., 2002)
- Effect of massage on low back pain (Furlan et al., 2008)
- Massage for infants (Underdown et al., 2006)
- Massage for mechanical neck disorders (Haraldsson et al, 2006)

Although the Cochrane reviews are known sources, other journals also publish reviews. There are systematic reviews on massage therapy (Moyer et al., 2004), and a great deal of recent attention to massage and cancer (Ernst, 2009; Jane et al., 2008; Wilkinson et al., 2008).

● THE RANDOMIZED, CONTROLLED TRIAL

In clinical research, the prevailing standard in research design is the **RCT**, or the *randomized, controlled clinical trial*

(RCCT). The steps of an RCT are shown in Figure 6-1. There are several key features of an RCT:

- It is a prospective study, planned ahead.
- There is a control group or control condition, used for comparison, that does not receive the active treatment being tested.
- Research subjects are randomly assigned to either the control group or the active treatment group.

Prospective Study

A clinical trial, by definition, requires planning. An RCT is prospective: it looks forward, not back. Researchers plan to study future behavior, not past behavior (as in a *retrospective study*). In the case of a massage study, investigators plan a massage intervention to see how it will affect the sample. This is different from, say, a study that examines a group of people who have well-managed symptoms of a chronic disease, and interviews them about whether they've used massage therapy in the past 6 months.

Control Group or Control Condition

Another essential component of a controlled trial is a control group or control condition. In clinical research on massage, medication, or any other therapy, a **control group** is a group of people who does not receive the therapy being tested. The same outcomes are measured in the control group to provide a comparison for the effects of the treatment (see Figure 6-1). Suppose 100 people receive back massage and their pain is relieved over the course of the study. How can one tell whether most of them would have gotten better anyway, without the massage? Without a comparison, the evidence for massage providing back pain relief would not be very strong. In fact, most of the time, back pain tends to improve on its own.

If this same study were done in a controlled fashion, some of the subjects would receive massage, and some would not. The massaged group is called the **active treatment** group or *experimental group*, the group of subjects that receives the treatment being tested. By comparing them to the control (non-massage) group, one can get a sense of whether they would have gotten better even without the massage.

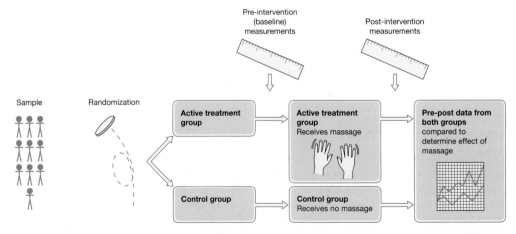

FIGURE 6-1. A RCT of massage therapy. Research subjects are randomly assigned to the massage or control group, using the electronic equivalent of the flip of a coin. Measurements are collected from both groups at baseline and after the intervention, and data from both groups are compared to determine any effect of massage.

If researchers observe that both the control and the active treatment groups improve by about the same amount, it suggests that the massage had no effect. On the other hand, if the difference in the two results is significant, then the improvement in pain is probably a true effect of massage.

A **control condition** is a research condition experienced by participants in a control group, to provide a comparison to the active treatment being tested. During the control condition, often subjects receive only **usual care (UC)**, also called *standard care (SC)*, the typical medical care for their condition. In a medical setting, UC includes all the normal ways in which patients are treated, with medications, procedures, and so on.

In some massage studies, control groups get another kind of treatment, such as imagery aimed at relaxing muscles. To be sure that massage effects aren't just a function of a caring interaction or the good nature of a massage practitioner, researchers might make the control condition a visit, with no touch (Post-White et al., 2004; Smith et al., 2002). If a visit turns out to be just as productive as a massage, a friendly volunteer might be capable of achieving the same positive results as a trained massage therapist.

Another investigator might ask whether the movement in most massage strokes is important, and compare non-moving touch with moving touch (Kutner et al., 2008). Yet another researcher might compare less skilled touch, for example, from massage students, nurses, or lay people, to touch from professional massage therapists, to see if the training makes a difference in the outcome. As the profession advances, more research will appear comparing different types of massage protocols for a given problem, helping to determine the best practice, and the massage elements that are most important in a therapeutic outcome.

Researchers incorporate control conditions differently, and different types of control conditions are possible. Some of these possibilities are:

- Parallel design
- Crossover design
- Wait-list control
- Attention control
- Sham control (or placebo)

PARALLEL DESIGN

One of the most common RCT designs is a **parallel design**. In this case, the research subjects in the control condition and others in the active treatment go through their respective conditions and measurements in parallel (see Figure 6-1). They are usually assessed at the beginning to obtain baseline measurements of the outcomes of interest. In a parallel design, because the control group does not receive the active treatment, research subjects from that group may be more likely to drop out of the study, leading to a loss of data.

CROSSOVER DESIGN

In a **crossover design**, all the participants in the study have the same experience, receiving the full active treatment as well as the control condition, and cross over from one condition to the other at some point. In a crossover design, shown in Figure 6-2, each study subject serves as his or her own control, and data are collected for both conditions. In this case, the subjects may be randomized, but only to determine the *order* in which they receive massage therapy and the control condition. For those receiving the massage intervention first, there may be a "holding period" before their control data are collected, so that the effects of the massage don't carry over into the control period. Crossover designs have many advantages, in that the control and active treatment groups are the same people, and each person generates two sets of data. A crossover design also satisfies any ethical concern over one group being denied treatment.

In a crossover study of foot massage in a hospital (Grealish et al., 2000), inpatients were assessed on three different evening occasions: on two evenings, they received a 10-minute foot massage and were measured before and afterward. On a third night, they received no massage intervention, but had quiet time for the same time period and were measured before and after the quiet time. These patients "crossed over" from one condition to the other. Figure 6-2 shows a crossover design; compare it to the parallel design in Figure 6-1.

WAIT-LIST CONTROL

In a **wait-list control** design, everyone in the study receives some form of active treatment, but one group, the control group, has to wait until the end of the study to receive it. It starts as a parallel design, with an active treatment group and a control group, and any baseline measurements.

After they complete their measurements, those in the control group receive some form of active treatment. This could be a lesser intervention, such as only a single massage in a study where active treatment subjects received a several-week course of massage therapy (Figure 6-3). On the other hand, some researchers add the wait-list control subjects to the active treatment group at that point, and they receive the full dose, with the usual data collection. This yields an active treatment group that is larger than the control, but it generates more data. In either case, the wait-list control is an appealing design, because it provides a kind of "consolation prize," or incentive for the control subjects to complete the study. Data collection can suffer when control subjects, dissatisfied with their group assignment, drop out of the study.

ATTENTION CONTROL

In an **attention control**, researchers attempt to answer the question, "How much of massage therapy benefit comes from the skilled touch, and how much of it is due to the attention that the therapist gives the client?" In an attention control, the group receives some other form of attention, such as the friendly visit, described above, being read to, or otherwise being given attention. This can also reduce the loss of data due to subjects dropping out of the study.

THE PLACEBO EFFECT AND THE SHAM CONTROL

Choosing the right control condition takes some thought on the part of a researcher. By far one of the most difficult controls to provide in massage research is a placebo. A **placebo** gives the suggestion of an active treatment; it is a substance (such as a sugar pill) or procedure that is designed to resemble the active treatment, but has no known therapeutic effect. The **placebo effect** is a positive effect attributed to a participant's expectation that she or he will be helped—that is, from simply believing in the potential for improvement.

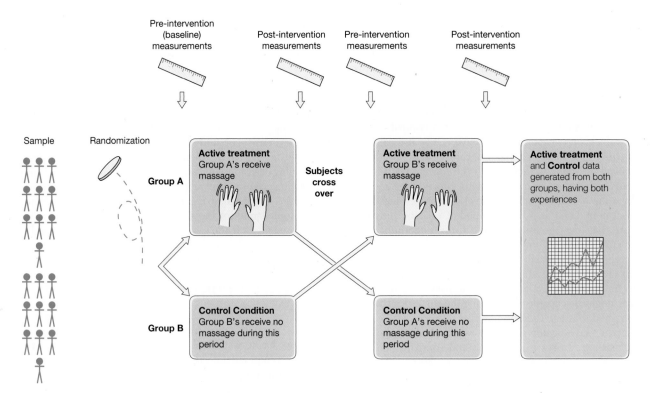

FIGURE 6-2. A crossover design in a massage therapy RCT. In contrast to a parallel design, research subjects in a crossover design experience both the control and massage condition, but in different sequences. The order is determined at random. After a subject experiences the first condition, measurements are collected and the subject proceeds to the second condition. Measurements are repeated for the second condition. When crossing over, subjects may have to wait a minimum "washout period" for the effects of the previous condition to wear off.

The placebo effect, or *nonspecific effect*, is not a specific response to the active treatment. In order to isolate the placebo effect, researchers often use a **sham control** or *sham condition*. The sham control is a substance or procedure that may be similar to the active treatment, but missing a key feature of the active treatment. In a sham acupuncture session, needles are placed, but not at the therapeutic points. A sham is designed to lead the subject into thinking he or she is receiving something valuable. This is difficult to do in massage therapy. How do you make a person think he or she is being massaged, when he or she's not? There is no obvious sugar pill here.

Some massage modalities are more conducive to sham procedures than others. Modalities with highly choreographed protocols, such as reflexology, acupressure, and manual lymph drainage, can be tested against a sham protocol that violates the correct sequence or placement. Specialized protocols are mysterious to most clients, so they can't tell the difference between an actual therapy and a placebo. On the other hand, with Swedish massage, more familiar to recipients and more variable in protocol, it's harder to "fool" the client.

Random Assignment of Study Subjects

Another key element of the RCT is randomization. This refers to the assignment of study subjects to their groups. Group assignment is random, that is, generated by the electronic equivalent of a flip of a coin. Neither the subject nor the researcher has a choice about which group the subject is assigned to. If entering a crossover study, each subject goes through all the interventions, but the *order* of the interventions is random. In the three-night foot massage study, discussed

previously, some patients crossed over twice, from foot massage to quiet time to foot massage. The sequence of the single control and two experimental evenings was determined by a random process so that different patients received the interventions in different sequences.

Randomization also helps produce control and experimental groups that are comparable at the outset, by mixing in any elements in the sample and distributing them evenly between groups. For example, suppose a number of unusually relaxed people enroll in a massage study, in which the experimental treatment is a weekly massage over 4 weeks.

Because researchers hope for equivalent groups, they would want these unusually relaxed subjects to be evenly distributed over the two groups so that they don't confound, or muddy the results. A **confounding variable** accentuates or obscures the apparent size of a treatment effect. It makes it hard to determine clear cause and effect. In this example, the relaxed subjects might have especially favorable responses to massage, because they are already relaxed, and are open to massage and its positive effects. Or they might have unfavorable responses to massage, because they are already so relaxed that massage cannot relax them much further. If too many of these subjects are assigned to one group or another, they might artificially enhance or diminish the apparent effect of massage, and randomization removes their choice in the matter.

It is impossible to completely keep a sample perfectly "clean," the groups perfectly balanced, or a study free of confounding variables, but their influence can be minimized as much as possible. Randomization can help limit this problem.

Randomization is also a vital feature in reducing bias in a study. **Bias** is any type of influence in a study that leads to error

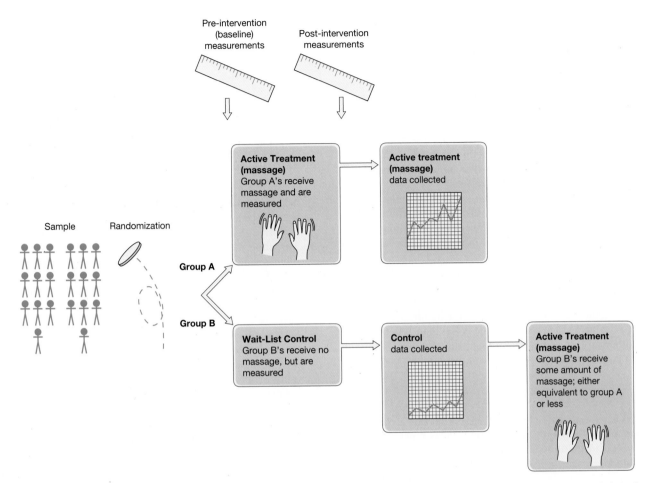

FIGURE 6-3. A wait-list control design in a massage RCT. After control subjects have completed the control condition and their data have been collected, they are given the active treatment.

by favoring one outcome over another. Bias can come from the investigators and the participants. By randomizing, neither the investigator nor the research subject can decide which group the subject is assigned to—the control or active treatment group. If research subjects were given a choice and the treatment was promising, and not uncomfortable, most people would choose to be in the active treatment group. In fact, many people enroll in a study with that hope. Their expectations could skew the results in favor of the treatment. Knowing a research subject's bias, an investigator might be tempted to enroll them in the active treatment, to contribute to favorable results. Instead, randomization distributes that bias across both groups.

Blinding

Another way of reducing bias is by **blinding**, or concealing the group assignments of the research subjects from the investigators or from the research subjects, or both. In **single-blind** studies, the subjects themselves are blinded. Their lack of knowledge about the treatment they are receiving (or not) may diminish the placebo effect, because neither group knows whether they are receiving the active treatment. This can, in kind, limit the influence of their personal bias on the outcome. This is easy to implement when there is an obvious placebo such as a sugar pill, because the pill looks like an active treatment. As discussed earlier, it is more difficult to achieve this in a massage study.

In a **double-blind** design, both researchers and participants are in the dark about group assignment. It can be difficult to

blind everyone on a study staff: a massage therapist providing the treatment knows whether or not she is providing massage. So researchers blind whomever they can blind. For example, the data collector, who takes measurements after the session, can enter the room with the study subject and take measurements without knowing whether a massage or control condition took place. If the participant doesn't reveal the intervention she just had, then observer bias can be reduced. Ideally, researchers describe the blinding process in the published research paper.

● SAMPLE SIZE

The number of people enrolled in a study, whether small or large, is called the sample size, expressed as the letter n. Many studies in massage therapy are too small to be convincing. If a sample size is too small, it increases the chance of the sample being atypical in some way, not truly reflecting the population of interest. For example, suppose a researcher chooses a sample size of 10 for a study on massage and symptom relief in multiple sclerosis (MS). With such a small sample, there is a chance that seven or eight of those would be unusual in some way—they might be under remarkable stress, or exceptionally averse to massage, or have other factors that make their MS symptoms hard to relieve. This would leave only two or three "average" subjects with MS. Any one of these factors might diminish the influence of massage in this sample of 10, where a larger, less skewed sample could demonstrate the true effect of massage. On the other hand, other factors might artificially amplify the apparent effects of massage. And the small sample size, less likely to reflect the average MS patient, makes it difficult to generalize the results, to the larger population of patients.

Studies with larger numbers are less vulnerable to these influences, and it is easier to generalize from them. They are also more expensive to carry out, and less common than small studies. In any field, research begins with small studies and grows, over the years, to larger ones. In fact, many of the studies in massage are pilot studies. A **pilot study** is a small, exploratory study designed to begin answering a simple research question, scout the territory, determine whether research in the area is feasible, provide direction for further inquiry, and gain funding for larger, more substantial studies.

Many of the studies in massage therapy are pilot studies. Even if they suggest robust massage benefits, the numbers are not usually large enough to draw firm conclusions. At the same time, small studies are vital in supporting further study and gaining visibility for massage.

There is no magic number that designates a credible study. Researchers consider many factors, including the expected effect of massage, when determining an appropriate sample size. In general, research with several hundred subjects is more convincing than a sample that is less than 100. But there are other aspects of research design that are also important, and a large sample size does not compensate for poor design.

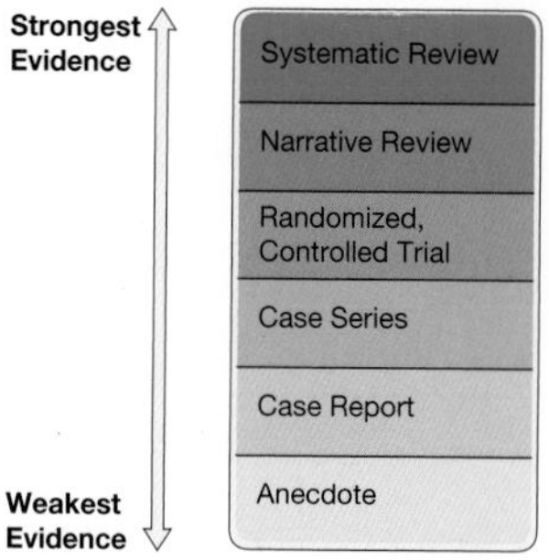

● LEVELS OF EVIDENCE

In evidence-based practice, evidence is ranked according to a hierarchy of strength and credibility. This ranking is called the **levels of evidence**. The systematic review is at the top of the hierarchy, shown in Figure 6-4. There are many levels of evidence. The main ones, from weakest to strongest, are listed below with a massage therapy example:

1. *Anecdote.* A single, informal story from clinical practice, such as a client whose headache is relieved after a massage session, or a series of sessions. This evidence is the weakest in strength, at the bottom of the hierarchy.
2. *Case report.* A formal account, written by a practitioner, of a single client's background, presentation, treatment, and outcomes. A case report might tell the story of a client whose chronic headaches reduced in frequency and severity after a course of massage sessions.
3. *Case series.* A formal write-up of several case studies, typically with similarities in presentation and treatment, that helps highlight similarities and differences among the cases. Several clients with chronic headaches, the therapist's treatment approach, and outcomes would be discussed in a case series on headaches.
4. *RCT (see description, this chapter).* Massage treatments are tested on a group of study subjects with chronic head-

FIGURE 6-4. Levels of evidence.

aches, and data are collected with symptom questionnaires. Randomization produces two groups: a massage group and a control group, receiving UC for headaches.
5. *Narrative review (see description, this chapter).* A researcher reviews the literature on massage and headaches and publishes his or her impressions of themes that emerge in the studies, the strength of the research designs, and the direction that the evidence seems to be leaning. No quantitative methods are used.
6. *Systematic review (see description, this chapter).* A researcher collects studies on massage and headaches using predetermined screening criteria. The evidence is analyzed using strict statistical methods (meta-analysis), and the strength of the studies and the direction of evidence are used to formulate a conclusion about massage and headaches. This type of evidence is considered the strongest.

The first three levels of evidence are observational, and can be gathered from a therapist's notes on her own clinical practice. The second three levels are analytical and quantitative. These projects are more calculated and planned, involving a lot of additional thought and expertise.

Even though the first three levels of evidence—anecdote, case report, and case series—are clinical observations, they can include formal measurement of outcomes. Therapists typically ask their clients about responses to treatment and can document these responses using various scales and symptom checklists in the literature (see "Visual Analogue Scale," this chapter). Such measurement tools help therapists notice trends or patterns in their practices and keep track of how clients are doing.

The levels of evidence provide a visual reminder that a single RCT does not necessarily prove something. Even though much of the massage research is in RCT form, the RCT has to be well designed and implemented to be taken seriously. And it takes a number of good RCTs, pooled in a systematic review, to make firm statements about a therapy's effectiveness. Of all of the levels of evidence, the most persuasive conclusion comes from a systematic review.

Tracking Massage Research

Most massage therapists have an interest in a special population of clients, or in certain clinical problems and successes. By checking the research literature on those topics, a therapist may find shared interest, inspiration, and support for her work. To check for systematic reviews and studies, scout established databases on the Internet. Usually, searching for "massage therapy" and a topic of interest yields a number of results. Each of the databases, below, is a unique research resource:

- *PubMed.* This searchable index of medical research is provided by the U.S. National Library of Medicine at the National Institutes of Health. It is possible to retrieve research articles as recent as the current month. Type in "massage therapy" and a topic of interest, such as dementia or arthritis.
- *The Massage Therapy Foundation.* This nonprofit organization provides a database of research articles that are not all indexed on PubMed, as well as other resources on

massage research, education, and community service. The foundation publishes, online, the open-access *International Journal of Therapeutic Massage and Bodywork*, which includes research as well as articles on clinical practice and massage education.

- *The Cochrane Collaboration*. Full text systematic reviews are available for purchase, and summaries in plain language are free.
- *The NIH RePORT (Research Portfolio Online Reporting Tools)*. The RePORTER database is an index of active research projects in the United States, funded by the National Institutes of Health. Unlike the other databases of published research, this resource catalogues research projects that are still in progress. Typing in "massage therapy" and a topic of interest yield listings of projects, names of investigators, locations, and short summaries of the research in process.
- *Clinicaltrials.gov*. This registry includes active clinical trials in the United States and at least 170 other countries. It serves as a clearinghouse for publicly and privately funded projects.

Although finding research citations is relatively easy using the Internet, retrieving the full text articles can be trickier. A portion of papers are available for free on the Internet, but many require more digging: paying for document retrieval services, using a medical library, or asking a health care provider to pull the paper from a hospital or clinic library. Some people write to the first author listed on a paper to request a reprint.

While not all massage therapists will actively participate in research, it is important to acknowledge the research available in the literature. One way to think about research is as a consumer. Any taxpayer is a consumer of research, because some tax revenue goes to government-funded medical research. As recognition of complementary and alternative medicine (CAM) therapies grows, more funding goes to CAM research, and taxpayers can evaluate publicly tended studies. Although many people think evaluating research is the domain of scholars and funding organizations, massage professionals can do it, too. Several excellent books are available to help massage therapists use and design research (Travillian, 2011; Menard, 2009; Hymel, 2006; Field, 2006). Research literacy is frequently discussed in professional journals.

Approaching Clinical Work as a Form of Research

In various ways, active massage therapists are already performing research themselves. They are already learning from their clients. Therapists study their clients' responses to massage, and try to determine the treatment that will optimize the outcome. With a curious mindset and a few simple, standardized measurement tools, a massage therapist can enhance this learning process.

● USING COMMON MEASUREMENT TOOLS

Easy-to-use checklists and scales, common to research and practice, can be used before and after a session to get a sense of how the client is responding to massage therapy. These are called **pre-post measurements**, and they can also be used periodically over a course of treatment. Pre-post measurements, also called *before and after* measurements, enhance the therapist's documentation, and focus the therapist's attention on what is and isn't working.

The Visual Analogue Scale

A visual analogue scale (VAS) is a numerical scale that provides a system for a client's self-report of symptoms. They come in various formats, but a VAS is usually a simple line, 10 cm long, with only the endpoints labeled as anchors: 0 and 10 (Figure 6-5). The endpoints are also labeled with a symptom or experience, such as pain, anxiety, relaxation, or fatigue. The respondent draws a hatch mark on the line that indicates how her symptom is at the moment. Later, the researcher measures the line with a ruler to see where the hatch mark appears, and the number is likely to be returned as a decimal, such as "7.1" or "5.3" In clinical practice, the VAS is easier to use with pre-labeled hatch marks added at numbers 1, 2, 3, and so on (see Figure 4-2).

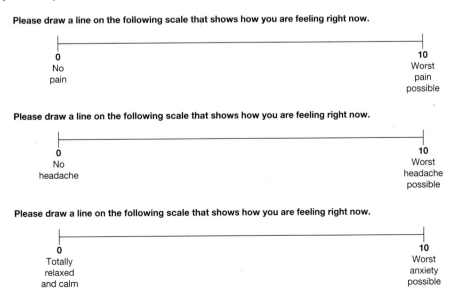

FIGURE 6-5. Samples of the VAS. Many symptoms and internal experiences can be described in a VAS.

The Verbal Rating Scale

The **verbal rating scale (VRS)** is a verbal version of the VAS, another way to self-report symptoms or internal experiences. A VRS takes less time than a VAS, because it is a natural part of conversation before and after a massage, and it does not require pen and paper to complete.

Here is an example: On a scale of 0–10, with 0 being no pain and 10 being the worst pain possible, how do you rate your pain in this moment?

Here is one on relaxation and anxiety: On a scale of 0–10, with 0 being totally calm and relaxed and 10 being the worst anxiety possible, how do you feel right now?

Often the response to a VRS is a whole or half-number, such as 4 or 7½. Other fractions or decimals are unlikely. Research on VASs and VRSs suggests that similar data are generated from the two formats (Cork et al., 2004).

VASs and VRSs are quick and convenient to use for symptoms such as pain, fatigue, nausea, depression, alertness, or any internal experience.

Other Measurement Tools

In addition to VASs and VRSs, a massage therapist can find measurement tools for just about any symptom or experience. On the Internet, by using search terms such as "clinical research," "checklist" or "questionnaire," "symptom," and a topic of interest, a therapist can locate symptom checklists, and common scales for many symptoms. Standardized tools are available for parameters such as daily function, anxiety, and even spiritual quality of life. By looking around at massage research, a therapist can find measurement tools for his or her clinical interests.

● REMAINING OPEN TO FINDINGS

One of the most important traits in a researcher is the ability to be open to different outcomes. This is true in clinical practice, too. Even the most results-oriented therapist recognizes that it is possible to become too narrow in focus, or too carried away with outcomes. Many wonderful things happen in massage when you are not trying too hard. By using an approach that is too goal oriented, a therapist may miss other important information.

Regular questions about symptoms and scales may appeal to many clients, but can put off others who prefer massage as a retreat, rather than another goal-oriented experience. For some people, answering questions or rating symptoms can be stressful; a sensitive therapist can determine who might want to evaluate her own experience, and who needs a break from it. During some of the most profound human experiences of illness, injury, and other life crises, many people would rather be ministered to instead of questioned and fixed. By reading a client's cues, a therapist can be of service in multiple ways.

● DOCUMENTING AND SHARING CLINICAL WORK

Therapists who document these things closely, using SOAP notes or some other consistent format, can learn much from their practice. When interesting things emerge in the practice, therapists should write them down! Even a small amount of feedback, such as the following, may evolve into a whole system or care plan:

> I worked certain muscles at their attachments to the occiput, and focused especially on the sternocleidomastoid (SCM) attachments. I followed this with 10 minutes of massage to the shoulders and back. The client reports that her headache eased during the massage and went away within an hour after the session. The client has been headache-free for 2 weeks.

Enough careful observations such as these, along with supporting information, may also be shaped into a short article for a trade journal, thereby inviting dialogue from readers. A therapist can use the resources of the Massage Therapy Foundation to develop a case report from her observations. By attending professional conferences, then sharing case reports with other therapists, and inviting feedback, therapists can find support to further their clinical work.

Massage therapists hear many stories from their clients—compelling stories of symptoms, successes, athletic performance issues, and all of the challenges people face in their bodies as they go about their days. While the clinical work doesn't need to stop and wait for science, good documentation of clinical work will help contribute to the science of massage therapy.

How Research is Used in This Text

Every effort is made to include thoughtful massage claims and careful use of research throughout this book. There are several places to find these:

1. In Massage Research sections, in Parts II and III;
2. In Possible Massage Benefits sections, in Parts II and III;
3. In the discussion of massage and circulation (see "Increased Circulation," Chapter 2);
4. On Decision Trees, whenever "circulatory intent" is used instead of "circulatory massage," to reflect the stated purpose of massage rather than an evidence-based fact.

For each medical condition in this book, a brief summary of relevant massage research appears in the Massage Research section. If the relevant massage research is indexed in PubMed, the Massage Therapy Foundation database, or the NIH RePORTER database at the time of this writing, it appears in this section. If nothing appears in these databases, then

that is also noted in this section. Therapists are advised to recheck resources periodically, as more research may have been initiated or published since this text was completed. Also, there may be ongoing or soon-to-be-published research that is not indexed, so it is good to search regularly for a topic of interest.

If a few studies or reviews are published on a condition, they are referenced by last name and date. If there are too many studies on a condition to list, a few selected studies are referenced. The full research citations are in the online bibliography.

Under each full discussion of a medical condition, the Possible Massage Benefits section is devoted to the benefits of massage that may or may not have been established by research, or may never be studied in formal research. Instead, common sense and clinical experience tell us how we might help someone with a skin condition, a heart condition, HIV/AIDS, or MS.

These summaries of benefits also come from client testimonials or the author's clinical observations over the years. Often therapists know how helpful massage can be, simply because clients tell them, or because clients continue to come for massage. Few people need research to convince them that they need to schedule another session; their own experiences tell them so.

The Limitations of Research

Research evidence is highly valued in the medical world, and using established scientific methods to study massage continues to yield interesting and useful perspectives on massage therapy. Still, research cannot tell us everything about massage.

As compelling as research is, its focus on cause and effect reflects a Western thought process, and a linear approach to the search for truth. Not all human experiences lend themselves to this framework. Indeed, some experiences of massage—relief of pain, care, connection, nurturing, healing—are some of the deepest, most personal and multidimensional experiences possible. Some of the nuances of massage therapy might never be captured in massage research. Research has its place; but, by studying things too closely, it also has the potential to reduce an individual story to pieces that ignore the wholeness of the experience.

Telling Stories

Every practitioner has an anecdote to tell, even after only a few months in practice. Personal experience is powerful. Even if no research supports massage for a certain condition, a therapist may have a single story or a handful of stories to share from his or her practice. One therapist could tell about a client's chronic headaches improving, or someone else's back pain getting better. Another therapist might tell about increased mobility, or improved sleep. If the therapist carefully guards her clients' confidences, withholding any identifying information, she may share these stories, and people respond to them. When someone asks, "How can massage help me?" he or she might be more interested in a single account of massage therapy than a battery of studies.

At some point, research, a growing collection of stories, may tell us much more about massage than we already know. But as limited as our present evidence-based knowledge is, we do see massage at work in people's lives every day. After massage, many people are more at ease in themselves, and feel more clearly seen, heard, and known. The support of massage can be carried out the door, toward whatever challenges the client faces next. Quiet, unassuming massage can do wonders for people as they move their bodies through their lives. These are things that we know in our minds, but also in our hearts and hands.

SELF TEST

1. Describe four ways that research can support the massage profession.
2. Define best practice research. How can it influence the practice of massage?
3. List three common claims made about massage that are not supported by research. How can massage therapists more correctly summarize the state of knowledge about each of the claims?
4. What is the difference between a narrative review of research and a systematic review? Define each term. Which one is a higher level of evidence?
5. Where can a therapist find a database of published massage research in the medical literature? Which organization publishes systematic reviews of medical research? Where can a therapist locate research studies that are currently in progress?
6. Why is a control group important in clinical research on massage? Give an example.
7. What is the difference between a wait-list control, an attention control, and a crossover design?
8. Why can it be challenging to provide a sham control, or to blind the research subjects, in massage therapy research?
9. Suppose you have a question about whether and how a client's low back pain is responding to massage after several weekly sessions. Formulate the question to your client in VAS and VRS formats.
10. What is the difference between a case report and a case series? Where do they appear on the levels of evidence?

 For answers to these questions and to see a bibliography for this chapter, visit http://thePoint. lww.com/Walton.

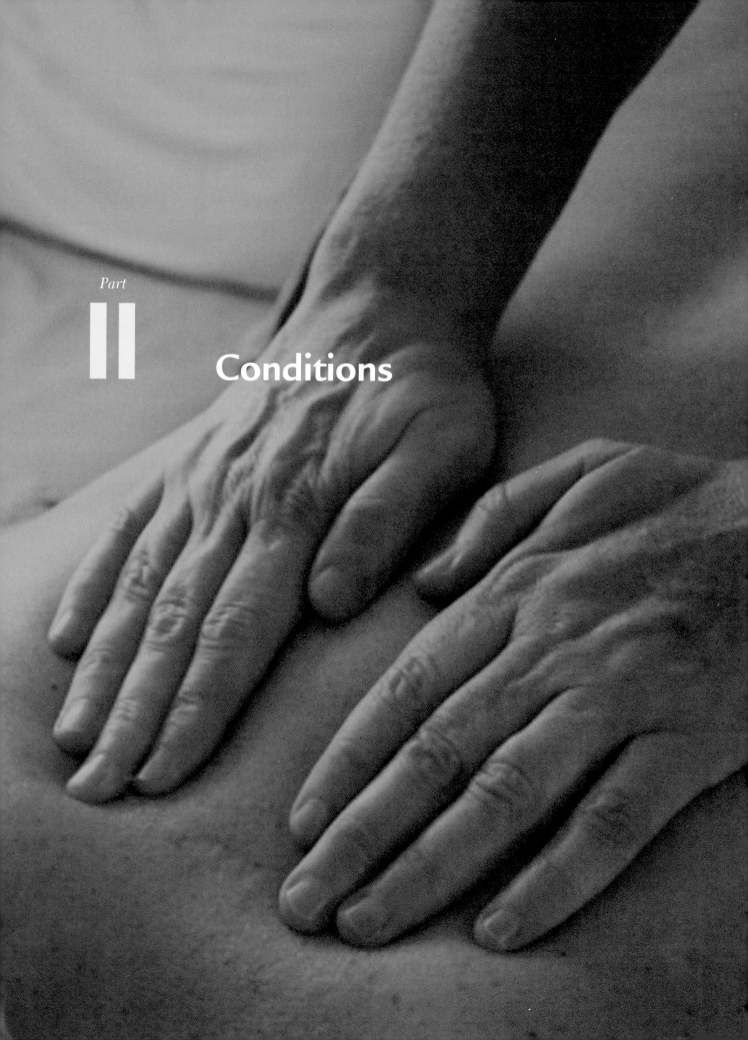

Part

II

Conditions

Depth must be hidden. Where? On the surface.

—HUGO VON HOFMANNSTHAL

Of all the systems of the body, perhaps the one that is most familiar to a massage therapist's hands is the integumentary system. The skin is the body's surface. It protects what lies beneath, cleanses the body, prevents water loss, and provides a barrier to infection. While working through the skin to the muscles and fascia beneath, therapists notice changes in client skin temperature, color, and texture over time.

This vital body system, which functions to help keep the rest of the body healthy, can itself be challenged—externally, by sources of infection, injury, and allergy, and internally, by hormonal and genetic factors. Therapists are responsible for considering the health of their own skin, as well as that of their clients, when making massage decisions.

The conditions introduced in this chapter represent a spectrum of common skin conditions, which include inflammation, infection, and breaks in the skin. Skin conditions often involve a specific type of **lesion**, a general term describing any change in tissue that makes it different from its normal state. Although a lesion can occur in any tissue, it is most visible on the skin, and is particularly apparent when it is open and the skin is no longer intact.

From such close, sustained contact with the skin, a massage therapist is often the first to notice a lesion on a client's skin that needs attention from a physician.

Such sustained skin contact can heighten a therapist's concern when infection is a possibility. Often, infection control practices can be borrowed from nursing and physical therapy, since nurses and PTs also touch the skin a great deal during patient care.

In this chapter, four conditions are discussed at length. The conditions are:

- Psoriasis
- Acne
- Oral and genital herpes (herpes simplex 1 and 2)
- Scabies

In addition, a full discussion of **eczema** (atopic dermatitis, or AD), including a Decision Tree, may be found online at http://thePoint.lww.com/Walton.

Conditions in Brief addressed in this chapter are: **Acne rosacea**, **athlete's foot** (tinea pedis), **basal cell carcinoma**, **boils**, **cellulitis**, cuts and **abrasions**, **folliculitis**, **hives** (urticaria), **impetigo**, **jock itch** (tinea cruris), **lipoma**, **lice** (pediculosis), **melanoma** (malignant melanoma), **methicillin-resistant** *Staphylococcus aureus* (MRSA), **moles**, **nail fungus** (tinea unguium), **poison ivy/oak/sumac**, **pressure sores** (decubitus ulcers), **ringworm** (tinea corporis), **shingles** (herpes zoster), **skin tags**, **squamous cell carcinoma**, **sunburn**, and **warts** (verrucae vulgaris).

General Principles

Skin lesions can come from many conditions, and several principles can be applied from Chapter 3: the Inflammation Principle, the Ask the Cause Principle, and the Waiting for a Diagnosis Principle. Along with these principles, three new principles are introduced:

1. The Body Fluid Principle. *If it's wet and it's not yours, don't touch it.* Borrowed from emergency medicine, this serves as a reminder that body fluids can transmit infection from person to person, even when there are no symptoms of infection. This is particularly relevant to fluid from open lesions on the skin.
2. The Open Lesion Principle. *Do not make contact with an open lesion.* This is not only an extension of the Body Fluid Principle, designed to protect the therapist from infection, it also protects the client from microorganisms entering the open skin. Regardless of the cause of the lesion, avoid making skin-to-skin contact. Also avoid touching an open lesion

with a gloved hand or massage lubricant. Open lesions, regardless of the cause, are vulnerable to dirt and **normal flora** (bacteria and other resident microorganisms on the skin) that can be introduced by direct contact. Therapists must be careful to minimize the transmission of known and undiagnosed infections.

3. The Ask If It's Contagious Principle. *Before making contact with a client's body, find out whether a skin lesion is contagious and how it is spread.* Some contagious conditions, caused by viruses, fungi, bacteria, or parasites, could be passed to the therapist by contact. If it is inflamed, painful, or itchy, there is an additional red flag. Other conditions, such as poison ivy, are not caused by microorganisms, but any plant oil remaining on the skin could be transmitted elsewhere on the client, or to the therapist, causing a rash (see "Follow-Up Questions About Infection," Chapter 4).

Psoriasis

In **psoriasis**, the cycle of skin cell growth is accelerated—from the normal time frame of 28–30 days to just 3–4 days. As a result, layers of skin cells in various stages of growth "pile up," giving the skin a thickened appearance.

● BACKGROUND

Psoriasis seems to be caused by a problem in the immune system involving overactive cells, inflammation, and the rapid formation of new skin cells. The most common type of psoriasis is *plaque psoriasis* (80% of cases). It often occurs in cycles: periods of flare-ups and remission. The flare-ups are triggered by stress, hormonal changes, injury to the skin, some prescription drugs, and a compromised immune system.

Signs and Symptoms

As shown in Figure 7-1, psoriasis can look like a dramatic, distinct, scaly rash. It is raised, with silver and red scales. Psoriasis tends to appear on the elbows, knees, scalp, and trunk, but it can develop anywhere. It may be accompanied by pain, itching, or cracking of the skin.

Complications

Plaque psoriasis has fewer complications than rarer forms. Rarer forms, such as *guttate, pustular, inverse,* or *erythrodermic psoriasis* are characterized by serious lesions and a more complex clinical picture. Other complications may be present, such as open and weeping lesions, inflammation, and fever.

Psoriatic arthritis develops in about 25% of cases, usually well after the skin lesions have appeared. This form of arthritis causes swelling, pain, and stiffness, usually in hands, knees, and feet, sometimes the spine. Fingers and toes can be so swollen that they have a "sausage-like" appearance. Psoriatic arthritis can be extremely painful. It can also appear without any corresponding skin lesions.

Treatment

Treatment depends on the type of psoriasis. Treatments typically interrupt the accelerated cycle of growth and the pile-up of skin cells, reducing inflammation. **First line therapy** refers to the initial treatment approach for a condition; if the treatment fails or stops working, subsequent treatments are called **second line therapy**, and so on. For psoriasis, first line therapy is **topical** creams, applied to the skin surface at the site. Ultraviolet light therapy is also used. Psoriasis is treated with anti-inflammatories, topical corticosteroids (see chapter 21), and, in some cases, a variety of stronger oral or injected medications with varying side effects. Often, treatments are rotated, in which an oral treatment will be used for a number of months, then stopped while a topical treatment is used. This can give the individual's body a break from some of the side effects of stronger oral medications.

Topical preparations are administered as a single type of medication or a combination of medications. Most of these have minimal side effects except for skin irritation. These include: coal tar, salicylic acid, anthralin, calcipotriene (a synthetic vitamin D_3), retinoid, and steroid medication.

Systemic medications may be used along with topical preparations. A **systemic medication** is any drug that affects the whole body, by being distributed through the bloodstream. There are several ways to administer a drug systemically, but the typical routes are oral, by injection into the muscle or skin, or by introducing it directly into a vein through an **intravenous (IV)** line. Systemic drugs for psoriasis include retinoids (such as Soriatane), cyclosporine (Neoral), methotrexate, and **biologic therapy**, also called *immunotherapy*. Biologic therapy acts on the immune system to turn down the inflammatory mechanisms that cause psoriasis.

Most systemic drugs for psoriasis act on the immune system in some way; in higher doses, cyclosporine is used to prevent tissue rejection, and methotrexate and biologic therapies are used in the treatment of cancer and other conditions. Although they are monitored closely, these drugs come with numerous possible side effects and complications, and individuals are monitored closely for toxic effects, which can include kidney damage, liver damage, and elevated blood pressure. Biologics can cause mild flu-like symptoms and respiratory infection.

● INTERVIEW QUESTIONS

1. What kind of psoriasis is it?
2. Where is it?
3. Does it itch or hurt?
4. Do you want some kind of massage or contact over the area?
5. How does the area respond to contact, pressure, or friction?
6. How does the area respond to lubricant? Do you have a preferred lubricant that you use there?
7. Does the skin in the area tend to crack?
8. Is there any arthritis associated with the psoriasis?
9. How is your psoriasis or psoriatic arthritis treated?
10. Are there any side effects or reactions to treatment? Tell me whether your treatment affects your skin, kidney function, or liver function.

● MASSAGE THERAPY GUIDELINES

Plaque psoriasis is the most common form that the therapist will encounter in practice. If a client is unsure how to respond to question 1, ask if their doctor said that it is a common

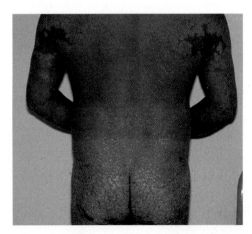

FIGURE 7-1. Psoriasis. (From Goodheart HP. *Goodheart's Photoguide to Common Skin Disorders,* 2nd ed. Philadelphia: Lippincott Williams and Wilkins, 2003.)

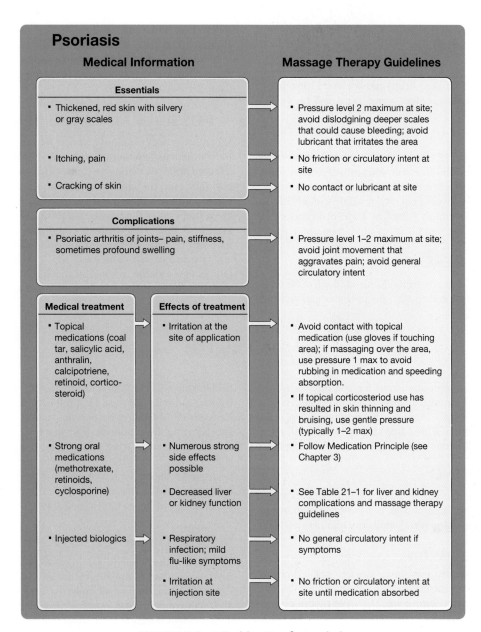

FIGURE 7-2. A Decision Tree for psoriasis.

form—plaque psoriasis. If the client has another type of psoriasis, ask for more details about signs, symptoms, and complications such as open, weeping lesions, inflammation, and fever. Adapt to open skin (see Figure 7-2), and follow the inflammation principle. Medications for other psoriasis types tend to be stronger than those for plaque psoriasis. Investigate your client's condition for these signs, symptoms, and complications. See the bibliography online at http://thePoint.lww.com/Walton for places to look for more information.

Questions 2–7 guide you to a possible pressure, friction, lubricant, or contact restriction at the affected site. If the area is painful or itchy, then friction and circulatory intent are contraindicated at the site. If the area is simply thickened and red, gentle massage at a maximum pressure level of 2 may be welcome, but avoid aggravating the condition; use a lotion or oil that does not irritate the area. If too much massage pressure causes peeling away of the scales of psoriasis, it may cause bleeding. If there is cracking of the skin, then contact and lubricant are contraindicated over the area.

Question 8 is used to identify psoriatic arthritis. If a client has psoriatic arthritis, it can be very painful and swollen, in some cases similar to rheumatoid arthritis (see Chapter 9). Use gentle pressure (2 max), if any, on affected areas, and avoid joint movement that aggravates discomfort. Also, avoid general circulatory intent during a flare-up of psoriatic arthritis, as the client may feel unwell.

Questions 9 and 10 about treatment can identify one or more of a range of medications. If topical medications are used, contact at the site may be contraindicated altogether because of irritation at the site of application, or because the condition itself is severe. If contact is not prohibited, and is welcome, then avoid rubbing in topical medication and speeding up the absorption; a pressure level 1 is the maximum to use at the site. Also, use gloves when contacting the area to avoid absorbing the medication into the skin of the hands.

If the client is taking oral medications for psoriasis, follow the Medication Principle from Chapter 3. In particular, be alert for diminished kidney or liver function. See Table 21-1 for relevant signs, symptoms, and massage therapy guidelines for renal and liver toxicity.

The Medication Principle. Adapt massage to the condition for which the medication is taken or prescribed, and to any side effects.

If the client is using injected biologics, the newer therapies for psoriasis, ask about flu-like symptoms or respiratory infections. If either of these is present, they are likely to be mild, but it is still a good idea to avoid general circulatory intent. Always avoid friction and circulatory intent at a recent injection site until the medication has had plenty of time to be absorbed.

● MASSAGE RESEARCH

As of this writing, there are no randomized, controlled trials, published in the English language, on psoriasis and massage indexed in PubMed or the Massage Therapy Foundation Research Database. The NIH RePORTER tool lists no active, federally funded research projects on the topic in the United States. No active projects are listed on the clinicaltrials.gov database (see Chapter 6).

● POSSIBLE MASSAGE BENEFITS

If contact is not contraindicated, it may feel good to the client to feel the massage therapist's hands simply resting directly on affected areas, or through a drape. Firm pressure without friction may help the client manage the itching and pain of psoriasis, and reach the underlying muscles without irritating the area. Remember that stress is a psoriasis trigger, so any massage work that reduces stress could play a role in preventing flare-ups. Finally, lesions can be quite distinct and dramatic, and a cause of self-consciousness. A therapist can offer not only compassionate, respectful touch, but also a gentle, unalarmed demeanor as the lesions are uncovered in the session.

Acne Vulgaris

Acne vulgaris is the scientific name for common acne; the name distinguishes it from a related condition, *acne rosacea* (see Conditions in Brief). Acne is the eruption of pimples caused by the interaction of the oil-producing glands of the skin, hormones, normal flora on the skin, and the immune response.

● BACKGROUND

Acne lesions most often occur on the face and the shoulders, but can appear on other surfaces, as well. It is most common in adolescents, but younger children and adults can also develop acne.

Signs and Symptoms

Acne can range in severity, presenting as a few isolated **comedones** (whiteheads or blackheads) to the deepest lesions, inflamed areas known as *cystic acne*. The most severe presentation can be painful and cause scarring.

Complications

Psychosocial issues including poor self confidence and self esteem are common, especially with severe acne.

Treatment

Mild acne is treated topically with over-the-counter preparations aimed at drying up oil, removing dead skin cells, or killing bacteria. **Over the counter (OTC)** refers to medications that are available without a prescription. Acne preparations contain benzoyl peroxide, salicylic acid, or other ingredients. These have few side effects: at most, some people experience uncomfortably dry or irritated skin. If OTC topicals are not effective, acne is treated with prescription topicals: antibiotics and retinoids. These also tend to cause few side effects, but peeling, irritation, and increased photosensitivity may occur. Often, combinations of topical preparations are used with success.

If topical preparations do not work, systemic medications may be tried, such as antibiotics, retinoids, and oral contraceptives. Oral antibiotics (such as tetracycline, erythromycin) may be prescribed, but may be required for months or years for maintenance. These can cause increased photosensitivity, mild nausea, and mild diarrhea. Oral retinoids such as Accutane may have side effects such as dryness and joint pain. Because they can also affect the liver, periodic liver function monitoring is part of the therapy. There is a risk of severe birth defects, and women of childbearing age are urged to use two forms of birth control while taking oral retinoids. Oral contraceptives are used when hormonal imbalances play a role in acne. These medications may cause weight gain and breast tenderness, among other side effects.

● INTERVIEW QUESTIONS

1. Where is the acne? Is it mild, moderate, or severe?
2. Have you had massage over the area before? How does the area respond to contact, pressure, and different lubricants?
3. If you are treating it, how?
4. How does the treatment affect you?

● MASSAGE THERAPY GUIDELINES

In general, be sensitive to possible effects of acne on body image, especially if it is severe, or if scarring remains years later.

An area of acne is an area of inflammation, and friction or circulatory intent may aggravate the inflammation. And although there is no absolute maximum pressure level for acne, the pressure should be gentle at the site. Some lubricants may irritate the area and worsen the acne, as well. Question 1 helps establish the location and severity of the inflammation.

That said, some individuals will want contact or even deep pressure on the muscles that are deep to the region of acne. This is especially true on the shoulders or back. Individual preferences for lubricant can vary. Some want lotion instead of oil, or even very little lubricant at all because of their experience that it aggravates the acne. Some clients prefer lots of lubricant, to ease friction on the area.

Requests for pressure in the affected area must be considered carefully. For example, a gentle amount of pressure at levels 1 or 2 might aggravate inflammation for one client, and should be avoided. However, it might not aggravate the inflammation for another client, and could relax the underlying muscles. In determining the best pressure, take into account the severity of the acne: Pressure level 3 might be fine around mild acne, but not for cystic acne. In general, resist requests for pressure in the 3–5 range, and find alternative ways to work with the muscles. Joint movement is not contraindicated, so stretching, positional release techniques, focused pressure between blemishes, and deep pressure elsewhere will serve the client better than direct pressure on the lesions. In any case, avoid contact and lubricant at the site of open skin.

Question 2 adds an additional consideration: whether the client has received massage over the affected area, and if so, whether it aggravated the acne. If this is the case, use the Previous Massage Principle in planning the session, along with other factors described above.

> *The Previous Massage Principle. A client's previous experience of massage therapy, especially massage after the onset, after the diagnosis, or during a flare-up of a medical condition, may be used to plan the massage.*

Side effects from acne medications are usually mild. If, from questions 3 and 4, you determine that topical medications are still present on the skin surface, avoid rubbing them in and speeding up the absorption; a pressure level 1 is the maximum to use at the site. Also, use gloves when contacting the area to avoid absorbing the medication into the skin of the hands.

If the skin is irritated or dry, use gentle pressure (1–2 maximum) and avoid friction at the treatment site.

If oral antibiotics cause nausea or diarrhea, only slight adjustments are needed as shown in the Decision Tree (Figure 7-3). For stronger side effects of oral medications such as retinoids or contraceptives, patients are carefully monitored for tolerance. It is a good idea to ask the four medication questions about oral retinoid therapy. If the client

is experiencing dryness, avoid friction if it causes discomfort. If there is joint pain, it is usually mild, but avoid strong joint movement in any case. In theory, the effect of oral retinoids on liver function would contraindicate general circulatory intent, but in practice, a client's liver function is monitored closely by the physician, and medications are modified or stopped if liver function is compromised. See Table 21-1 for further guidelines for liver effects. Oral contraceptives can lead to tender breasts and might call for a change in position during massage.

● MASSAGE RESEARCH

As of this writing, there are no randomized, controlled trials, published in the English language, on acne and massage indexed in PubMed or the Massage Therapy Foundation Research Database. The NIH RePORTER tool lists no active, federally funded research projects on the topic in the United States. No active projects are listed on the clinicaltrials.gov database (see Chapter 6).

● POSSIBLE MASSAGE BENEFITS

Stress can cause acne to flare, or aggravate an episode. For instance, a small study suggests that students with acne tend to have more severe flare-ups during final exam periods (Zeitlin et al., 2000). Another small study observed that massage at exam time can lower stress (Chiu et al., 2003). These studies are far from conclusive, but one might consider them together and begin to build a theory for massage therapy lowering stress and thereby preventing acne flare-ups. This theory is worth testing, in the research and clinical worlds.

Acne can cause acute self-consciousness, especially when it is on the face, and especially in adolescents. People with acne may experience ridicule or even unsolicited advice from others about how to treat it. Against this backdrop, the quiet acceptance and nonjudgmental touch of a massage therapist can be especially welcome.

Oral and Genital Herpes (Herpes Simplex 1 and 2)

Herpes simplex viruses are common viruses, divided into two types: herpes simplex 1 and 2. **Herpes Simplex Virus 1 (HSV-1)** causes cold sores or fever blisters on the face. Because the sores are often in or around the mouth, it is sometimes called **oral herpes**, but lesions can appear anywhere on the face, including the nose. Most people are exposed to HSV-1 as children, through casual contact such as sharing utensils or towels.

About 90% of individuals have been exposed to HSV-1 and have the antibodies to it, but just 10% of them develop the symptoms at the initial infection. **Primary infection** is the development of symptoms after the first exposure to an infectious agent. Once established, the virus stays in the body, remaining in a dormant state in nerve cells until it is activated again, often by stress, sun exposure, a menstrual period, or fever from another condition. These **recurrent infections**, or repeating flare-ups, tend to produce milder symptoms than the primary infection. They usually occur at the same site as the first infection, or at a site nearby.

Herpes Simplex Virus 2 (HSV-2), or **genital herpes**, is also common. It causes uncomfortable blistering of the skin, but it usually occurs below the waist. In contrast to the casual

contact that results in HSV-1 transmission, HSV-2 is usually sexually transmitted. HSV-2 lesions appear in the genital and anal area, buttocks, and upper thighs, although they can also appear on the face, as there is cross-infection that occurs during oral-genital sex.

There is significantly more stigma attached to genital herpes than oral herpes, and people are often reluctant to talk about it. This stigma persists, despite the large number of people infected: about 30% of adults in the United States have been exposed to HSV-2, and about one in six experience outbreaks.

● BACKGROUND

Both HSV-1 and HSV-2 are transmitted from person to person through the blister fluid, but a person does not have to have an outbreak to transmit the virus to another person. In fact, most of the time, HSV is transmitted while the carrier is **asymptomatic**, with no visible symptoms. In the transmission of HSV, **the incubation period**, the period after primary infection and before symptoms develop, is 2–20 days. This delay makes it difficult to trace the point of infection.

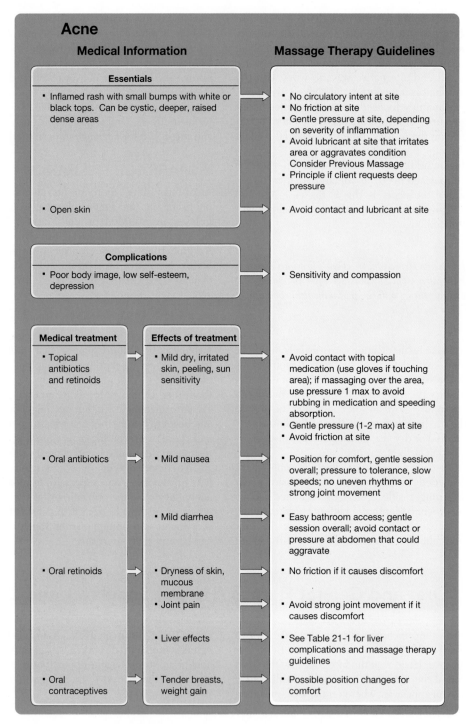

FIGURE 7-3. A Decision Tree for acne.

Signs and Symptoms

Both HSV-1 and HSV-2 outbreaks may begin with burning, tenderness, tingling or itching in the area, followed by the formation of red bumps or blisters (Figure 7-4). The blisters have clear fluid, and they rupture, ooze, and even bleed before healing over in a crust. The crust eventually peels off, and the reddened, healing skin beneath fades with time. It is often painful or tender until it heals.

In HSV-2, sores on the urethra may cause painful urination. Flu-like symptoms such as swollen lymph nodes, headache, fever, and muscle aches may be present. In both cases, recurrent outbreaks tend to be milder than the primary outbreak, and many people experience milder outbreaks with the passage of years. Some people never experience recurrence, or do not experience a second outbreak until decades after the primary infection.

Complications

In someone who is **immunocompromised**, meaning having a weakened immune system, both kinds of herpes can cause severe or prolonged outbreaks, with fever, chills, and severe lesions. Conditions such as HIV, organ transplant, or cancer therapy

FIGURE 7-4. Oral and genital herpes (herpes simplex 1 and 2). (A) Oral herpes presents as a cold sore or fever blister, usually on the mouth. (B) Genital herpes, shown here on the sacrum, can appear outside the genital and anal area in some cases. (A: From Rubin E, Farber JL. *Pathology*, 3rd ed. Philadelphia: Lippincott Williams and Wilkins, 1999. B: From Goodheart HP. *Goodheart's Photoguide to Common Skin Disorders*, 2nd ed. Philadelphia: Lippincott Williams and Wilkins, 2003.)

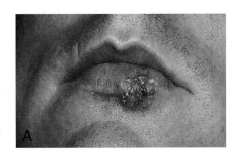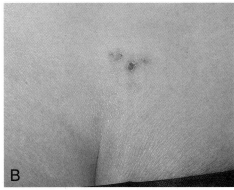

suppress the immune system, so that some cases of herpes can even be life threatening. In addition, newborns are highly vulnerable to herpes I infection, and people with active lesions are advised to avoid handling them. Transmission of HSV-2 from a pregnant woman with genital herpes to her baby during childbirth can be serious and life threatening for the newborn.

A serious complication of HSV-1 infection is *ocular herpes*, when the virus has been transferred to one or both eyes. Ocular herpes can usually be treated successfully to prevent a further serious complication, scarring of the surface of the eye and resulting blindness.

Herpes whitlow or *herpetic whitlow* is a complication of HSV infection that is particularly relevant to massage therapists. Blisters form on an individual's finger when blister fluid enters small cracks in his or her skin, often at the cuticle, as shown in Figure 7-5. An individual can contract herpetic whitlow by touching his or her own blister fluid, or someone else's. Health care workers who are in contact with saliva or open lesions are at risk for developing herpes whitlow. Children who suck their thumbs while they have fever blisters can also develop herpes whitlow. Recurrent infection is rare in herpes whitlow, but both primary and recurrent episodes require covering with a bandage to prevent transmission.

Treatment

There is no cure for HSV-1 and HSV-2, so infection is lifelong. Oral herpes sores are common and the sores are minor, so many people simply tolerate them until they go away. Prescription treatment is reserved for more severe cases of oral herpes, or for genital herpes. Prescription antiviral medications may be used to reduce the severity and frequency of outbreaks and decrease the chances of HSV-2 transmission to a sexual partner. A mainstay of antiviral medication is acyclovir, famciclovir, and valacyclovir, although not all of these are used in all forms for herpes simplex. Topical acyclovir may be used for recurrent cold sores, and can cause mild burning and discomfort at the site of application. All three drugs are available in oral form, used for recurrent genital herpes. In the dosages for HSV, the side effects of these drugs tend to be mild. They include nausea, headache, and diarrhea. Some people experience dizziness or lightheadedness while taking these drugs.

● INTERVIEW QUESTIONS

1. Are you having a herpes flare-up currently? If so, where are the lesions located?
2. Are the blisters open and weeping? Are the blisters dry or crusting over?

3. Do you have any other symptoms, or complications? If so, how have they affected you?
4. Are you on any medication for it?
5. Are there any side effects or reactions to medication?

● MASSAGE THERAPY GUIDELINES

When herpes lesions are on the face, they are usually obvious, providing a visible answer to questions 1 and 2. Genital herpes lesions on the buttocks or upper thighs might also be visible. To prevent transmission of the infection, or introducing another microorganism into a vulnerable area, avoid making direct contact with your hands or massage lubricant. Regardless of the status of the infection—open, weeping, crusted over, or healing—avoid contact and lubricant at the site. As always, handle linens carefully before laundering.

The Open Lesion Principle. **Do not make contact with an open lesion.**

While it's easy to avoid contact with a visible lesion, the fluid from open lesions is also a concern for the massage therapist.

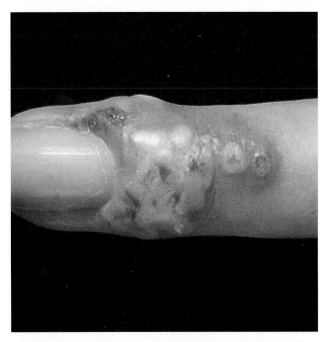

FIGURE 7-5. Herpes whitlow. (From Goodheart HP. *Goodheart's Photoguide to Common Skin Disorders*, 2nd ed. Philadelphia: Lippincott Williams and Wilkins, 2003.)

During massage of a client with herpes, there is a real possibility of contracting herpes whitlow, especially during a flare-up. Avoid contact with blister fluid, no matter where it appears on the skin, linens or clothing. Logical areas to avoid include the face and the hands, but since most people tend to touch their own lesions and can transfer the fluid from the fingers to other areas of the body, the safest approach to a session with a client with herpes lesions is to use gloves for the entire session.

Although herpes virus cannot survive well outside the body, health care workers who handle oral secretions or come in close contact with lesions use gloves to avoid transmission. Because massage therapists make skin-to-skin contact for a sustained amount of time, a case can be made for glove use throughout the session. Gloved hands can still transfer virus from place to place on the client's body, but the barrier prevents it from passing to the therapist's hands.

> **The Body Fluid Principle.** *If it's wet and it's not yours, don't touch it.*

There is a slippery slope in infection control. As mentioned earlier, HSV-1 can be transmitted even when there are no lesions, and 90% of adults have been exposed, so one could argue that therapists should use glove for *all* clients to protect their hands from the virus. Likewise, an argument can be made that massage therapists with a cold sore should cancel all of their appointments for 10 days to avoid transferring the virus to his or her clients. But these would be extreme measures.

Although it is easy to become alarmed about infection when working in skin-to-skin contact, common sense and careful standard precautions—steps that all health care workers take to minimize infection—protect therapists. In standard precautions, therapists practice the same infection control measures with all clients, as any client (or therapist) can carry and transmit infection, often while asymptomatic. In particular, good hand care to reduce cuts, thorough handwashing, and judicious use of gloves will all lower the chances of infection. Remember that infection goes both ways. If you have herpes simplex in any form, never touch a client with any surface (such as a bare hand, gloved hand, or any clothing) that has touched your own blister fluid. Where possible, cover exposed lesions. And if you are seeing immunosuppressed clients, remember that herpes exposure can be very unsafe during this time, and offer them the opportunity to reschedule until your lesions have healed.

Most cases of HSV-1 are mild and pass quickly; at worst, they are annoying and unsightly. But both HSV-1 and -2 can be chronic, painful, and aggravating, and have complications. If the client mentions flu-like symptoms in response to question 3, avoid general circulatory intent and use gentle pressure overall—level 2 maximum. Higher pressures and circulatory intent can be too vigorous for most people during active infection. Your massage should be supportive rather than challenging.

If the client mentions active ocular herpes, or active herpes whitlow, treat it the same as any other HSV-1 outbreak, by steering clear of the fluid and sores. Blindness from ocular herpes does not, by itself, require any adjustment in the elements of massage.

If the client reports frequent or severe outbreaks, it is important to ask follow-up questions about any conditions that compromise immunity. Ask gently, something like, "Sometimes herpes lesions are severe when there are other things going on. Is there anything else going on that weakens your immune system?" Adapt the massage to HIV/AIDS (see Chapter 13), strong cancer therapies (see Chapter 20), or organ/tissue transplant (see Chapter 21). If the client's immune system is weak, lesions may be present over a wider area: for example, lesions that are typically confined to the genital area can appear on the buttocks or inner thighs.

The prevalence of herpes simplex 1 and 2 highlights the importance of *always* asking the clients about skin integrity and any lesions. Also, always inspect the skin before massaging. Do not work under the edge of a drape, without visually checking the skin first! Work through the drape rather than under it, where possible. Given the stigma and confusion surrounding herpes, your client may or may not disclose genital herpes. But an open lesion is an open lesion and should be treated with caution, no matter what its cause or where it is located.

Questions 4 and 5 may raise side effects of antiviral medications; these are important to ask about, even though they tend to be mild in the treatment of herpes simplex. As with any topical medication, avoid direct contact with topical acyclovir. Since topicals tend to be applied at the lesion site, this guideline is taken care of by avoiding the lesions themselves.

Massage adjustments for headache, mild nausea and diarrhea, and possible responses to oral antivirals are noted in the Decision Tree (see Figure 7-6). Dizziness or lightheadedness may also occur with these medications. Whenever a client complains of dizziness or lightheadedness, it's important to be gentle in repositioning, use slow speeds, and use even rhythms throughout the session. A gradual transition to standing at the end of the massage is also in order.

● MASSAGE RESEARCH

As of this writing, there are no randomized, controlled trials, published in the English language, on HSV and massage indexed in PubMed or the Massage Therapy Foundation Research Database. The NIH RePORTER tool lists no active, federally funded research projects on the topic in the United States. No active projects are listed on the clinicaltrials.gov database (see Chapter 6).

● POSSIBLE MASSAGE BENEFITS

HSV-1 and HSV-2 have a recognized stress component. Many people get flare-ups when they are run-down and under stress. It seems plausible that massage, as an important self-care measure, could help people minimize the effects of stress.

Scabies

Scabies is a highly contagious parasitic skin infection, caused by a small mite. Worldwide, the number of cases occurring each year is estimated at 300 million. Although it occurs in epidemics in group settings such as hospitals, nursing facilities, and schools, it can affect any age, ethnic group, and socioeconomic class. Contrary to public perception, scabies is not associated

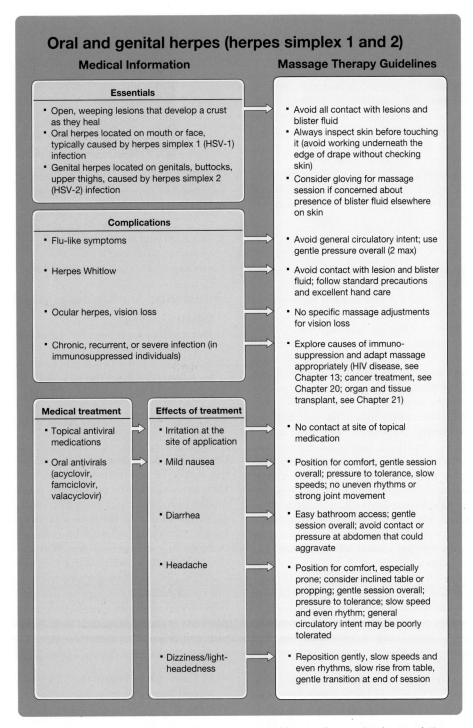

FIGURE 7-6. A Decision Tree for oral and genital herpes (herpes simplex 1 and 2).

with poor hygiene. It is spread by skin-to-skin contact and by contact with clothing and bedding.

● BACKGROUND

The scabies skin reaction is an allergic response to the mite. The first time an individual is infested with scabies, he or she is asymptomatic for the first 2–6 weeks, making it difficult to trace the time and place of exposure. Then the allergic response develops. The second time an individual becomes infested, the timeline is shorter: he or she has already been sensitized and is likely to develop an allergic reaction within hours of contact.

Signs and Symptoms

The signature symptom of scabies is intense itching. Scratching can cause a rash (Figure 7-7). The mite burrows under the skin, laying eggs that trigger the allergic reaction in the host. The burrow marks can sometimes be seen as thin marks on the skin, but are often obliterated by marks from scratching. The mite prefers cracks and folds of skin, so the itching can be anywhere, but it is often between fingers and toes, in the gluteal fissure and genitals, at the waist, in the elbows, and under the breasts in women. Itching may be worse at night or after a hot bath. It can persist for several weeks after the mites have been killed, as the bodies of the mites linger and continue to trigger an allergic reaction.

Complications

Reinfestation with scabies, a common occurrence, may be considered a complication. Also, because of the strong urge to scratch, open skin can develop quickly in scabies. In some cases, this leads to a **secondary infection**, in which a second infection closely follows the first. In scabies, the secondary infection is often impetigo (see Conditions in Brief).

Crusted scabies, a severe condition in which the number of mites can exceed 1 million on an affected individual, occurs in immunocompromised patients. Crusted lesions appear over large areas of the body.

Treatment

In the United States and United Kingdom, first-line therapy for scabies is a prescription cream containing permethrin (Elimite), which is applied to the skin and left on overnight and is then washed off. It is repeated one week later. Additional or alternative treatment may be necessary if it does not kill the mites, or if reinfestation occurs through continued contact with scabies mites. Household members and others in close contact with the individual are also treated, even if they are asymptomatic. They are treated on the same day, so that the mite is not passed back and forth between people. Children are typically cleared to return to school the morning after the first treatment has been applied and washed off.

Permethrin has few side effects, limited to a temporary increase in itching, swelling, and redness on application. Second-line therapy is lindane cream (Kwell), a stronger drug with neurotoxic effects in children that make it less safe. Other gentler topical treatments are used as well. A systemic drug, ivermectin, may be prescribed in stubborn cases. Ivermectin can cause nausea and drowsiness. Secondary infections from scratching, such as impetigo, are treated with antibiotics (see Impetigo, Conditions in Brief).

Linens, clothing, and towels are bagged in plastic bags for at least a week, or washed in hot water and dried on high heat the day after treatment has begun. It is not necessary to treat pets, or to fumigate homes or furniture, but vacuuming carpets and upholstery is encouraged. Antihistamines may be prescribed for itching, and in severe cases, corticosteroid cream may be used.

Itching can persist for several weeks after the mites have been killed, as the bodies linger and incite allergic reaction. If itching persists for longer than 2–3 weeks after the initial treatment, individuals should see a doctor again, because an alternative treatment may be needed.

● INTERVIEW QUESTIONS

Questions for clients with scabies can be used to determine when it is safe for a client to reschedule after a scabies episode. Questions about undiagnosed itching are just as important: they can help a therapist assess the likelihood of scabies when a situation arises during the massage session.

Questions for Clients with Scabies

1. Has this condition been seen by a doctor?
2. How have you treated it, and when? Were your close contacts and household members treated at the same time?

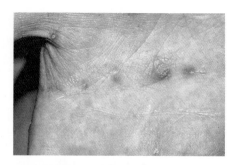

FIGURE 7-7. Scabies. (From Goodheart HP. *Goodheart's Photoguide to Common Skin Disorders*, 2nd ed. Philadelphia: Lippincott Williams and Wilkins, 2003.)

3. What did your doctor tell you about preventing the spread of scabies to others?
4. Did your doctor say it has resolved?

Questions for Undiagnosed Itching

1. Where is the itching?
2. Has it spread from one place to another on your skin?
3. Is it worse at night or after a hot bath or shower?
4. Is anyone else in your household, or among your close contacts, complaining of the same itching?
5. Have you spoken to your doctor about it?

● MASSAGE THERAPY GUIDELINES

There is a single massage therapy guideline for scabies: all contact with skin, clothing, and linens is contraindicated until the individual has been successfully treated, reinfestation from the individual's environment is unlikely, and both the individual and the physician are sure that it is no longer contagious. The Decision Tree is clear on this point. Questions 1–4, for use with a client who has been diagnosed with scabies, are designed to learn whether the client has followed up on scabies appropriately and is no longer at risk of transmitting it.

A therapist considering rescheduling a client after his or her first treatment for scabies may be inclined to do so the next day, because individuals are cleared to return to school or work on the morning after the first treatment. But massage involves more sustained skin contact than these daily activities, and there are compelling reasons to delay a session for additional few weeks:

- You may not feel comfortable providing massage until the second treatment, a week later, has been completed.
- It can take longer than 1 week to be sure that the treatment was successful.
- Even with successful treatment, it can take a few weeks to prevent reinfestation from an individual's environment.
- Persistent itching for several weeks after successful treatment could make massage unwelcome.

These massage precautions for diagnosed scabies are clear, but a client who complains of itching, without a diagnosed cause, presents an equally serious scenario. Questions 1–5 about undiagnosed itching can help a therapist assess the likelihood of scabies and evaluate his or her own tolerance of the risk. Here, knowing the cause of the itching is important: recall the Ask the Cause Principle from Chapter 3. Scabies is only one cause of itching, but scabies infection has particularly heavy consequences for massage practice; it can lead to weeks of time out of work.

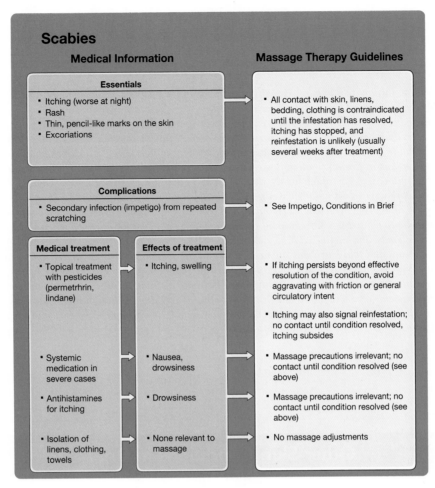

FIGURE 7-8. A Decision Tree for scabies.

In line with this concern, give serious consideration to a client's complaint of itching. Use the follow-up questions to weigh the risk of skin-to-skin contact. Be particularly cautious if the itching is in the classic scabies body areas, or if the client answers affirmatively to questions 2–4. If you need guidance, contact your physician or public health department.

> *The Ask If It's Contagious Principle.* **Before making contact with a client's body, find out whether a skin lesion is contagious and how it is spread.**

If you suspect that a client has scabies, find a sensitive, respectful way to postpone the session or to end a session that has already begun. Wash your hands carefully, paying extra attention to the folds of your skin and your fingernails. Carefully remove linens from the table (do not shake them out), bag them, and set them aside. Call your physician or health department to determine how to clean the linens and your own clothing. Call a physician immediately about getting preventive treatment, as well as preventing the spread of the mite in the building. Recall that the incubation period is several weeks, and an individual can infect others during that asymptomatic time. Therapist's Journal 7-1 tells two stories about scabies in massage practice.

If a recent client tells you that he has developed scabies since he saw you, or if you develop scabies, contact your health department for guidance about how and whom to contact about a possible outbreak and receiving preventive treatment. Ask the health department nurse or your physician about when it is advisable to resume massage practice.

● MASSAGE RESEARCH

As of this writing, there are no randomized, controlled trials, published in the English language, on scabies and massage indexed in PubMed or the Massage Therapy Foundation Research Database. The NIH RePORTER tool lists no active, federally funded research projects on the topic in the United States. No active projects are listed on the clinicaltrials.gov database (see Chapter 6).

● POSSIBLE MASSAGE BENEFITS

Because scabies is highly infectious, there is no case for massage during infestation. However, scabies can be isolating, embarrassing, and provoke strong feelings of disgust or revulsion. Once the infestation has cleared and a client returns to massage, a therapist can offer compassion and reassuring touch.

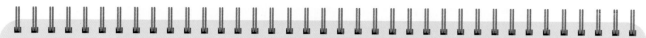

THERAPIST'S JOURNAL 7-1 *Scabies, Touch, and Caution*

I remember a colleague, Jordan, telling a hair-raising story. One of his practice clients called him a few weeks after a session and told him she found out she had developed scabies.

Jordan had already begun to itch a bit in the area of the waistband of his jeans, but he hadn't thought anything of it. This phone call scared him and he saw his doctor the next day. A quick test revealed the mites. Jordan was in the awkward position of calling all the clients he had seen after his client with scabies. He told them about the incident and urged each one to see a doctor. Jordan treated himself twice with permethrin cream according to his doctor's instructions. He also bagged and cleaned all of his linens, drying them on high heat. He lost a week's worth of income, and returned to massage work a few days after his second treatment.

Another massage therapist, Ana, who was also a nurse, had worked a lot in long-term care and was familiar with the spread of scabies in institutional settings. One evening she was draping her client for a session when she noticed the client furiously scratching his hands. She questioned him and learned that he was quite uncomfortable, especially after hot showers.

Ana took a deep breath and told her client she needed to end the session right then, and strongly urged the client to see his physician. Without diagnosing, she told the client of her concern about scabies. After he left, Ana carefully folded up the linens, put them in a garbage bag, and added her own clothing to the bag that night, just to be sure. She stored them in her basement for a week. She saw her physician the next day. Although it was unpleasant, she used the permethrin, and never developed scabies. She checked with her health department to be sure she'd handled the situation safely and returned to massage a couple of days later.

Tracy Walton
Cambridge, MA

Other Skin Conditions in Brief

ACNE ROSACEA

Background	• Inflammation caused by bacteria; usually on the face, sometimes neck, chest, scalp, ears. • Flare-ups triggered by stress, diet, extreme temperature exposure. • Treatments include topical and oral antibiotics, retinoids (see "Acne vulgaris," this chapter).
Interview Questions	• Flare-up? Where? Treatment? Effects of treatment?
Massage Therapy Guidelines	• No friction, circulatory intent at the site. • Use gentle pressure (pr 1 max), nonaggravating lubricant at the site. • No direct contact with topical medication. • See "Acne vulgaris," this chapter, for medication side effects and massage therapy guidelines.

ATHLETE'S FOOT (TINEA PEDIS)

Background	• Fungal infection forming in dark, warm, moist interdigital areas. • Causes dry skin, burning, itching, scaling, blisters, cracking, pain. • Treated with OTC powders, oral and topical antifungal drugs. • Side effects of oral antifungals include GI upset, headache, impaired liver function (rare; well-monitored).
Interview Questions	• Where? Cracked or open skin? Topical treatments? Oral treatments? Effects of treatment?
Massage Therapy Guidelines	• No contact or lubricant at the site of inflammation; interdigital areas are easy to avoid during massage.

- If hands make contact by mistake, wash carefully before continuing. Routinely leave feet for last, or wash hands after foot contact, before moving to other areas of the body.
- For people at risk, avoid applying oil or lotion near interdigital areas, which can hold moisture and favor fungal growth.
- For side effects of oral antifungal drugs, follow the Medication Principle (Chapter 3), including position changes for headache or GI upset; see Table 21-1 for liver complications.

BASAL CELL CARCINOMA

Background	• Mild form of skin cancer, typically resolved with excisional biopsy or other surgical procedure. • Topical chemotherapy or immune response modulators (IRMs) such as Imiquimod used, with skin irritation common; numerous strong side effects possible.
Interview Questions	• Where? When removed? • Other treatment? Effects of treatment?
Massage Therapy Guidelines	• No friction or circulatory intent at the site until removed (see "Surgery," Chapter 21). • Follow the Medication Principle (see Chapter 3) for topical chemotherapy and IRM medications.

BOILS

Background	• Staph infection spread by contact; causes extremely painful eruptions on the skin, producing systemic symptoms such as fever, tender lymph nodes, chills, and fatigue. • Treated with topical antibiotics, compresses, and lancing to drain pus.
Interview Questions	• Where? Open Skin? Swelling or pain? Fever, chills or fatigue? • Worsening, or improving? • Treatment? Effects of treatment?
Massage Therapy Guidelines	• Safest, most conservative approach: Reschedule session, regardless of severity of symptoms, avoiding contact with the client until diagnosed and resolved. • Less conservative approach: Provide massage, but with no contact at the site; no general circulatory intent during fever, chills or fatigue, and until symptoms have significantly improved for 3–4 days. • Less conservative approach is advised only if the client has reported the boil to his or her physician and boil is MRSA-negative (see "Methicillin-resistant *Staphylococcus aureus*," Conditions in Brief, this chapter). • In either case: Wash and dry linens carefully on high heat, and avoid contact at the site until incision heals.

CELLULITIS

Background	• Common bacterial skin infection; inflammation forms at the site, sometimes with fever and small spots on the surface of reddened skin; frequently on lower legs (but can appear anywhere), caused by staph or strep. • Can lead to blood poisoning and be life threatening. • Treated with oral or IV antibiotics; side effects usually mild (diarrhea, nausea, abdominal pain, headache, dizziness, rash).
Interview Questions	• Where? Worsening, or improving? Has the doctor said that it is resolving? • Treatment? Effects of treatment?

| Massage Therapy Guidelines | • Avoid contact at the site until resolved.
• No general circulatory intent or heavy pressure overall (2–3 max) until symptoms have significantly improved for 3–4 days, fever and chills are absent, and the physician states that it is resolved.
• Strongly urge the client to report signs and symptoms to the physician if unreported.
• Adapt massage to the side effects of antibiotics (see Table 21-1). |

CUTS AND ABRASIONS

Background	• Injury to skin caused by trauma.
Interview Questions	• Where? How and when did it happen? • Worsening or improving? Other areas injured? • Open skin? Pain or swelling?
Massage Therapy Guidelines	• No contact or lubricant at the site of open skin. • Gentle pressure (1 max) around site if recent, or if bruises are red, blue, or purple; follow up on other injuries that might have occurred. • If bruising is severe or widespread, or it involves the lower extremities, consider DVT Risk Principles (see Chapter 11).

FOLLICULITIS

Background	• Bacterial, fungal, or viral infection of hair follicle, skin surrounding hair follicles; may be superficial, or in more serious cases, deep. • Causes clusters of red bumps around hair follicles, tenderness, itching, blisters that burst and crust over, swelling, and scarring. • Treatments include warm compresses, topical and oral antibiotics or antifungals, antiviral medication, retinoids, and lancing to cause drainage.
Interview Questions	• Where? Worsening or improving? Has the doctor said that it is resolving? • Treatment? Effects of treatment?
Massage Therapy Guidelines	• Avoid contact at the site until resolved. • No general circulatory intent or heavy pressure (2–3 max) until symptoms have significantly improved for 3–4 days, fever and chills are absent, and the physician states that it is resolved. • Strongly urge the client to report signs and symptoms to the physician if unreported. • Follow the Medication Principle (see Chapter 3); adapt massage to the side effects of medications (see Table 21-1).

HIVES (URTICARIA)

Background	• Raised red welts, frequently itchy; usually a reaction to certain foods or drugs. • Treatment usually includes antihistamines, which may cause drowsiness. Oral corticosteroids, other medications used for stubborn cases.
Interview Questions	• Where? When did it start? Identified trigger? Effects of lubricant? • Chronic or acute? Worsening or improving? • Treatment? Effects of treatment?
Massage Therapy Guidelines	• Gentle pressure (1 max) surrounding the site. • If onset is recent (last few days) or condition still acute, avoid general circulatory intent. • If trigger is not clear, be cautious with overall pressure, friction; use a lubricant known not to trigger or aggravate reaction. • If medication causes drowsiness, slow rise from the table at the end of the session. • Adapt massage to the effects of oral corticosteroids (see "Corticosteroids," Chapter 21), other medications (see Table 21-1).

IMPETIGO

Background	• Highly contagious bacterial infection, caused by a strain of staph or strep, that produces rounded, oozing lesions; lesions crust over. • Often on hands and face; can occur as a result of open skin in dermatitis. • Rare but serious complications include kidney inflammation, cellulitis (see Conditions in Brief, this chapter) and methycillin-resistant *Staphylococcus aureus* (MRSA) (see Conditions in Brief, this chapter). • Usually clears in 2–3 weeks on its own, but may be treated with oral or topical antibiotics to prevent complications.
Interview Questions	• Where? When did it start? Treatment? • Has your doctor said that it is no longer contagious—are you cleared to return to work or school?
Massage Therapy Guidelines	• General contact contraindicated until physician verifies no longer contagious, usually 24 hours after treatment is started. • Contact public health department or consult physician if unsure about communicability. • Adapt massage to the effects of antibiotics (see Table 21-1).

JOCK ITCH (TINEA CRURIS)

Background	• Fungal infection affecting genitals, anus; can also appear on inner and upper thighs, and buttocks. • Causes dry skin, burning, itching, scaling, blisters, cracking, and pain. • Treated with topical and oral antifungal medication; side effects of oral antifungals include GI upset, headache, impaired liver function (rare; well-monitored)
Interview Questions	• Flare-up? Does it appear anywhere else, such as the upper thighs or buttocks? • Topical treatments? Oral treatments? Effects of treatment?
Massage Therapy Guidelines	• Site of jock itch is typically outside the therapist's scope of practice, but take extra care to avoid contact with the area if working on muscle attachments in the region; for example, at ischial tuberosity. • For any side effects of antifungal drugs, follow the Medication Principle (Chapter 3), including position changes for headache or GI upset; see Table 21-1 for liver toxicity (rare).

LIPOMA

Background	• Flattened lump of fat cells, usually less than 2" in diameter, in a capsule in the subcutaneous layer of neck, back, shoulders, arms, thighs. • Moves with finger pressure; can be tender; usually removed surgically.
Interview Questions	• Where? Have you reported it to your doctor? Has it been diagnosed?
Massage Therapy Guidelines	• If diagnosed as lipoma, be careful with pressure (2 or 3 max in most cases) at the site; do not disturb capsule. • As with any lump or mass, if unreported or self-diagnosed, urge medical referral and avoid contact at the site until diagnosed.

LICE (PEDICULOSIS)

Background	• Infestation by mites that causes intense itching and small red bumps on the scalp (head lice), body (body lice), and pubic area (pubic lice). • Spread by contact with skin, clothing, furniture, and belongings.

- First line therapy is OTC lotions and shampoos, then prescription lotions and shampoos (malathion, lindane) if needed; repeat treatment at 7–10 days after initial treatment.
- Possible side effects include skin irritation (common) and seizures (rare). Household decontamination requires laundering linens and clothing on high heat, isolating nonwashable items for two weeks, vacuuming.

Interview Questions	• When did you develop it? Did you see a doctor for it? • Treatment? When? Effects of treatment? • Any symptoms since treatment? Has the doctor stated that it is no longer contagious? • Anyone else in household, or other close contacts, infested?
Massage Therapy Guidelines	• Avoid contact with skin, clothing, and linens until the infestation is resolved and the individual is no longer being re-infested from the environment, for example, decontamination for at least two weeks. • Investigate the side effects and complications of treatment; follow Medication Principle (Chapter 3) and see Table 21-1 for common side effects.

MELANOMA (MALIGNANT MELANOMA)

Background	• Most aggressive form of skin cancer; can occur in the skin, eye, or mucous membranes such as the mouth and anus. • Typically presents as changes in an existing mole (becoming asymmetric, nonuniform border, color change, enlarging diameter). • Tends to metastasize to lungs, liver, brain, and bone, but can also spread to GI tract, adrenal glands, and spleen. • Treated with surgery, radiation therapy, chemotherapy, biologic/immunotherapies, and others. • Numerous, strong side effects are possible (see Chapter 21)
Interview Questions	• For change in appearance of a mole: Are you aware of the mole? I see that it appears a little different (describe change); are you aware of any changes? Have you spoken to your doctor about this mole? • For diagnosed melanoma: See interview questions for cancer, Chapter 20 for follow-up questions which should highlight bone metastasis, vital organ involvement, lymph node removal/lymphedema risk, and biologic therapy/immunotherapy.
Massage Therapy Guidelines	• If any changes in moles, or other skin changes are noted, avoid contact, bring them to the client's attention, and encourage an urgent medical referral within the next day or two. • With diagnosed melanoma, no direct massage pressure at/over active tumor site; review Cancer, Chapter 20, for massage therapy guidelines for cancer and cancer treatment, with extra attention to metastasis to bone, spleen, and liver (see "Filter and Pump Principle," Chapter 3), lymphedema risk, and effects of treatment.

METHICILLIN-RESISTANT *STAPHYLOCOCCUS AUREUS*

Background	• Infection of skin and other tissues by strain of staph bacteria that is resistant to many antibiotics; spread by skin-to-skin contact. • Most infections occur in hospitals, but some occur in the community. • Skin lesions look like pimples, boils, or spider bites. • Complications occur when bacteria move to deeper tissues, causing pneumonia, damaging heart valves, joints, and other tissues. • Treatment includes drainage of lesions, vancomycin and other antibiotics; side effects of vancomycin tend to be mild and include nausea, vomiting, chills, rash, hypotension. • Renal failure and other serious side effects possible but rare, more likely with IV administration (well monitored).

Interview Questions	• Where? Open Skin? Covered with a bandage? • How does it affect you? Swelling or pain? Fever, chills, or fatigue? • Worsening or improving? • Treatment? Effects of treatment?
Massage Therapy Guidelines	• Avoid general circulatory intent until resolved. • Avoid skin-to-skin contact with the site, which should be covered with a bandage, by gloving for massage. • Follow standard precautions and wash and dry linens carefully on high heat. For any side effects of antibiotics, follow the Medication Principle (Chapter 3) and see Table 21-1.

MOLES

Background	• Benign (non cancerous) clusters of pigmented skin cells that produce spots that are darker than their surroundings; can be raised.
Interview Questions	• Where? Any changes?
Massage Therapy Guidelines	• Avoid heavy pressure at the site; massage over benign moles is permissible, but be careful not to catch on them if raised. • Observe for changes that could signal skin cancer; urgent medical referral if changes occur in shape, color, diameter, border (See "Melanoma," Conditions in Brief).

NAIL FUNGUS (TINEA UNGUIUM)

Background	• Fungal infection of nailbed; toenail more commonly affected than fingernail, causing thickened, dull, crumbling nail. • Can spread from nail to nail, but less likely to spread from person to person. Topical treatments used, but oral antifungal drugs usually needed for effective treatment,
Interview Questions	• Where? Treatment? Effects of treatment?
Massage Therapy Guidelines	• Wash hands carefully if contact with nail occurs, to avoid spreading it to other nails during the session.

POISON IVY, POISON OAK, POISON SUMAC

Background	• A type of contact dermatitis, caused by allergy to plant oil. • Includes inflammation, itching and blistering; begins with a red, warm, extremely itchy rash, followed by the formation of blisters that crust over. • Develops 8–48 hours after initial exposure, but new areas of rash can continue to appear as plant oil continues to absorb, or with repeated contact with oil on clothing, pets, garden tools. Healing takes up to 10 days. • Inhaled plant oil (e.g., after burning brush) can cause lung inflammation and severe skin rash. • Treated with mild OTC preparations and antihistamines, which may cause drowsiness; oral corticosteroids in severe cases.
Interview Questions	• Where? Has it spread on your body since your initial reaction? • When did you develop the rash? Contact or inhaled? Getting worse or better? • Is it showing up in more areas, beyond the initial rash? • Are you still picking up plant oil from pets or other people in your home? Has anyone else in your household, or close contacts, developed it since your initial reaction? • Treatment? Effects of treatment?
Massage Therapy Guidelines	• Avoid contact with plant oil; establish as well as possible whether plant oil is still present on the skin.

- Avoid all contact with skin and clothing as long as there is any chance of plant oil being present, since individuals can re-expose himself or herself through repeated contact in the environment.
- No contact or lubricant over lesions or topically treated areas until lesions heal, scab over, and resolve.
- If rash is due to inhaled plant oil, general circulatory intent is contraindicated until resolved.
- Slow rise from table if the client is drowsy from antihistamines; see Chapter 21 for massage guidelines for corticosteroids.

PRESSURE SORES (DECUBITUS ULCERS)

Background	• Skin and tissue damage from sustained pressure in the same position (usually wheelchair or bed), impairing blood circulation; common areas are back and sides of head, ears, scapulae, spine, sacrum, buttocks, iliac crest, greater trochanter, knee, ankles, heels, toes. • Ranges from red, itchy, painful skin (stage I) to crater-like wound, loss of skin, and damage to the surrounding tissues, for example, muscle and bone (stage IV). • Complications include infection (cellulitis, septic arthritis, osteomyelitis, gas gangrene, sepsis), which can be life-threatening. • Treatment: dressings, cleaning, removal of dead tissue. Surgery and reconstruction for serious cases.
Interview Questions	• Where? How severe is it? Is it wrapped in a dressing? • How should we modify your position so that you do not have any pressure on it during the massage? • Have you had any complications? Have you had to be treated for infection? • Treatment? Effects of treatment?
Massage Therapy Guidelines	• When working with someone at risk, *always* inspect tissue before making contact with it in a session. • Adjust positioning and bolstering in accordance with nursing practices for the patient. • Circulatory intent at preulcer site might be helpful to prevent pressure sores, but avoid friction and pressure at and around existing sores. • Avoid contact and lubricant over open areas. Work around dressings. • Urge the client to report any worsening sore or sign of infection, including fever, immediately to physician; no general circulatory intent if infection develops.

RINGWORM (TINA CORPORIS)

Background	• Common, highly contagious fungal infection, typically produces small, clearly defined, round red patches of itchy rash. • Spreads easily from one body area to another through scratching and touch; communicable to others through touch, clothing, linens. • Treated with OTC topical creams that clear infection in 3–4 weeks; stubborn cases clear quickly with oral antifungals; side effects of oral antifungals include GI upset, headache, impaired liver function (rare; well-monitored)
Interview Questions	• Where? When? Any medical evaluation? Resolved? • Treatment? Effects of treatment?
Massage Therapy Guidelines	• Avoid general contact and contact with clothing and linens until condition resolved and no longer contagious; postpone all contact until at least 1 week after symptoms resolve. • For side effects of oral antifungal drugs, follow the Medication Principle (Chapter 3), including position changes for headache or GI upset; see Table 21-1 for liver toxicity (rare).

SHINGLES (HERPES ZOSTER)

Background	• Inflammation, strong pain, and skin lesions in a dermatome, caused by reactivation of chicken pox virus (varicella-zoster).
	• Extremely painful lesions with fever, fatigue, and muscle ache; blisters form, break, and crust over in 2–7 days, although pain can last for weeks after blisters heal.
	• Often triggered by stress, can worsen with immunosuppression.
	• Complications include hearing and vision loss when face is affected, and postherpetic neuralgia (PHN), in which pain persists for months or years after shingles episode.
	• Treatment includes antivirals such as Acyclovir (see "Herpes Simplex," this chapter, for side effects) and pain medications.
Interview Questions	• When? Open lesions, or dry and crusted? Any fever, fatigue, chills?
	• Any complications? Any residual pain?
	• Treatment? Effects of treatment?
Massage Therapy Guidelines	• Avoid contact with rash and blister fluid. Avoid all contact if you have not had chicken pox.
	• Most people with shingles are in too much discomfort to want massage.
	• Avoid general circulatory intent until lesions have resolved. Gentle pressure overall, to tolerance—most prefer 2 or 3 maximum while acute, or if affected by PHN.
	• Adapt massage to the side effects of medications (see Decision Tree for oral and genital herpes, Figure 7-6, for antiviral drugs; see Chapter 21 for analgesics).

SKIN TAGS

Background	• Soft, benign growths of skin tissue that often form on neck, armpits, or genital area.
	• Treatment includes surgery, freezing, and cauterizing, typically with minor side effects (irritation, bleeding).
Interview Questions	• Where? Are any irritated or bleeding? Any recent treatment for them?
Massage Therapy Guidelines	• Client interviews do not usually disclose skin tags. Avoid catching or pulling on them during the massage, as they are vascular and can bleed.
	• If recently treated, avoid contact over the area until healed.

SQUAMOUS CELL CARCINOMA

Background	• Slow-growing skin cancer that forms on the skin or in mouth as a bump with flat reddish patches, some scaly, with a crusted surface; eventually becomes an open lesion as it extends into the underlying tissue.
	• Can metastasize to lymph nodes and distant organs if untreated, although this is rare.
	• Generally resolved with surgical procedures including Mohs surgery, a layer-by-layer surgical removal that minimizes injury to the surrounding tissue; may also be treated with radiation, laser therapy, freezing, or topical chemotherapy.
	• All treatments cause some local irritation; chemotherapy can cause severe inflammation of the area.
Interview Questions	• Where is it/was it on your body? Confined to that area, or found in other areas?
	• Treatment? Effects of treatment?
Massage Therapy Guidelines	• No contact at the site until resolved with treatment and area of treatment has healed; no contact with topical treatments.
	• If metastasized, or if the client is in cancer treatment, review "Cancer," Chapter 20.

SUNBURN

Background	• Inflammation from overexposure to sunlight or tanning equipment; resolves in several days, with skin sensitivity that may linger for weeks. • Treated with OTC topical preparations with anesthetics and with oral analgesics.
Interview Questions	• Where? How long ago? Is there still pain or irritation? Any peeling?
Massage Therapy Guidelines	• Avoid friction and circulatory intent at the site until resolved. • If pain has subsided but dry skin is peeling, some stroking with pressure (2 max) may be well tolerated at the site.

WARTS (VERRUCAE VULGARIS)

Background	• Raised skin growth caused by a viral infection; can become open and bleed. • Can be spread from one place to another on an individual's skin; infrequent spread from person to person; more common in children and immunosuppressed individuals than in healthy adults. • Treated with chemical peeling agents, freezing, and burning/cutting with laser treatment; side effects usually minor irritation as the area heals.
Interview Questions	• Where? Isolated, a few, many? Sore? Open? • Treatment? Effects of treatment?
Massage Therapy Guidelines	• Use cautious pressure if the wart is sore; be careful not to catch or pull on it during massage; avoid contact if the skin is open or there are topical treatments; • In theory, contact is contraindicated at the site because of the possibility of the spread of virus; in practice, some people develop warts more readily than others; warts not highly communicable; are an annoyance more than a real danger.

SELF TEST

1. Compare the Open Lesion Principle and the Body Fluid Principle. How are they related?
2. Explain the Ask If It's Contagious Principle.
3. Define first and second line therapy.
4. Compare systemic medication and topical medication.
5. Describe the symptoms of psoriasis. Where do they tend to appear on the body?
6. Explain two reasons why you might have to use gentle pressure for a client with psoriasis. In each case, is it a general precaution, or a site-specific one?
7. Describe two massage guidelines for a client who is receiving biologic therapy for psoriasis.
8. Describe three systemic medications for acne. What are the side effects of each?
9. Without using direct pressure, how could you relax a muscle that is deep to an area of severe acne?
10. What does the term "immunocompromised" mean? What causes it, and how can herpes simplex 1 and 2 appear in someone who is immunocompromised?
11. Compare herpes simplex 1 and herpes simplex 2. List similarities and differences in areas affected, symptoms, and treatments.
12. Describe herpes whitlow. How is it relevant to the massage therapist? How can a therapist prevent it?
13. Why might you wear gloves while massaging a client with open lesions, even while avoiding the affected area?
14. A person who has completed an overnight treatment for scabies is typically cleared to return to school or work the next day. Why wouldn't that be an appropriate time to resume massage therapy?
15. If a client is experiencing itching and is scratch-ing an area, but has received no formal diagnosis for the condition, what questions should you ask about it?

 For answers to these questions and to see a bibliography for this chapter, visit http://thePoint. lww.com/Walton.

Chapter

8 Muscle and Soft Tissue Conditions

What matters is this: you can look at a scar and see hurt or you can look at a scar and see healing. Try to understand.

—SHERI REYNOLDS

The scaffold of the body—the skeleton—is supported by skeletal muscles and other soft tissues such as ligaments, tendons, adipose tissue, and layers of fascia. Massage therapists handle all of these as they work. When these structures become injured or compromised in some way, changes are necessary in the way therapists work.

Muscles and other soft tissue injuries are a natural consequence of human movement, and often more than one structure is injured in a single episode. Overuse, overstretching, stepping on uneven ground, and collisions make soft tissue injuries part of the landscape of massage therapy.

Several injuries are introduced in this chapter, along with some systemic diseases, to reflect a range of conditions. Conditions affecting the bones and joints are introduced in Chapter 9.

In this chapter, four conditions are discussed at length. The conditions are:

- Soft tissue injuries (strain, sprain, tendinopathy, and tenosynovitis)
- Whiplash
- Fibromyalgia syndrome (FMS)
- Muscular dystrophy

Conditions in brief addressed in this chapter are Baker cyst, bursitis, compartment syndrome, cramp, myositis ossificans, plantar fasciitis, and shin splints.

General Principles

Numerous principles from Chapter 3 apply to the conditions in this chapter. Because so many of these conditions involve injury, massage therapists rely on the Pain, Injury, and Inflammation Principles to work with them. In particular, the Inflammation Principle is appropriate when a client has had a recent injury, the inflammation persists, or the structure continues to be reinjured. The Unstable Tissue Principle is also relevant after an injury, or in the event of pain. As such, therapists are careful not to aggravate an injury in its acute phase.

Two new principles are introduced in this chapter. Although they appear to contradict each other, the Respect Muscle Splinting Principle and the Pain-Spasm-Pain Principle provide useful counterpoints to guide massage therapy:

1. The Respect Muscle Splinting Principle. *Do not try to eliminate muscle tension that may be protecting an area of injury, pain, or disease.*

    Once an individual experiences pain from an injury, the body responds with a reflexive contraction of skeletal muscle around the area. In effect, muscle spasm splints the area; the body immobilizes the structure or part, protecting it from overstretching, irritation, and reinjury while it heals. If too much of this protective spasm is released in a single session, the client might feel better temporarily, but the area becomes more vulnerable to reinjury. In response, muscles return to their previous, chronically contracted state, or seem to rebound, the spasm becoming worse than before. An overzealous approach to relaxing muscle can result in the opposite of the intended effect. Instead, a gradual approach is advised, in which a muscle is gently coaxed out of spasm over a course of treatment.

2. The Pain-Spasm-Pain Principle. *Relief of excess muscle tension around an injured or painful area may lead to pain relief, apart from the original cause of the pain.*

    This principle describes the pain relief that may be possible, once a vicious cycle of pain and spasm is arrested. For simplicity, we use the term pain-spasm-pain cycle in this text. In actuality, the cycle includes three steps: pain, spasm, and ischemia, shown in Figure 8-1.

The cycle begins when injury and/or stress on an area cause pain. Reflexive muscle spasm restricts blood flow to the tissues, a process known as ischemia. With ischemia, the tissues in the area become hypoxic, starved of oxygen, and this causes more pain. The increased pain causes further spasm, and the cycle continues for weeks, months, or years. An injury often initiates the cycle, as in the reflexive muscle splinting, described above. Muscle splinting has its place, but it has a downside when it is too strong, or goes on for too long.

Besides injury and stress, other things, too, can initiate the pain-spasm-pain cycle: a disease process, a painful medical procedure, or referred pain from an internal organ. The cycle can start with muscle tension from emotional stress, or cold weather that causes an individual to hunch his or her shoulders. Although the exact mechanisms are yet to be worked out, massage therapy may interrupt the cycle at several points:

1. Reducing muscle spasm
2. Relieving ischemia by increasing circulation to tissues at the site (see Chapter 2)
3. Relieving emotional stress that can initiate or compound the cycle

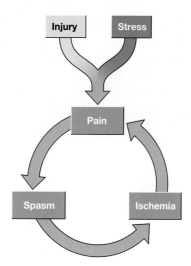

FIGURE 8-1. The pain-spasm-pain cycle. Pain leads to muscle tension, which impedes blood flow to tissues in the area (ischemia), depriving them of oxygen. This leads to further pain, which propagates the cycle.

The longer a cycle continues, the harder it is to tell how much pain is due to the original event, and how much is due to spasm. Often, a person can answer this question once a course of massage therapy has relieved his or her pain.

The Respect Muscle Splinting Principle and the Pain-Spasm-Pain principle may seem to contradict, but they work well in tandem, like two guard rails defining a road, with one on each side. Together, they guide therapists to release excess muscle tension, but not all at once, to leave any functional tension in place. They serve as a reminder that the original injury or event responsible for muscle splinting may, itself, be a cause for caution. Used well, these two principles can help a therapist provide techniques safely, while maximizing their effectiveness.

The pain-spasm-pain cycle may explain why, even without specialized techniques, basic relaxation massage can be helpful in injury healing, as Therapist's Journal 8-1 relates. Simple muscle tension responds well to massage, and therapists can alleviate a great deal of pain and stiffness, along with its consequences.

In the area of soft tissue injury treatment, some educators in the massage profession teach deeper pressures and stronger joint movements, outside of the massage therapy guidelines in this chapter. The variety of massage therapy approaches to soft tissue injury raises important questions: When should stronger techniques be used? How should they be used? And, most importantly: What qualifies practitioners to use them? How much training and clinical supervision is needed to practice them safely? As of this writing, there is little consensus among US massage therapists on standards of massage practice and education in injury work. Instead, a range of approaches are taught and practiced. With good specialized training in injury assessment and treatment, many advanced practitioners can work more with more focus, depth, and specificity than the limits suggested in this chapter. The guidelines introduced here are good reminders for all therapists, but are primarily designed for providers of basic relaxation massage.

Soft Tissue Injuries (Strain, Sprain, Tendinopathy, Tenosynovitis)

Injuries to soft tissue occur as a result of trauma, overstretch, and overuse. There are several types of soft tissue that can be injured, but the principal injuries are muscle strain, ligament sprain, tendinopathy, and tenosynovitis.

● BACKGROUND

The common types of soft tissue injuries are distinguished and defined as follows:

Muscle **strain** is an injury to muscle fibers, caused by too much pull on the muscle fibers or musculotendinous junction. It is commonly called a muscle pull. Muscle strains are often sudden, occurring in sports, or as a consequence of heavy lifting. A chronic strain can also occur from prolonged, repetitive use.

A **sprain** is an injury to ligament fibers that typically occurs when stress on a joint overstretches the ligament, for example, when a person pivots or lands incorrectly in sports, or steps into a hole while walking. Sprains are often the result of twisting at a joint.

Tendinopathy is a general term that describes injury and irritation of tendon. Two conditions that fall under this category are **tendinitis**, injury with an acute inflammatory component, and **tendinosis**, degeneration of the tendon without inflammation. Until recently, the pain of most tendon injuries was ascribed to inflammation, and thought to be tendinitis. Current understanding of tendon injuries suggests that many people have symptoms of tendinitis but no local inflammation or white blood cell involvement (Kahn, 2005). The tendon has simply degenerated, is not inflamed, and tendinosis is a more accurate term. Causes of this degeneration and weakening of the tendon include overuse, aging, repeated corticosteroid injections, trauma and underlying disease.

For those tendons that pass through a synovial sheath—for example, at the wrist, the thumb, the biceps muscle, or the ankle—both the tendon and the sheath can become inflamed. This condition is called **tenosynovitis**, and it is caused by repetitive movements and trauma. It can also be due to underlying disease such as rheumatoid arthritis, gout, diabetes, or gonorrheal infection.

Signs and Symptoms

In medicine, the challenge of diagnosing a soft tissue injury is twofold: first, there is a fair amount of symptom overlap between the three conditions. Second, typically more than one structure is injured at one time, and all can simultaneously be causing symptoms: swelling, pain, stiffness, and loss of strength, to varying degrees.

With an understanding of overlapping symptoms, a therapist is in a good position to work safely. Many people self-diagnose and self-treat their soft tissue injuries, and seek massage for first-line therapy. By being aware of the range of structures that might be injured, a massage therapist can refer a client for a proper medical diagnosis and treatment.

MUSCLE STRAIN

Muscle strains are classified into three grades. In **grade 1 strain** (mild), a few fibers are torn, there is some pain or tenderness, but

THERAPIST'S JOURNAL 8-1 *Massage After the Porch Accident: Therapy or Relaxation?*

It could have been a terrible accident: a second-floor porch peeled away from its moorings, dropping half a dozen people to the sidewalk below. But somehow, no one broke a bone or injured a spinal cord. Instead, people at this ill-fated gathering were left with sprains, strains, and plenty of bruises. They were dazed and traumatized, with sore backs and hips and heads.

And plenty of muscle tension.

Somehow two-thirds of them found their way to me for massage therapy, some for many months after the accident. This incident happened early in my career, before I learned SOAP charting (at the time, few massage therapists were documenting that way). I'd never coded for insurance, or written up a formal report for an insurance company or a court. I'd never worked with clients in litigation.

I got help from a co-treating therapist, from the clients' lawyer, and from reading all I could, so I picked up the paperwork steps pretty quickly. It was challenging, though, because I was not the most technically-oriented massage therapist. I did not have advanced training for clients with injuries, and was not experienced in working with scar tissue or rehabilitative work. In short, I provided relaxation massage.

Those of us who do relaxation massage are sometimes dismissed, because it is considered less than medical massage, orthopedic massage, or even therapeutic massage. These terms are yet to be clearly defined and universally understood in the profession, but they still carry the weight of our biases and assumptions.

As a provider of relaxation massage for the porch clients, my approach was, first, to wait for a physician's visit and negative x-rays in each case. My protocol: listening carefully for tension, respecting its role in splinting after trauma, and gently coaxing it free wherever it didn't seem useful. I used very gentle joint movement at first, to avoid overstretching anything. Later, as things loosened up, I used more stretching and extending the range of motion at each joint.

I continued to follow this plan with a few of these clients, through a long healing process and eventual litigation. I worked with them as they gradually released excess tension, received chiropractic care to realign their bodies, and resumed the physical demands of their lives. This included adjusting to a new worldview—one in which a porch cannot always be counted on to support body weight.

Looking back on that time, I wonder about the language in our field—it could use some clarification. A course of relaxation massage therapy turned out to be therapeutic, especially as an adjunct to other modalities. The role of muscle spasm in healing—to protect an injury as it heals—is well established, but at some point, spasm outlives its usefulness, and becomes a habit. Even beginning therapists, practicing relaxation massage, can bring about therapeutic change. As the profession grows, I hope that we choose ways to define ourselves and our work that are clear and precise, but not too limiting. Often healing knows no bounds, and it happens outside of the language you impose upon it.

Tracy Walton
Cambridge, MA

no loss of muscle strength or function. **Grade 2 strain** (moderate) involves a significant number of fibers, with stronger pain and some loss of muscle function. In **grade 3 strain** (severe), the muscle has completely ruptured, with loss of function. There may be bruising. Usually, there is severe pain, aggravated by movement and relieved by rest. Swelling is not usually noticeable in muscle strain unless it is severe.

Strains are common in the muscles of the low back (lumbar strain) or posterior thigh (hamstring pull). With extensive use, as in racquet sports, they can also occur in the forearm and hand.

LIGAMENT SPRAIN

Like muscle strains, ligament sprains are also classified in three grades. **Grade 1 sprain** (mild), involves stretching of the ligament fibers, or microscopic tears. It tends to take 1–2 weeks to heal. In **grade 2 sprain** (moderate), larger tears are present in a significant number of fibers, and healing usually takes 6 weeks. A grade 2 knee ligament sprain is shown in Figure 8-2. In **grade 3 sprain** (severe), complete rupture of the ligament occurs, and healing takes 6 months or more.

When acute, a sprain produces swelling, pain, and stiffness. Discoloration from bruising, warmth, and redness may also be present, depending on severity. But the cardinal sign of a sprain is pronounced swelling, which distinguishes it from other soft tissue injuries. The swelling from a sprain persists into the subacute period. Persistent swelling is especially likely in an ankle sprain, where gravity favors the pooling of fluid. The intense symptoms of a sprain, especially the swelling, can mask other injuries such as a fracture of bone in the area.

Sprains occur most often in the lateral ankle; they are also common to knees, fingers, the sacroiliac joint, and the neck.

TENDINOPATHY

Tendinopathy and muscle strain symptoms are similar, but stronger symptoms are usually present in tendinopathy. A key diagnostic indicator is pain, especially upon resisted movement of the involved muscle. Pain may also occur with stretching, and there is stiffness in the involved joint.

In the acute phase, tendinopathies may show heat and swelling, but the swelling is not usually remarkable unless it is an ankle injury. The pain and stiffness usually persist into the

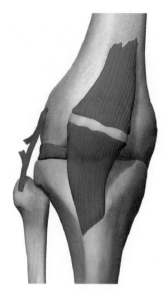

FIGURE 8-2. Grade 2 ligament sprain. Fibers of the lateral collateral ligament are torn.

subacute phase of the condition. Classic tendinitis injuries are named by their locations, as in achilles tendinitis, rotator cuff tendinitis, and tennis elbow (medial epicondylitis).

TENOSYNOVITIS

Tenosynovitis includes all of the inflammatory symptoms of tendinitis, and may also include a grinding sound, crepitus, with movement. It may be difficult to flex the joint, but even more difficult to extend it again. Tenosynovitis can occur wherever tendons are surrounded by synovial sheaths: the finger flexors (called trigger finger), the thumb (also called de Quervain tenosynovitis), the wrist, ankle, and long head of the biceps muscle.

Complications

A common complication of soft tissue injury is reinjury, compounded problems, and loss of function of an injured area. Weakening and tension in soft tissues reduce the ability to bear weight or carry a load. To address the soft tissue problem, the body lays down scar tissue quickly, but not neatly. This scar tissue is called fibrosis. Instead of laying fibers down in the same direction as the injured tissue, scar formation is in all directions. As shown in Figure 8-3, this haphazard organization is weaker than the original structure, as different layers of tissue become adhered to themselves, other layers, and unrelated structures nearby. Scar tissue causes pain and leaves the tissue more vulnerable to injury, the next time the structure is overstretched or overused.

Although all tissues are subject to the pitfalls of scar tissue, muscle strains tend to do the best healing, with the fewest complications. A sprained ligament is more serious: the structure is less elastic than muscle or tendon, and is made of dense fibers with little blood supply. This leaves a sprained ligament in a stretched position, no longer stabilizing the joint. It is vulnerable to recurring injury, which can worsen each time. Joint instability, resulting from the sprain, allows bones to slide and grate against each other, a condition that favors osteoarthritis (see Chapter 9) over time.

Tendinopathies, in which tendons weaken over time, lead to reinjury and a chronic condition of pain, stiffness, and loss of function. If the structure weakens too much, it can lead to rupture. Then, disordered scar tissue interferes with the natural movement and sliding of tendons across other structures, or through their tendon sheaths, leading to long-term pain and immobility.

Treatment

All three types of injuries cause pain, and are treated with OTC analgesics—medications that relieve pain. Of these, nonsteroidal anti-inflammatory drugs (NSAIDs) are commonly used. This class of medications acts against inflammation, fever, and pain (see "NSAIDs," Chapter 21). NSAIDS have numerous side effects and complications. These are often mild, but tend to be more problematic in older adults. Side effects include gastrointestinal upset, drowsiness, dizziness, and headache.

A mainstay of home treatment for soft tissue conditions is RICE, which stands for rest, ice, compression, and elevation. Rest from the aggravating activity prevents further injury to the area. Ice and compression are used to keep swelling and hypoxic damage to tissues in check. Elevation helps limit fluid pooling in the tissues of an extremity, and therefore reduce swelling. Protection or support provided by taping, a splint, or a brace may also be used, depending on the injury. The RICE approach is a conservative treatment; when done properly, there are few side effects.

While rest is essential, movement is also important to soft tissue healing. A gradual, thoughtful return to movement, working within pain tolerance, is vital. It is especially important to begin moving a joint in a sprain, to avoid scar tissue formation. Eccentric contractions are important to tendon regeneration. Movement helps exert tension on fibers, so that tissue rebuilds in an ordered, aligned fashion, rather than the chaotic disposition of scar tissue. Stretching is especially important for tendon and muscle injuries, to align scar tissue and give integrity to the healing structure.

The right balance of rest and exercise is important, as too much exercise can reinjure structures, causing or worsening inflammation. In the best situation, physical therapy provides the supervised return to exercise that a person needs after a soft tissue injury.

Corticosteroid injections may be used for pain relief and to deinflame an area, but this treatment is falling out of favor for two reasons: first, because it can cause further tissue degeneration, and second, because it does not help noninflammatory conditions such as tendinosis.

Treatment for tenosynovitis may include treatment for an underlying condition, such as antibiotics for infection. If these conservative measures are not successful, or if the structure has completely ruptured, surgical repair may be necessary. In tenosynovitis, the synovial membrane may need to be split surgically, to allow movement of the tendon inside the sheath.

● INTERVIEW QUESTIONS

1. Have you seen your doctor for it? Is there a diagnosis? Is it classified as mild, moderate, or severe?
2. Where is it?
3. When and how did you injure it? (See "Follow-Up Questions About Injuries," Chapter 4)

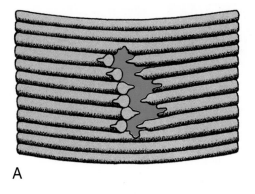

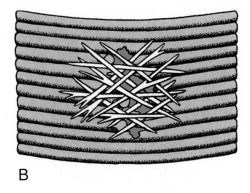

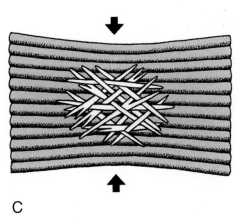

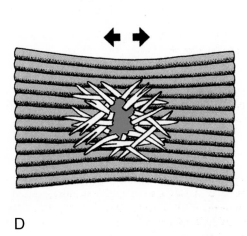

FIGURE 8-3. Scar tissue formation in soft tissue injuries. (A) Injured structure. (B) Scar tissue accumulates. (C) Scar tissue contracts: structural weak spot. (D) New injury at the site of scar tissue. (Adapted from Werner R. *A Massage Therapist's Guide to Pathology*, 4th ed. Philadelphia: Lippincott Williams and Wilkins, 2009.)

4. What are your symptoms? Is the condition acute or chronic? Do symptoms tend to recur?
5. Do you have pain? Does it hurt to use it, move it, or put weight on it? If you have pain, can you describe your pain? (See "Follow-Up Questions About Pain," Chapter 4)
6. Does the condition seem to be improving, worsening, or staying the same?
7. How is it being treated?
8. How do treatments affect you?

● MASSAGE THERAPY GUIDELINES

Massage therapists working with soft tissue injuries are more likely to help them heal (see "Possible Massage Benefits," this chapter) than aggravate them. There are many different massage therapy approaches to injury treatment; most of them require advanced professional training. In contrast, the guidelines presented here focus on massage care during the acute phase, and are designed to avoid overtreatment of a condition. For this purpose, guidelines for all four conditions—strain, sprain, tendinopathy, and tenosynovitis—are similar, and are grouped together on the Decision Tree in Figure 8-4.

The Pain, Inflammation, and Injury Principles (see Chapter 3) should be applied to each injury scenario. The follow-up questions about injuries and pain (see Chapter 4) should be used to determine when to apply these principles.

Although many people self-diagnose and self-treat their soft tissue injuries, and seek massage before seeking medical care, a therapist should view this common scenario with caution. There is a strong argument for avoiding pressure above level 2, friction, circulatory intent, and joint movement at the site of a soft tissue injury without a physician's diagnosis (question 1). This case can easily be made for acute cases, but can be argued for subacute situations as well. Soft tissue symptoms can mimic other serious conditions, such as a bone fracture or a blood clot.

If the client has seen a physician, question 1 may bring up additional information about the severity of the condition. If the client is self-diagnosing or self-treating, and the condition hasn't improved in 1–3 days, encourage him to report it to his physician to receive appropriate medical care. Soft tissue conditions tend to improve noticeably over time. Worsening symptoms, strong pain that limits use, new symptoms, pain with movement, neurological symptoms, and recurring

Soft Tissue Injuries (strain, sprain, tendinopathy, tenosynovitis)

Medical Information

Massage Therapy Guidelines

Essentials

- Muscle Strain: tear in muscle fibers, ranging from a few fibers (Grade 1, mild) to complete rupture (Grade 3, severe); pain with movement, loss of function (mild and severe cases), swelling and warmth (severe cases)

- Ligament sprain: tear in ligament fibers, ranging from a few fibers (Grade 1, mild) to complete rupture (Grade 3, severe); all grades feature pronounced swelling, pain, stiffness; warmth, redness, bruising likely in grades 2 and 3

- Tendinopathy: injury with inflammation (tendinitis) or non-inflammatory degradation of a tendon (tendinosis); pain on resisted movement of involved muscle, pain on stretch of tendon, stiffness

- Tenosynovitis: inflamed tendon and synovial sheath; pain, swelling, heat, stiffness, crepitus

- Physician's diagnosis necessary to rule out serious conditions (bone fracture, blood clot) before using friction, circulatory intent, pressure >2, or joint movement at site, whether acute or subacute

- During acute phase (pain, stiffness, swelling), avoid friction, circulatory intent at site (unless MT has training in advanced injury work and is working as part of a health care team); use gentle movement at site to tolerance

- During acute phase (pain, stiffness, swelling), use gentle pressure at site (pr 1-2 max, depending on tolerance); pressure exception: if mild or moderate muscle strain, careful massage with pr 3 max permitted at site if well tolerated, results monitored each session, pressure can increase in small increments to level 4 or 5 over course of treatment if well tolerated

- When subacute, re-introduce circulatory intent, deeper pressure levels, stronger movements in increments; physician consultation strongly advised, especially if multiple injuries present

- Consider Pain, Injury, and Inflammation Principles (see Chapter 3)

- Avoid joint movement that produces pain or overstretches injured tissue; special caution with neck, low back injuries

- If lower extremity injury, consider DVT Risk Principles (see Chapter 11)

- If self-diagnosed or self-treated, encourage medical referral; if pain is severe or unstable, mobility is limited, other symptoms occur, or condition is not improving 1-3 days after injury or aggravation of symptoms, strongly encourage medical referral

Complications

- Formation of scar tissue with weakened tissue, chronic symptoms, re-injury, rupture

- Osteoarthritis (from sprain and unstable joint)

- Follow guidelines for acute phase, above, especially for joint movement; medical referral if unreported

- See Osteoarthritis, Chapter 9

Medical treatment / Effects of treatment

Medical treatment	Effects of treatment
- OTC analgesics (NSAIDs)	- Numerous side effects possible, most mild, see Chapter 21 - GI disturbances - Headache - Drowsiness, dizziness
- Rest, ice, compression, elevation (RICE)	- Few side effects; none relevant to massage
- Corticosteroid injections	- Thinning of tissue at area
- Surgery	- See Surgery, Chapter 21, for side effects, complications
- Treatment of underlying disease (for tenosynovitis, gout, rheumatoid arthritis, others)	- Treatments for gout, rheumatoid arthritis, gonorrhea, etc.

- See NSAIDs, Chapter 21

- See Table 21-1 for common GI side effects and massage therapy guidelines
- Position for comfort, especially prone; consider inclined table or propping; gentle session overall; pressure to tolerance; slow speed and even rhythm; general circulatory intent may be poorly tolerated

- Reposition gently, slow speed and even rhythm, slow rise from table, gentle transition at end of session

- No significant massage adjustments

- Until medication absorbed, use gentle pressure (2 max); avoid circulatory intent at injection site
- Gentle movement and pressure at site if tissue integrity compromised

- Follow the Procedure Principle; see Surgery, Chapter 21.

- Use the Medication Principle or Procedure Principle, as necessary

FIGURE 8-4. A Decision Tree for soft tissue injuries.

injury are all red flags. (see "Follow-Up Questions About Pain, Follow-Up Questions About Injuries," Chapter 4).

> *The Physician Referral for Pain Principle. If a client's pain has specific qualities, such as sharp, stabbing, radiating, or shooting pain, or if the pain is accompanied by tingling, numbness, or weakness, refer the client to a physician.*

That being said, questions 2–6 provide key background information, and help to establish whether the injury is chronic or acute. In the acute phase, avoid all of the massage elements described above, in order to avoid aggravating inflammation. Continue this approach if reinjury has occured. Therapists with injury treatment skills often use deep transverse friction in order to bring about a therapeutic inflammation, bring down scar tissue, and help the tissue mend with integrity. This approach requires good assessment skills and a clear diagnosis, and should not be attempted casually.

An exception to the pressure caution is in diagnosed muscle strain: Pressure level 3 may be a good starting pressure, and a gradual increase in pressure to level 4 or 5 may be exactly what is needed over time. Most therapists can work on a lumbar or hamstring strain safely at level 3, taking care to position the client well and monitor the results over time.

Although sprains benefit from a fair amount of movement to keep the joint flexible, the pronounced swelling of a sprain makes it especially likely to mask another serious condition. Movement at the joint is best done in close communication with the physician or as part of a health care team. If ligaments of the neck are sprained, see "Whiplash," this chapter.

Once a soft tissue injury enters the subacute phase—any inflammation has subsided, and the symptoms have significantly and steadily been improving—stronger massage elements may be helpful. Some muscle tension is still needed to stabilize the area, and protect it from further injury as the tissue heals. Obviously, joint movement should not overstretch an area. But stronger massage and movement can remove excess, unnecessary tension, interrupting the pain-spasm-pain cycle.

> *The Pain-Spasm-Pain Principle. Relief of excess muscle tension around an injured or painful area may lead to pain relief, apart from the original cause of the pain.*

In most soft tissue injuries, pressure and movement can be increased in increments, while monitoring a client's response over a course of treatment. Strains, sprains, and tendinitis may all benefit from this gradual increase. Sprains may respond especially well to increasing friction, pressure, and circulatory intent at the site during the subacute phase, and movement of the joint is useful to help healing. However, tendinosis, with a less clear acute-subacute delineation, may feature symptoms that come and go. Because it's less clear whether tendinosis is getting better, stronger massage elements are offered cautiously.

If osteoarthritis forms at this site, see chapter 9. If the injury affects a lower extremity, consider the DVT Risk Principles (see Chapter 11). Recent research (van Stralen et al., 2008) suggests that minor soft tissue injuries to the lower extremity may elevate the risk of blood clots. As always, stay alert for DVT symptoms and consider a client's DVT risk factors when working with the thighs and lower legs.

Most clients will respond to questions 7 and 8 with conservative treatment: mild analgesics and RICE. If the client is taking NSAIDs, mild side effects are possible; massage guidelines for some common side effects are described on the Decision Tree in Figure 8-4. If the client reports any additional side effects of treatments, refer to "NSAIDs," Chapter 21.

If the client has had a corticosteroid injection, limit pressure and circulatory intent at the injection site until the drug is absorbed. Pressure and movement should also remain gentle (in the 1–2 range) if multiple corticosteroid injections have been done at a site over time, leading to thinning of tissue.

If the problem was corrected surgically, see Chapter 21 for massage guidelines after surgery. If another underlying disease is also being treated (as in diabetes, for tenosynovitis), adapt the session to the medication or procedure being used, as well as the underlying condition.

● MASSAGE RESEARCH

At the time of this writing, the effects of massage on specific soft tissue injuries are difficult to isolate in the body of literature. Studies do not often delineate between strains, sprains, and tendinopathies. Instead, most studies focus on the more general topic of musculoskeletal pain without isolating a clear diagnosis or cause. Enough studies exist for a Cochrane review on low back pain (Furlan et al., 2008). The authors looked at massage for nonspecific low back pain, which means back pain with no detectable cause. This classification opens up the study to many possible causes such as soft tissue injury, an inflammatory process, or osteoporosis. The reviewers concluded that massage might be beneficial for people with low back pain. It specifically identifies subacute (lasting 4–12 weeks) and chronic (lasting longer than 12 weeks) back pain, and found that massage was more likely to be helpful when combined with exercises and education than when used alone. Reviewers noticed more favorable outcomes with eastern massage than with classic Swedish techniques, but noted that this needed confirmation. One Cochrane review looked at deep transverse friction massage and tendinitis (Brosseau et al., 2002) and found the available studies inconclusive. Although the data are not yet published at the time of this writing, at least one large RCT has compared relaxation massage and focused, structural massage in chronic low back pain (Cherkin et al., 2009).

● POSSIBLE MASSAGE BENEFITS

With a course of treatment, or even an occasional single session, massage therapists have observed improvement in symptoms of soft tissue injuries. Clients report less restriction, freer movement, and less pain. Skilled massage, often with deep pressure and a fair amount of specificity, seems to have an impact. Whether symptom relief turns out to be a true effect of massage will have to wait for more research. Best practice for injuries will no doubt emerge from the profession in the coming years, and our understanding of the mechanisms of massage will grow. At that time, some of the theoretical foundations of the massage profession—well-placed friction can reduce adhesions, and circulatory intent can reduce swelling—may be borne out, as well. The interest in massage for pain is building, and perhaps future studies will identify a role for massage with specific injuries.

Whiplash

Whiplash is a collection of injuries to the neck from a sudden sharp movement, as in a motor vehicle collision. The neck is thrown into hyperextension and hyperflexion in a manner that resembles the lash of a whip.

● BACKGROUND

Many soft tissues can be injured in a single accident, including muscles and ligaments. In particular, supraspinous and intertransverse ligaments are often sprained. The sternocleidomastoid muscles, scalenes, and splenius cervicis are often strained. Joint capsules and disks may be damaged, and the motion can throw cervical vertebrae out of alignment.

Signs and Symptoms

Signs and symptoms often take a day or two to begin manifesting, and some symptoms can take weeks to intensify. Symptoms include neck and shoulder pain, stiffness, and muscle spasm, which set off the pain-spasm-pain cycle. Irritation to nerves can cause headaches, dizziness, blurred vision, and difficulty in swallowing. Fatigue is common.

Complications

Radiculopathy occurs when injuries compress and irritate nerve roots in the area, causing nervous system symptoms. If whiplash is accompanied by numbness, tingling, severe pain, or motor weakness in the shoulders or arms, the situation could be serious. Chronic whiplash problems can persist, such as headaches, pain in the neck and lumbar area, fatigue, and problems sleeping, plus tingling in the upper extremities.

Treatment

Right after an accident, emergency responders immobilize the neck to prevent further injury until doctors can determine the extent of the damage. If there is no fracture, the pain of whiplash can be treated with analgesics, anti-inflammatories, and possibly muscle relaxants. Some practitioners use cold therapy to de-inflame tissues.

Neck collars, used to immobilize and support the neck, are falling out of favor in the treatment of whiplash. Instead, the value of returning to movement is becoming clear, and patients are urged to do so as soon as they can tolerate it. Range of motion exercises such as neck rotation may be recommended as early as 4 days after the accident. Physical therapy may be prescribed to help move and strengthen the area; ultrasound and other techniques are also used. Spinal manipulation, provided by an osteopath or chiropractor, may facilitate healing.

● INTERVIEW QUESTIONS

1. When did the injury occur? (See "Follow-Up Questions About Injuries," Chapter 4)
2. Describe your symptoms: mild, moderate, severe? Are they easy to manage?
3. If you have pain, can you describe your pain? (See "Follow-Up Questions About Pain," Chapter 4)
4. What aggravates and relieves your symptoms? Does movement of your neck in any direction aggravate your symptoms? If so, is the pain sudden or stabbing?
5. How stable does the area feel?
6. Are there complications of your whiplash? Any severe pain, tingling, weakness, or headaches?
7. Have you seen your doctor and received a diagnosis?
8. How is it being treated?
9. How does treatment affect you?

● MASSAGE THERAPY GUIDELINES

Because whiplash is a collection of strains and sprains, many of the guidelines for soft tissue conditions can be applied. However, an additional layer of caution is in order because of the heightened vulnerability of the neck, and the proximity to the spinal cord and nerve roots. Although most whiplash injuries heal in a matter of weeks, some persist and become disabling, and injuries to neck structures can be serious.

Review the Pain, Injury, and Inflammation Principles before working directly with the area. In particular, note whether litigation or insurance claims are pending. If so, provide cautious massage, and document it well.

> *The Claim or Litigation Principle.* **If a client's recent injury involves an insurance claim or litigation, do not complicate the clinical picture with massage that could aggravate the condition.**

Recall that significant time lags are possible between the injury and the development of symptoms. Often a minor car accident seems inconsequential at first, and the individual may brush off the need to see a doctor. But symptoms may first appear, and continue to develop, over weeks following an accident. Strongly encourage an urgent medical referral if the client hasn't seen his or her doctor yet. With a client who comes in after an accident, complaining of minor stiffness, be cautious. Without a physician's diagnosis, ruling out fracture and other problems, it is nearly impossible to provide massage safely; instead, limit pressure to level 1, and provide no movement at all. The guidelines below assume a physician's diagnosis is in place.

Questions 1–6 provide important background on the injury and a context for the role of massage. Together with the follow-up questions from Chapter 4 about injuries and pain, they provide good coverage of possible massage issues.

If symptoms are acute, hard to manage, or unstable, massage pressure should remain in the 1–2 range. Any movement should be extremely gentle. This goes for complications of whiplash, as well, when neurological symptoms are present, or when whiplash syndrome has set in. In these cases, medical consultation is needed for anything stronger. Position the neck comfortably in a neutral position.

> *The Stabilization of an Acute Condition Principle.* **Until an acute medical condition has stabilized, massage should be conservative.**

Whiplash

Medical Information	Massage Therapy Guidelines

Essentials

- Cervical strains and sprains, caused by sudden impact; usually from rear-end collision

- Injury to joints, disks, vertebrae

- Acute phase: moderate to severe pain, unstable pain, neurologic symptoms (headaches, dizziness, tingling, motor weakness), stiffness

- Reduced ROM (acute and chronic)

- Consider all Pain, Injury, and Inflammation Principles (Chapter 3)

- If unreported to physician, urgent medical referral; without physician's diagnosis, avoid movement at neck and limit pressure to level 1 max until fracture, joint injury, disk injury ruled out (follow Recent Injury Principle, Claim or Litigation Principle)

- Avoid friction at site (unless MT has advanced injury training and works as part of an integrated health care team)

- Use gentle pressure at site (pressure 1-2 max, depending on tolerance), gentle movement at site; position for comfort and neutral neck; medical consultation required for stronger work

- At all times: avoid joint movement that produces pain or overstretches injured tissue; wait for client's ROM to return to normal before moving joints at site; medical consultation advised

Complications

- Pain, tingling, motor weakness from injury

- Whiplash syndrome: ongoing neck and lower back pain, headaches, fatigue, sleeping problems

---

- Follow guidelines for acute phase and reduced ROM, above

- Follow guidelines for acute phase and reduced ROM, above

Medical treatment | Effects of treatment |

- OTC analgesics (NSAIDs)

  - Numerous side effects possible, most mild, see Chapter 21

  - GI disturbances

  - Headache

  - Drowsiness, dizziness

- Muscle relaxants

  - Drowsiness, dizziness
  - CNS suppression
  - Constipation

- Physical therapy

  - Side effects, complications unlikely

- Spinal manipulation

  - Side effects, complications unlikely

- See NSAIDs, Chapter 21

- See Table 21-1 for common GI side effects and Massage Therapy Guidelines

- Position for comfort, especially prone; consider inclined table or propping; gentle session overall; pressure to tolerance; slow speed and even rhythm; general circulatory intent may be poorly tolerated

- Reposition gently, slow speed and even rhythm, slow rise from table, gentle transition at end of session

- See OTC analgesics, above

- Gentle pressure overall
- Gentle pressure at abdomen (level 2 max); medical referral if client has not had a bowel movement for several days

- No contraindications; consult with PT to ensure coordinated care

- No contraindications; consult with practitioner to ensure coordinated care

FIGURE 8-5. A Decision Tree for whiplash.

Some therapists have advanced skills in injury treatment, with training in whiplash, and may be able to do deeper, more focused work safely than a basic practitioner. Both basic and advanced practitioners are advised to work in collaboration with a client's physician. (See Figure 5-2, Chapter 5 for physician correspondence about a client's whiplash). In either case, document closely to reinforce that the work was done safely.

Once the injury is healing well, the client's range of motion has significantly improved, and the area is stable, less caution may be needed. Deeper pressures in the 3 and 4 ranges may be possible, but keep the attention to the area brief, monitor the client's responses over time, and increase pressure in small increments. Joint movement should also be cautious; do not do joint movement that overstretches the area, or produces pain. In most cases, massage therapists should not be stretching the neck; this should be left to other practitioners such as a physical therapist. Allow the splinting muscles to release gradually over a course of massage treatment, rather than forcing them in a single session.

The Respect Muscle Splinting Principle. **Do not try to eliminate muscle tension that may be protecting an area of injury, pain, or disease.**

If a particular client has received symptom relief from massage in the past, make an attempt to approximate the previous massage methods used. A client's physical therapist can be a helpful guide for the massage therapist in terms of joint movement and pressure.

Questions 8 and 9 determine whether there are other treatment modalities or medications. Medications that are commonly used in whiplash—NSAIDs and muscle relaxants—have some side effects. The Decision Tree in Figure 8-5 lists some of the side effects and massage guidelines; others may be found in Chapter 21. If the client is using any manual therapies such as physical therapy, osteopathy, or chiropractic care, communication with those practitioners can enhance the client's care, and prevent working at cross-purposes.

● MASSAGE RESEARCH

At the time of this writing, there is little research, published in the English language, focused on massage and whiplash. Research reviews tend to focus on multiple modalities, grouped under search terms such as "manipulation" or "conservative treatment" (Verhagen et al., 2007). Given that whiplash can involve multiple injuries and multiple tissue types, research on multiple treatment approaches makes sense.

One Cochrane review of massage therapy surveyed mechanical neck disorders, those thought to be due to simple, minor strains and sprains (Haraldsson et al., 2006). Reviewers found studies of uneven quality and concluded that there was insufficient evidence to say whether massage is helpful. Clearly, more research is needed on massage and whiplash, and whiplash in general.

● POSSIBLE MASSAGE BENEFITS

Although earlier therapy for whiplash used an immobilizing neck collar, it is now recognized that neck movement is essential to healing from whiplash. By easing muscle spasm, massage has the potential to facilitate movement, and to remove restrictions to blood circulation in the healing tissues. By disrupting the pain-spasm-pain cycle, massage may relieve pain. Done carefully and well, massage may help reduce the role of muscle tension in whiplash symptoms.

Advanced practitioners with specialized assessment and treatment skills may be able to facilitate deeper healing in whiplash. Ideally, they have good training, supervised clinic experience, and continued access to instructors and mentors, as well as strong bonds with the client's health care team.

Fibromyalgia Syndrome

The term fibromyalgia syndrome (FMS), also known as *fibromyositis* or *fibrositis* (or fibromyalgia for short), describes a group of chronic pain conditions characterized by widespread pain in muscles, fatigue, weakness, and sleep disturbances. FMS pain is experienced throughout the body, rather than in one particular region. There are nine pairs of characteristic tender points, located at or near the occiput, lower cervical area, second rib, trapezius, supraspinatus, lateral epicondyle, gluteal muscles, greater trochanter, and medial knee (Figure 8-6).

● BACKGROUND

Fibromyalgia is poorly understood, because no abnormality is visible in the affected muscles. The cause is unknown. Triggers may include physical or emotional trauma, an infectious agent such as a virus, or even sleep disturbances. The signs and symptoms overlap with those of many other conditions, some of which are inflammatory conditions, including lupus. However, there is no true inflammation with fibromyalgia.

Signs and Symptoms

The cardinal symptom of fibromyalgia is pain, and it spans a wide spectrum. Some patients describe it as achy, throbbing, burning, or flu-like. It is often worse in the morning. The pain is chronic, persistent, and diffuse, or widespread. It is experienced as soreness, stiffness, or a deep ache in the muscles. It may also include numbness and tingling. The pain often concentrates in the tender point areas. People with FMS may have very low pain tolerance, and may feel pain in response to other stimuli such as cold or pressure.

Other symptoms of FMS include debilitating fatigue and low energy, often also described as a constant flu-like experience. Fatigue ranges from mild to incapacitating, interfering with daily activities, and no amount of daytime or nighttime rest alleviates it. For a fibromyalgia diagnosis, the following minimum criteria are used:

- The person has experienced chronic pain for at least 3 months.
- At least 11 of the 18 characteristic tender point locations are active; in response to minimal pressure from a finger, the person feels significant, diffuse pain.
- The active tender points are all not concentrated in one place; some from each body quadrant are represented.
- The person experiences persistent fatigue.
- The person awakens tired and stiff in the morning, as sleep is nonrestorative.

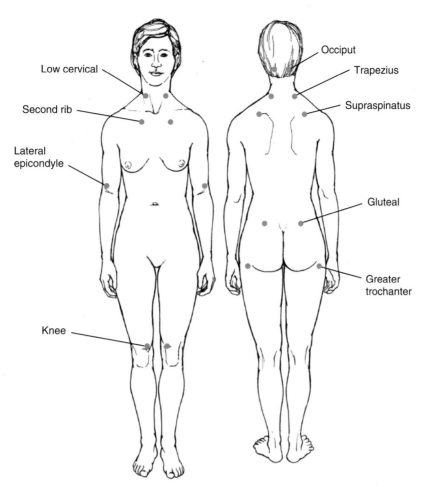

FIGURE 8-6. Tender points in fibromyalgia syndrome (From Werner R. *A Massage Therapist's Guide to Pathology*, 2nd ed. Philadelphia: Lippincott Williams and Wilkins, 2002.)

There is significant overlap between FMS and several other conditions. This means that people with fibromyalgia might also have other conditions diagnosed (*comorbidities*), or the conditions simply share symptoms. The two most common comorbidities are irritable bowel syndrome (see Chapter 15) and chronic fatigue syndrome (CFS). **Chronic fatigue syndrome (CFS)** is characterized by chronic fatigue along with memory and concentration difficulties, sore throat, tender lymph nodes, muscle and joint pain, and other symptoms.

There is also some overlap in symptoms between FMS and rheumatological diseases, such as lupus and rheumatoid arthritis. Many of the same symptoms are produced by these diseases, although they are inflammatory conditions, and there is no inflammation associated with the pain of fibromyalgia. Some cancers, HIV infection, and Lyme disease have similar symptoms.

People with FMS may also have migraine headaches (see Chapter 10), TMJ syndrome (see Chapter 9) and restless leg syndrome. **Restless leg syndrome** is a condition of uncomfortable sensations, usually in the lower legs, occurring at night in bed, that are relieved by leg movement. There is symptom overlap between FMS and hypothyroidism (see Chapter 17), multiple chemical sensitivities, candidiasis (yeast overgrowth), and celiac disease (see Chapter 15).

The prognosis for FMS is variable. Some people's symptoms improve; others worsen or remain the same for months or years after the onset.

Complications

One common complication of fibromyalgia is depression (see Chapter 10). Another is sleep loss, which can be part of a vicious cycle. Poor sleep aggravates other symptoms, which, in turn, interfere with sleep. The resulting fatigue worsens the psychological complications of the disease.

Feelings of frustration and despair are common, because a firm diagnosis can take a long time; there are no definitive imaging tests or laboratory markers. People with fibromyalgia visit an average of five physicians before obtaining a FMS diagnosis. Due to the disease's invisibility, it can be profoundly isolating.

Treatment

Milder cases of fibromyalgia may respond to lifestyle changes and stress reduction. In the United States, pregabalin (Lyrica), an antiseizure drug, is the first FDA-approved medication for fibromyalgia treatment. Another antiseizure medication, gabapentin (Neurontin), is also used. Side effects of these antiseizure drugs, also called *anticonvulsants*, may include sedation, dizziness, swelling in the lower legs, and weight gain. However, most people taking these medications tolerate them well.

Low-dose antidepressants are used for FMS to relieve depression and pain, improve sleep, relax muscles, and activate the release of endorphins. Because nonrestorative sleep is a problem in people who have FMS, a low-dose sedating antidepressant may be used before bedtime. A less sedating or more activating antidepressant such as sertraline (Zoloft) or fluoxetine (Prozac) may be used in the morning.

NSAIDs are also used for pain relief in fibromyalgia, even though there is no inflammatory element in FMS to act upon. However, NSAIDs can be useful in combination with other drugs. Acetaminophen (Tylenol) may help. Side effects tend to be mild (see "NSAIDs," Chapter 21). An opioid analgesic called tramadol (Ultram), in an extended-release preparation, is used for pain flare-ups, or to give the person a break from antidepressant use for several weeks. Its long-term use is discouraged. Tramadol can cause dizziness, diarrhea, and sleep disturbances when used for chronic pain as in fibromyalgia.

● INTERVIEW QUESTIONS

1. How long have you had symptoms of fibromyalgia? When were you diagnosed?
2. What are your symptoms? What are your specific tender point areas? Can you describe your pain? (See "Follow-Up Questions for Pain," Chapter 4)
3. How do your symptoms respond to touch? To pressure? To stretching? To different positions? Are there other stimuli or triggers?
4. How are you sleeping? Do you know how your sleep is affected by massage?
5. Do your symptoms appear in cycles, with good and bad times of day, week, or month?
6. How is your condition being treated?
7. How does the treatment affect you?

● MASSAGE THERAPY GUIDELINES

The client's answer to question 1 may suggest a significant time period between the date of onset and the date of diagnosis, since people often experience symptoms for months or years before obtaining a diagnosis. You'll also find out whether a physician's diagnosis is part of the picture, as people often self-diagnose.

In response to questions 2–5, be prepared for a range of client presentations. In mild cases, clients are highly functional but have some ongoing pain. Some clients tolerate and benefit from a stronger massage without aggravating tender point pain. But in most moderate or severe cases, clients are hypersensitive to mild stimuli, and such pressure on the tissues may activate debilitating pain and fatigue.

Take care not to overtreat at first, avoiding pressure that is too strong. An overall pressure of 1–2 is the best for a client who reports moderate to severe pain. An overall pressure of 3 may be possible for a client with mild symptoms, with a history of good tolerance of massage pressure. Over a course of treatment, you may be able to increase the overall pressure to level 4, with good results.

When asking about symptoms, pay attention, first, to the involved muscles and the pain levels. Ask the client to point to the areas, which may be tender upon gentle palpation and painful with even more pressure. Record these points and avoid any pressure, stretch, joint movement, or other stimuli that might cause pain. Be mindful of any positions or other factors (even cold or heat) that might aggravate pain.

For tender points, pressure level 1 or 2 is a good start for most clients, until you find out how each point responds to massage. If using joint movement, introduce it slowly so that the involved muscles are not overstretched. If the client has moderate or severe pain, it's a good idea to use slow speeds and even, predictable rhythms.

If the client mentions other symptoms such as headache or irritable bowel syndrome, guidelines for those conditions may be found in other chapters; see the Decision Tree, Figure 8-7, for specific locations. If the client reports restless leg syndrome, massage is unlikely to aggravate it, although it makes common sense to follow the same guidelines as for sleep problems, below.

Question 4 about sleep should be helpful in designing the session. The answer to Question 5 about cyclical symptoms might help in this regard. Massage with activating and stimulating effects should be confined to earlier in the day, and more sedating approaches may be used toward bedtime.

Be sensitive to the psychological and psychosocial complications of fibromyalgia. If a client seems depressed, see Chapter 10 for signs and symptoms, and thoughtful interview questions that can help you to make a good medical referral. He or she may feel frustrated and desperate after rounds and rounds of medical appointments, perhaps without success or help, for a long time. Sensitivity and compassion are in order even if the client chooses not to discuss his or her emotions explicitly. As with any chronic illness, do not rush in to judge, hypothesize, speculate, or offer advice about the condition; it's likely that client's heard it all before. Stick to massage therapy, being a good witness and companion for his or her health journey, and offer whatever simple support you can provide in the context of massage.

Questions 6 and 7 may yield treatments with side effects that require massage adjustments, principally for antidepressant and pain medications. Adapt the session to the effects of antiseizure medication, low dose antidepressants, NSAIDs, or opioid analgesics. Massage therapy guidelines for antiseizure medications are fairly straightforward, listed in the Decision Tree in Figure 8-7. Note the different uses of antidepressants: low dose for pain, which causes milder side effects, and full dose for depression, which causes stronger side effects. Side effects and massage guidelines for low doses are discussed in Table 10-1; see "Depression," Chapter 10, for full dose treatment and its effects. Opioid analgesics have numerous side effects (see Chapter 21), although low doses of these medications are used in fibromyalgia.

● MASSAGE RESEARCH

Research on massage therapy and fibromyalgia is limited. Only a small RCT suggests massage to reduce fibromyalgia pain, increase sleep, and reduce anxiety and depression (Field et al., 2002). One research review found only modest research support for massage in fibromyalgia (Tsao, 2007); another found moderate research support for it (Schneider et al., 2009). One study looked at fibromyalgia and massage with a mechanistic approach, evaluating urine samples along with subjective stress measures (Lund et al., 2006). The authors did not make conclusive statements about massage, but called for more research.

At the time of this writing, the National Center for Complementary and Alternative Medicine (NCCAM) is funding a study of the mechanisms of massage therapy in normal volunteers, designed to untangle some of the physiological effects of massage, and the relief it seems to provide for a broad range of conditions, including fibromyalgia. Clearly, research interest in massage is growing, and additions to the literature may come at any moment.

Fibromyalgia (FMS)

Medical Information	Massage Therapy Guidelines

Essentials

- Bodywide chronic, persistent pain for at least 3 months, persistent fatigue, nonrestorative sleep, tiredness and stiffness on rising

- Tenderness on palpation at 11 of 18 tender points; low pain tolerance; hypersensitivity to pressure, cold

- Other conditions such as headaches, restless leg syndrome, irritable bowel syndrome, TMJ syndrome, chronic fatigue syndrome

→ Conservative massage at first, monitor results; do not overtreat; if pain moderate or severe, gentle pressure overall (pr 1-2 max), slow speed, even rhythm

→ Gentle pressure (pr 1-2 max) on involved muscles; do not overstretch during joint movements; monitor results at first; use deeper pressure only if initial responses are favorable

→ Adapt to signs, symptoms, and treatments for each condition (see Headache, Chapter 10; IBS, Chapter 15; TMJ syndrome, Chapter 9)

Complications

- Depression

- Sleep loss

- Frustration, despair

→ See Chapter 10

→ Toward end of the day, use sedating strokes; at beginning or middle of day, use stimulating strokes that increase energy

→ Sensitivity; compassionate, nonjudgmental listening

Medical treatment	Effects of treatment	
- Lifestyle changes, stress reduction	- None relevant to massage	→ - No massage adjustments
- Anti-seizure medication	- Sedation, dizziness	→ - Reposition gently, slow speed and even rhythm, slow rise from table, gentle transition at end of session
	- Swelling in lower legs	→ - No circulatory intent at site; use gentle pressure at site, 2 max
	- Weight gain	- No significant massage adjustments
- Low dose antidepressants	- Numerous side effects possible, most mild, see Table 10-1	→ - See Table 10-1
- OTC analgesics (NSAIDs)	- Numerous side effects possible, most mild, see Chapter 21	→ - See NSAIDs, Chapter 21
	- GI disturbances	→ - See Table 21-1 for common GI side effects and massage therapy guidelines
	- Headache	→ - Position for comfort, especially prone; consider inclined table or propping; gentle session overall; pressure to tolerance; slow speed and even rhythm; general circulatory intent may be poorly tolerated
	- Drowsiness, dizziness	→ - Reposition gently, slow speed and even rhythm, slow rise from table, gentle transition at end of session
- Opioid analgesics	- Numerous side effects possible, see Chapter 21	→ - See Opioid Analgesics, Chapter 21

FIGURE 8-7. A Decision Tree for fibromyalgia syndrome.

● POSSIBLE MASSAGE BENEFITS

Many clients with fibromyalgia seek massage. Therapists report easing pain, relaxing symptomatic muscles, and improved sleep. Both exercise and stress relief are encouraged for people with fibromyalgia to help ease symptoms. However, exercise is often the last thing an individual feels like doing, because of the pain and fatigue of FMS. Common sense suggests that massage therapy can support whatever level of exercise the client can maintain, by relaxing muscles, preventing injury, and promoting body awareness. The emotional support of the therapist, combined with skilled touch, has the potential to make the disease less isolating for the individual experiencing it.

Muscular Dystrophy

Muscular Dystrophy describes a group of conditions, all involving progressive muscle weakness. They are usually inherited conditions that most often affect males. The two most common are Duchenne (affecting 1 in 3,600 boys born) and Becker (affecting 3 in 100,000 boys born). Other, less common types of muscular dystrophy affect both males and females.

● BACKGROUND

Muscles have a structural protein called dystrophin, needed to contract. When genes responsible for muscular dystrophy are expressed, the dystrophin does not function. In Duchenne muscular dystrophy (DMD), dystrophin production is severely impaired, and it causes a severe, rapid progression or disease. In Becker muscular dystrophy (BMD), dystrophin is still partly functional; the disease is milder and progresses more slowly. Poor dystrophin production leads to muscle contracture. Contracture is a term describing the permanent shortening and often shrinking of soft tissue. When it occurs in muscle tissue, it leads to compressed and fixated joints, impaired movement, and uneven pull on the skeleton, pulling it out of alignment.

Signs and Symptoms

The condition typically causes changes in gait, difficulty pulling up from a sitting position, and then weakness in other muscles. In Duchenne muscular dystrophy (DMD), early signs generally involve the lower extremities, including a developmental delay in walking. Later, falling, difficulty walking, and difficulty climbing stairs occurs, and between ages 3 and 7, a waddling gait. The calves become pseudohypertrophic, noticeably enlarged with connective tissue and fat. Pseudohypertrophy is the enlargement of an organ or tissue as its functional tissue is replaced by fatty or fibrous tissue.

As the condition advances, upper body effects include weakness in shoulder muscles and formation of contractures in muscles around joints, making extension difficult. The ability to walk is usually lost during this time, by age 13 at the latest. The muscle groups affected in DMD are shown in Figure 8-8. Enlargement of the heart accompanies most cases of DMD.

In Becker muscular dystrophy (BMD), signs and symptoms tend to appear in puberty, the weakness is milder, and the worst effects are on the pelvis and lower extremities. A person with BMD is less likely to need the use of a wheelchair than a person with DMD.

Some people with muscular dystrophy—about a third of those with DMD—have learning disabilities. They may struggle with attention, verbal learning, and emotional interactions. A few individuals have more serious developmental delays.

There are several other muscular dystrophies that are less severe, with less pronounced weakness, later onset, and more focused areas of disease. In many cases, the effects on activities of daily living are minimal.

Complications

Complications of muscular dystrophy include scoliosis, a lateral curvature of the spine which becomes more pronounced as the disease progresses. Scoliosis can cause pain and motor difficulties, and severe malformation can impair lung function.

Muscle weakness can also give rise to breathing problems, making the person susceptible to pneumonia. This is compounded by dysphagia, difficulty in swallowing. Problems in the later stages of the disease occur when individuals aspirate food and saliva, drawing it into the airway and setting the stage for respiratory infection. Osteoporosis can lead to bone fracture, with the most serious consequences in the spine. In some cases, the heart muscle becomes weak and enlarged, and this cardiomyopathy can lead to heart failure; people with muscular dystrophy also experience heart arrhythmias (see Chapter 11). For most people with DMD, death occurs in the 20s or early 30s; those with BMD tend to live past their 40s and 50s.

Treatment

There is no cure for muscular dystrophy. As with many motor disorders, physical therapy is prescribed for strength and flexibility, and massage is used to prevent disabling contractures. Assistive devices such as braces, walkers, and wheelchairs help people with mobility, and breathing assistance with assisted ventilation is begun at night, then expanded to daytime as breathing problems progress. People with muscular dystrophy sometimes have surgery to treat severely contracted muscles.

Corticosteroid medication (such as prednisone) can be used to help the person maintain strength, as it has been observed to prolong the ability to walk. However, its use is controversial because of the effects of prolonged use. For this reason, it is usually used only in severe cases.

● INTERVIEW QUESTIONS

1. What kind of muscular dystrophy do you have?
2. Which muscles are affected? How?
3. How does it affect your mobility?
4. If you have muscle pain, where is it? Please describe the pain (see "Follow-Up Questions for Pain," Chapter 3).
5. Is your spine affected in any way, or the stability of your bones? Any osteoporosis?
6. Is your breathing affected?
7. Is your swallowing affected?
8. Does it affect your heart function? Is the effect significant?
9. What positions are comfortable for you? Which muscles do you use to position and reposition yourself?
10. What kind of treatment have you received? How does treatment affect you?

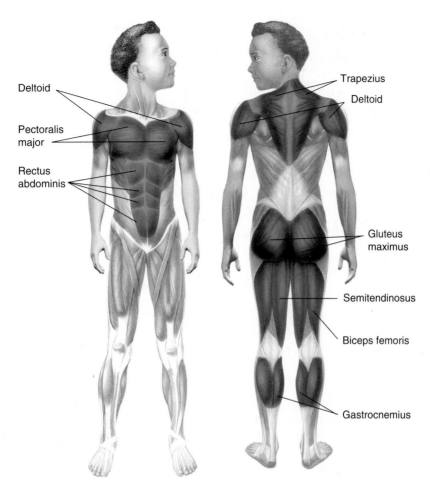

FIGURE 8-8. Muscle groups affected in Duchenne muscular dystrophy. (Asset Provided by Anatomical Chart Company.)

● MASSAGE THERAPY GUIDELINES

The massage plan depends on the extent of the client's symptoms and any mobility impairment. Contractures typically respond favorably to massage and movement. Any need for assistance in massage positioning should become clear in the interview. Questions 1–3 help highlight these matters, and whether the client's lower extremities are affected. If the client's lower extremities are immobilized, then consider the DVT Risk Principles (see Chapter 11).

More serious complications of MD are addressed by questions 4–8. Scoliosis may be present, which could require a positioning adjustment. Osteoporosis calls for gentle pressure overall, likely in the 1–3 range (see "Osteoporosis," Chapter 9). Find out if bone and spine stability is a concern; consult with the client's physician before attempting pressure level 3, especially on the back.

If breathing or swallowing is impaired, adjust massage positions for client comfort and safety. With many breathing problems, lying flat, whether prone or supine, can cause difficulty and anxiety. For ease of both breathing and swallowing, an inclined position may be the best. Raising one end of the table may be sufficient, or bolstering the upper body with pillows. The sidelying position can help discomfort, and a seated position may be ideal. A client with a tracheostomy or other breathing device may require position modifications to avoid compressing the tubing or equipment.

If the client's heart function is compromised, find out whether the impairment is significant, and review Chapter 11 for related issues in congestive heart failure and arrhythmia. Apply the Activity And Energy Principle to determine whether general circulatory intent is advisable, and consult the physician if there is still a question. Figure 8-10 shows areas on the body affected in muscular dystrophy, along with the corresponding massage therapy guidelines.

The client's answer to question 9 can reinforce positioning decisions, and identify the most heavily used muscles, that are likely to benefit from massage. Question 10 will trigger answers such as surgery, corticosteroid medication, or even heart medication if there is cardiomyopathy.

If the client has had surgery to release a tendon, do not resume stretching at the joint until it is stable; consult the physician for guidance. If surgery was performed to straighten and fuse the spine, be gentle with pressure until it has stabilized; again, consult the physician for guidance. The risk of major complications after surgery is heightened for patients with muscular dystrophy, so that massage in the early weeks after surgery may need to be extremely gentle. Adjustments to heart problems, lung complications, and infection may be necessary. See "Surgery," Chapter 21 for massage therapy guidelines for recent surgery.

If the client is taking prednisone, note that high doses may be used, with strong side effects. See "Corticosteroids," Chapter 21 for effects of prolonged use, because

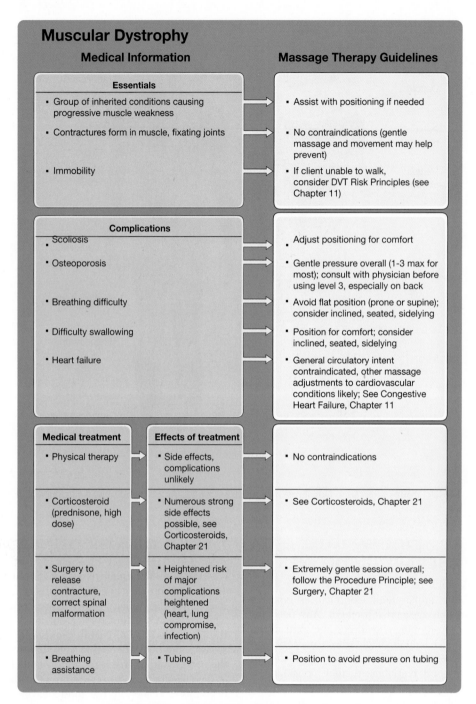

FIGURE 8-9. A Decision Tree for muscular dystrophy.

adaptations in pressure, general circulatory intent, and joint movement may be in order. If the client is using breathing assistance, be careful not to compress the tubing while positioning the client. Finally, see Chapter 11 for any pertinent treatment of cardiovascular conditions, and adapt massage accordingly.

● MASSAGE RESEARCH

As of this writing, there are no randomized, controlled trials, published in the English language, on muscular dystrophy and massage indexed in PubMed or the Massage Therapy Foundation Research Database. The NIH RePORTER tool lists no active, federally funded research projects on the topic in the

United States. No active projects are listed on the clinicaltrials.gov database (see Chapter 6).

● POSSIBLE MASSAGE BENEFITS

Physicians often recommend massage therapy and physical therapy to keep the muscles as functional as possible. Judicious use of massage may help slow down the progression of contracture formation, especially earlier in the disease. This could help ease the significant pain caused by contracture and spinal malformation. Functional and flexible muscles support people in maintaining movement and exercise as long as possible. This can be invaluable to people with the condition. Skilled touch could also provide great benefit to clients with muscular dystrophy, by supporting body image and body awareness.

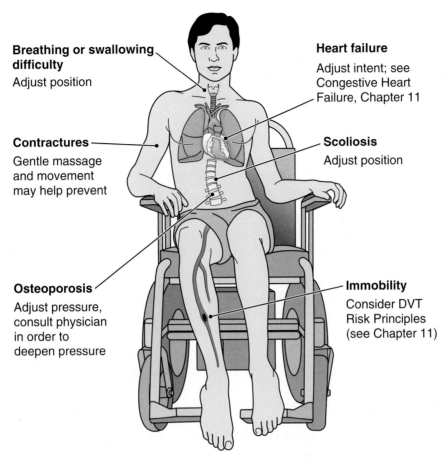

Breathing or swallowing difficulty
Adjust position

Contractures
Gentle massage and movement may help prevent

Osteoporosis
Adjust pressure, consult physician in order to deepen pressure

Heart failure
Adjust intent; see Congestive Heart Failure, Chapter 11

Scoliosis
Adjust position

Immobility
Consider DVT Risk Principles (see Chapter 11)

FIGURE 8-10. Muscular dystrophy: Selected clinical features and massage adjustments to consider. Specific instructions and additional massage therapy guidelines are in Decision Tree and text.

Other Muscle and Soft Tissue Conditions in Brief

BAKER CYST

Background	• Synovial membrane at knee forms a pouch that extends posteriorly into popliteal area. Can accompany meniscus tears or arthritis. • Rupture produces acute pain in calf, temporary swelling, DVT-like signs and symptoms. • Treated with needle aspiration for drainage, corticosteroids, and surgical removal in stubborn cases.
Interview Questions	• Have you seen a doctor about it? Diagnosis? Is it thought to be large? • Swelling, coolness, or clamminess in lower leg? Any other joint issues in the area? • Treatment? Effects of treatment?
Massage Therapy Guidelines	• At all times, no pressure at the site in popliteal fossa. • If undiagnosed, especially if lower leg is cold, clammy, or swollen, follow DVT Risk Principles (Chapter 11); urgent medical referral. • If arthritis is also present, adapt to arthritis type (see Chapter 9). • See "Corticosteroids," "Surgery," Chapter 21.

BURSITIS

Background	• Inflammation of bursa, caused by overuse, trauma, some types of arthritis; in rare cases, caused by infection. Commonly appears in shoulder, elbow, hip, and knee.

- Causes throbbing, deep, burning pain when acute, and soreness to touch or compression when chronic. Acute phase lasts several weeks.
- Stiffness may occur; swelling, warmth, and redness occur if superficial, or if caused by infection.
- Treated with rest, NSAIDs, corticosteroid injection, aspiration of excess fluid, injected antibiotics (all office procedures), and surgical removal of bursa.
- Physical therapy with exercises used to resume movement, correct imbalances to prevent recurrence.

Interview Questions	• Where? Symptoms? When did symptoms start? Improving, worsening, or staying the same? Acute or chronic? Have you seen a doctor about it? Diagnosis? • What positions are comfortable for you? • Treatment? Effects of treatment?
Massage Therapy Guidelines	• Avoid friction, circulatory intent at the site. Limit pressure at the site—even pressure level 1 and 2 can be painful when acute. • Avoid passive movement when acute; limit to gentle movement when chronic. • Adjust position for comfort. • If client presents with swelling, warmth, and redness, but has not reported it to a physician, encourage urgent medical referral; may need antibiotic injection to clear infection in bursa. • Adapt massage to the effects of analgesics, such as GI upset, dizziness, drowsiness, headache (see Chapter 21); for surgery, follow the Procedure Principle, see Chapter 21.

COMPARTMENT SYNDROME (EXERTIONAL COMPARTMENT SYNDROME)

Background	• Muscles in a compartment expand to fill their fascial sheath, causing inflammation and compression on nerves, blood vessels, and muscles within the compartment. • Often involves anterior lower leg, but can appear in thighs, upper arms, forearms, and hands; can lead to tissue death and damage to nerves, vessels, and muscles. • Pain aggravated by activity, relieved by rest; can also cause numbness, weakness, and foot drop. • Treatment with rest, physical therapy, orthotics to adjust biomechanics, massage; surgery to split or remove fascial restriction is widely accepted as most effective treatment.
Interview Questions	• Where? Have you seen a doctor about it? Diagnosis? Considered acute or chronic? • Treatment? Effects of treatment?
Massage Therapy Guidelines	• If acute, symptoms unreported to physician, immediate medical referral indicated—de-inflammation may be necessary to prevent tissue death; if chronic, unreported, urgent medical referral. • If acute, avoid friction, and circulatory intent at site; gentle pressure at site, level 1 max; do not aggravate inflammation. • If chronic, cautious pressure and circulatory intent may be okay depending upon the level of inflammation, but consult physician for input. • For surgery, follow the Procedure Principle, see Chapter 21.

CRAMP ("CHARLEY HORSE")

Background	• Acute, involuntary, painful tightening of skeletal muscle fibers due to inadequate fluid and electrolyte supply. • Contributing factors: pregnancy, vigorous exercise, dehydration, or CV disease. • Treated with hydration, vitamin D and E supplementation, mineral supplementation, stretching. • Systemic cramps (in more than one area) treated with emergency IV fluids.
Interview Questions	• Where? In one area, or all over? Chronic problem? Known cause? Any CV condition?

Massage Therapy Guidelines	• If cramps are systemic, immediate medical referral. • If chronic, adapt to any contributing factors (see Cardiovascular Conditions, Chapter 11). • If acute, sustained pressure or stretch of involved muscle may relieve.

MYOSITIS OSSIFICANS

Background	• Formation of bone-like fragments between layers of muscle tissue; caused by trauma, bleeding into muscle or fascia; often in brachialis, quadriceps muscles. • Dense mass of tissue causes pain, limits joint movement. Can take months or years to reabsorb. • Treated with rest, stretching to regain ROM, strengthening exercises; surgical removal for persistent, severe cases, but often recurs months after surgery.
Interview Questions	• Where? Symptoms? Acute or chronic? • When was initial injury? Any restrictions on movement? • Treatment? Effects of treatment?
Massage Therapy Guidelines	• Learn and record the location of lesion and limit pressure around site (1 max for most); too much pressure could damage soft tissue by pressing it against fragments. • During acute phase, follow any joint movement restrictions; gentle stretching may be well tolerated in chronic phase. • Consider DVT Risk Principles (see Chapter 11). • See Chapter 21 for massage guidelines after surgery.

PLANTAR FASCIITIS

Background	• Pain in arch of foot, isolated to attachment of plantar fascia to calcaneous, or extending forward to ball of foot; may be accompanied by bone spur. • Traditionally thought to be caused by inflammation of the structure, but recent data suggest that degradation of tissue is the cause. • Treated with rest, ice, stretching, NSAIDs, corticosteroid injection, and surgery (rare cases)
Interview Questions	• Where? When did problem begin? Inflamed (swelling, warmth)? • Have you seen a doctor? Diagnosis? Any bone spur? • Treatment? Effects of treatment?
Massage Therapy Guidelines	• If signs of inflammation or severe pain, avoid friction, circulatory intent, medium pressure (pressure 2 max) at the site; if not inflamed, massage with deep pressure at the site, passive dorsiflexion may be helpful. • At all times, avoid pressure above level 2 at attachment to calcaneous to avoid pressing on bone spur (may be undiagnosed). • If the condition is not improving, and client has not already reported it to the doctor, encourage medical referral.

SHIN SPLINTS

Background	• Collection of injuries causing mild or severe pain to anterior or posterior lower leg; aggravated by movement. • Can be due to compartment syndrome (this chapter), stress fracture, muscle strain (this chapter), or periostitis; multiple injuries possible. • RICE treatment usually recommended, and OTC analgesics; surgery for some cases of compartment syndrome and nonhealing stress fracture.
Interview Questions	• Where? When did problem begin? Worsening or improving? Inflamed? • Have you seen a doctor? Diagnosis? • Treatment? Effects of treatment?

Massage Therapy
Guidelines

- Massage guidelines depend on cause: more caution is necessary for stress fracture or compartment syndrome; less caution for periostitis, muscle strain.
- Urgent or immediate medical referral if swelling, heat, or redness is present, indicating possible stress fracture or compartment syndrome (this chapter); medical referral indicated if pain does not improve after 1–3 days with rest.
- Pressure, circulatory intent, and friction contraindicated at the site if inflamed; if improving and not visibly/palpably inflamed, heavier pressure levels, circulatory intent, and friction likely to be helpful; gentle movement indicated.
- See Chapter 21 for analgesics, surgery, and massage therapy guidelines.

SELF TEST

1. Explain the pain-spasm-pain cycle, and the role that ischemia and hypoxia play in the cycle. How can a massage therapist intervene in the cycle?
2. Compare tendinitis, tendinopathy, and tendinosis. Which one, until recently, was thought to be the cause of most tendon pain?
3. Compare sprain and strain. Which is characterized by swelling? Where do the two types of injuries tend to occur? Which one tends to heal with the fewest complications?
4. In the grading of strain and sprain, which one involves complete rupture of the structure? Which grade involves only small tears or over-stretching of the tissue?
5. When working with a client with an acute soft tissue injury, which massage elements should be avoided at the site? How does this change in the subacute phase?
6. List and explain each element of the RICE regimen. How does each element help soft tissue injury?
7. How are massage guidelines for whiplash different from those for other sprains and strains? Why are they different?
8. Suppose you work with a client with whiplash for a period of several months after the accident. What factors should

guide you to limit pressure to levels 1-2, and to use only extremely gentle joint movement? When should pressure and joint movement be limited even further?
9. Is the use of massage with whiplash supported by research? Describe any existing RCTs or research reviews on the topic.
10. List the tender points in fibromyalgia. How should massage be adjusted at these sites?
11. How can massage therapy be adapted to sleep problems in fibromyalgia?
12. How can a therapist be sensitive to the psychosocial complications of fibromyalgia?
13. How can massage be adapted to someone with breathing difficulties, as in advanced muscular dystrophy?
14. If muscular dystrophy is advanced, what other non-muscle structures may be affected, and what are the massage adjustments in each case?
15. How is massage thought to be helpful to clients with muscular dystrophy?

 For answers to these questions and to see a bibliography for this chapter, visit http://thePoint. lww.com/Walton.

Skeletal System Conditions

I have no history but the length of my bones.

—ROBIN SKELTON

The skeletal system gives the body form, stability, and levers for purposeful movement through space. When disease or injury compromises the skeletal structures, the effects on movement can be powerfully felt. And even though the skeletal system is capable of regeneration and repair, a person can often point to the site of an old fracture decades later, noting some residual stiffness or vulnerability. Bones tell us stories of the past.

Some skeletal system conditions involve a disease process, such as osteoarthritis, osteoporosis, and cancer. Others are a result of injury, as bones and joints are injured along with soft tissue. In Chapter 8, injuries and disease of soft tissue are addressed. This chapter picks up where Chapter 8 leaves off, at the surface of bone and in its depths.

In this chapter, four common conditions are discussed at length. These are:

- Osteoarthritis (OA)
- Osteoporosis
- Fracture
- Herniated Disk (Disk Disease)

Conditions in Brief addressed in this chapter are **Ankylosing spondylitis, Psoriatic arthritis, Rheumatoid arthritis, Septic arthritis, Avascular necrosis, Bone cancer, Bunion** (hallux valgus), **Gout** (gouty arthritis), **Lyme disease, Osteomyelitis, Paget disease** (osteitis deformans), and **Temporomandibular joint disorders.**

General Principles

There are no skeleton-specific massage principles to use with bone pathologies, but for conditions due to injury, several principles from Chapter 3 apply here. The Pain, Injury, and Inflammation Principles are all useful, especially the Inflammation Principle and the Unstable Tissue Principle.

The Pain-Spasm-Pain Principle (Chapter 8) is a theory that explains the pain relief that occurs even when massage cannot directly correct the source of pain. No matter what the condition, the intent to relax muscle can be welcome, indeed. After a massage, a client with a skeletal system condition may discover that a meaningful portion of his or her pain is gone and can be ascribed to muscle tension, rather than the underlying injury or disease.

In some skeletal conditions, such as fracture, the risk of thrombosis is elevated. In these cases, refer to Chapter 11 in order to use the DVT Risk Principles described there.

Osteoarthritis

In **osteoarthritis (OA)**, inflammation and damage to the synovial joints occur through normal aging, injury, and repeated use of the joints over time. The experience of osteoarthritis is familiar to many people as they age, and almost everyone has some amount of osteoarthritis by age 70.

● BACKGROUND

Another name for osteoarthritis is *degenerative joint disease*. Typical joints affected by osteoarthritis are the fingers, thumbs, the vertebrae of the neck and low back, the hips, knees, and feet (especially the big toes). Figure 9-1 shows the distribution of common sites of osteoarthritis in the body.

Signs and Symptoms

Osteoarthritis can be asymptomatic, but the most obvious symptom is deep, aching joint pain. The pain is aggravated by movement (especially weight-bearing movement if weight-bearing joints are affected) and is often relieved by rest. Wet weather can also worsen arthritis pain. As the condition advances, pain may even be felt at rest and at night. Osteoarthritis limits movement, and stiffness is common, especially after periods of inactivity. The stiffness generally subsides after about a half hour of movement. A common complaint is joint stiffness in the morning on rising. **Crepitus**, a grinding sound, sometimes accompanies movement.

Swelling is not typical of OA, but if it does appear, it's usually mild, even in acute cases. Osteoarthritis changes the shape of the bones in several ways. Joint spaces narrow. Joint enlargement may occur, along with the formation of **bone spurs**, or *osteophytes*, at the edges of the joint. These overgrowths of bone tissue are not painful but may irritate neighboring structures such as nerves or bone. Enlargement of the joints in osteoarthritis is sometimes called *nodes*. In the

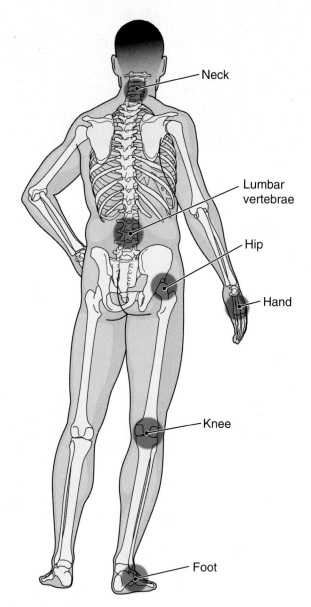

FIGURE 9-1. Common sites of osteoarthritis.

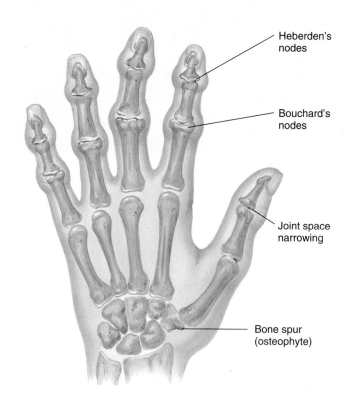

FIGURE 9-2. Osteoarthritis in joints of the hand.

hand, these are called *Heberden nodes* and *Bouchard nodes*. Massage therapists may notice these arthritic changes in their hands, after years of doing massage. These changes are shown in Figure 9-2.

In osteoarthritis, symptoms and diagnostic findings often disagree. An individual with no symptoms may have significant arthritic changes on an X-ray, while another might have negative X-ray findings but significant symptoms.

Complications

Complications of osteoarthritis occur when signs and symptoms persist or worsen. This can impair movement. Movement supports health at all levels, and when individuals find it difficult to move, they become deconditioned, losing strength and endurance. They can then suffer declines in cardiovascular health and balance and can become overweight. This can make movement even harder and contribute to overall poor health.

In severe cases, arthritic changes cause pressure on surrounding nerves, accompanied by pain, numbness, or tingling in the area supplied by these nerves. For example, osteoarthritis of the cervical spine can cause symptoms down the arm, or changes in the lumbar spine can cause symptoms down the thigh or lower leg.

Treatment

Exercises aimed at improving flexibility and building strength are beneficial in osteoarthritis. The goal is to strike a balance, so that movement increases flexibility and strength but does not worsen symptoms. To that end, low-impact exercises, such as swimming and other types of water exercises, are often recommended.

Medications for pain relief include NSAIDs and other analgesics, and low doses of muscle relaxants. In general, these tend to have mild side effects, although they have stronger side effects in older adults, the population most likely to take them for osteoarthritis. Prescription cox-2 inhibitors (see Chapter 21) such as Celebrex have been used for osteoarthritis, but their use is limited because of serious cardiovascular and gastrointestinal side effects.

Capsaicin, a pain-relieving derivative of red pepper, may be applied topically to a painful arthritic area, with few side effects beyond temporary skin irritation. Heat therapy, cold therapy, and massage are aimed at pain relief and increasing flexibility around affected joints. Dietary supplements include glucosamine and chondroitin, which have some research support but are still being evaluated.

With acute osteoarthritis that includes swelling and other signs of inflammation, the swelling may be drawn off with a needle, or **aspirated**. This is followed with an injection of corticosteroid medication into the joint, but because corticosteroids can thin tissue, the joint has to be rested for a while. A synthetic form of **hyaluronate**, a protective, lubricating component of connective tissue, may be injected into the joint weekly for several weeks, to provide pain relief. Although it is still being studied, individuals report pain relief that can last several months.

If conservative treatment fails and diagnostic tests show significant erosion of the cartilage, surgical joint replacement is suggested. Hip and knee joint replacements are common and have high success rates.

● INTERVIEW QUESTIONS

1. Where is it located?
2. Has a doctor diagnosed it? Is it clear that it is osteoarthritis, not rheumatoid arthritis or any other type of arthritis?
3. What are your symptoms? What aggravates and relieves them?
4. Would you classify your pain as mild, moderate, or severe? Does it limit your activities in any way? (See "Follow-Up Questions about Pain," Chapter 4)
5. Do you have any pain, tingling, or numbness? Has your doctor said it's due to the arthritis?
6. Do you have any bone spurs or visible changes in the affected joints?
7. How is it being treated?
8. How does treatment affect you?

● MASSAGE THERAPY GUIDELINES

Questions 1-6, together with the Follow-Up Questions about Pain (see Chapter 4), establish important background on the client's condition. If the client reports swelling, follow the Inflammation Principle.

> *The Inflammation Principle. **If an area of tissue is inflamed, don't aggravate it with pressure, friction, or circulatory intent at the site.***

In the absence of swelling, massage right at the site may be beneficial. By reducing muscle tension, you may provide the client with a good deal of pain relief. Make sure your pressure is lighter over the joint itself—in most cases, pressure levels 2 and 3 are well tolerated. Limit joint movement in the session if it causes any pain.

Some individuals have more than one type of arthritis. Question 2 will help you determine whether additional guidelines should be followed for other types of arthritis; these are addressed in the Conditions in Brief table. This question also helps establish whether the condition is self-diagnosed. Self-diagnosis is common because people often expect arthritis as they age and often don't complain about it when it happens. Although it would be ideal to have a firm diagnosis for every condition you encounter in practice, it is unlikely. Review the different types of arthritis in the Conditions in Brief table, and make a medical referral for symptoms of other types.

Questions about symptoms can take the conversation in several directions. If the client mentions neurologic symptoms such as sharp pain, tingling, or numbness and hasn't brought it to his or her physician's attention, encourage an urgent medical referral. Avoid pressure, joint movement, and positions that produce or aggravate neurologic symptoms.

If the client states that arthritis limits his or her activities, be alert for a decline in general health. Look for diseases of aging and inactivity, such as cardiovascular conditions, and

adapt massage to them (see Chapter 11). Question 6, about bone spurs, highlights areas where slightly gentler pressure and joint movement are in order. You do not want to irritate surrounding soft tissues by pressing them into a bone spur.

Some arthritis treatments may influence the massage plan. Common side effects for arthritis medication appear in the Decision Tree (Figure 9-3). Massage therapy guidelines may be found for most other side effects in Table 21-1. Other arthritis treatments, including heat, cold, exercise, glucosamine, and chondroitin, carry few side effects. When correctly used, they have little impact on the massage.

If the joint was aspirated and corticosteroid medication was injected, joint movement should be avoided until the joint is stable again. If joint replacement surgery was recent (in the last 3 months), follow the Procedure Principle, staying alert for possible complications and massage precautions (see "Surgery," Chapter 21).

● MASSAGE RESEARCH

As of this writing, there is little evidence favoring massage therapy for people with osteoarthritis. However, two small RCTs are of interest. In a study published in the *Archives of Internal Medicine*, a well-regarded medical journal, 68 adults with OA of the knee were given 8 weeks of Swedish massage. Half of the group received the intervention at the outset of the study, and half served as a wait-list control for 8 weeks, then received the intervention (Perlman et al., 2006). When compared to the control condition, massage was associated with improvements in pain, stiffness, function, ROM, and other parameters.

Because massage therapists depend heavily on the health and function of their own hands, a study on massage and osteoarthritis of the hand is of interest. Twenty-two adults with OA of the hand were randomized to usual care or to four 15-minute hand massage sessions over 4 weeks (Field et al., 2007). The massage group also received instruction in daily self-massage of the hand. Compared to the controls, the authors noted less pain in the massaged hands, as well as increased grip strength. They also found less anxiety and depressed mood in the massage group.

These two small studies, and a smattering of others, are all we have on massage and osteoarthritis, and we are a long way from conclusive research in this area. Further study, which was suggested in both papers, will be important to determine whether massage has a role in treating people with osteoarthritis.

● POSSIBLE MASSAGE BENEFITS

Although research is not yet conclusive on the benefit of massage for people with OA, massage around affected joints is often recommended. By easing pain due to muscle tension, aiding flexibility, and supporting activity, massage therapy can be a wonderful support to people with arthritis. As such, it should be included part of any rehabilitation and maintenance program aimed at managing arthritis. Even though massage cannot and should not penetrate deep into the joint where the source of pain is, it may provide symptom relief, in keeping with the Pain-Spasm-Pain Principle (see Chapter 8).

> *The Pain-Spasm-Pain Principle. **Relief of excess muscle tension around an injured or painful area may lead to pain relief, apart from the original cause of the pain.***

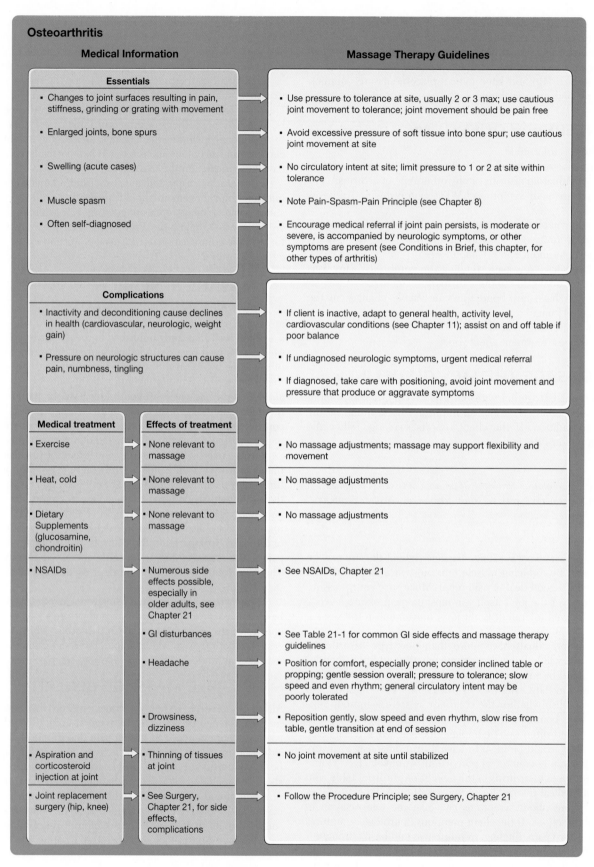

Osteoarthritis

Medical Information

Massage Therapy Guidelines

Essentials

- Changes to joint surfaces resulting in pain, stiffness, grinding or grating with movement

- Enlarged joints, bone spurs

- Swelling (acute cases)

- Muscle spasm

- Often self-diagnosed

- Use pressure to tolerance at site, usually 2 or 3 max; use cautious joint movement to tolerance; joint movement should be pain free

- Avoid excessive pressure of soft tissue into bone spur; use cautious joint movement at site

- No circulatory intent at site; limit pressure to 1 or 2 at site within tolerance

- Note Pain-Spasm-Pain Principle (see Chapter 8)

- Encourage medical referral if joint pain persists, is moderate or severe, is accompanied by neurologic symptoms, or other symptoms are present (see Conditions in Brief, this chapter, for other types of arthritis)

Complications

- Inactivity and deconditioning cause declines in health (cardiovascular, neurologic, weight gain)

- Pressure on neurologic structures can cause pain, numbness, tingling

- If client is inactive, adapt to general health, activity level, cardiovascular conditions (see Chapter 11); assist on and off table if poor balance

- If undiagnosed neurologic symptoms, urgent medical referral

- If diagnosed, take care with positioning, avoid joint movement and pressure that produce or aggravate symptoms

Medical treatment	Effects of treatment	
• Exercise	• None relevant to massage	• No massage adjustments; massage may support flexibility and movement
• Heat, cold	• None relevant to massage	• No massage adjustments
• Dietary Supplements (glucosamine, chondroitin)	• None relevant to massage	• No massage adjustments
• NSAIDs	• Numerous side effects possible, especially in older adults, see Chapter 21	• See NSAIDs, Chapter 21
	• GI disturbances	• See Table 21-1 for common GI side effects and massage therapy guidelines
	• Headache	• Position for comfort, especially prone; consider inclined table or propping; gentle session overall; pressure to tolerance; slow speed and even rhythm; general circulatory intent may be poorly tolerated
	• Drowsiness, dizziness	• Reposition gently, slow speed and even rhythm, slow rise from table, gentle transition at end of session
• Aspiration and corticosteroid injection at joint	• Thinning of tissues at joint	• No joint movement at site until stabilized
• Joint replacement surgery (hip, knee)	• See Surgery, Chapter 21, for side effects, complications	• Follow the Procedure Principle; see Surgery, Chapter 21

FIGURE 9-3. A Decision Tree for osteoarthritis.

Osteoporosis

In **osteoporosis**, the bones become "thinned" and weakened by the slowing of mineral deposition over time. This leaves bones vulnerable to fracture.

● BACKGROUND

Loss of bone strength occurs increasingly in older adults, especially in Asian and Caucasian women of slight frame. Risk factors include age, family history, poor dietary calcium and vitamin D, menopause, and other hormonal changes. Other conditions can also cause osteoporosis, such as Cushing disease, hypothyroidism, diabetes mellitus (see Chapter 17), and chronic kidney failure (see Chapter 18). Prolonged corticosteroid therapy can also thin the bones.

Signs and Symptoms

Osteoporosis is often not obvious until a notable fracture has occurred. A loss of height is one sign, and pronounced *kyphosis*, or "dowager hump," is another.

Complications

The most serious concern and complication of osteoporosis are a bone fracture. A **pathologic fracture** results from a force that ordinarily would not cause a bone to break. In osteoporosis, pathologic fractures, also called *osteoporotic fractures*, can occur anywhere, but they commonly occur in the hip, wrist, and spine (Figure 9-4). The proximal humerus is another vulnerable site.

Fractures, especially of the hip, can profoundly impair independence, causing pain and suffering. Small compression fractures accumulate in the vertebrae, and they collapse. Collapsed vertebrae become wedge shaped, changing the shape of the spine, as shown in Figure 9-5. Compression fractures diminish height and contribute to the characteristic stooped, kyphotic posture of osteoporosis. These compression fractures may be asymptomatic, but often they cause severe pain and discomfort.

Unfortunately, like any injury, an injury from osteoporosis is likely to limit an individual's activities. Without physical activity, thinning bones can be weakened further, initiating a downward spiral of bone loss and inactivity. For this reason, educational programs, medical devices, and support aimed at fall prevention are high priorities for individuals with advanced osteoporosis, whose fall risk is often compounded by weakened muscles, compromised reflexes, and poor balance.

Treatment

Osteoporosis prevention campaigns target modifiable risk factors, such as nutrition (more dietary calcium plus the vitamin D needed to absorb it) and weight-bearing activity. Bone density measurements are used to monitor osteoporosis so that it can be addressed before fracture occurs.

Most people with osteoporosis are prescribed medications called **bisphosphonates**, which encourage bone mineralization. Some bisphosphonates are taken orally, and some by IV infusion. Common bisphosphonates are alendronate (Fosamax), risedronate (Actonel), ibandronate (Boniva), and zoledronate (Zometa). Even with bisphosphonates, bone density is unlikely to return to earlier peak levels, but it can improve considerably, effectively reversing osteoporosis and reducing the risk of pathologic fracture. Oral bisphosphonates cause heartburn and stomach upset in many people, especially when lying down after a dose. They must be taken with a large amount of water, away from food, and most people take them in the morning.

Because of these restrictions and uncomfortable side effects, adherence rates are low with these drugs, and most patients stop taking them on schedule after a year of use. IV bisphosphonate infusion, on an annual or quarterly schedule, bypasses the GI tract and associated side effects. However, repeated high doses of bisphosphonates have resulted in jaw problems, especially in people who receive bisphosphonates as part of cancer treatment (see Chapter 20).

Hormone therapies are considered for some people with osteoporosis. For years, **hormone replacement therapy (HRT)** was given to women after menopause to prolong the favorable effects of estrogen on bone mineralization. This treatment

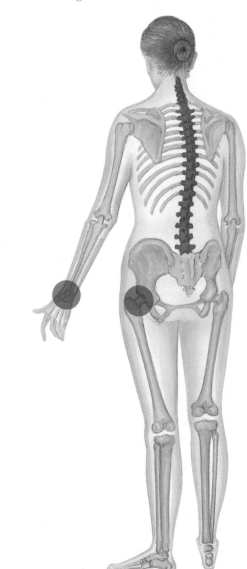

FIGURE 9-4. Areas at risk of pathologic fracture in osteoporosis.

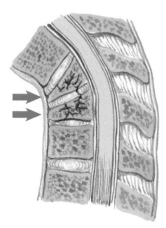

FIGURE 9-5. Compression fractures in vertebrae, caused by osteoporosis. Arrows point to two vertebral bodies that have fractured, compressed, and become wedge shaped, leading to loss of height and a stooped posture.

fell out of favor once significant side effects and life-threatening complications of HRT became clear. It is now rarely used, in part, because bisphosphonates are highly effective.

Bone repair progresses more slowly in people with osteoporosis, so fractures take a long time to heal. Some fractures are treated surgically: If a hip is fractured, the joint can be replaced. With a wrist fracture, surgery is performed or the area is immobilized so that bone union can occur.

Compression fractures in the spine may be treated with **vertebroplasty**, in which an acrylic-based "bone cement" is injected into each vertebra. This procedure has few side effects. Improving the spine's structural integrity can relieve pain and reduce the risk of further fracture.

● INTERVIEW QUESTIONS

1. How long has it been since you were diagnosed with osteoporosis?
2. Is it caused by another condition or medication, or is it bone thinning over time?
3. Does your doctor say it's improving or getting worse? Do you have regular bone density tests?
4. What are your usual daily and weekly activities?
5. Do any of your health care providers—doctors, nurses, physical therapists, or occupational therapists—express concern about the stability of your bones, or about your balance?
6. Have you had any bone fractures, especially in the last few years? If so, has your doctor attributed any of them to osteoporosis?
7. Have you lost any height because of osteoporosis? Has your spine changed in any way?
8. Does your osteoporosis cause you any pain? (See "Follow-Up Questions About Pain," Chapter 4)
9. How has your osteoporosis been treated?
10. How does treatment affect you?

● MASSAGE THERAPY GUIDELINES

With osteoporosis, your primary concern is the stability of the bones and their susceptibility to pathologic fracture. The interview questions are organized to identify that concern, respecting the **Unstable Tissue Principle.**

> *The Unstable Tissue Principle. If a tissue is unstable, do not challenge it with too much pressure or joint movement in the area.*

Gentle joint movement may be required, with cautious stretching, ROM, or rocking. Take care not to pull or push on the bones while working the muscles.

Questions 1 and 2 establish the background of the condition. In particular, note whether the cause is just the natural progression of age, or if osteoporosis is secondary to something else, such as prolonged corticosteroid treatment over time (see Chapter 21), or another disease. Often if the cause is corrected, the osteoporosis resolves, as well. Conditions causing osteoporosis are typically serious enough to require additional massage therapy guidelines. Investigate conditions such as Cushing disease, hypothyroidism, diabetes mellitus (see Chapter 17), and chronic kidney failure (see Chapter 18).

Taken together, Questions 3–8 help assess the appropriate pressure and caution in joint movement. There are no absolute guidelines for pressure in osteoporosis, and how gently to go is relative, but the 1–3 range is likely for most clients, at least in the most vulnerable areas (see Figure 9-4).

At one end of the osteoporosis spectrum are people with severe osteoporosis, at high risk of fracture, who should receive pressure in the 1–2 range. At the other end of the spectrum are mild cases—people whose current risk of fracture is only slightly elevated, who can safely sustain pressure level 3 and possibly 4. At this end are people who are reversing the condition through exercise, nutrition, and preventive medication. In many cases, people make significant improvements in bone density by taking these steps.

Without being able to see or assess bone stability, how can you determine where your client fits on the spectrum? In the interview, listen, watch for, and ask about the following:

- A history of bone fracture, attributed to osteoporosis;
- Loss of height or changes in the shape of the spine;
- Osteoporosis that is worsening;
- Limited physical activity or movement;
- The client's doctor or other health care professional expresses concern about the client's balance or risk of falling;
- The client's doctor or other health care professional expresses concern about the client's bone density or fracture risk.

If any of this information emerges in the interview, use gentle joint movement and limit pressure to level 1 or 2 in the initial session. A medical consultation is advised before going any deeper, especially on the back. Consult the physician, or communicate with a client's physical therapist for equivalent physical therapy concerns.

This approach may lead to a session that is too cautious for some client presentations, but it is very safe. In an ideal situation, massage pressure is customized to the client's preference, tolerance, and safety, but a physician's input is necessary for the latter.

> *The Shred of Doubt Principle. If there is a shred of doubt about whether a massage element is safe, it is contraindicated until its safety is established. When in doubt, don't.*

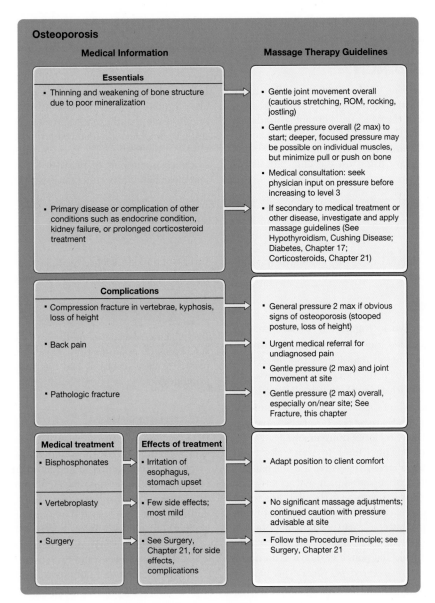

FIGURE 9-6. A Decision Tree for osteoporosis.

You can be less cautious with clients at the other end of the spectrum, with the following features: good activity levels; a track record of improving the condition with diet, activity, and treatment; and a low level of fracture risk. Regular and recent physician evaluations, with favorable test results, are the best indicators of this success. In this case, pressure 3 would be fine, and some clients could tolerate and benefit from higher pressure without injury. Again, physician input is advised before advancing the pressure.

People often come to massage therapy to seek relief from back pain. If clients with osteoporosis complain of back pain, they have not reported it to their physician, or there is any question about their bone stability, then resist the impulse to address the pain with heavy massage pressure or strong joint movement. Instead, encourage an urgent medical referral; for the moment, limit the pressure on the back to levels 1 or 2. In this case, you design the session for the worst-case scenario—pathologic fracture—until the physician rules it out. If fracture

is discovered, with or without pain, continue with this gentle approach (see "Fracture," this chapter).

> *The Waiting for a Diagnosis Principle. If a client is scheduled for diagnostic tests, or is awaiting results, adapt massage to the possible diagnosis. If more than one condition is being investigated, adapt massage to the worst-case scenario.*

Questions 9 and 10 about treatment will inform you about medications or surgeries that may require massage adaptations. In particular, people who take oral bisphosphonates are told to avoid lying down for 30–60 minutes after taking the drug, to avoid irritating the esophagus. If providing massage during that window of time, adjust the client's position accordingly. If the fracture was treated with a surgical procedure, see "Surgery," Chapter 21 for relevant massage therapy guidelines. Vertebroplasty does not tend to produce many side effects or complications that concern massage therapy, but common sense suggests continued caution with pressure in the area.

● MASSAGE RESEARCH

As of this writing, there are no randomized, controlled trials, published in the English language, on osteoporosis and massage indexed in PubMed or the Massage Therapy Foundation Research Database. The NIH RePORTER tool lists no active, federally funded research projects on the topic in the United States. No active projects are listed on the clinicaltrials.gov database (see Chapter 6).

● POSSIBLE MASSAGE BENEFITS

Exercise is central to osteoporosis prevention and prevention of complications. In persons with osteoporosis, exercise is used to prevent falls and fracture by building strength, flexibility, and balance. Even without a body of research evidence, a reasonable argument can be made for the role of massage in supporting movement and exercise. Massage has the potential to keep muscles flexible and enhance body awareness; both of these are vital in preventing falls. Perhaps future studies will generate evidence in support of massage for smooth, fluid movement, and clear benefit for individuals with osteoporosis.

Fracture

A **fracture** is a break in a bone. Unless the bones are especially vulnerable, it takes a great deal of force to break the bone.

● BACKGROUND

Types of fractures are shown in Figure 9-7. A shattered or crushed state of bone is called a **comminuted fracture**. A **greenstick fracture** is a pattern similar to the break in a young stick or branch, in which the bone does not break all the way through. In an **oblique fracture**, the line of break runs at an angle to the length of the bone. A **spiral fracture** spirals down the bone, and a **transverse fracture** separates the length of the bone into two pieces transversely.

All of these types of fracture tend to show clearly in diagnostic tests. In contrast, a **stress fracture**, a small, hairline crack in the bone produced by repeated or heavy activity, may be less clear. Stress fractures often appear in the tibia, as a result of overtraining, and can pose a challenge in the diagnosis of shin splints (see Chapter 8). Hairline cracks can occur in other bones, too, especially when osteoporosis puts the bones at greater risk.

When a broken bone breaks the skin, it is known as an **open fracture** (formerly called a *compound fracture*). This type of fracture is more likely to occur in a bone that lies close to the surface of the skin, such as the tibia, than in a deeper bone. A fracture that does not break the skin is called a **closed fracture**.

Signs and Symptoms

In the acute phase, a bone fracture causes all of the signs and symptoms of inflammation, plus bleeding and bruising. The pain is usually severe. A bad fracture can produce tingling or numbness.

Complications

With an open fracture, infection can occur, as microorganisms move into the open wound. Depending on the structures involved, osteomyelitis or septic arthritis may occur, and the infection can be serious (see Conditions in Brief).

Delayed union describes a fracture in which two pieces do not join in the expected amount of time. This can prolong healing, but delayed union fractures typically heal eventually without medical intervention. A **nonunion fracture** occurs when the gap between the two structures does not fill at all.

Delayed union and nonunion fractures happen for various reasons, including failure to set the bone properly, or a delayed

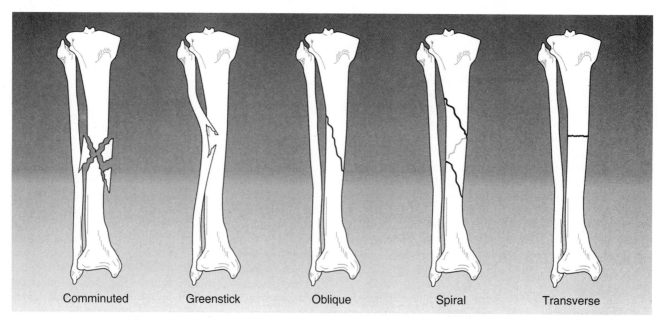

Comminuted   Greenstick   Oblique   Spiral   Transverse

FIGURE 9-7. Types of fracture. (From Willis MC. *Medical Terminology: The Language of Health Care*, 2nd ed. Philadelphia: Lippincott Williams and Wilkins, 2005.)

diagnosis, which can make treatment difficult. Poor health also can keep broken bones from resealing. Diabetes mellitus, steroid medication, poor nutrition, osteoporosis, and cigarette smoking can be associated with poor bone healing.

Fracture can also be complicated by *compartment syndrome* (see Chapter 8). It may occur when the swelling produced by a fracture is contained within a closed soft tissue compartment, and pressure develops on nerves and vessels in the area. When compartment syndrome occurs with a fracture, it produces severe pain, sensation changes, weakness, and skin changes. Tissue death can occur within hours in acute cases.

Some fractures cause *deep vein thrombosis (DVT)*, a serious complication that can lead to *pulmonary embolism (PE)*, a life-threatening condition (see Chapter 11). DVT and PE are more common in fractures of the hip or pelvis than in other areas, of the body, and PE is one of the most common and serious complications of fracture in this area. Trauma, immobilization, and swelling all contribute to the risk.

When bones fracture, they release marrow to the surrounding area. In some cases, fat droplets escape to the bloodstream and *embolize* (are carried in the blood), then obstruct capillary beds in the lungs or other areas. This is called **fat embolization syndrome (FES)**, and it typically occurs in the first few days after a closed fracture to a long bone, pelvic bone, or rib. The droplets are numerous and often smaller than the blood clot of DVT and can be more widely disseminated.

Symptoms of FES are similar to PE (see Chapter 11). In addition, rash on the chest, neck, shoulders, and axillae may appear. If fat is present in circulation to the brain, confusion, behavioral changes, and coma result. This condition can cause death in severe cases, but it is often **self-limiting**, meaning it tends to run its course and resolve on its own. The risk of FES is minimized by rapid immobilization and treatment of a fracture.

Treatment

The type of initial care of a fracture depends on its severity and location. The bone fragments must be immobilized, often with a cast, splint or sling, accompanied by ice and elevation to reduce swelling. Pain management is achieved with acetaminophen at first; aspirin and other NSAIDs are avoided at first because they aggravate bleeding. Stronger analgesics may be used if stronger pain relief is required.

The pieces of bone are realigned if necessary, to orient them properly for healing. In simple cases, this can be achieved manually. The term **fixation** is used to describe the immobilization of bone fragments. A cast or splint is an example of *external fixation*. In more complex cases, surgery may be required, with *internal fixation*: the placement of hardware such as screws or plates to hold the fragments in place. Often this placement is permanent. In some cases, internal fixation also includes elaborate external hardware, shown in Figure 9-8. Surgery may also involve the placement of a bone graft, obtained from another part of the body, to fill in the gaps between the fragments.

If the fracture is open, prophylactic antibiotics are administered to prevent infection. **Prophylactic** is a term for treatment designed to prevent a problem rather than treat one that already exists. An area of open fracture may need to be surgically cleaned, called **debridement**, to remove any foreign material and contaminated or dead tissue from the area. This limits the movement of microbes into the wound.

Most simple fractures heal in 6–8 weeks and, if they take longer, nonunion is suspected and addressed. Other complications of

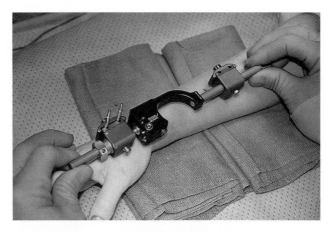

FIGURE 9-8. Treatment of a fracture by fixation. External and internal hardware help keep bone fragments in place, facilitating union. (From Koval KJ, Zuckerman JD. *Atlas of Orthopedic Surgery: A Multimedial Reference*. Philadelphia: Lippincott Williams and Wilkins, 2004.)

fracture are treated if they arise. Treatments for DVT and PE are described in Chapter 11. Minor cases of fat embolism syndrome are treated with oxygen therapy through a face mask. Severe cases are treated in an intensive care unit (Figure 9-9).

● INTERVIEW QUESTIONS

1. Where is the fracture? When did it occur? (See "Follow-Up Questions About Injuries," Chapter 4)
2. Is there swelling, pain, warmth, redness, or bruising in the area? (See "Follow-Up Questions About Pain," Chapter 4)
3. According to your doctor, has it healed well? Has healing been delayed, or incomplete?
4. Has your doctor verified complete union of the bone?
5. Do you feel any lingering vulnerability or stiffness in the area?
6. Do you feel any muscle tension, or changes in your movement patterns, as a result of the fracture?
7. Did your doctor say this was a mild, moderate, or severe fracture? Did he or she tell you it was serious for any reason, such as its location, extent, or possible complications?
8. Have you had any other complications from the fracture?
9. How has it been treated? Have you been receiving any sort of therapy for it?
10. How have treatments affected you?

● MASSAGE THERAPY GUIDELINES

Massage adjustments for a fracture are straightforward: use only the gentlest pressure—maximum level 1 for most, and 2 for some—at a fracture site until it has healed. Avoid all joint movement, as well.

The benchmark for stronger work at the site is when the physician has verified complete union of the fracture, devices are removed, and bruising and inflammation have subsided. At that point, pressure and movement should be introduced gradually, and adjusted to the client's tolerance. The client's answers to Questions 1–4 will help you determine when it is time to introduce these elements, and an external fixation device, still barricading the area, is an obvious sign that it is not yet time. Once the area has healed, the client's answers to Questions 5 and 6 help you identify goals for a course of massage treatment (see "Possible Massage Benefits").

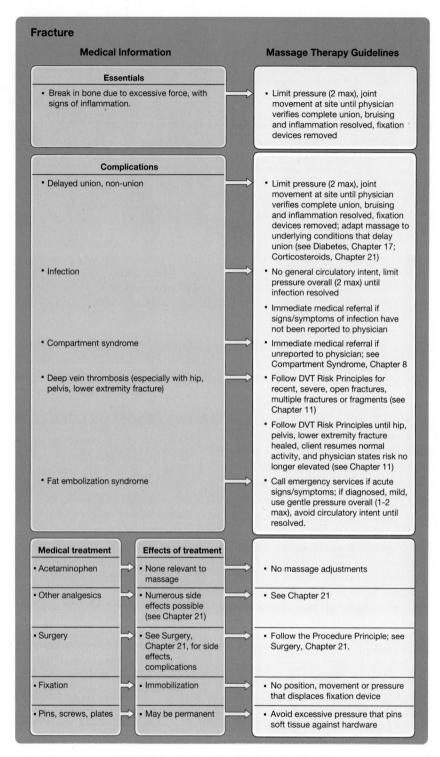

FIGURE 9-9. A Decision Tree for fracture.

Questions 7 and 8 identify possible complications. If there is delayed union or nonunion, adjust the massage in the same way you would for a fracture that is still healing. Investigate any other conditions that contribute to delayed union, including diabetes or corticosteroid treatment. Apply appropriate massage guidelines to these conditions (see "Diabetes," Chapter 17; see "Corticosteroids," Chapter 21).

In the case of an open fracture, a client may be experiencing side effects of antibiotics and massage should be adapted to those (see Table 21-1). Although it's infrequent, if signs of

infection appear after an open fracture, an immediate medical referral is in order. For diagnosed infection, avoid general circulatory intent, and limit the overall pressure to level 2 until it resolves.

A severe trauma invites caution, especially if it was recent. A fracture that was open, recent, or severe requires all of a client's resources for healing and calls for a gentle session overall. Chances are that such a trauma caused soft tissue injuries, bruising in other areas, and symptoms at other sites, as well.

THERAPIST'S JOURNAL 9-1 *A Fracture, Years Later*

I have a client in her mid-sixties who fell asleep while driving, and her car hit the guard rail on the highway. No one else was hurt, nor was she hurt particularly badly, considering how tragic it could have been. Her seat belt held her fast, saving her life but fracturing her left clavicle. She did not need surgery. She wore a sling, she iced it liberally. After the bruising had faded and her physician had pronounced the union complete, I was able to gently massage the area. She was in a fair amount of pain. I massaged her pectorals, used quiet energy holds on her shoulder, and gently moved it through its range. For weeks, we continued with this pattern and she continued, in exercise classes, to stretch. About a year and a half later, she suddenly stopped complaining of pain in the area. Now, 8 years later, she'll occasionally come in with stiffness when she's "slept wrong," and all of the above massage approaches seem to help. All in all, her shoulder seems content, and she's pretty happy with it.

As I've worked with her over time, I've noticed two things. First, our bones hold our history. With specific provocation, such as the wrong sleeping position, they are prompted to remind us what happened long ago. It's a sobering return to that early story. Second, the innate ability of our bones to pull themselves back together under the right conditions and return to work is remarkable. Quietly, behind the scenes, they reinvent themselves! Major advances in orthopedic medicine clear a path for some of the harder healing. When I hold my client's shoulder with my hand, closing my fingers around her scapula, I am reminded what good comes when everything does its work: the seat belt, our helpers, the ice pack. And most of all, the bone.

Tracy Walton
Cambridge, MA

The Compromised Client Principle. If a client is not feeling well, be gentle; even if you cannot explain the mechanism behind a contraindication, follow it anyway.

Be alert for serious complications, such as compartment syndrome, DVT, and fat embolization. If the client shows signs of compartment syndrome, he or she needs to see a physician right away (see "Compartment Syndrome," Chapter 8). Because of the incidence of DVT following fracture, there is a strong case for abiding by the DVT Risk Principles anytime a fracture is recent, severe, open, involves multiple fragments or bones, or involves any structure in the pelvis or lower extremity. DVT risk isn't an exact science, but it's reasonable to continue to follow the principles until the fracture has healed, the client has resumed normal activity, and the physician agrees that the DVT risk is no longer elevated (see Chapter 11).

Emergency services should be called if there are acute signs or symptoms of FES. However, if the condition has already been diagnosed and is mild and self-limiting, massage may be provided with limited pressure (1–2) overall, and no circulatory intent. A medical consultation is advised in this case.

Massage therapy guidelines for fracture treatment are clearcut: acetaminophen has few side effects, but stronger analgesics such as NSAIDs or opioids may; these are addressed in Chapter 21. Obviously, take care not to displace any external fixation device, and if internal hardware is present, avoid heavily pressing soft tissue against it. See "Surgery," Chapter 21, for massage therapy guidelines for clients who have had recent surgery.

● MASSAGE RESEARCH

As of this writing, there are no randomized, controlled trials, published in the English language, on fracture and massage indexed in PubMed or the Massage Therapy Foundation Research Database. The NIH RePORTER tool lists no active, federally funded research projects on the topic in the United States. No active projects are listed on the clinicaltrials.gov database (see Chapter 6).

● POSSIBLE MASSAGE BENEFITS

Fractures leave behind muscle tension, pain, stiffness, and postural imbalances. Discomfort can linger for years after union has occurred, and the site of a fracture may still be sore and weak months later as the bone continues to remodel. A massage therapist is well positioned to help with these problems, especially when working in collaboration with the client's medical team. Massage can support physical therapy, ease pain, keep the muscles in the area flexible, and thereby support the client's movement and exercise. Therapists can also focus on other muscles that were pressed into service during rehabilitation—muscles on the opposite side may be tense from overuse. Therapist's Journal 9-1 tells a story of massage therapy with a client with a fracture.

Herniated Disk (Disk Disease)

A *herniation* describes a general event in which a structure protrudes into a place it is not supposed to be, through an abnormal opening. Commonly called a slipped disk, a **herniated disk** occurs when the intervertebral disk or a portion of it extends outside its usual space, into the spinal canal. *Disk disease* is a general term that describes a breakdown in disk structure that occurs from trauma, or in response to aging. The **nucleus pulposus**, or elastic core of the disk, becomes smaller and harder over time. The protective capsule of the disk, called the **annulus fibrosus**, becomes worn and torn with age. When these structures thin and harden over time, the disk becomes more susceptible to injury and to movement outside its customary space.

● BACKGROUND

A common occurrence in low-back injuries, a herniated disk can also occur in the cervical spine. Thoracic herniated disks are less common because of the stability of the spine afforded by the rib cage.

In a severe herniation, the disk structure may weaken under pressure and tear open, forcing the contents of the disk into the spinal canal. This is known as a **ruptured disk**.

Signs and Symptoms

A herniated disk becomes a problem when it presses on the spinal cord or nerve root, as shown in Figure 9-10. Depending on where it presses, it can cause pain. A disk problem can cause *local pain* at the site, or radicular pain. **Radicular pain** is pain that is referred along the sensory distribution of a nerve when the nerve root is compressed or irritated. If this occurs in the cervical area, radicular pain and other symptoms may appear in the shoulder, upper arm, and scapula as well as local symptoms in the neck. In a cervical herniated disk, radicular pain can be aggravated by coughing, neck flexion, or neck rotation. Tingling, known as **paresthesia**, may occur, along with numbness or loss of motor function.

If a disk herniates in the lumbar area, the symptoms include severe local pain in the low back, and radicular pain to one or both hips and lower extremities. This pain distribution down the buttock and side or back of the lower extremity is called **sciatica**. The pain in this area is also aggravated by coughing, laughing, straining, or sitting for long periods. Numbness and tingling occur in the legs and feet.

Complications

Complications of a herniated disk are indistinct from the severe symptoms, described above. When chronic, lower level symptoms do not respond to conservative (nonsurgical) treatment, it is considered a complication.

A rare, serious complication of a lumbar herniated disk occurs with a chronic pressure on the spinal cord itself, or, in the lumbar area, the *cauda equina*—the bundle of nerve extensions below the spinal cord. In **cauda equina syndrome**, compression of these nerves leads to increasing pain, loss of bowel or bladder function, problems with sexual function, and numbness in the groin, medial thighs, and low back. Compression of these structures is a medical emergency, as continuous pressure can lead to paralysis.

Treatment

Conservative treatment includes rest, heating pads and warm baths, pain-relieving medications (NSAIDs), massage, and resuming movement as soon as possible. For an acute herniated disk, 1–2 days of rest are often recommended, along with pain medications. This conservative treatment gets most people—about 60%—back to functioning in 1–2 weeks. After 6 or 8 weeks, about 90–98% of people are fully functioning.

If milder drugs are not effective for pain relief, muscle relaxants or opioid analgesics (see Chapter 21) may be used. In some cases, epidural and spinal nerve injection of corticosteroid medication is done, to reduce inflammation. This seems to help some people feel better, although the evidence for it is inconclusive. The side effects are severe headache, increased back and leg pain, and dizziness.

Physicians want patients to resume movement, especially walking or swimming, as soon as possible to avoid deconditioning. Support may be provided through physical therapy and lifestyle modifications, including weight loss where needed.

If conservative measures are not effective, various levels of surgery can be performed. A **diskectomy** is the removal of a herniated disk, followed by surgical fusion of the surrounding vertebrae. A less invasive procedure is the drawing out of the nucleus pulposus through a small incision.

● INTERVIEW QUESTIONS

1. Where is the disk herniation?
2. How long have you had it? Was there just one episode, or do you have flare-ups over time? (See "Follow-Up Questions About Injuries," Chapter 4)
3. What are your symptoms? Do you have pain, tingling, numbness, or weakness? (See "Follow-Up Questions About Pain," Chapter 4)

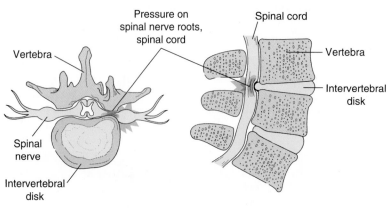

Pressure on spinal nerve roots, spinal cord

Spinal cord

Vertebra

Vertebra

Spinal nerve

Intervertebral disk

Intervertebral disk

Superior view of vertebra

Sagittal view of spine

FIGURE 9-10. Herniated disk. (From Willis MC. *Medical Terminology: The Language of Health Care*, 2nd ed. Philadelphia: Lippincott Williams and Wilkins, 2005.)

4. Does the area feel stable or unstable to you? Are position changes, movement, daily activities, and exercise okay, or do these activities worsen the condition? Is your doctor concerned about the stability of the area?
5. Are there positions, such as sleeping positions, which make you more or less comfortable?
6. How has your herniated disk been treated? How does treatment affect you?

● MASSAGE THERAPY GUIDELINES

The most pressing massage therapy concern is arriving at the best pressure, position, and level of joint movement for the client with a herniated disk. To that end, questions 1–5 are combined with "Follow-Up Questions About Pain and Injury" (see Chapter 4). The Pain, Injury, and Inflammation Principles are helpful here.

The massage therapy guidelines here are focused on the critical 6–8 weeks after injury.

In general, a medical consultation is advised when working during the acute phase of it, or in the 6–8 weeks following the event. Questions 2 and 3 will help identify the progression of the condition. Question 4 about stability is important, to establish how careful you have to be. Bear in mind that the age of the individual has an impact on stability; most herniated disks occur in 35–55 year olds, but the older the individual, the less stable the area is likely to be. In general, if the condition is healing well and the client's stability and function are increasing, less caution is necessary.

The best positions are the most neutral ones. Question 5 should elicit some guidance from the client. Most people with lumbar disk issues are comfortable in the prone position with slight padding at the waist and ankles but may feel stiffness in the low back after a short while. A client with a herniated cervical disk may be comfortable prone in a face cradle, but small adjustments in the height and angle of the face cradle are likely to make a significant difference in comfort. A well-supported side-lying position is usually best for cervical and lumbar disk conditions.

Because small movements in the area can cause pain, give good thought to the best pressure at the site, and limit the intentional and unintentional movements of joints. Recall that joint movement during a massage can be intentional, as in imposing a stretch, and it can be unintentional, as in the natural rotation of the cervical spine as the shoulders are massaged and rocked with pressure. Slight movement of adjacent joints occurs at pressure levels 3 and above (see "The Pressure Scale," Chapter 2).

With these cautions in mind, the safest pressure at the site for an acute condition is levels 1–2 because there is no movement. In practice, a pressure level 3 may be well tolerated in the lumbar area, but level 2 may be best in the cervical area. Modify pressure even further for a client in severe pain, is experiencing disk disease symptoms for the first time, or is having trouble managing the condition.

> *The New, Unfamiliar, or Poorly Managed Pain Principle.* **Massage for a client with new, unfamiliar, or poorly managed pain should be more conservative than massage for a client with a familiar, well-managed pain pattern.**

Caution is best for intentional joint movement, as well. Because movement caused a shift in the disk in the first place, avoid any movement or stretch that puts the spine into the positions that cause the injury. At minimum, flexion and rotation are a concern, but additional movements may be important to avoid, as well.

By easing muscle spasm in the area, you can support the work of a manual therapist such as an osteopath, physical therapist, or chiropractor who is attempting to reestablish proper alignment. This argues for communication with the rest of the health care team. Work gradually to ease muscle tension. It may be needed to stabilize the area and should not be addressed all at once.

> *The Respect Muscle Splinting Principle.* **Do not try to eliminate muscle tension that may be protecting an area of injury, pain, or disease.**

Ask at each session about the client's symptoms, and be alert for changes. If a client has pain or numbness in the arms or legs, worsening symptoms, or weakness, encourage the client to report it to his or her physician. Weakness and "electric shock" sensations are serious red flags. If a client complains of numbness or pain in the saddle configuration—groin, medial thighs, and buttocks—he or she should seek immediate medical attention for possible cauda equina syndrome.

Adapt massage to any medications the client is taking to manage pain. Common effects of muscle relaxants and NSAIDs are in the Decision Tree (see Figure 9-11). Other side effects are in Chapter 21 along with effects of opioid analgesics.

If the client received an injection of corticosteroid in the last several days, adapt to potentially strong side effects, such as a temporary increase in back and leg pain, with gentler pressure overall and limited joint movement. Severe headache is addressed in Table 21-1 and in Chapter 10. If a client has had recent surgery, see "Surgery," Chapter 21, for massage therapy guidelines.

● MASSAGE RESEARCH

As of this writing, there are no randomized, controlled trials, published in the English language, on herniated disk and massage indexed in PubMed or the Massage Therapy Foundation Research Database. The NIH RePORTER tool lists no active, federally funded research projects on the topic in the United States. No active projects are listed on the clinicaltrials.gov database (see Chapter 6).

There are two Cochrane reviews that may be relevant: one on neck pain (Haraldsson et al., 2006) found insufficient evidence in support of massage, though the abstract did not specify the inclusion of disk disease in the review. Another review, on nonspecific low back pain (Furlan et al., 2008), found that massage might be helpful. But the second review is on massage and back pain with no detectable cause. Whether some of the studies in this category included subjects with symptomatic, undiagnosed herniated disks is unclear. Future massage trials, focused on diagnosed disk disease patients, will provide valuable information to the massage profession.

Herniated Disk

Medical Information	Massage Therapy Guidelines

Essentials

- Extension of intervertebral disk material into spinal canal
- Often causes pressure on spinal cord or nerve roots
- Common in lumbar spine, less common in cervical spine, rare in thoracic spine

→

- Follow the Pain, Injury, and Inflammation Principles
- Position client with spine in neutral, comfortable position (consider sidelying)
- Limit joint movement (intentional and unintentional)

Complications

- Pain, can radiate to associated extremities
- Numbness, tingling
- Weakness

- Muscle spasm

- Cauda equina syndrome (rare): numbness/pain in "saddle" configuration, loss of bowel and bladder control

→

- See above guidelines for position, joint movement; limit pressure
- Medical referral if neurologic symptoms haven't been reported to physician
- Follow the Respect Muscle Splinting Principle, once stabilized, note Pain-Spasm-Pain principle
- Immediate medical referral if signs/symptoms have not been reported to physician

Medical treatment	Effects of treatment	Massage Therapy Guidelines
• Conservative treatment: rest 1-2 days, heating pads, warm baths, gentle exercises	• Few side effects or complications	• No massage adjustments
• NSAIDs	• Numerous side effects possible, especially in older adults, see Chapter 21	• See NSAIDs, Chapter 21
	• GI disturbances	• See Table 21-1 for common GI side effects and massage therapy guidelines
	• Headache	• Position for comfort, especially prone; consider inclined table or propping; gentle session overall; pressure to tolerance; slow speed and even rhythm; general circulatory intent may be poorly tolerated
	• Drowsiness, dizziness	• Reposition gently, slow speed and even rhythm, slow rise from table, gentle transition at end of session
• Muscle relaxants	• CNS depression	• Gentle pressure overall (2 or 3 max)
	• Reduced muscle tone	• Avoid stretching; do not attempt to increase ROM
	• Constipation	• Gentle pressure at abdomen (2 max); medical referral if client has not had a bowel movement for several days.
	• Drowsiness, dizziness	• Reposition gently, slow speed and even rhythm, slow rise from table, gentle transition at end of session
• Opioid analgesics	• Numerous side effects possible (see Chapter 21)	• See Chapter 21
• Corticosteroid injections (spinal, epidural)	• Increased pain in back, lower extremities	• Gentle pressure overall (1-2 max), avoid general circulatory intent, limit joint movement
	• Severe headache	• See Table 21-1
• Surgery	• See Surgery, Chapter 21, for side effects, complications	• Follow the Procedure Principle; see Surgery, Chapter 21

FIGURE 9-11. A Decision Tree for herniated disk.

POSSIBLE MASSAGE BENEFITS

Some muscle spasm is to be expected in a herniated disk because of muscle splinting. Once the injury has stabilized, massage in the area, using medium and deep pressure levels, may interrupt the pain-spasm-pain cycle and bring about considerable relief. Massage may also support the work of other manual practitioners in reestablishing good alignment. By facilitating exercise and increasing body awareness, massage may help prevent reinjury, a high priority for anyone who has experienced a herniated disk.

Other Skeletal System Conditions in Brief

ANKYLOSING SPONDYLITIS

Background	• Autoimmune condition of spine and large joints (hips, knees, shoulders); inflammation causes episodes of back pain and stiffness, damage and eventual fusion of vertebrae. • In some cases, mild eye inflammation, heart valve inflammation. • Breathing problems occur with stiffness of costovertebral (rib-vertebra) joints; stooped posture develops as a way to relieve pain; increased vulnerability to respiratory infection. • Vulnerability to vertebral fracture, cauda equina syndrome (see "Herniated Disk [Disk Disease]," this chapter). • Treated with NSAIDs, disease-modifying antirheumatic drugs (DMARDs), corticosteroids, biologics, with some strong side effects.
Interview Questions	• How long have you had it? Symptoms? Which joints affected? • Aggravating and relieving factors? What are your most comfortable positions? • Any complications or effects on eyes, heart, breathing? • Any fracture history? • Treatment? Effects of treatment?
Massage Therapy Guidelines	• During flare-up, or if spine stability questionable (fracture history or physician concern), use gentle pressure (2 max), very gentle joint movement at the sites. • Adjust positioning and bolstering for comfort. • Massage of muscles near affected sites may facilitate flexibility, breathing. • Investigate pulmonary, cardiac complications, adapt massage accordingly. • Adjust massage to side effects and complications of medications (see "NSAIDs," "Corticosteroids," Chapter 21; see "Biologic Therapy," Chapter 20). Investigate side effects of DMARDs, which can be strong (Wible, 2009); work gently overall. Consult Table 21-1 for massage guidelines for immunosuppression and other side effects.

ARTHRITIS, PSORIATIC

Background	• Chronic, autoimmune inflammation of joints, ligaments, tendons, and fascia; causes intense pain at joints; features flare-ups and remissions. • Associated with psoriasis (see Chapter 7), although some do not have any symptoms of psoriasis. • Treated with corticosteroid injections at joint, methotrexate and other disease-modifying antirheumatic drugs (DMARDs), biologics, combination therapies. • Numerous, strong side effects of drugs possible (see Chapter 21).
Interview Questions	• Where? In flare-up now? Symptoms? When was last flare-up? • Comfortable positions? Massage history? • Treatment? Effects of treatment?
Massage Therapy Guidelines	• During flare-up, use caution to avoid aggravating pain at affected joints; pressure level 1–2 maximum at site; avoid joint movement that aggravates pain; avoid general circulatory intent. • During remission, continue gentle pressure at affected sites; if possible, use massage history to gauge tolerance near affected areas; position and bolster for comfort. • Adjust massage to side effects and complications of principal medications (see "Corticosteroids," Chapter 21; see "Biologic Therapy," Chapter 20). Investigate side effects of DMARDs, which can be strong (Wible, 2009); work gently overall. Consult Table 21-1 for massage guidelines for immunosuppression and other side effects.

ARTHRITIS, RHEUMATOID

Background	• Chronic, autoimmune inflammation of joints; results in joint injury and destruction over time; characterized by flare and remission periods. • Begins with small, distal joints in hands, wrists, ankles, feet, and progressing to larger, proximal joints. • Causes flare-ups of pain, stiffness, redness, and heat at joints; fever, fatigue, muscle pain. • Complications include disability, inflammation and destruction of skin, muscles, vertebrae, heart, vessels; severe cases involve destruction of vertebrae with neurologic complications. • Treated with NSAIDs, corticosteroids, disease-modifying antirheumatic drugs (DMARDs), biologics, combination therapies. • Numerous, strong side effects of drugs possible (see Chapter 21).
Interview Questions	• Where? In flare-up now? Symptoms? When was last flare-up? • Comfortable positions? Massage history? • Treatment? Effects of treatment?
Massage Therapy Guidelines	• No general circulatory intent during flare-up; position and bolster for comfort. • Gentle pressure to tolerance, no circulatory intent at affected sites during flare-up. • During remission: If joints damaged, disfigured, use gentle pressure (1–2 maximum); massage may help muscle tension, soreness. • Adjust massage to side effects and complications of principal medications (see "NSAIDs," "Corticosteroids," Chapter 21; see "Biologic Therapy," Chapter 20). Investigate side effects of DMARDs, which can be strong (Wible, 2009); work gently overall. Consult Table 21-1 for massage guidelines for immunosuppression and other side effects.

ARTHRITIS, SEPTIC

Background	• Infection in joint capsule through open fracture, surgery, implants. • Acute joint inflammation with spread of organism to bloodstream; intense joint pain, redness, heat, swelling, fever. • Joint damage may occur if treatment delayed; complications of infection can be fatal; treated with antibiotics.
Interview Questions	• Where? When was onset? Has doctor said infection is resolved? • Symptoms of inflammation? Fever? • Treatment? Effects of treatment?
Massage Therapy Guidelines	• No general circulatory intent; gentle pressure overall (2 max) until infection resolved. • Limit pressure (2 max), friction, joint movement, circulatory intent at affected site until inflammation is resolved. • After resolution, massage may help ease muscle tension at site and restore function. • Adjust massage to side effects of antibiotics (see Table 21-1).

AVASCULAR NECROSIS

Background	• Interrupted blood flow to bone, occurring in femoral head (most common), wrist, knee, shoulder; causes pain, loss of ROM. • Secondary to another condition such as vascular spasm (Raynaud disease), embolization of fat (due to pancreatitis), sickle-cell anemia (occlusion by damaged red blood cells). • Treated with NSAIDs, bisphosphonates; irreversible damage due to bone death usually necessitates surgical bone transplant, reshaping, joint replacement.
Interview Questions	• Where? Symptoms? Cause? • According to doctor, how stable is area? Any medical restrictions on movement or activity? Comfortable positions? • Treatment? Any surgery? Effects of treatment?
Massage Therapy Guidelines	• Limit pressure and avoid joint movement at affected site if any chance of joint instability; use caution when moving joint into massage position. • Investigate primary cause and adapt massage session accordingly. • Adapt massage to NSAIDs, bisphosphonates (see "Osteoporosis," this chapter), or to recent surgery (see Chapter 21).

BONE CANCER, PRIMARY

Background	• Cancer that *begins* in the bone (for cancer that has *spread*, or metastasized to bone from another primary site such as breast or prostate, see "Bone Metastasis," Chapter 20). • Bone is uncommon site of primary cancer but is more common in children than in adults. • Can be asymptomatic or cause pain, swelling, tenderness at the site; weakening of bone structure can lead to pathologic fracture; can metastasize to other organs, especially lungs.
Interview Questions	• Where is (or was) it in your body? Is it malignant or benign? What are your symptoms? • Any complications? Is cancer present only in the bones, or in other organs such as lungs? Any history of fracture? • Describe your activity level, or movement habits, day to day and week to week? Does your doctor support your activity level? Any medical restrictions on movement or activity? Are any of your health care providers (doctors, nurses, physical therapists, occupational therapists) concerned about the stability of your bones? • Treatment? Effects of treatment?
Massage Therapy Guidelines	• Review "Cancer," Chapter 20, for massage therapy guidelines for cancer and cancer treatment; no direct massage pressure at/over active tumor site. • Be careful with joint movement and pressure at site where bone stability is in question; pressure level 1 or 2 may be maximum; to determine appropriate pressure, joint movement, seek medical consultation (especially if history of pathologic fracture). • Check in regularly about changes in bone stability. • Adapt to any cancer spread to other organs; if metastasis to lungs, effects similar to primary lung cancer; see Lung Cancer, Chapter 14. • Adapt to effects of cancer treatments (see Chapter 20; "Surgery," Chapter 21). • Massage or simple touch may ease bone pain; note Pain-Spasm-Pain Principle.

BUNION (HALLUX VALGUS)

Background	• Misalignment of medial aspect of proximal phalanx of big toe produces protrusion, stretching of joint capsule, callus. • Osteoarthritis, bone spur, and bursitis can develop at protrusion, causing inflammation and intense pain, aggravated by walking. • Treated with change in footwear, corticosteroid injection at joint, surgery to remove bunion, fuse joint, reshape bones.
Interview Questions	• Where? Symptoms? Acute or chronic? • Treatment? Effects of treatment?
Massage Therapy Guidelines	• Avoid friction, circulatory intent at site when acute. • Limit pressure (and possibly contact, depending on level of tenderness) at site when acute; massage of regional muscles may ease pain, stiffness, especially when chronic. • Adapt to side effects, complications of corticosteroid injection at site, surgery (see Chapter 21).

GOUT (GOUTY ARTHRITIS)

Background	• Inflammation in the foot, usually in big toe, causing severe pain. • Sharp uric acid crystals press on joints and soft tissue. • Strong associations with kidney stones and CV conditions, including hypertension, atherosclerosis, and stroke. • Treated with NSAIDs (except aspirin) and colchicine, which may cause peripheral neuropathy (see Chapter 10).
Interview Questions	• Where? When did it start? More than one episode? • Any CV conditions or medications? Any history of kidney stones, high blood pressure, atherosclerosis, or stroke? • Treatment? Effects of treatment?

Massage Therapy Guidelines	• No contact or joint movement at site of gouty joint; clients with gout are unlikely to let you near affected joints; any massage at all may be unwelcome.
	• For client with gout history, investigate CV conditions; consider DVT Risk Principles and Plaque Problem Principle (see Chapter 11); if cardiac disease present, medical consultation may be necessary before providing massage with general circulatory intent.
	• Adapt massage to effects of treatments (see "NSAIDs," Chapter 21; "Peripheral Neuropathy," Chapter 10).

LYME DISEASE

Background	• Bacterial infection, from tick bite, causes arthritic condition with other symptoms.
	• Symptoms occur in stages: flu-like symptoms (fever, night sweats, swollen lymph nodes, generalized achiness, fatigue), CV symptoms (dizziness, fainting due to heart problems), neurological symptoms (headache, stiff neck, weakness in extremities and trunk, cognitive difficulties, sleep disorders), Lyme arthritis (joint inflammation, often in knees, elbows, shoulders).
	• Chronic symptoms can continue over years; mechanisms poorly understood.
	• Treated with oral or IV antibiotics; common side effects include nausea, mild diarrhea, fatigue.
Interview Questions	• When did you first have symptoms? When was it diagnosed? Current symptoms? Symptoms over the course of the disease?
	• Any neurological or CV complications? Any joints affected?
	• Treatment? Effects of treatment?
Massage Therapy Guidelines	• General circulatory intent contraindicated for flu-like symptoms
	• If dizziness, fainting present, reposition gently and encourage slow rise from table at end of session. For more serious heart problems, see Chapter 11.
	• Adapt massage to neurologic symptoms: Use cautious pressure at site of headache, stiff neck, weakness, and position for comfort; for other neurological symptoms, see Chapter 10.
	• Schedule and design massage appropriately for sleep disorders: sedative approach at end of day, activating/stimulating earlier in day.
	• For inflamed joints, limit pressure at site to 1–2; use cautious, pain-free joint movement. If infection resolved, but arthritis remains, massage with heavier pressure and movement at site may be helpful in reducing tension, stiffness, pain.
	• Follow Compromised Client Principle (see Chapter 3).
	• Adapt massage to effects of antibiotics (see Table 21-1).

OSTEOMYELITIS

Background	• Bacterial or fungal infection of bone and marrow, can be localized or systemic.
	• Usually caused by trauma to nearby soft tissue during injury, open fracture, surgery; individuals with poor circulation, immunosuppression are vulnerable.
	• Occurs less commonly when microorganisms from infection of heart, urinary tract, or upper respiratory tract move through bloodstream, establish infection in bone.
	• Symptoms include severe pain, swelling, redness, high fever and chills; can be acute or chronic (milder symptoms).
	• Can destroy bone, cause joint deformity, collapse of bone structure, arthritis, or septicemia (blood poisoning).
	• Short- or long-term treatment with antibiotics; surgical procedures include debridement, removal of fixation devices, tissue graft, amputation.
Interview Questions	• Where? When? Currently acute, chronic, or resolved?
	• Symptoms? Fever, chills, pain, swelling, redness?
	• Treatment? Effects of treatment?
	• Comfortable and uncomfortable positions? Activity restrictions?

Massage Therapy Guidelines	• For acute and chronic cases, or lingering symptoms, general circulatory intent contraindicated. • Gentle pressure at site (1 max), limit joint movement; position and bolster for comfort; no contact at open lesion. • For chronic cases, during recovery, follow Activity and Energy Principle (see Chapter 3). • If condition resolved and you are working as part of a health care time, site-specific massage may be indicated to address muscle tension, restore function.

PAGET DISEASE (OSTEITIS DEFORMANS)

Background	• Degenerative bone disease in which highly mineralized bone structure is broken down and replaced by fibrous, eventually brittle tissue; lesions become enlarged, weakened, with vast networks of vessels. • Often occurs in one bone; most common in spine, cranium, pelvis, long bones of the lower extremity. • May be asymptomatic or produce pain that worsens at night, is not relieved by movement or rest; skin temperature may increase near site, as vascularization occurs. • Complications include pathologic fracture, osteoarthritis near affected joints, disfigurement, compression of adjacent nerves or spinal cord. • Blood calcium levels may be disrupted; in severe cases with multiple or large lesions, heart failure may occur. • Treatment with bisphosphonates, analgesics, exercise, physical therapy.
Interview Questions	• Where? When diagnosed? Symptoms? Any pain? Complications? • Instability? Activity level? Does your doctor support your activity level? Any medical restrictions on movement or activity? Are any of your health care providers (doctors, nurses, physical therapists, occupational therapists) concerned about the stability of your bones? • Any comfortable or uncomfortable positions?
Massage Therapy Guidelines	• Limit pressure (2 max) and joint movement at affected sites until bone stability is determined; consult physician about best pressure levels. • Position and bolster for comfort. Adapt to osteoarthritis at adjacent joints (see "Osteoarthritis," this chapter). • Avoid general circulatory intent if heart function is compromised. No general circulatory intent if complications include heart failure. • Adapt massage position, scheduling to bisphosphonates when necessary (see "Osteoporosis," this chapter). Adapt to effects of analgesics (see Chapter 21).

TEMPOROMANDIBULAR JOINT DISORDERS (TMJD)

Background	• Umbrella term for jaw problems, causing popping and clicking, difficulty opening and closing mouth, difficulty chewing and swallowing; symptoms also include pain in jaw, neck, shoulder, ear; headache. • Interplay of multiple factors contribute to or trigger TMJD, including derangement of joint, trauma, osteoarthritis, rheumatoid arthritis, teeth grinding, spinal imbalances, and emotional stress. • Treated with dental splints (e.g., night guard), heat, cold, physical therapy, including ultrasound and massage; drug treatments include muscle relaxants, NSAIDs; surgical procedures include arthroscopic surgery, joint replacement.
Interview Questions	• Symptoms? When diagnosed, by whom? Pain in other areas besides jaw? • Treatment? Effects of treatment?
Massage Therapy Guidelines	• Many people self-diagnose; urge medical referral if client has not already reported condition to physician or dentist. • Massage could help with excess tension in jaw, neck, head, and shoulders, but before using pressure level 3 or above at jaw, consult treating physician, dentist, physical therapist, chiropractor, or other provider, in order to coordinate care.

SELF TEST

1. Describe the differences between osteoarthritis and osteoporosis in terms of the tissues affected, presence or absence of inflammation, complications, and massage therapy guidelines.
2. Regarding osteoarthritis pain, is it felt during activity or at rest? Explain.
3. Describe the research that supports the use of massage with people with osteoarthritis. Does it clearly establish a benefit of massage for people with osteoarthritis?
4. Osteoporosis often goes unrecognized until a complication occurs. Explain the common complication of osteoporosis.
5. Which massage pressure levels are appropriate for a client with visible spine changes due to osteoporosis?
6. If a person with osteoporosis comes to you for relief of back pain, how should you work with her or him that day? What information do you need from the client to proceed?
7. Explain the massage guideline for a client who is taking oral bisphosphonates for osteoporosis.
8. A client comes to you with a recent fracture with delayed union. What are the possible causes of the delay?

9. What information is needed from the client's physician before using pressure or movement in the area of a fracture?
10. Compare two types of embolization that can complicate a fracture: Which types of fracture give rise to each one? What are the consequences of each, and how should you respond to the risk?
11. How could massage therapy help a person who is recovering from a fracture?
12. Define local pain and radicular pain. Describe the areas of local pain and radicular pain in a herniated cervical disk. Describe, as well, for a herniated lumbar disk.
13. Describe the cautious use of movement required for a client with an acute herniated disk, including intentional and unintentional movements. How does pressure need to be adjusted?
14. What are the symptoms of cauda equina syndrome? What is the appropriate response to a client who reports these symptoms?
15. How could massage therapy be helpful to a person with a herniated disk? Is massage benefit supported by research in this case?

 For answers to these questions and to see a bibliography for this chapter, visit http://thePoint. lww.com/Walton.

Our nervous systems are not self-contained; they link with those of the people close to us in a silent rhythm that helps regulate our physiology.

—TIAN DAYTON

Against the landscape of a fast-paced, stress-filled information age, massage therapists offer quiet and relaxation. But even more may be going on, deep below the surface interactions of hands and tissues. Skilled touch seems to have profound effects on people: evening out inner rhythms and smoothing out human interactions. Massage therapy is a rhythmic give and take between two nervous systems. It goes beyond the fleeting electronic connections and hurried conversations that fill many people's days, restoring balance and wholeness to the human form.

This underground process engages the nervous system, the network of hidden wiring that processes every interaction.

Nervous system disorders and conditions have numerous causes. Nerve pathways can be injured, crowded out by other structures in the body, or subject to destruction by inflammation and scarring. The effects are often widely felt. Damaged sensory nerves can cause pain, tingling, burning, or even the absence of any sensation at all. Impaired motor nerves can cause abnormal skeletal muscle movement, weakness, or the irregular action of cardiac muscle, smooth muscle, or glands.

If the effects are in the *somatic nervous system*, sensation changes or motor weakness are apparent. If the effects are

in the *autonomic nervous system*, functions such as bladder or bowel control, blood pressure or temperature regulation are affected. When the brain is involved, seizures or cognitive impairments may occur, along with disturbances in sensation and movement. In general, conditions that affect the central nervous system–the brain and spinal cord–are more serious than conditions that affect the pathways of the peripheral nervous system (PNS).

The following five conditions, four of which involve the central nervous system (CNS), are discussed in depth in this chapter, with full Decision Trees:

- Multiple sclerosis
- Parkinson disease
- Stroke
- Depression
- Peripheral neuropathy

In addition, a full discussion of cerebral palsy, including a Decision Tree, may be found online at http://thePoint.lww.com/Walton. Conditions in brief are anxiety (anxiety disorder), addiction (chemical dependency), alcohol intoxication, Bell palsy, brain tumor (primary) and metastatic brain disease (secondary), carpal tunnel syndrome, dementia/Alzheimer disease, encephalitis, cluster headache, migraine headache, tension headache, meningitis, polio and postpolio syndrome, reflex sympathetic dystrophy (complex regional pain syndrome), seizures/seizure disorders, spina bifida, spinal cord injury (SCI), and trigeminal neuralgia (tic doloreux).

General Principles

No single principle is practiced with all neurological conditions, but several basic principles from Chapter 3 are frequently applied. Because a massage therapist is often working in unknown, unpredictable territory with nervous system conditions, the Previous Massage Principle and the Where You Start Isn't Always Where You End Up Principle

are commonly used. The therapist uses a client's track record of massage, or the client's responses to massage over time, to guide the session. And because sensation is sometimes compromised in nervous system conditions, the Sensation Principle and the Sensation Loss, Injury Prone Principle are also applied.

Multiple Sclerosis

Multiple sclerosis (MS) is a chronic, progressive, autoimmune condition that damages the myelin sheath around certain nerves in the CNS, in a process called demyelination. MS is one of several *demyelinating diseases*. The destruction

and scarring of the myelin tissue lead to plaque formation at the site. A plaque is a thickening or hardening of tissue. MS symptoms and signs depend on the location of plaque, and the functions of the affected area, in each case.

● BACKGROUND

Most cases of MS are diagnosed between the ages of 20 and 50. Symptoms often manifest in cycles of relapse and remission, as myelin sheaths are damaged, repaired, then damaged again; the damage may be cumulative. Remissions can bring a full return to baseline or absence of symptoms, or they can be partial. Relapses of symptoms are often called exacerbations, and some people call them flare-ups.

There are four main types of MS, based on symptom patterns over time: relapsing-remitting, primary progressive, secondary progressive, and progressive-relapsing. Many people with MS switch from a relapsing-remitting pattern, in which symptoms completely disappear after an episode, into another more progressive pattern over time, in which episodes worsen each time, or are no longer punctuated by remissions. In the primary progressive pattern, symptoms begin to increase at the onset of the first symptoms; in the secondary progressive pattern, distinct episodes are followed by a gradual increase in symptom severity. In the progressive-relapsing pattern, a steady increase in symptoms occurs over time, with episodes of aggravated symptoms. Figure 10-1 shows the characteristic symptom patterns and resulting disability in the four main types of MS.

In most symptom patterns, people function at high levels for many years, and the disease does not tend to shorten life expectancy. Although it is associated with progressive disability, 70% of individuals with MS will not need a wheelchair, and about 40% experience no significant effect on normal activities. Medications can improve function and slow the progression of MS for many people.

Signs and Symptoms

In newly diagnosed patients, symptoms tend to include motor weakness in the limbs, partial or complete vision loss with eye pain, and sensation changes called paresthesia (abnormal, spontaneous, usually nonpainful sensations such as tingling, burning, pricking, or buzzing) in the trunk, extremity, or on one side. Numbness may be present, and some people experience tremor.

Clinical features of MS include disturbances in bowel and bladder function, such as constipation, urinary incontinence, frequency and urgency, or partial urinary retention due to poor bladder control. Spasticity, or a state of resistance to passive movement in muscles, is a result of CNS damage. Spastic muscles are stiff, with increased tone, attributed to an overactive stretch reflex. Spasticity worsens when a limb is moved too quickly and can be aggravated by various stimuli, including touch that is too hard or soft. Ataxia, or the inability to coordinate voluntary movement, can also be present, resulting in a staggering gait. Disabling fatigue is a common complaint of people with MS, and vertigo or vomiting may occur. Less commonly, difficulties occur with memory or attention.

Nearly half of people with MS experience pain. Some MS pain is neuropathic, arising directly from nervous system dysfunction. This pain often has a burning, shooting, or gnawing quality. MS pain is also musculoskeletal in origin, resulting from spasm, postural changes, changes in body use due to spastic muscles, and disability. In addition to steady pain, some pain is position dependent: A good portion of people experience Lhermitte sign, an electric sensation that shoots down the body when the neck is flexed.

Episodes of MS can be triggered or aggravated by a rise in core body temperature from hot or humid weather, saunas, or hot baths. However, symptoms tend to recede when the body temperature returns to normal.

Complications

Any of the earlier symptoms can worsen as MS advances. Progressive disability can occur, as seen in Figure 10-1. If MS limits movement, inactivity causes a loss of muscle tone, resulting in deconditioning. All the problems that attend inactivity, such as loss of bone density, shallow breathing, and poor posture, are possible complications. If MS symptoms interfere with the

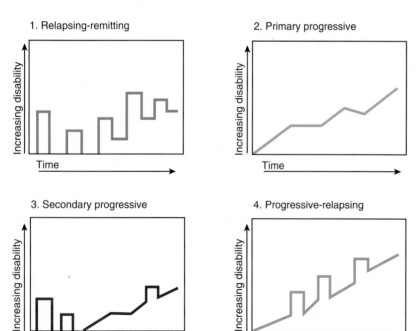

FIGURE 10-1. Progression of symptoms and disability in MS. The four main types of MS feature discrete episodes of relapse and remission, steady worsening symptoms, or a combination.

ability to walk, there is a risk of pressure sores (see Conditions in Brief, Chapter 7), as with any disability that limits movement.

Later, less common complications of MS include mania and dementia. Seizures are possible but rare. Bladder problems (partial retention of urine) develop into urinary tract infections (see Chapter 18).

Treatment

Many medications are used to treat MS. They vary according to the symptom pattern. Some medications are used to modify the course of the disease; others are used to manage symptoms. Brief courses of corticosteroids are used to manage symptoms during acute exacerbations. They ease the CNS inflammation that causes the range of symptoms. However, they have strong side effects and complications with repeated use (see "Corticosteroids," Chapter 21).

Interferon-β and glatiramer acetate are used to prevent exacerbations. As *immunomodulators*, they disrupt the normal course of the disease, decreasing the frequency of exacerbations and slowing disease progression. Both drugs can cause reactions at the injection site, and glatiramer acetate (Copaxone) can cause shortness of breath and flushing immediately after the injection. Interferons can cause flu-like symptoms, but the side effects tend to decrease over time. Because liver toxicity can be a complication, patients are monitored for liver function. These disease modifiers are more beneficial when taken early in the course of the disease. They are not appropriate for all symptom patterns, however, and other drugs may be needed.

Because of their immunosuppressant effect, a few drugs normally used in cancer chemotherapy, such as mitoxantrone and cyclophosphamide, are used for severe MS. People taking these drugs are subject to some of the side effects of chemotherapy (see Chapter 20). Plasma exchange, also reserved for severe, intractable cases, may be done to remove the circulating antibodies that are thought to be responsible for the disease. In this process, whole blood is withdrawn, the plasma is separated out and purified, and the suspension of cleansed blood is returned to the individual. The benefit of plasma exchange in MS is controversial, but the procedure tends to be well monitored and well tolerated. Side effects after the procedure may include reduced resistance to infection and blood clotting problems (either poor blood clotting because of heparin used during the treatment, or an elevated risk of thrombosis).

Symptom management is achieved with a host of medications. Spasticity and pain are high priorities, as are urinary problems. Among the medications for spasticity are muscle relaxants (baclofen, diazepam, tizanidine, dantroline). Botulinum toxin (Botox) may also be used, injected directly into spastic muscles, with few side effects.

For MS pain that is due to nervous system dysfunction, low doses of antiseizure medications may be used: gabapentin and clonazepam. Low-dose tricyclic antidepressants (TCAs) are a class of drugs originally developed for the treatment of depression (this chapter), but some, such as amitriptyline, are used in lower doses for neuropathic pain. Muscle relaxants, antiseizure drugs, and antidepressants are commonly used for other nervous system conditions, as well. These medications and massage therapy guidelines are summarized in Table 10-1.

NSAIDs and other analgesics are used for musculoskeletal pain, and antispasmodics such as oxybutynin for bladder problems. Fatigue, cited as the most disabling symptom in people with MS, is treated with amantadine (Symmetrel), fluoxetine (Prozac), CNS stimulants such as methylphenidate, and a waking agent called modafinil (Provigil).

Some medications used for MS can control more than one symptom: for example, a single drug may help both spasticity and pain, or another, such as imipramine (a TCA), helps both pain and bladder problems.

Physical therapy (PT), occupational therapy (OT), and speech therapy are used in MS to preserve function and daily activities. A primary focus of therapy is preserving the patient's ability to walk.

● INTERVIEW QUESTIONS

1. When was your diagnosis of MS? How long have you had symptoms?
2. Are you currently experiencing symptoms? Do you have flare-ups and remissions, or is it chronic?
3. What are your symptoms, if any? Do they include any sensation changes, weakness, or uncomfortable neck movement? If you have pain, can you describe it? (See "Follow-Up Questions About Pain," Chapter 4)
4. If you are having symptoms now, how have they responded to massage in the past? Describe any massage that affected you positively or negatively.
5. How are you being treated for MS and symptoms?
6. How do the treatments affect you? Any side effects you're experiencing currently?
7. Do you have any positioning preferences for massage? Are you comfortable on your back, front, or side, for example?
8. Do you experience temperature sensitivity?

● MASSAGE THERAPY GUIDELINES

While it is not the only trigger of MS symptoms, stress can trigger and aggravate symptoms. Focus your efforts, where possible, on reducing stress, relieving pain and other symptoms, and facilitating movement.

The client's answers to Question 1 indicate how familiar the client is with his or her condition, and whether he or she has established patterns of symptoms. In general, the more familiar clients are with their condition, the more reliable the information they provide; however, people who have been diagnosed for a long time may be so accustomed to their symptoms that they forget to mention them all. You may also decide to ask what type of MS the client has, although current symptoms are more relevant to massage than what might be expected in the future.

Questions 2 and 3 help you get the current clinical picture. If needed, ask about specific symptoms on the Decision Tree, such as spasticity and sensation changes, to determine the best massage pressure and joint movement. Question 4 might provide some history of how the symptoms respond to massage; use the Previous Massage Principle (see Chapter 3) to plan elements like position, joint movement, and a starting pressure.

Use special care with clients who experience spasticity and pain. Spasticity can be aggravated massage that is too light or too deep. In general, a moderate level 3 is a good starting pressure for zones of spasticity, using full, firm hand contact. While stretching is beneficial to spastic muscles, it can also worsen spasticity and should be attempted cautiously at first. Move joints slowly, and apply strokes with even, predictable rhythm as well as slow speeds. As always, client feedback is essential throughout the session.

If the client reports pain, use a few of the Pain Questions from Chapter 4 to learn more about it. Nerve pain and unstable pain would usually direct you to a medical referral, but in the case of diagnosed MS, chances are that the symptoms were already reported long ago. The treating physician likely already knows about the neuropathic pain, a familiar element of the disease. If the client's pain is neuropathic, be more cautious with joint movement and pressure until you know how it responds to massage. If the pain seems to be muscular, approach it as you would approach any muscle tension. A verbal rating scale (VRS) or visual analogue scale (VAS) can be a useful tool to use at each session, to monitor the effects of massage (see Chapter 6).

In question 3, neck movement is mentioned in order to address Lhermitte sign. If the client experiences this unpleasant sensation, avoid joint movement at the neck that is likely to provoke it. Finally, if there are areas of sensation loss, follow the Sensation Principle and Sensation Loss, Injury Prone Principle (see Chapter 3).

Recall the variability in MS presentations. While some clients have no symptoms at all, others could have a number of things going on, with different treatments and responses.

TABLE 10-1.	**MEDICATIONS FOR SYMPTOM RELIEF IN NERVOUS SYSTEM CONDITIONS**[a]
Muscle Relaxants	
Generic Names (Brand Names)	Baclofen (Clofen, Lioresal), diazepam (Diazepam, Valium), tizanidine (Zanaflex), dantrolene (Dantrium)
Uses	Relief of pain Relief of spasticity
Selected Side Effects	CNS depression, drowsiness, muscle weakness, GI upset
Massage Therapy Guidelines	• In general, for muscles with weakness/reduced tone: Use gentle pressure overall (level 2 or 3 maximum); avoid stretching; do not attempt to increase ROM • For CNS depression/drowsiness: Reposition gently, use slow speed and even rhythm, slow rise from table, gentle transition at end of session • For GI upset: Adjust position for comfort; use gentle pressure at site
Antiseizure Medications (Anticonvulsants)	
Generic Names (Brand Names)	Older drugs: Phenobarbital (Luminal), phenytoin (Dilantin), carbamazepine (Tegretol), gabapentin (Neurontin), valproic acid (Depakote) Newer drugs: lamotrigine (Lamictal) pregabalin (Lyrica), oxcarbazepine (Trileptal), topiramate (Topamax), zonisamide (Zonegran), clonazepam (Klonopin)
Uses	Prevention of seizures (full dose) Relief of pain (low dose)
Selected Side Effects	Drowsiness, dizziness, fatigue, decreased cognition, forgetfulness, headache, GI upset, gait disturbances
Massage Therapy Guidelines	• For drowsiness, dizziness, gait disturbances: Reposition gently, use slow speed and even rhythm, slow rise from table, gentle transition at end of session • For fatigue: Gentle session overall • For headache: Position for comfort, especially prone; consider inclined table or propping; gentle session overall; pressure to tolerance; slow speed and even rhythm; avoid headache trigger; general circulatory intent may be poorly tolerated • For GI Upset: Adjust position for comfort; use gentle pressure at site
Tricyclic Antidepressants (TCAs)	
Generic Names (Brand Names)	Amitriptyline (Elavil, Endep), imipramine (Tofranil), nortriptyline (Allegron, Pamelor), desipramine (Norpramin)
Uses	Relief of depression (full dose; see "Depression," this chapter) Relief of pain (low dose)
Selected Side Effects	Side effects usually mild in low doses: drowsiness, dizziness, hypotension, constipation, weight gain
Massage Therapy Guidelines	For drowsiness, dizziness, hypotension: Reposition gently, use slow speed and even rhythm, slow rise from table, gentle transition at end of session For constipation: If abdominal tenderness present, or no bowel movement in 72 hours, limit pressure at site (1 max), make medical referral; otherwise, gentle abdominal massage (2 max) may be helpful

[a]Many drugs can be used to relieve more than one symptom. Not all medications are listed here. Not all drugs in a class cause all side effects, and some are mild or infrequent at low doses. Brand names are listed in parentheses next to the generic or nonproprietary name.

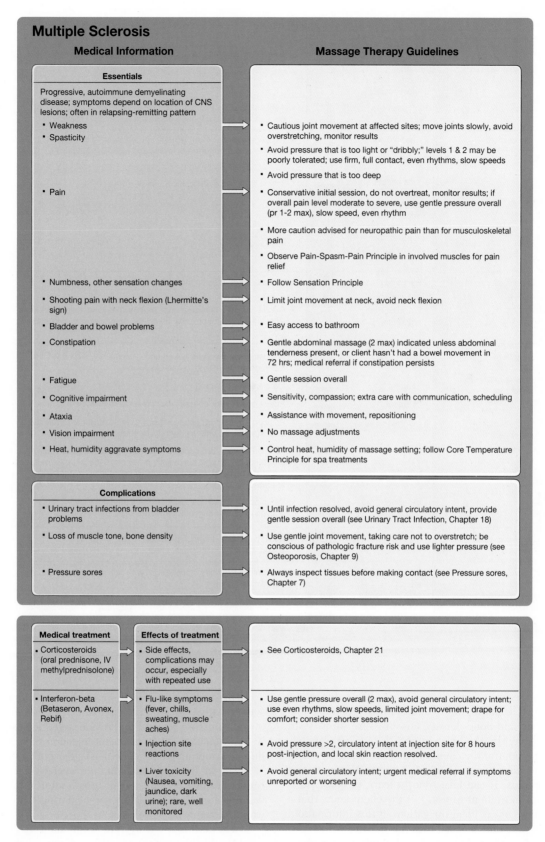

FIGURE 10-2. A Decision Tree for MS. Of the numerous MS drugs, drug classes, and side effects, only selected information is shown. Drugs include antiseizure medication (gabapentin, clonazepam, phenytoin), TCAs (amitriptyline, desipramine, imipramine), SSRIs (sertraline, fluoxetine), NSAIDs, amantadine, modafinil (Provigil), muscle relaxants (baclofen, dantrolene, diazepam, tizanidine), botulinum toxin (Botox), oxybutynin, bethanechol, tamsulosin, natalizumab (Tysabri), cyclophosphamide, and methylphenidate (Ritalin). Some drugs for MS have strong side effects. Not all drugs cause all side effects, and not all side effects are shown. Use the Four Medication Questions (see Chapter 4), Table 21-1, and appropriate texts (Wible, 2009) to plan massage for clients who are taking these and other medications.

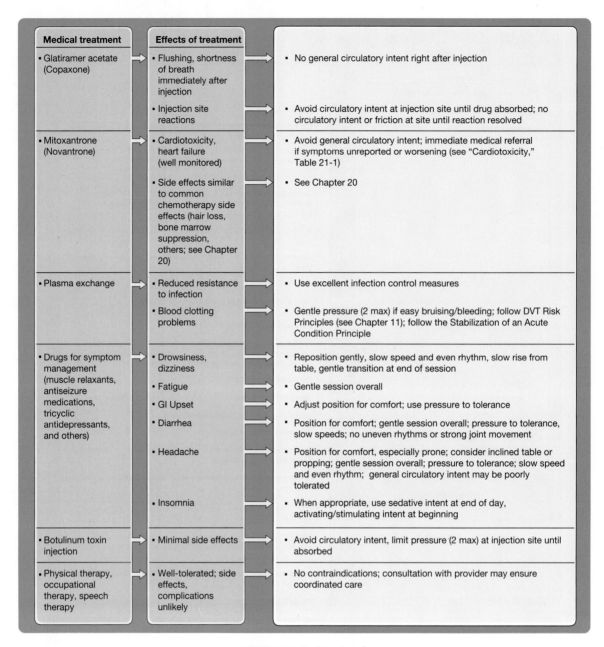

Medical treatment	Effects of treatment	
• Glatiramer acetate (Copaxone)	• Flushing, shortness of breath immediately after injection	• No general circulatory intent right after injection
	• Injection site reactions	• Avoid circulatory intent at injection site until drug absorbed; no circulatory intent or friction at site until reaction resolved
• Mitoxantrone (Novantrone)	• Cardiotoxicity, heart failure (well monitored)	• Avoid general circulatory intent; immediate medical referral if symptoms unreported or worsening (see "Cardiotoxicity," Table 21-1)
	• Side effects similar to common chemotherapy side effects (hair loss, bone marrow suppression, others; see Chapter 20)	• See Chapter 20
• Plasma exchange	• Reduced resistance to infection	• Use excellent infection control measures
	• Blood clotting problems	• Gentle pressure (2 max) if easy bruising/bleeding; follow DVT Risk Principles (see Chapter 11); follow the Stabilization of an Acute Condition Principle
• Drugs for symptom management (muscle relaxants, antiseizure medications, tricyclic antidepressants, and others)	• Drowsiness, dizziness	• Reposition gently, slow speed and even rhythm, slow rise from table, gentle transition at end of session
	• Fatigue	• Gentle session overall
	• GI Upset	• Adjust position for comfort; use pressure to tolerance
	• Diarrhea	• Position for comfort; gentle session overall; pressure to tolerance, slow speeds; no uneven rhythms or strong joint movement
	• Headache	• Position for comfort, especially prone; consider inclined table or propping; gentle session overall; pressure to tolerance; slow speed and even rhythm; general circulatory intent may be poorly tolerated
	• Insomnia	• When appropriate, use sedative intent at end of day, activating/stimulating intent at beginning
• Botulinum toxin injection	• Minimal side effects	• Avoid circulatory intent, limit pressure (2 max) at injection site until absorbed
• Physical therapy, occupational therapy, speech therapy	• Well-tolerated; side effects, complications unlikely	• No contraindications; consultation with provider may ensure coordinated care

FIGURE 10-2. (*Continued*)

Review the Decision Tree (see Figure 10-2), for other symptoms such as ataxia, bowel and bladder problems, loss of muscle tone and bone density, and pressure sores. With clients who have MS, therapists report that several sessions are needed to monitor the client's responses to massage, and determine which massage elements seem to aggravate and relieve symptoms. It can take time to learn the best pressure and joint movement to use. Let the client know that a course of treatment is ideal for gathering this information, and providing the best that massage has to offer.

Questions 5 and 6 could prompt a lot of information about treatment and effects. Here, be mindful of how individualized treatments are. Medications are used to modify the course of MS, prevent relapses, or manage symptoms; these medications can affect different people differently. Many are shown in the Decision Tree (see Figure 10-1); some are discussed here.

If the client is on interferon and is experiencing flu-like symptoms, avoid general circulatory intent and limit the overall pressure to level 2. Provide a gentle session overall. Avoid circulatory intent at recent injection sites, and adapt to flu-like symptoms with gentle massage overall.

If, as in the case of glatiramer acetate, the medication causes flushing or shortness of breath after an injection, you will avoid general circulatory intent during that time (and it would probably be unwelcome).

If chemotherapy drugs are used, such as mitoxantrone or cyclophosphamide, review the effects of chemotherapy in Chapter 20, and ask the client specifically how the medication affects him or her. If the client reports symptoms of cardiotoxicity, see Table 21-1.

A host of drugs are used for symptom management. Selected side effects of these drugs are grouped on the Decision Tree (see Figure 10-2), along with massage guidelines. In addition, Table 10-1 lists specific effects of muscle relaxants, antiseizure drugs, and low-dose TCAs. Learn all you can about how each drug affects the client, and if needed, adapt massage to the effects. If you encounter a drug or side effect that is not listed here, follow the Medication Principle by asking the four medication questions (see Chapter 4).

> *The Medication Principle.* **Adapt massage to the condition for which the medication is taken or prescribed, and to any side effects.**

The question about positioning preferences could elicit information about limitations due to pain or assistive devices. The last question will alert you to adjust the ambient temperature for comfort. See "Cool Down the Waiting Room," online, for the consequences of an overheated massage setting. In the spa and any other setting, follow the Core Temperature Principle for clients with MS whose symptoms are aggravated by heat.

> *The Core Temperature Principle.* **Avoid spa treatments that raise the core temperature if a client's cardiovascular system, respiratory system, skin, or other tissue or system might be overly challenged by heat, or if there are comparable medical restrictions.**

Some individuals may also be sensitive to local heat applications, such as hot packs or hot stones.

● MASSAGE RESEARCH

Research is spotty on massage therapy and MS. A small controlled trial of 24 subjects suggested improvements in anxiety, depressed mood, self-esteem, and body image from massage (Hernandez-Reif et al., 1998). Another group tested a course of reflexology versus sham reflexology in 53 subjects and found symptom improvements in the treatment group that seemed to endure 3 months after the treatment ended. (Siev-Ner et al., 2003).

At the time of this writing, there are no Cochrane reviews on the topic, and just one older systematic review appears to have been published (Huntley and Ernst, 2000). The reviewers looked at CAM therapies for people with MS, and found no conclusive research support for them. Although all works suggest further study, the NIH RePORTER tool lists no active, federally funded research projects on this topic in the United States. No active projects are listed on the clinicaltrials.gov database (see Chapter 6).

Although the available research does not provide an evidence base for massage benefit, several studies in the United Kingdom, Poland, the United States, and other countries suggest that many people with MS actively use CAM therapies, and massage therapy figures prominently in their choices (Esmonde and Long, 2008; Fryze et al., 2006; Marrie et al., 2003; Nayak et al., 2003; Olsen 2009). This interest suggests something is happening, but *what* is unclear. A natural next step in research is a closer look at the therapeutic outcomes. MS has numerous symptoms and complications. Some good research could lie ahead.

● POSSIBLE MASSAGE BENEFITS

People with MS are choosing massage therapy for good reasons. Physicians encourage massage as part of self-care: for relief of muscle tension, relief of constipation, stress reduction, and overall well-being. In particular, clients' anecdotal reports of easing pain and spasticity are encouraging. As more therapists work with people with MS, and more patients report the results of their work, massage therapy may begin to take a firm place in the ongoing care of people with MS.

Parkinson Disease

Parkinson disease (PD) is a progressive degenerative disease of the CNS, specifically in a region of the brain known as the **basal ganglia**, the area that that regulates coordinated muscle movements and postural changes.

● BACKGROUND

In PD, dopamine is not released from the neurons in normal quantities. **Dopamine** is a neurotransmitter associated with many functions, including skeletal muscle movement, behavior, cognitive function, and well-being. (Because of its role in well-being, dopamine is often measured in massage studies.) Reduced dopamine levels in PD lead to various movement problems.

PD is distinct from Parkinsonism, although the two disorders share many of the same features. **Parkinsonism** is a complication of another disease, such as viral encephalitis, toxicity from certain drugs, or repeated trauma to the head.

Signs and Symptoms

PD has four major features:

1. A **Tremor**, or involuntary shaking movement in one or more limbs at rest.
2. Increased muscle tone or rigidity in the trunk or limbs (the area is stiff, even with passive movement).
3. **Bradykinesia**, or slowness of voluntary movement.
4. Poor balance.

A typical feature of PD is a shuffling gait, without the usual swinging arm movement. PD can make it difficult to initiate movement, change positions, sit down or rise from sitting.

Another characteristic, due to muscle rigidity, is a blank facial expression, with minimal blinking, difficulty swallowing, and possible drooling. This "masklike" face can make the person appear hostile or depressed, even if he or she does not feel that way. The masked facial expression can make social connections difficult (Figure 10-3).

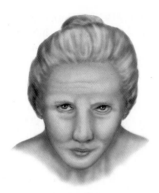

FIGURE 10-3. Lack of facial expression in PD. Facial muscle rigidity results in a "masklike" appearance.

Pain and fatigue are common in people with PD. The pain may be felt as a diffuse achiness, along with weakness and fatigue. Both stress and fatigue can aggravate the tremor of PD. The tremor occurs at rest, but it lessens with voluntary movement and disappears completely during sleep. Other symptoms include oily skin on the face and scalp, with dry skin elsewhere, and constipation.

Complications

Disability develops as PD advances, progressively interfering with mobility. Activities of daily living become harder to perform, and difficulty swallowing and eating make malnutrition a risk. Injuries from falls occur, from slowed voluntary movements and reflexes.

Depression and confusion are possible complications, and individuals feel a great deal of anxiety as the disease progresses, and in the anticipation of worsening symptoms. Late complications include dementia, which occurs in about half of individuals with PD.

Treatment

The focus of medication for Parkinson disease is to restore the inadequate dopamine, and prevent its breakdown. Various approaches to therapy are summarized in Table 10-2, along with selected side effects.

A mainstay of PD treatment is the use of synthetic **precursors**, or forerunners, of dopamine: levodopa and carbidopa. These drugs are taken in combination, because carbidopa prevents the breakdown of levodopa by enzymes in the body. Carbidopa also minimizes side effects of levodopa. These medications are highly effective in reducing symptoms, but after 5 years of use, about half of individuals experience lapses in effectiveness, or *on-off phenomenon.*

When levodopa becomes less useful, **dopamine agonists** may be used to increase its effectiveness. These drugs, which mimic the action of dopamine, may also be used earlier to delay the use of levodopa. Additional medications for PD include low doses of *monoamine oxidase inhibitors (MAOIs),* which supplement levodopa, and **catechol o-methyltransferase (COMT) inhibitors,** which prevent its breakdown. β-**Blockers** are used to control tremor (see "Hypertension," Chapter 11).

Medications for PD cause some side effects. These include blood pressure changes, dizziness, drowsiness, nausea, and dry mouth. Constipation can be a problem. Particularly troublesome side effects are nightmares and hallucinations.

If drug treatment is no longer effective, electrodes are surgically implanted in the basal ganglia. This is called *deep brain stimulation (DBS).* These electrodes are connected to a pulse generator, implanted in the chest (typically below the clavicle). This procedure can reduce involuntary movements and help with initiating movement.

● INTERVIEW QUESTIONS

1. How long have you been diagnosed with PD?
2. What are your symptoms?
3. What do your muscles and joints feel like, where?
4. What are comfortable positions (e.g., when sleeping)?
5. Describe any treatments or medications you are taking.
6. How do treatments and medications affect you?

● MASSAGE THERAPY GUIDELINES

In massage therapy, your typical goals are addressing the client's stress, pain and rigidity, and easing side effects of medications, where possible. There are no specific massage adjustments for tremor. Pain and rigidity can be approached with gentle pressure and joint movement initially. If the client responds well, it may be appropriate to gradually increase these elements over a course of treatment. Shorter sessions may be in order at first, until the client's tolerance is established. Depending on the severity of symptoms, extra time may be needed before and after the massage for checking in, dressing and undressing, and positioning the client.

Difficulties with speech and expression might make the interview a challenge for someone with PD. If the client has difficulty communicating, listen carefully, with a relaxed, unhurried demeanor. Many people appreciate shortened questions that are easy to answer. The questions above are the minimum needed for a well-designed session, but can be re-worded; for example, questions 2 and 3 can be asked with a list of symptoms in a yes/no format for ease of answering. Be alert for nonverbal cues. Be receptive to the client's answers without pressuring him or her, and focus on your own breathing, breathing easily while you wait for the client to respond.

Together with your own observations, the client's responses to questions 1–3 give you a sense of how severe and advanced his or her condition is, and the appropriate strength of the first session. Many people with PD function at a high physical level, continuing to lead active lives, and could take stronger massage. In later disease and more severe symptoms, gentler work is in order. Much could be learned from the client's previous massage experiences.

> *The Previous Massage Principle. A client's previous experience of massage therapy, especially massage after the onset, diagnosis, or flare-up of a medical condition, may be used to plan the massage.*

Question 4 may cue you to the need for extra supports: a chest pillow for the prone position, or head support for the supine position. To accommodate a stooped posture, the side-lying position may be best, or a slight incline for someone with difficulty swallowing.

If poor balance and movement difficulties heighten the client's fall risk, you may need to stay in the treatment area and

TABLE 10-2.	MEDICATIONS FOR PARKINSON DISEASE[a]		
Type of Medication	**Generic Names (Trade Names)**	**Use**	**Selected Side Effects**
Precursors to Dopamine	Levodopa, taken in combination with carbidopa to support and reduce levodopa's side effects (Sinemet)	Replacement of dopamine	Involuntary movement, nightmares, BP changes, heart palpitations, flushing, constipation, nausea, drowsiness
Dopamine Agonists	Bromocriptine (Parlodel), pergolide (Permax), pramipexole (Mirapex), ropinirole (Requip)	Delay use of levodopa (early in disease); support use of levodopa (later in disease)	Drowsiness, BP changes, nausea, swelling, hallucinations
MAOIs	Selegiline (Ataptryl, Carbex, Eldepryl, Selpak)	Help prevent dopamine breakdown	Nausea, dizziness, confusion, dry mouth, abdominal pain
COMT Inhibitors	Entacapone (Comtan), tolcapone (Tasmar)	Prevent levodopa breakdown; extend time between levodopa doses	Nausea, involuntary movements, diarrhea, back pain; tolcapone linked to liver damage
Anticholinergic Drugs	Benztropine (Apo-Benztropine, Cogentin), trihexyphenidyl (Apo-Trihex, Trihexy-2, Trihexy-5), TCAs	Substitute for levodopa (early disease); supplement levodopa (later disease)	Drowsiness, dry mouth, blurred vision, dizziness, constipation, urinary difficulties, confusion, hallucinations
β-Blockers	Propranolol (Inderal)	Reduce tremor	Hypotension, drowsiness, dizziness, weakness, fatigue, depression, insomnia, cold hands and feet

[a]Not all medications are included in this table, nor all side effects of each. Not all medications cause all side effects. Brand names are listed in parentheses next to the generic or nonproprietary name.

assist in undressing and dressing, and moving on and off the table. If stepping up to a massage table is too difficult, you can work with the client in the seated position next to the massage table, leaning his or her upper body and head forward on a few pillows.

Most other massage adjustments for PD are good common sense: If the client experiences pain or fatigue, massage may be able to help. Start with gentle pressure initially, monitoring tolerance. If the client is fatigued, consider a shorter session, or scheduling sessions for good times of day or evening. If the client has oily skin in some places, drier in others, modify the amount of lubricant you use. If the client has constipation, see Chapter 15. More symptoms and complications are shown in the Decision Tree (see Figure 10-4).

If the client's mobility is limited, a general health decline is likely. Ask about osteoporosis (see Chapter 9) and consider cardiovascular problems, including deep vein thrombosis (DVT) (see Chapter 11). Also be alert for pressure sores (see Chapter 7). Watch for apparent weight loss, and gently mention a referral to the client's doctor for nutrition support if you can. Some of the major massage guidelines for PD are shown in Figure 10-5.

Be alert for side effects of medication, which can be considerable. In particular, drowsiness, dizziness, and a drop in BP call for heightened attention and assistance in rising from the table. Constipation may be relieved by massage; see Chapter 15. If the client experiences hallucinations or nightmares, sensitive, caring communication in order and massage may help with disrupted sleep. Be sure to refer the client to his or her doctor if these side effects have not been reported.

Review Table 10-2 for an expanded list of side effects. If you encounter a side effect that is not addressed here, check Table 21-1 for massage therapy guidelines. Give good thought to how massage might ease certain side effects, such as back pain, nausea, and cold hands and feet, and, if appropriate, ask the client to rate these symptoms before and after the session, and over a course of massage treatment.

If the client has had surgery for deep brain stimulation, follow the Procedure Principle (see Chapter 3). Learn the location of the pulse generator and extension, and use cautious pressure in those areas in the chest and neck. If the client is seeing a PT, OT, or speech therapist, consider working in collaboration with the provider in order to ensure coordinated care.

● MASSAGE RESEARCH

Research on massage and PD is limited. Only a few small studies are available at the time of this writing. From a non-controlled pilot study on seven people with widely ranging symptom severity, investigators observed that eight, weekly 1-hour sessions of deep massage were well received. They noted improvements in walking and other parameters (Paterson et al., 2005). An RCT of neuromuscular therapy in 36 subjects found improvements in motor symptoms, including tremor, in the massage group compared to a music relaxation control (Craig et al., 2006). Another small RCT compared massage and progressive muscle relaxation in 16 people with PD, and saw improved function and sleep in the massage group (Hernandez-Reif et al., 2002). Finally, one study looked at several weeks of spa therapy (Brefel-Courbon et al., 2003) that suggested benefit for people with PD. These studies do not add up to conclusive support for massage in PD, but they suggest a compelling area for more research.

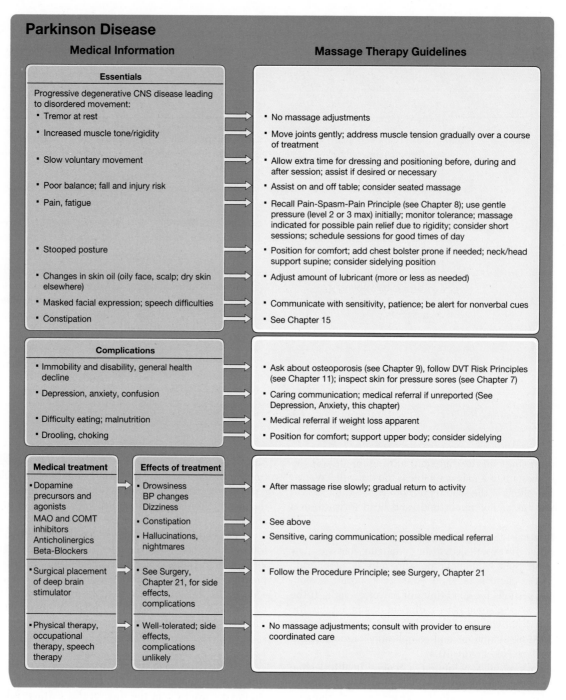

FIGURE 10-4. A Decision Tree for Parkinson disease. Of the numerous PD drugs and side effects, only selected information is shown. Some drugs for PD have strong side effects. Use the Four Medication Questions (see Chapter 4), Table 21-1, and appropriate texts (Wible, 2009) to plan massage for clients who are taking these and other medications.

● POSSIBLE MASSAGE BENEFITS

PD is a long-term, debilitating, and demoralizing illness, and massage has the potential to be of great benefit. Reduced mobility can contribute to fatigue and muscle ache, and massage therapy may provide some relief. Tremor is thought to be aggravated by stress, and relaxation massage could offer an important stress relief. Constipation arises from the condition itself, and from some medications.

Gentle abdominal massage may provide symptom relief. Sleep disturbances are common and may be helped by massage therapy.

As with any degenerative disease, stress, anxiety, and depression compound the problems that individuals and families face. A person who is grappling with the effects of PD is a good candidate for the caring touch of massage.

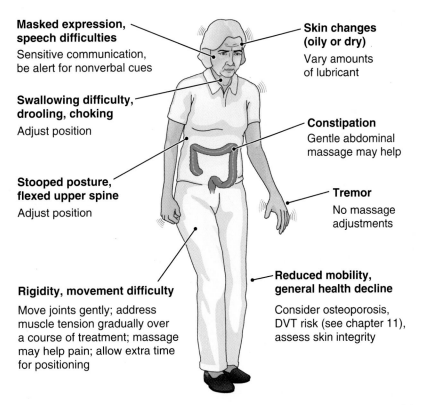

Masked expression, speech difficulties
Sensitive communication, be alert for nonverbal cues

Swallowing difficulty, drooling, choking
Adjust position

Stooped posture, flexed upper spine
Adjust position

Rigidity, movement difficulty
Move joints gently; address muscle tension gradually over a course of treatment; massage may help pain; allow extra time for positioning

Skin changes (oily or dry)
Vary amounts of lubricant

Constipation
Gentle abdominal massage may help

Tremor
No massage adjustments

Reduced mobility, general health decline
Consider osteoporosis, DVT risk (see chapter 11), assess skin integrity

FIGURE 10-5. Parkinson disease: selected clinical features and massage therapy guidelines.

Stroke (Cerebrovascular Accident)

A **stroke**, also known as a cerebrovascular accident (CVA), is a common injury to brain tissue, caused by interrupted blood flow to one or more parts of the brain. The effects can range from mild disability to severe disability and even death.

● BACKGROUND

In developed countries, the incidence of stroke is staggeringly high. Although more common in older adults, stroke also affects younger adults and children, and the sheer number of strokes in the general population makes it vital for massage therapists to be prepared.

Because stroke incidence is so high, education and research are increasing, raising public awareness about stroke prevention and recognition. A stroke, now often referred to as a "brain attack," calls attention to the seriousness of the symptoms, which, like those of a heart attack, require immediate medical attention. Patient education materials make it easy for massage therapists to learn more about stroke.

A common complication of other cardiovascular conditions, stroke affects 700,000 Americans each year, 300,000 Canadians, and 150,000 people from the United Kingdom. In the United States, 200,000 of the 700,000 strokes occur in people with a previous history of stroke. About 5.7 million stroke survivors are alive today in the United States.

A stroke is often preceded by **atherosclerosis**, a disease of the linings of the arteries (see Chapter 11). When this condition narrows the arteries serving the brain, it is called *cerebral artery disease*. When a stroke occurs, the flow of blood to the brain is disrupted by one of three general processes, shown in Figure 10-6. The processes involve either ischemia or hemorrhage,

and the types of stroke are commonly referred to as "clots or bleeds." **Ischemic strokes**, which account for about 80% of all strokes, occur when arteries to the brain are blocked.

There are two types of ischemic stroke. In a **thrombotic stroke** or *cerebral thrombosis*, atherosclerotic **plaque** forms in an artery directly at the trouble site (Figure 10-6). In arteries, plaques are composed of cholesterol, other fatty substances, calcium deposits, and blood cells. These can rupture and lead to thrombus (clot) formation at the site, narrowing the artery and blocking blood flow to a region of brain tissue. In an **embolic stroke** or *cerebral embolism*, a clot originates somewhere else "upstream" in the circulatory system, such as the heart or a larger artery in the neck; the clot or its fragments break loose, lodging in a smaller cerebral artery. Atrial fibrillation can be an underlying cause of an embolic stroke; a blood clot can form in the heart, then loosen and embolize to an artery of the brain.

In **hemorrhagic strokes**, which account for about 20% of all strokes, a cerebral vessel wall weakens and ruptures, sending its contents into the brain tissue. This type of stroke is called a bleed. The loose blood compresses the surrounding brain tissue, causing swelling. A hemorrhagic stroke can result from **intracerebral hemorrhage (ICH)**, when a blood vessel within the brain breaks, or from a **subarachnoid hemorrhage**, in which an artery near the meninges (the tissues covering the brain) ruptures. Hemorrhagic strokes stem from two types of weakened vessels—an **aneurysm** and a congenital problem called **arteriovenous malformation (AVM)**, a cluster of weak, tangled blood vessels.

A number of strokes are *cryptogenic*, meaning the exact source of the stroke has not been identified. Some of these

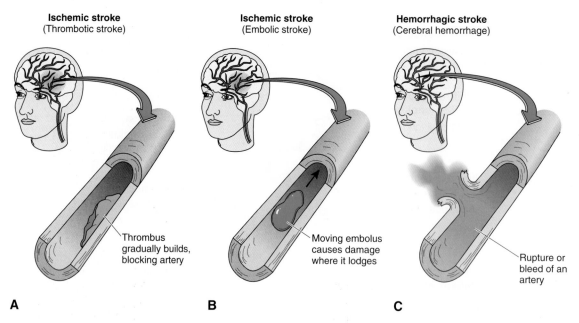

Ischemic stroke
(Thrombotic stroke)

Ischemic stroke
(Embolic stroke)

Hemorrhagic stroke
(Cerebral hemorrhage)

Thrombus
gradually builds,
blocking artery

Moving embolus
causes damage
where it lodges

Rupture or
bleed of an
artery

A **B** **C**

FIGURE 10-6. Comparison of ischemic and hemorrhagic stroke. (A) and (B) show two causes of ischemic stroke: thrombosis and embolism. In thrombotic stroke (A), a clot forms at the site of plaque in an artery serving the brain, narrowing the vessel and ultimately blocking it. In embolic stroke (B), a clot originates from another artery, embolizes, and lodges in a cerebral artery. In hemorrhagic stroke (C), no clot is involved but an artery ruptures, losing blood to surrounding brain tissue and producing swelling.

strokes are thought to be caused by DVT in a lower limb. In some people, an abnormal opening between the right and left heart called **patent foramen ovale** allows passage of a venous clot to the arterial side of the systemic circulation (see "Deep Vein Thrombosis," Chapter 11).

When tissues of the brain are damaged during a stroke, there is no way to repair or regenerate them. However, other intact areas of the brain can compensate and perform the function of the damaged tissue.

A **transient ischemic attack (TIA)** is also called a mini-stroke. A TIA is a minor, temporary ischemic stroke, and symptoms tend to last a few minutes or up to 24 hours, then disappear without doing permanent damage. A TIA is a warning of a possible major stroke, and stroke prevention steps should be taken whenever a TIA occurs.

Signs and Symptoms

The signs of a stroke are important for everyone to know. The signs and symptoms often come without warning, or they may develop over hours or days. They are:

- Confusion or difficulty understanding
- Difficulty speaking or slurred speech
- Vision change, such as blurred, double, or decreased vision, in one or both eyes
- Dizziness, or loss of balance
- Difficulty with walking or coordination
- Severe headache with no known cause
- Numbness or weakness in an arm or a leg, or on the face (often on one side)

Even if these signs and symptoms fade in a few minutes or a few hours, the person may have experienced a TIA and should see a physician immediately.

An easy way to remember the most common, recognizable stroke symptoms is the mnemonic *FAST*:

- Face—Sudden weakness, vision that is blurred, double, or compromised
- Arm—Sudden weakness or numbness of one or both
- Speech—Difficulty speaking; slurred or garbled speech
- Time—The importance of rapid emergency response

There are two important emergency responses to the signs of a stroke. The first is to call emergency services immediately. Time is of the essence, to minimize loss of brain tissue. Call even if the person protests, which is common during a stroke, or if the person has a history of a TIA "mini-strokes" and downplays the situation. The second step is to note the time that the sign or symptom occurred, as this question will be asked later and the answer is vital to determining the best treatment. Noting the time of onset can be lifesaving. In an emergency situation, if the person vomits, the head should be turned to the side to avoid choking. The person should not eat or drink.

Complications

In stroke, the distinction between disease essentials (signs and symptoms) and complications is blurred. Because of the broad effects a stroke has across body systems, any sign or symptom can also be considered a short-term complication. In this chapter, signs and symptoms are considered part of the acute event, and complications are functional problems that linger and become chronic or progressive afterward.

The functional loss from a stroke depends on the area of the brain affected. The impairment may be partial or complete, and may be temporary or permanent. The outlook is most favorable with limited injury to brain tissue, rapid treatment response, and good rehabilitation resources.

Because the brain's right hemisphere governs functioning of the left side of the body and vice versa, many of the effects of a stroke are *contralateral*, on the opposite side. Common complications are:

- *Speech and language problems.* Slurred speech, or **dysarthria**, may occur. If a language center in the brain is affected, **aphasia**, or difficulty with speaking (*expressive language*) and understanding speech (*receptive language*) may occur. Reading and writing are also affected.
- *Cognitive problems.* In addition to confusion and memory loss, difficulty concentrating and focusing are common. It can be difficult to recognize familiar faces, or to recall names of objects. Simple arithmetic can be challenging. Distinguishing between yes and no, right and left, and other things can become difficult.
- *Vision impairment.* Vision changes are often on one side. The person may have trouble seeing things on that side, and may seem to ignore food on that side of the plate, or bump into things on that side of the room.
- *Difficulty swallowing, aspiration.* **Dysphagia**, or difficulty swallowing, can occur, as well as **aspiration**, the accidental inhalation of food or fluid into the lungs. This can lead to a serious chest infection, **aspiration pneumonia**.
- *Paralysis and weakness.* Paralysis typically occurs on one side of the body, called **hemiplegia**. **Hemiparesis** is weakness or partial paralysis on one side of the body. Both hemiplegia and hemiparesis may be confined to the face, an arm, a leg, or the entire side. In a classic hemiplegia pattern, shown in Figure 10-7, the upper limb is fixed in the adducted position, with flexion at elbow and wrist. The lower limb shows plantar weakness or partial paralysis.
- *Spasticity.* High muscle tone makes muscles tight, and it places joints in fixed positions.
- *Falls.* Weakness, spasticity, loss of coordination, poor balance, confusion, and agitation can result in falls. A person is considered to be a **fall risk** if this is the case.
- *Functional disabilities.* A person may be able to regain functions of swallowing, walking, dressing, and other activities. As "Massage After a Mild Stroke" describes, this recovery may happen rapidly (see online). On the other hand, in severe cases, assistive devices may be needed, or the person may be in bed much of the time.
- *Pain.* This may be due to **central pain syndrome**, causing steady background pain, which is deep, burning, aching, or cutting. Background pain may be punctuated by sudden, excruciating bursts of pain. When weakness in the shoulder and hand is accompanied by strong pain, it is called **shoulder-hand syndrome (SHS)**. These two pain syndromes are poorly understood, and both can be significantly debilitating, interfering with PT and other elements of rehabilitation.
- *Other sensation changes.* Sensations of cold, tingling, throbbing, and skin reactions to light touch may occur, such as itching, burning, or a crawling feeling. Discomfort, prickly sensations, and other strange sensations are common when sensory areas of the brain are affected by a stroke. The person might feel numbness in the skin, or extra sensitivity.
- *Bowel and bladder incontinence.* Loss of bladder and bowel control may occur, but these are typically short lived, and these functions are frequently recovered soon after the acute event. If they persist, urinary tract infections can become a recurrent problem.
- *Deep vein thrombosis (DVT).* Both **deep vein thrombosis (DVT)** and **pulmonary embolism (PE)** can develop after a stroke, in part because of the immobility caused by paralysis. Moreover, some of the same conditions that produce ischemic strokes also produce blood clots in other areas (see Chapter 11).

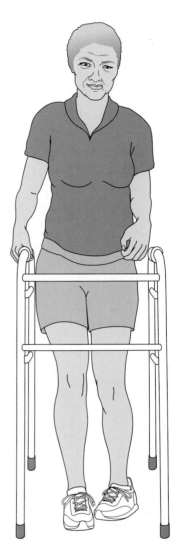

FIGURE 10-7. Hemiplegia in stroke. This is a typical body position of a person who has had a stroke on the right side of the brain.

- *Pressure sores.* Also called **decubitus ulcers**, these lesions can form over bony landmarks after immobilization (see Conditions in Brief, Chapter 7).
- *Unusual emotional responses.* Outbursts of laughter, crying, or swearing may occur at unusual moments, seemingly, "the wrong times." Uncontrolled anger or aggression may arise.
- *Depression and anxiety.* Feelings of sadness and deep depression are common after a stroke and often warrant psychotherapeutic and pharmacologic intervention. Anxiety is common, especially with significant loss of function. Fearfulness and cautiousness may manifest in difficulty in trying new things. Both anxiety and depression can persist long after the acute event.

Treatment

Treatment of a full-blown stroke depends on the type of stroke. It is critical to determine the type of stroke because a certain treatment could worsen the situation if it is not appropriate. A hemorrhagic stroke is treated quite differently from an ischemic stroke. In a hemorrhagic stroke, treatment efforts focus on preventing bleeding, and in treating an ischemic stroke, the goal is to prevent clotting.

An ischemic stroke is treated by techniques that removed the obstruction and restore blood flow. Emergency treatment, if begun within 3 hours of the initial incident, may include the use of **thrombolytic** drugs that break down the clot. These strong drugs, also called "clot busters," include *tissue plasminogen activator* (*TPA*), and are administered intravenously. This approach has significant risks, including bleeding, that may outweigh the benefits, so the timing of beginning treatment is critical. This is one reason it's so important to time the onset of symptoms.

Various surgery options are used to prevent or treat stroke. As in any surgery, possible complications include infection, bleeding, and clotting (see Chapter 21), and sometimes there is risk of another stroke. A surgical procedure for ischemic stroke is called **carotid endarterectomy**. The carotid artery is opened, and plaques that narrow the artery are removed. Filters are placed to catch any plaque or clot fragments released during the procedure because the incision itself could initiate a stroke.

Another surgical procedure for ischemic stroke is **angioplasty**, the placement of a balloon-tipped catheter in the narrowed artery, with a stent to keep it open (see Chapter 11). A **catheter embolectomy** may be performed, in which a catheter is threaded into the artery and used to remove clots. Thrombolytic drugs can be administered locally through the catheter.

To surgically treat a hemorrhagic stroke, an aneurysm may be clipped; a clamp is placed at its base to prevent it from bursting or bleeding. In an **aneurysm embolization**, a catheter is used to maneuver a coil into the aneurysm, causing clotting and effectively walling it off from the circulation (see "Aneurysm," Chapter 11).

If an AVM is causing the stroke, it might be removed surgically. If it's too deep or too large to operate, radiation or embolization may be directed at the cluster of vessels.

Recovery begins immediately for many people after a stroke, and the most rapid recovery typically occurs during the first 3 months. The process usually continues for 6–12 months, and many stroke survivors experience improved function in the years following the original event.

After treatment of an acute stroke, **stroke rehabilitation** starts—a multipronged approach to maximizing stroke recovery. Individuals use education, counseling, and physical interventions to restore function and facilitate returning to active and productive living as much as possible. These skills are typically recovered first: sitting, balancing while sitting, then standing, then walking. Typically, the leg of the affected side begins to improve before the hand on that side. Symptoms tend to worsen after a minor illness or a busy day, even if recovery is steady.

Stroke recovery and rehabilitation depend on the area of the brain affected. The rehabilitation team may include a physician, a nurse, physical therapist, occupational therapist, speech therapist, psychotherapist, and dietitian. A PT teaches the patient sitting and walking, and challenges the patient to move between different activities. An OT teaches the patient activities of daily living, including bathing, cooking, writing, and using the toilet. Speech therapist helps with swallowing, language, and communication. A psychotherapist, psychopharmacologist, and chaplain may also be involved, supporting emotional and spiritual quality of life. In general, rehabilitation hinges on early treatment and good social support. Rehabilitation may take place in a rehab unit in a hospital or a separate rehabilitation facility, a subacute care unit, on an outpatient basis, in the home, or in a long-term skilled nursing facility.

Treatment of a TIA or full-blown stroke includes therapy to prevent a future stroke. Diagnostic tests are used to determine the nature of the problem, and stroke prevention is aimed at preventing thrombosis or rupture of an aneurysm. For someone at risk of thrombotic stroke, maintenance doses of anticoagulant or antiplatelet medications are prescribed over the long term. For a person known to be at risk of hemorrhagic stroke, antihypertensive medication is used to reduce pressure on unstable vessel walls and thereby help prevent future strokes. In both thrombotic and hemorrhagic stroke, drugs for lowering cholesterol and blood pressure may be used over the long term (see Chapter 11 for effects of treatments).

● INTERVIEW QUESTIONS

1. When did your stroke occur?
2. Have things stabilized since the stroke? Have you recovered partially or completely?
3. What was the cause? Was it a clot or a bleed?
4. How does (or did) the stroke affect you? Which side of your body is affected?
5. Do you have any difficulty communicating? Are there any changes in memory or concentration?
6. Do you have any changes in your vision? How and where?
7. Are there any effects on swallowing? Are there positions that are more comfortable or less comfortable for you?
8. Do you have any difficulty with movement? Is there any paralysis, weakness, or spasticity? Do you have any problems with balance or history of falling?
9. Do you have any pain?
10. Do you have any changes in sensation?
11. Do you have any bladder or bowel control issues that make bathroom access important?
12. How is your skin? Are there any areas where it is open or irritated?
13. Has your doctor or nurse discussed any risk of blood clots (DVT) with you?
14. Are there any complications? Effects of the stroke on your skin, muscles, sensation, or movement?
15. How was your stroke treated? Was there any follow-up treatment?
16. How does the treatment affect you?

● MASSAGE THERAPY GUIDELINES

Depending upon the client's status and ability to reliably answer questions, you might need to interview a caregiver or family member. Be prepared to be flexible. You might want to reword or simplify certain questions for some clients, or alter questions for caregivers or members of the health care team.

Because a stroke usually involves atherosclerosis, review Chapter 11 for relevant principles: The Plaque Problem Principle, DVT Risk Principles, and the CV Conditions Often "Run in Packs" Principle. Apply these principles with clients known to be at *risk* of stroke as well as those with a *history* of it.

> *The Plaque Problem Principle. If atherosclerosis is identified, or is likely to be present, use cautious pressure and joint movement at all arterial pulse points. In particular, limit pressure to level 1 at or near the carotid arteries.*

Because your client's risk of recurrent stroke is likely to be elevated (and lifelong), become familiar with the signs of a stroke. Also see "Warning Leaks" for a story of a therapist correctly recognizing the warning signs in a guest at her spa (online at http://thePoint.lww.com/Walton).

Questions 1–2 establish the client's status. Recall that some early stroke symptoms resolve over time. Refer to Figure 10-9 for common clinical features of stroke. Patients are often considered stable within 24–48 hours of the acute event, at which point they can be discharged to a rehab facility or to the home. Still, in the first few days and weeks thereafter, the patient is learning about the effects of the stroke and adapting to them. Therefore, you should work extremely gently for a few weeks, well within the massage guidelines, and monitor the results. This is a good time to communicate with the client's doctor. Follow the Stabilization of an Acute Condition Principle.

> *The Stabilization of an Acute Condition Principle. Until an acute medical condition has stabilized, massage should be conservative.*

Question 3 about a clot or a bleed is basic information, but it may lead to little change in the massage design. Your adaptations are similarly cautious in each case because even the different kinds of strokes share risk factors such as hypertension and atherosclerosis (see Chapter 11). Cardiovascular conditions often appear in groups. Whether it was a clot or a bleed, always follow the Plaque Problem Principle.

Question 4 is a general overall question about the essentials and complications of a stroke; allow for the possibility that a stroke in the past does not currently affect the client's function. With any stroke history, continue to follow the DVT Risk Principles and Plaque Problem Principle, as both may be necessary for some time, or indefinitely (see Chapter 11). And recognize that DVT is itself a complication of stroke.

Also use question 4 to anticipate which side might require massage adaptations, reinforced by your observations of the client and the information in questions 5–14. Massage therapy guidelines for these stroke complications are in a Decision Tree in Figure 10-8. You can ask question 5 earlier in the interview, or while scheduling the session over the phone. Determine whether you need to provide information to caregivers if the client is unable to answer. If the client has aphasia, try to have just one-on-one conversation, with minimal distractions, rather than including others. Give the client plenty of time to speak, and allow him or her to speak for himself or herself rather than rushing in. If memory or concentration is affected, the client might be easily distracted, or he or she might struggle with tasks that used to be simple. The client may need help remembering appointments or following instructions. But be sure to speak in a normal tone of voice (unless there is hearing loss) and at an adult level. Whenever communication or cognition is compromised, be alert for nonverbal cues.

If the client has experienced vision changes (question 6), ask which side. When talking with the client, face the unaffected side. Notice whether the vision impairment affects ease of movement; be sure to clear a path to the massage table or bed, and provide assistance getting there if needed. Let the client know when you are beginning to touch, move, or massage the side that he or she cannot see.

If there is difficulty with swallowing, the client could be at risk of aspirating his or her own saliva. Position changes may be in order, avoiding the flat supine position in favor of an inclined or a seated position.

Question 8 gets at any movement problems caused by spasticity or hemiparesis. If muscles are spastic, review the effects of spasticity (see "Multiple Sclerosis," this chapter). Any time there is spasticity, it's important not to overwork or overstretch the affected muscles. Pressure that is too light or too deep may aggravate spasticity, and slow speeds and even rhythms are in order, with full hand contact. Limit the duration and joint movement in the area until you are sure how the muscle responds to the work, then increase in small increments, preferably with input from the client's doctor or PT.

If the client has balance problems, be alert as he or she moves and transfers to the massage table or bed. If the client has an identified fall risk and is in nursing or home care, check with the facility or staff about the procedures for reducing falls, and observe them. There may be specific nursing precautions to follow, such as protocols for side rails on a bed or a call for assistance whenever repositioning the client.

Question 9 addresses the issue of pain following a stroke. The pain can take many forms, ranging from mildly distracting to completely debilitating. Before beginning the session, ask whether certain positions aggravate or relieve symptoms and avoid them. A client with SHS may benefit from massage at the site, but begin with conservative pressure and movement, and monitor results over time. If pressure or joint movement is poorly tolerated, simply holding the area with soft hands may be tolerated and welcome.

If pain takes the form of central pain syndrome, also proceed cautiously. Use similar caution, as well, with odd skin sensations, such as burning, crawling, and pain with light touch. In these cases, even the lightest touch may be unbearable. While touch and massage may bring relief, it is best to start conservatively.

> *The Where You Start Isn't Always Where You End Up Principle. Although a client's condition may call for a conservative initial massage, stronger elements may be appropriate in later sessions, after monitoring the client's response to massage over time.*

If you learn that sensation is impaired, do not use pressure that is too deep. Customize the pressure levels for each client, and monitor the results over time. Follow the Sensation Principle and the Sensation Loss, Injury Prone Principle (see Chapter 3). If unpleasant or painful sensations are present, take care not to aggravate them with massage.

Question 11 about bladder and bowel control can point to the need for easy bathroom access. Identify a clear path to the bathroom from the massage table. A client in the early days after a stroke, who is at risk of bladder or bowel incontinence, may be using adult diapers. Also, ask regularly about any urinary tract infection or other urinary problems, and adapt the massage accordingly (see Chapter 18).

Question 12 about skin could reveal problems with pressure sores, or strange sensations, such as prickliness, that would call for gentler pressure or even avoiding contact. If pressure sores are present, avoid contact or lubricant at sites of open skin (see "Pressure Sores," Chapter 7).

Question 13 about DVT risk may open up dialogue with the client and physician about the risk of using pressure on the legs or other at risk areas. Follow the DVT Risk Principles until such dialogue has occurred. In a person with a stroke history, there is a good argument for using the DVT Risk Principles indefinitely. If you notice signs of DVT, or your client complains of symptoms of the condition, you will need

Stroke

Medical Information	Massage Therapy Guidelines

Essentials

- "Brain attack:" injury to brain tissue from interrupted blood flow to brain; caused by ischemic (clot) and hemorrhagic (bleed) event in cerebral vessel; associated with common cardiovascular disease risk factors (hypertension, atherosclerosis)

- Transient ischemic attack (TIA), mini-stroke lasting less than 24 hours, no permanent damage; high risk of a major stroke

- Signs and symptoms of acute stroke:
  - Confusion, difficulty understanding
  - Difficulty speaking, slurring
  - Vision change (blurred, double, loss)
  - Dizziness, loss of balance
  - Difficulting with walking or coordination
  - Severe headache, no known cause
  - Numbness or weakness in arm, leg, or face (often on one side)

→ For stroke risk and stroke history, follow DVT Risk Principles, Plaque Problem Principle, CV Conditions Often "Run in Packs" Principle (see Chapter 11)

- Gentle overall session in first few weeks after acute event, until stabilized

→ Immediate medical referral if unreported; follow principles, above, for ongoing stroke risk

→ Emergency medical referral; note time of symptom onset; discourage eating or drinking; turn individual's head side to side if s/he vomits

Complications

- Speech and language problems

- Cognitive problems (confusion and memory loss, poor concentration, poor recognition of familiar faces and word retrieval, difficulty with arithmetic, distinguishing between yes and no, etc.)

- Vision impairment, often on one side

- Difficulty swallowing and aspiration

- Paralysis, weakness, spasticity, typically on one side (hemiplegia, hemiparesis)

- Falls, fall risk

- Functional disability

- Pain (central pain syndrome; shoulder-hand syndrome)

- Sensation changes (strange sensations and sensation loss)

- Bowel and bladder incontinence, urinary problems or infection

- Pressure sores

- Deep vein thrombosis, pulmonary embolism

- Unusual emotional responses (laughter, crying, swearing; uncontrolled anger or aggression)

- Depression, anxiety

→ Sensitivity, clear communication; minimize distractions, give client time to answer; direct questions to caregivers if necessary; be alert for nonverbal cues

→ Help with appointment reminders, sensitivity, clear communication, simple instructions; minimize distractions, give client time to answer; be alert for nonverbal cues; direct questions to caregivers if necessary

→ Face unaffected side when communicating with client; clear path to massage table/bed; assist if necessary; alert client before touching affected side

→ Position for comfort and avoiding aspiration of saliva

→ Cautious joint movement at affected sites; move joints slowly, avoid overstretching, begin conservatively, monitor results

- Avoid pressure that is too light, may be poorly tolerated; avoid pressure that is too deep; best starting pressure may be level 3

- Use firm, full contact, even rhythms, slow speed

→ Be alert for fall risk; follow nursing precautions for fall risk

→ Allow time and ask caregiver to help with transfer, position changes when necessary

→ Position appropriately to avoid aggravating; avoid pressure or joint movement at site that aggravate; begin conservatively, monitor results over time

→ Avoid aggravating unpleasant sensations at site; follow Sensation Principle and Sensation Loss, Injury Prone Principle (see Chapter 3) if numbness present

→ Easy bathroom access if necessary; see Urinary Tract Infection, Chapter 18

→ See Pressure Sores, Chapter 7

→ Follow DVT Risk Principles (see Chapter 11)

→ Take cues from caregivers on how to respond

→ See Depression, this chapter; see Anxiety, Conditions in Brief

FIGURE 10-8. A Decision Tree for stroke.

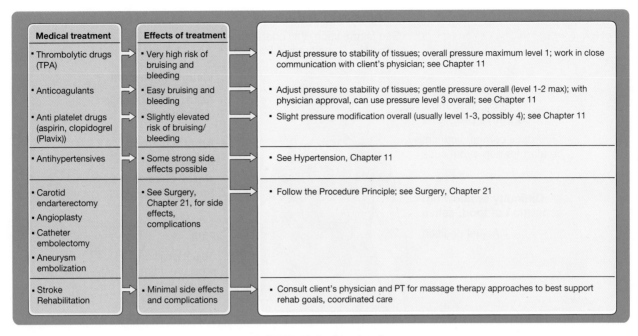

FIGURE 10-8. (*Continued*)

to make a medical referral (see "Deep Vein Thrombosis," Chapter 11).

Question 14 provides a chance to catch any complications or functional impairments that weren't captured in the previous ten questions. A stroke can have quirky and individually unique effects, so it's helpful to inquire about any in order to adapt the session. See the Decision Tree (Figure 10-8) for emotional responses in stroke.

Questions 15 and 16 about treatment can point to a number of massage adaptations. These are shown in the Decision Tree (see Figure 10-8). If ischemic stroke treatment involved recent thrombolytics, limit your pressure to 1 and work closely with the client's physician, as the tissues are *highly* unstable in this case. If anticoagulants are in use, then your overall pressure should be limited to a level 2, or 3 if the physician agrees. Antiplatelet medications such as aspirin usually require a small pressure adjustment, as these drugs do not significantly increase bruising or bleeding. The client's doctor or nurse is the best source of advice on massage pressure. If treatment for hemorrhagic stroke involves antihypertensive drugs, see Chapter 11 for massage adaptations to the side effects of these medications.

If the client had recent surgery for ischemic stroke (carotid endarterectomy, angioplasty, catheter embolectomy) or for hemorrhagic stroke (aneurysm embolization), then follow the massage guidelines for surgery (see Chapter 21). Question the client closely about any complications of surgery and adapt massage accordingly. If there is a past history (more than 3 months) of any of these surgeries, there probably isn't a need for specific massage adaptations beyond the ongoing ones for the stroke itself. But also be sure any medications are addressed, as some people may still be taking aspirin.

For a client in stroke rehabilitation, respect the goals and practices of the various health care professionals involved, and the policies of the residential facility where the massage takes place. It is wise to include the input of the physician, nurse, and PT regarding the massage care plan, so a consultation is advisable for the best coordinated care. The common clinical features of stroke and massage therapy guidelines are summarized in Figure 10-9.

MASSAGE RESEARCH

As of this writing, there is only one substantial randomized, controlled trial, published in the English language, on stroke and massage. Researchers in Hong Kong looked at elderly stroke patients' experiences of shoulder pain and anxiety, introducing daily 10-minute back massages for 7 days to see if there was any change in these parameters (Mok and Woo, 2004). There were 102 subjects in the study, and the control group received usual care. On the last day of the study, they found significantly lower scores in self-reported anxiety, heart rate, systolic BP, diastolic BP, and pain in the massage group, compared to the control group. The differences persisted 3 days later.

This study is compelling, but larger sample sizes and additional studies are necessary to more firmly establish any effectiveness of massage. Moreover, the massage was described as *slow-stroke back massage* (SSBM), a common term in the nursing literature. It is frequently described as a nursing intervention, and as a gentle, rhythmic back massage using long, flowing strokes at 60 strokes/minute (Elizabeth, 1966). This may be a more rapid rate of application than customarily applied in massage therapy, and may not reflect effects of other approaches.

POSSIBLE MASSAGE BENEFITS

A stroke can be a terrifying event, and even a mild stroke can be profoundly life changing. In that context, it is hard to argue against massage therapy for clients who have had a stroke. In fact, the potential of massage to contribute to stroke rehabilitation—a client's recovery and transition to the "new normal"—cannot be overemphasized.

Spasticity and weakness may worsen with stress, and massage is a well-recognized stress-reduction tool. The role of massage in reducing stroke symptoms such as pain, and supporting other therapeutic efforts, such as PT, OT, and speech therapy, has yet to be determined.

In the medical literature, there are many studies about stroke recovery and rehabilitation, with particular attention to

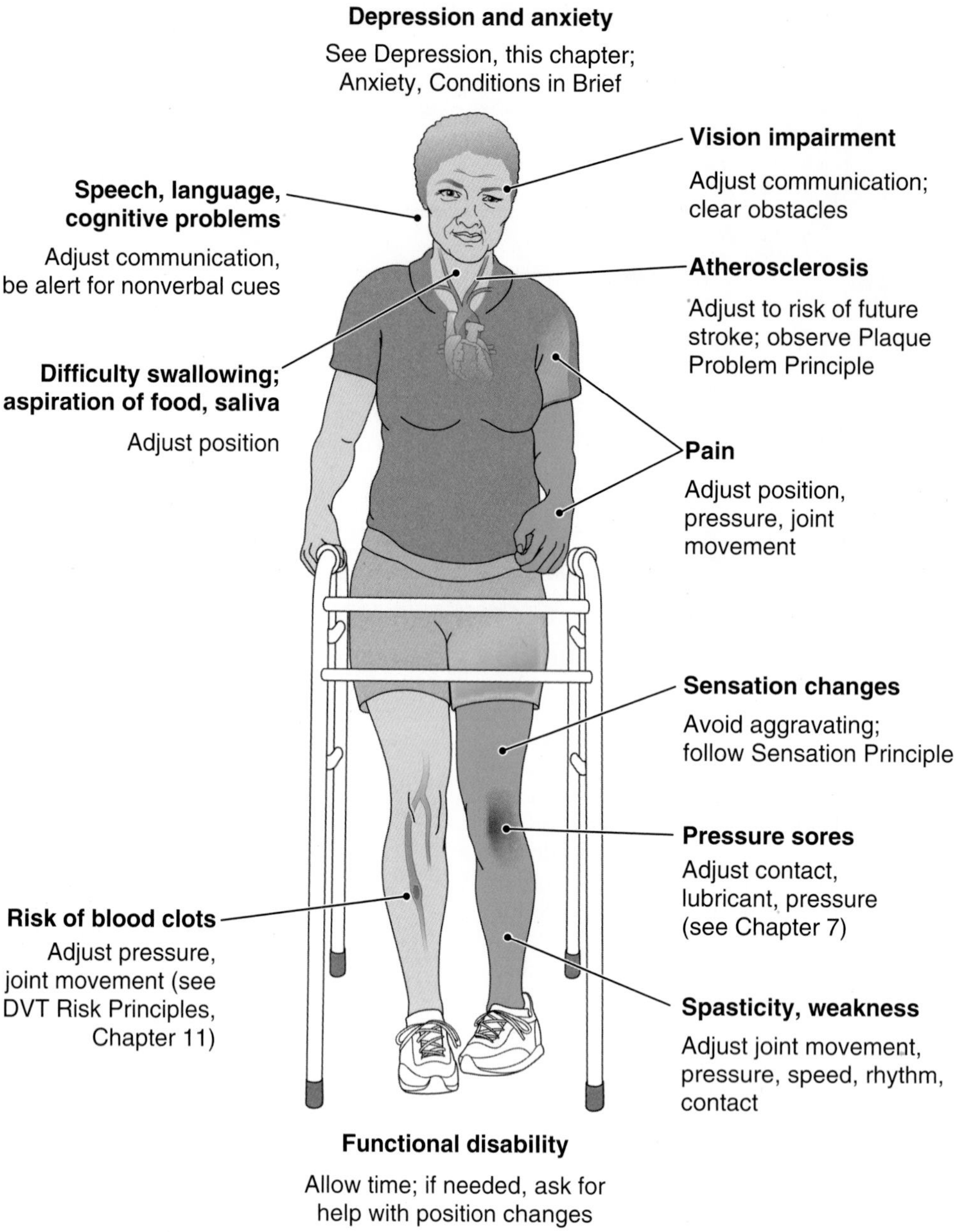

Depression and anxiety

See Depression, this chapter;
Anxiety, Conditions in Brief

Vision impairment

Adjust communication;
clear obstacles

**Speech, language,
cognitive problems**

Adjust communication,
be alert for nonverbal cues

Atherosclerosis

Adjust to risk of future
stroke; observe Plaque
Problem Principle

**Difficulty swallowing;
aspiration of food, saliva**

Adjust position

Pain

Adjust position,
pressure, joint
movement

Sensation changes

Avoid aggravating;
follow Sensation Principle

Pressure sores

Adjust contact,
lubricant, pressure
(see Chapter 7)

Risk of blood clots

Adjust pressure,
joint movement (see
DVT Risk Principles,
Chapter 11)

Spasticity, weakness

Adjust joint movement,
pressure, speed, rhythm,
contact

Functional disability

Allow time; if needed, ask for
help with position changes

FIGURE 10-9. Stroke: Selected clinical features and massage adjustments to consider. Specific instructions and additional massage therapy guidelines are in Decision Tree and text.

depression and anxiety. Interest in the role of social support is gaining research attention, and massage can be part of the support network. Massage therapy can provide wordless support when words are hard to come by, as when language and speech are affected by stroke. As well, the communication between therapist and client around the client's body, and the simple companionship of your hands, may provide support for a stroke survivor. Therapist's Journal 10-1 is a moving account of one therapist's relationship with a client during his last years of life.

Depression

Depression is the general name for several conditions characterized by sadness, apathy, low self-esteem, and guilt. There are acute, chronic, and intermittent forms, and depressive episodes can occur once, a few times, or many times in a lifetime. Different forms of depression often co-appear, in mixed anxiety-depression scenarios. At its worst, depression can be profoundly disabling, with far-reaching mental, emotional, behavioral, and physical effects. Often misunderstood, and historically misdiagnosed, depression is an experience that is much worse than "having the blues." Although a major loss, such as a job change or a death in the family, can trigger a period of depression, clinical depression is a disease; it is distinct from the sorrow and grief that naturally follows such a loss. Mental health campaigns have raised awareness about

THERAPIST'S JOURNAL 10-1 *Gentle Handling After a Severe Stroke*

My new client was 82 years old. He'd had a stroke 4 years before, and his wife had called me for a home visit. He lived most of the time in a hospital bed set up in his living room. A couple of times a day, his caregivers would help him into his wheelchair for meals.

The client's stroke had affected the right side of his brain, and he had no motor control of his left arm or leg. His left arm was in a splint. His speech, vision, and other senses were intact, although he was a man of very few words. I got most of his medical information from his wife.

The client's hips and knees were both flexed and stiff. His head was flexed forward and to the left. I had to work with him in the position he was in, and very gently. I did gentle kneading and stroking, some rocking and range of motion at his hips. I did a lot of work on his feet. My sessions were roughly half Swedish massage and half cranial-sacral work. Because position changes were hard on him, I only occasionally worked on his back. I used gentle pressure on his legs because of DVT risk.

I got the sense from the client that he had not always been well handled by his caregivers. He was afraid at first that he might be hurt. Once, I reached for his left arm, which he was holding tightly with his right hand. I reached and asked, gently, "Can I hold this?" He said, "You don't expect me to trust you with this, do you?" He was humorous about it, but I think there was truth in it, too. He needed gentle care.

This was a hard client situation for me. It frustrated me that there was so little communication. It wasn't that his speech was impaired; it was his reserve. There were no words, smiles, or thank you's that would indicate the massage was helping him. I never even had the sense that my work was softening his tissues or that he was making any improvement. I was frustrated and longed for more positive feedback. Once, I asked, "Is this helping you at all? Do you want me to continue to come back?" He said, simply, "Yes." No elaboration. His wife agreed.

I had to search my soul to be sure I was helping him, that I should be there. That my motives were good. I learned to settle with his simple feedback, "Yes." I had to rely on my sense that massage was giving him touch, one-on-one care, and attention, and that these were enough. It was a good exercise for me. And so we continued, week after week, for 2 years. Eventually, I found it easier on my body and my heart to see him every 2 weeks rather than weekly. Cutting back a bit allowed me to show up more easily and put my heart into my work. I always saw him at around 3:00 in the afternoon. Then his caregivers would help him into his wheelchair for tea at 4:00. This was his routine.

As the months went on, he began to talk a little. I learned some things about him. Some violent war stories. His courtship of his wife, years ago. His firm belief that there was no afterlife, no God. His life as a professor, and his habit of having tea with his students at 4:00. I began to treasure these glimpses into his long, interesting life. They helped my connection with him.

He began to develop blood clots. One day his wife called to cancel the session because hospice had just been started and they were going to be there that day. She said she would call to reschedule. A week later, after not hearing from her, I called to ask if I could stop by and see him. He had just passed away that morning. It was the first time I had ever lost a client.

A few months later I received an invitation to a memorial service held at his house. Of course, it was followed by tea at 4:00. I felt honored to be asked, and lucky to be there and meet the rest of his family. Also, since I'd missed saying goodbye to him, it was a chance for us to finish our work together.

I still think of him. Recently, I felt his presence around me. It was a strong feeling. I wondered, "Where is he now? How is he doing? And has he changed his mind about an afterlife?"

Kate Peck
Framingham, MA

its signs and symptoms, complications, and treatment, and the extent of the problem.

● BACKGROUND

The magnitude of depression in the population means that everyone is touched by it in some way, even if it is not in one's own experience. Massage therapists are no exception. Statistics vary, but it appears that about 18% of adults in the United States have had some sort of depressive disorder. Numbers are comparable in Australia, the United Kingdom, and in most other developed countries. The incidence of depression in children is also growing at an alarming rate.

Despite increasing awareness and education about depression, many people still believe it reflects personal weakness or lack of will. This misconception probably contributes to the fact that many cases are undiagnosed and therefore untreated. It is estimated that 80% of currently depressed individuals in the United States are not currently undergoing any form of treatment. About 41% of depressed women feel too embarrassed to seek help for depression, and a staggering 92% of depressed African-American men are not undergoing treatment. The prevalence of untreated depression means that it is highly likely that you will encounter clients with the condition in your massage practice. In Therapist's Journal 10-2, a practitioner describes how important it

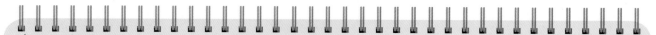

THERAPIST'S JOURNAL 10-2 *Keeping Company with a Client with Depression*

I first saw the patient at the front desk, trying to compose herself as she gave her insurance information and co-payments to the financial representative. Our cancer treatment center is an old house renovated with air conditioning, which makes it either too hot or too cold. She was shivering from cold and crying, struggling to compose herself. I brought her a heated blanket and stood behind her, gently rubbing her back as she completed the initial paperwork. It was the beginning of her journey of chemotherapy, surgery, and possibly radiation treatment.

As I waited with her, we talked about many things—about her occupation as a sales clerk in a store that I frequent, her upcoming wedding, the family members who were with her. She confided in me that she had a long history of clinical depression. I thought to myself how cancer treatment alone puts people at risk of clinical depression; starting out with a risk had to make it even harder. And so often, depression and anxiety occur together. I brought her something to drink and waited as she had blood taken. At times, she was tearful as she talked.

I asked her if I could give her a gentle shoulder massage while she waited to see the doctor. First I taught her a relaxation technique that I use with lots of patients, something to focus on while I massaged her shoulders. It's easy: Breathe in, think of a word, breathe out, think of another. Once she could do that, I massaged her hands for a few minutes until she was called into the examination room. I know the importance of patients telling their stories. So we talked. I listened.

A few days later I got a phone call from her. She wanted me there on her 1st day of chemotherapy. I was across the street at our other center, but told her to call me when they started and I would walk over. When I walked in and saw her face, her smile was so genuine, her eyes lit up, it amazed me how different she looked from a few days ago. I hardly recognized her.

To decrease anxiety in a cancer treatment center, this is what I do: bring blankets and refreshments. Talk about families and vacations and jobs. Share photos of grandchildren, commiserate over parenting challenges. Laugh. Give hugs for good news and extra hugs when the news is not so good. Depending on the patient, massage can also be done. It can calm someone's heart and put her on a beach somewhere. When there is a lot of anxiety and isolation, the personal contact of massage can offer a simple, brief diversion.

I never forget that each patient may come in with a host of preexisting conditions. In our work with people in cancer treatment, each patient comes in with a whole physical and emotional history. We can't forget or overlook these conditions. In the case of anxiety and depression, someone may need extra care. I am mindful of this as I work.

Toni Muirhead
Cooper City, FL

is to acknowledge a depression history even in someone with another condition.

Most types of depression seem to involve brain and endocrine imbalances. They are:

- **Major depressive disorder.** Also called *major depression*, this is continuous depression that lasts more than 2 weeks, and is marked by sadness or grief, the absence of pleasure or interest in activities that were once enjoyed, and feelings of guilt or worthlessness. Sleep, appetite, energy level, and concentration can be impaired. It can occur at any age, but the median age is 32. About 14.8 million adults in the United States are affected.

- **Dysthymia.** Also called *dysthymic disorder*, this is a more enduring, milder form of major depression. The symptoms are less severe and disabling than major depression, but they still affect function and feeling. Dysthymia typically persists 2 years or more. An individual may struggle with it for years, so that being chronically mildly depressed seems part of his or her personality. Dysthymic disorder affects about 3.3 million adults in the United States. The median age of onset is 31.

- **Bipolar disorder.** Also called *manic-depressive disorder*, this condition is characterized by mood swings between euphoria (mania) and depression. The extreme highs are characterized by feelings of exhilaration or irritability. Thoughts race,

and the person may talk excessively, or demonstrate impulsive behavior, such as risky driving, spending sprees, making high-risk investments or spur-of-the-moment travel plans. *Hypersexuality*, an excessive interest or involvement in sexual activity, is common. The depressive phase includes classic signs of depression, plus slow speech and poor coordination. The person with bipolar disorder cycles between these dramatic moods, often with normal moods in between. Some people with bipolar disorder have psychotic features, such as delusions or hallucinations. Bipolar disorder affects 5.7 million adults in the United States, or about 2.6% of the adult population. The median age of onset for this condition is 25.

- **Postpartum depression.** Also called *postnatal depression* this is a common condition affecting women within a month after giving birth. This is distinct from the "baby blues," which occurs after childbirth, typically peaks at 3–5 days, and tends to resolve in a few more days. While intense, the baby blues are short-lived. In contrast, postpartum depression lasts more than 2 weeks, and is a major depressive episode that affects 10%–15% of U.S. women after giving birth. It is not well recognized, and most patients still suffer 6 months later; 25% are still depressed 1 year later. Feelings of guilt and worthlessness related to motherhood are common, and a woman might focus an excessive amount of anxiety on her child's health and safety. Feelings of loss—of freedom, identity, control, and independence—are common. This chronic condition can cause delusions and suicidal tendencies. Postpartum depression can affect the mother's relationship with the child. *Puerperal psychosis* is a rare type of postpartum depression, occurring after 0.1–0.2% of births in the United States. The disorder usually appears in the first 4–10 weeks after birth, or later, at 18–24 months following delivery. Puerperal psychosis is marked by hallucinations and delusions, with some risk of suicide and infanticide.

- ***Seasonal affective disorder (SAD).*** This condition affects people in a seasonal pattern. During the winter months, when there is less natural sunlight, individuals with SAD feel lethargic, irritable, and depressed. They may have difficulty concentrating, weight gain, and poor sleep. SAD lasts about 5 months. At other times of the year, the mood is normal, or, in a fraction of individuals, insomnia, weight loss, and irritability occur during the spring and summer months. SAD is thought to affect about 6% of U.S. adults.

Signs and Symptoms

The signs and symptoms described above are specific features of specific conditions. In general, the two most central and recognizable symptoms of depression are a depressed mood and a loss of interest in usual daily activities. The mood may include persistent sadness, hopelessness, helplessness, and spells of crying. People who are depressed lose interest in activities and relationships that previously gave them enjoyment, or made them feel engaged and whole. Instead, they experience profound feelings of emptiness.

People with depression may also feel irritable, agitated, and restless. Sleep disturbances include insomnia, wakefulness in the early morning, and/or oversleeping. Fatigue and weariness are common, as are cognitive changes, such as difficulty with concentration, short-term memory, and decision making. Changes in weight result from overeating or loss of appetite. Loss of interest in sex is common.

Diminished participation in activities makes work, study, relationships, and general functioning difficult. Thoughts of death and dying may be intrusive, and physical symptoms may be present. These problems are classified as complications and are described below.

Complications

Physical complaints can also be caused or aggravated by depression. Headache and back pain are common, as are gastrointestinal disturbances such as indigestion, constipation, and diarrhea (see Chapter 15). When these conditions are associated with depression, treating them is difficult.

Substance abuse is a common complication of depression, as individuals attempt to self-medicate for depression. Drug and alcohol addiction are frequent, and for many people, depression and bipolar disorder remain undiagnosed until they receive treatment for substance abuse. See Addiction (chemical dependency), Conditions in Brief.

The most serious complication of any type of depression is attempted or completed suicide. Infanticide, a possibility in severe postpartum depression, is another devastating consequence. Suicide is a real risk in severely depressed individuals. In 2004, just a single year, 32,439 people in the United States committed suicide. About 90% of documented suicides had a diagnosable mental disorder, and depression is extremely common among this population. Women attempt suicide two or three times more often than men, but men are more likely

to succeed: four times as many men die by suicide as women. Men over the age of 70 are the most likely to commit suicide.

Suicidal behavior and risk factors include the following:

- A history of suicide attempts
- Expressed feelings, questions, jokes, or ideas about suicide
- A plan for suicide (the means, setting a time, rehearsing)
- Reckless behavior: unprotected sex, reckless driving, repeated accidents
- Agitated behavior (pacing, restlessness)
- Several nights of sleeplessness
- Self-inflicted injuries (cutting or burning oneself)
- Frequent mood changes, such as a sudden improvement after a period of depression
- Giving away possessions, making a will, "putting affairs in order"
- Saying goodbye inappropriately

Treatment

Treatments for depression primarily consist of medications and psychotherapy. Medications are often first-line therapy, followed by a short course of psychotherapy to identify and manage depression triggers.

Medications fall into several main classes of **antidepressants**: selective serotonin reuptake inhibitors (SSRIs), serotonin and norepinephrine reuptake inhibitors (SNRIs), norepinephrine and dopamine inhibitors (NDRIs), tricyclic and tetracyclic antidepressants, MAOIs, and stimulants. Bipolar disorders are treated with the mood stabilizer *lithium* and other medications.

Selective serotonin reuptake inhibitors (SSRIs) are often the first-line therapy for depression. **Serotonin** is a neurotransmitter that is associated with improved mood. Because they have few side effects, SSRIs can safely be tried and tested for effectiveness. SSRIs include the drugs Prozac, Paxil, Zoloft, Lexapro, and Celexa. Similar drugs called **serotonin and norepinephrine reuptake inhibitors (SNRIs)** keep both serotonin and norepinephrine available to the brain. Cymbalta and Effexor are examples of SNRIs. Another similar class of drugs, **norepinephrine and dopamine reuptake inhibitors (NDRIs)**, including the popular drug Wellbutrin, keep dopamine available. These classes of antidepressants are the newest on the market. Side effects include decreased sexual desire, nausea, headache, insomnia, jitteriness, orthostatic hypotension, drowsiness and sleepiness, anxiety, and constipation.

If these medications do not work, **tricyclic antidepressants** may be used, including amitriptyline, Elavil, Endep, Norpramin, Sinequan, Tofranil, Pamelor, Vivactil and Surmontil. These drugs tend to have more side effects than SSRIs. A similar drug class is *tetracyclic antidepressants*, of which only one (Remeron) is approved for use in the United States. TCAs are older drugs, with a slightly different mechanism of action than SSRIs, but they can be used for anything from mild to severe depression. Some side effects of tricyclic and tetracyclic antidepressants are drowsiness, dry mouth, constipation, hypotension, dizziness, headache, and blurred vision. Hypotension and drowsiness are often worse at the start of therapy. Sexual difficulties, urinary hesitancy, arrhythmia, and weight gain are possible.

Monoamine oxidase inhibitors (MAOIs) are used when other treatments have failed, because their side effects can be serious, and there are life-threatening interactions with certain foods and drugs. These drugs have been used at full dose for depression since the 1950s, and include Nardil, Parnate, and Marplan. Emsam is a new form of MAOI, delivered in the form of a transdermal patch. These drugs can interact with other antidepressants, with other drugs such as decongestants, or with aged or cultured foods such as wine, yogurt, pickles, or cheese. When these and other foods are consumed, MAOIs can lead to a dangerous rise in blood pressure called *hypertensive crisis*, so individuals are carefully educated about dietary restrictions when taking these drugs.

Side effects of MAOIs are the same as other antidepressants: headache, drowsiness, dry mouth, nausea, constipation, and diarrhea. Hypotension and dizziness/lightheadedness occur. Some of the more troubling side effects are restlessness, shakiness, sleep problems, urinary difficulties, and decreased sexual function.

Stimulants such as Ritalin, Concerta, Dexedrine, Dextrostat, and Provigil might be prescribed for someone with depression if other antidepressants can't be used because of another coexisting medical condition. Stimulants also might be prescribed in combination with other antidepressants. Side effects of stimulants are similar to other antidepressants. Among them are headache, insomnia, GI upset, and jitteriness.

For bipolar disorder, drugs are needed to combat both the mania and the depression. Bipolar has been challenging to learn how to treat over the years, as antidepressants may produce mania. At first, the only options for treating mania came in different forms of *lithium*, which is a mood stabilizer. Forms such as Carbolith, Duralith, and Ciablith-S are still used to treat the mania of bipolar disorder, but lithium has many side effects. Hypotension occurs, as does dizziness, drowsiness, weakness, changes in reflexes, rash, weight gain, nausea, loss of appetite, mild diarrhea, increased thirst, and increased urination. Restlessness, tremor, hypothyroidism, and skin rash are also possible.

Toxic side effects of lithium, cause for medical emergency, include muscle weakness and lack of coordination, nausea, vomiting and diarrhea, and slurred speech. Confusion and increased tremor are cause for concern, as well. The occurrence of these side effects could indicate a need for dose adjustment, and therefore immediate medical attention.

Other medications may be elected instead of lithium, including antiseizure drugs: Depakene, Depakote, Tegretol, and Lamictal. Depakote and Depakene are effective, but cause side effects such as drowsiness, dizziness, constipation, diarrhea, and weight gain. Tegretol and Lamictal, also antiseizure drugs, may be used. Both drugs cause dizziness. Tegretol causes drowsiness, stomach upset and vomiting, and headache. Lamictal may cause loss of balance, vision disturbances, and headaches. It can also cause serious rash if dose is increased too rapidly.

Antipsychotic drugs for bipolar disorder include Abilify, Risperdal, Seroquel, and Zyprexa. These drugs may increase a person's risk of diabetes, heart disease, and stroke. Common side effects include dry mouth, drowsiness, and blurred vision. Except for Abilify, these drugs may also cause rapid weight gain.

SAD is often treated with light therapy, to compensate for inadequate sunlight. The individual sits in front of a light box, which emits a very bright light, similar to natural sunlight. Light therapy has few side effects, and they tend to be mild, such as eyestrain and headache.

Medications for SAD include Wellbutrin, Paxil, Zoloft, Prozac, Celexa, and Effexor. Medications are started before the usual time of year when symptoms begin, until after they would usually subside.

Treatment for postpartum depression usually continues for at least a year, and medications are chosen carefully so that they do not affect the baby through breast-feeding. SSRIs are often used in postpartum depression.

In general, side effects of antidepressants appear soon after starting the medication, and well before symptom relief, which can often take 6 or 8 weeks. The side effects also tend to disappear as the individual's body becomes used to them.

When other treatments for depression fail, when suicide is a high risk, or when medications are contraindicated due to other medical conditions, electroconvulsive therapy, also known as electric shock therapy, may be tried. The mechanism of effect is unclear, though enough electrical current is used to cause a seizure. For some reason it brings about rapid relief of symptoms.

St. John's wort is an herb that is suggested to be effective for mild to moderate depression, as effective as TCAs. In severe depression and SAD, the evidence is less clear. It has few side effects but does have some interactions with other drugs and herbs that need monitoring.

● INTERVIEW QUESTIONS

1. How long have you had depression? How long has it been diagnosed or recognized?
2. Do you find that depression causes any physical effects? Do you have any physical symptoms such as headache or stomach upset?
3. How would you characterize its severity? Do your symptoms ebb and flow, or do they remain steady?
4. How is it treated? How long have you been treated? Do you feel the treatment has been helpful?
5. How does the treatment affect you?
6. Is there anything else you'd like me to know about it?

● MASSAGE THERAPY GUIDELINES

There are few concrete changes in hands-on techniques for clients with depression. While it is always a good idea to adapt the massage therapy session to the client's activity and energy level, there is a range of possible presentations: One client may come in who is physically debilitated by depression; another client, who is being successfully treated, could be very high functioning, with a good amount of energy. If a client reports symptoms of depression, but has not brought it to a physician or psychotherapist, or if diagnosed depression seems acute, a medical referral is in order.

Be gentle with the interview questions, and do not force them. While questions 2 and 5 will yield important answers for massage planning, for many clients, the entire list of questions may be too intimate, too soon, especially for a first session. A certain amount of nuance and finesse, as well as rapport with the client, is necessary before asking the full list. Explaining why the interview questions are necessary might help: "I typically have questions about any condition or treatment that has physical effects. If it's okay with you, I'd like to know how your depression or treatment affects you physically so that I can consider these in the massage session."

Questions 1–3, gently asked, establish the background of the condition. Get a sense of how mild or severe the client's condition is. More severe depression (question 3) or poorly treated depression should heighten your vigilance for complications and worsening disease. In both these cases, good communication with the treating physician or psychotherapist is advised.

Massage therapy guidelines are straightforward for most depression symptoms, but in the case of bipolar disorder, be sure extreme moods have stabilized before using strong massage. Typically, manic episodes are not a good time for massage. If the client has postpartum depression, fluctuating hormone levels may make her more or less sensitive to massage; provide a gentle massage overall until the client's tolerance is established. In some cases, communication with the client's psychotherapist may be in order. Also be alert for suicide risk, discussed below. These massage guidelines are shown in the Decision Tree in Figure 10-10.

The answers to questions 2 and 5 may indicate a low energy level: from the depression itself, from sleep problems causing fatigue, or from a medication that causes drowsiness. If this is the case, again, follow the Activity and Energy Principle (see Chapter 3); be gentler at first if the person's symptoms are acute. If the client's physical energy is being significantly sapped, that is one indicator of a more severe condition.

> *The Activity and Energy Principle. **A client who enjoys regular, moderate physical activity or a good overall energy level is better able to tolerate strong massage elements—including circulatory intent—than one whose activity or energy level is low.***

The complications of depression can be physical and emotional, and they are summarized in the Decision Tree. Question 2 might unearth some physical complications. If they are associated with depression, these symptoms might tend to be somewhat nonspecific in nature, and respond poorly to treatment. If the client has a headache, position him or her for comfort, especially if lying prone with a face cradle is uncomfortable. Sometimes an inclined table or other prop to raise the head and upper body helps lessen pressure on the head. Avoid any headache triggers that are identified, such as cold, heavy pressure, and so on. Consider the possibility that general circulatory massage is too much for someone with a headache, and work gently overall. If the client has back pain, begin with gentle pressure and joint movement to tolerance. Review the Physician Referral for Pain Principle in Chapter 3 to identify symptoms that might indicate a serious cause of pain. If the client mentions indigestion, constipation, or diarrhea, see the Decision Tree for massage guidelines, or Chapter 15 for a lengthier review of these conditions.

If the client has physical signs or symptoms that may signal untreated depression, a gentle referral can be supportive, in part because it conveys your sense that the client is worthy of help. Normalizing the condition can be useful: "Have you ever wondered if you are depressed? Has the idea ever come up for you?" Or, "We know depression can cause physical symptoms, too, and seeking help can resolve both physical and emotional aches and pains." But take care that by normalizing the condition, you do not dismiss its severity; someone experiencing profound pain might feel dismissed or take offense at a light tone or the phrase, "aches and pains."

Questions 4–5 focus exclusively on treatment. If the client is undergoing treatment, keep track of the medications and their effects, and follow appropriate massage guidelines. Recall that many side effects of antidepressants are temporary and tend to fade as the client becomes accustomed to the medication.

Massage therapy guidelines for common antidepressant side effects are relatively straightforward because they repeat across many classes of drugs and client situations. Only selected side effects are covered in the Decision Tree, and they are not repeated in entirety here. If your client complains of any additional side effects, not addressed here, look them up in Table 21-1.

Of note, antidepressants that cause drowsiness, sleepiness, dizziness, hypotension, and orthostatic hypotension all require a slow transition at the end of the massage: the client needs to rise slowly from the table and to slowly leave the massage setting, getting "ready for the road." If the client is taking an MAOI, ask whether they have experienced any spike in blood pressure, and how they recognize the symptoms of a spike. Ask them what they were taught about any emergency response. A hypertensive crisis is serious business and requires an emergency medical referral. An arrhythmia could also be serious, and a client should be urged to report any symptoms to his or her doctor.

If a client takes lithium for bipolar disorder, and complains of side effects, urge him or her to report it to his or her doctor. Lithium toxicity is serious and side effects must be monitored closely by the doctor. If side effects have been reported, then adjust the massage as you would any time a client presents with rash, nausea, nausea, drowsiness, and so on.

A client who has had recent electroconvulsive therapy for severe depression will usually have some lingering confusion and other symptoms if it was in the last day or so. Follow the Stabilization of an Acute Condition Principle, and wait until the effects of treatment have subsided and the person is reoriented before using massage. At that point, be conservative overall.

> *Stabilization of an Acute Condition Principle. **Until an acute medical condition has stabilized, massage should be conservative.***

Other side effects are listed in the decision tree, such as sun sensitivity from St. John's wort, an herbal preparation, or weight gain, or urinary hesitancy. These are unlikely to require any massage adjustments. If the client is undergoing psychotherapy, but his or her condition is not stable, communication with the psychotherapist may offer signs or symptoms to be alert for, as well as general support for massage therapy. Use the formats for physician communication to communicate with the client's psychotherapist, and obtain advance permission from the client beforehand (see Chapter 5).

Question 6 is an open-ended invitation to any other information that might come up. It could lead to the formal name of the condition, more about the client's history, or any role that massage has played in coping with the condition. Take care, in what you say and offer, to remain within the massage therapy scope. It is important that the massage therapist not substitute for other forms of appropriate therapy. Other massage therapy texts can help you make these distinctions (McIntosh, 2010).

Depression

Medical Information	Massage Therapy Guidelines

Essentials

- **Major depressive disorder**
  Sadness, grief, loss of pleasure, guilt, feelings of worthlessness, despair, sleep problems, loss of appetite, lack of energy, lack of concentration, withdrawal from activities, relationships

- **Dysthymia (dysthymic disorder)**
  Milder form than major depression; lasts two years or more

- **Bipolar disorder**
  Mood swings between mania (exhilaration, irritability, impulsiveness, racing thoughts, rapid speech) and depression

- **Postpartum Depression**

  - "Baby blues," temporary, peaks at day 3-5, resolves in several days
  - Postpartum depression, chronic, lasts more than 2 weeks, often 6-12 months
  - Puerperal psychosis (rare) onset 4-10 weeks or 18-24 months

- **Seasonal Affective Disorder**
  Depression in seasonal pattern (winter months), accompanied by weight gain, lethargy, poor sleep

For all:

- Medical referral if unreported, untreated, acute; immediate medical referral if unstable or client safety in question

- Follow Activity and Energy Principle (see Chapter 3)

- Communication with treating psychotherapist, physician where necessary (if acute or unstable)

- Gentle overall massage at first until tolerance established

For Bipolar disorder:

- If mood changes were recent, resistant to treatment, or acute, follow Stabilization of an Acute Condition Principle (see Chapter 3)

- Massage therapy is not recommended (and may not be welcome) during manic episodes

Complications

- Headache

- Back pain

- Constipation

- Diarrhea

- Indigestion
- Substance abuse
- Suicidal thoughts and feelings

- Position for comfort, especially prone; consider inclined table or propping; pressure to tolerance; avoid headache trigger; general circulatory massage may be poorly tolerated; work gently

- Gentle pressure, gentle joint movement to tolerance; follow Pain, Injury, Inflammation Principles (see Chapter 3) if pain increases

- Gentle abdominal massage (2 max) indicated unless abdominal tenderness present, or client hasn't had a bowel movement in 72 hrs; medical referral if constipation persists; see Constipation, Chapter 15

- Easy bathroom access; position for comfort; gentle session overall; pressure to tolerance; slow speeds; no uneven rhythms or strong joint movement; see Diarrhea, Chapter 15

- Position for comfort; consider inclined table or propping if reflux is a problem

- See Addiction, Conditions in Brief

- Seek help, advice, professional supervision for yourself from mental health crisis experts

- Strongly encourage medical/psychological referral for client (suicide hotline, mental health crisis line, trusted friend, psychotherapist)

- Avoid assessing suicidality; stay in massage therapy scope of practice; organize questions around goal of getting help for client

FIGURE 10-10. A Decision Tree for depression. Of the numerous antidepressant drugs, drug classes, and side effects, only selected information is shown. Some antidepressants and antipsychotics have strong side effects. Not all drugs cause all side effects. Use the Four Medication Questions (see Chapter 4), Table 21-1, and appropriate texts (Wible, 2009) to plan massage for clients who are taking these and other medications.

Medical treatment	Effects of treatment	
Antidepressants (SSRIs, SNRIs, NDRIs, TCAs, MAOIs, stimulants, others); antiseizure medications (for bipolar)	Nausea	Position for comfort, gentle session overall; pressure to tolerance, slow speeds; no uneven rhythms or strong joint movement
	Constipation	See above
	Diarrhea	See above
	Drowsiness/sleepiness	Reposition gently, slow rise from table, gentle transition at end of session
	Dizziness	Medical referral if unreported; reposition gently, slow speed and even rhythm, slow rise from table, gentle transition at end of session
	Hypotension	Reposition gently, slow rise from table, gentle transition at end of session
	Headache	Position for comfort, especially prone; consider inclined table or propping; gentle session overall; pressure to tolerance; slow speed and even rhythm; general circulatory intent may be poorly tolerated
	Insomnia	When appropriate, use sedative intent at end of day, activating/stimulating intent at beginning
	Jitteriness, restlessness	Use even rhythms, firm, moderate pressure; position for comfort; adapt to need to move, shift, change positions
	Anxiety	See Anxiety, Conditions in Brief
	Arrhythmia	Immediate medical referral if unreported, acute
	Hypertensive crisis (MAOIs)	If client reports severe, throbbing headache (possible spike in BP), emergency medical referral
	Blurred vision	Medical referral if unreported; no massage adjustments
	Dry mouth	Have drinking water available during and after massage
	Urinary hesitancy	No massage adjustments
	Reduced sex drive	No massage adjustments
	Weight gain	No massage adjustments
Lithium (for bipolar)	Side effects similar to antidepressants, above	See above
	Toxicity (including nausea, vomiting, diarrhea, drowsiness, muscle weakness, lack of coordination, tremor, ringing in ears, blurred vision)	Immediate medical referral if unreported; otherwise, adapt to individual side effect (see above, Table 21-1)
Antipsychotics (for bipolar) (Abilify, Risperdal, Seroquel, Zyprexa)	Drowsiness; dry mouth; blurred vision, weight gain	See above
	Increased risk of stroke, heart disease, diabetes	See Stroke, this chapter; Heart Disease, Chapter 11; Diabetes, Chapter 17
Psychotherapy	None relevant to massage	No massage therapy adjustments; communication with treating physician/psychotherapist may be advisable
St. John's wort	Sun sensitivity	No massage adjustments
Electroconvulsive therapy	Symptoms immediate (lasting a few minutes or hours):	Follow the Stabilization of an Acute Condition Princple
	Confusion, memory loss	Simple, sensitive communication
	Nausea, vomiting; headache	See above
	Muscle ache, jaw pain	Massage at site may be helpful, begin conservatively, gentle pressure

FIGURE 10-10. (Continued)

Although there are no specific questions about suicide on the interview list, think ahead about what to do if a client mentions suicide. Use the following guidelines:

1. *Get help for yourself.* Always get help and expert advice if you have even a small amount of concern about client's suicide risk; it is too large a burden to bear alone. Your client's safety and your own well-being are best served when you consult a professional.
2. *Encourage a medical or psychological referral.* If you are concerned about a client's safety, and worried about him or her being alone, then strongly encourage them to get help while still in your office—through a mental health crisis line, a trusted friend, or a psychotherapist.
3. *Avoid assessing suicidality.* Such skills are outside the scope of massage training and practice. Avoid asking a client about a suicide plan, history of suicidal thoughts or attempts, how long they have been feeling suicidal, and so on. Instead, organize your concern, questions, and reflective listening around the goal of helping the client accept a referral for help.

Here are some appropriate questions to ask your client:

- "Have you told anyone about these feelings? If so, how did they respond?"
- "Has there been any support or guidance for you during this time?"
- "Who else would you feel comfortable talking to about this? Can you imagine reaching out to someone by phone?"
- "I'm concerned about you. Many, many people have felt this way, and it's always cause for concern. There are some good resources for people when they're feeling this badly. There are good, skilled, nonjudgmental people who understand how you feel, and who can help you around the clock. You don't even have to tell them your name! May I share some resources with you?"

Although it's not up to you to assess a person's risk of suicide, it may become necessary to try and determine whether a given situation is acute and the person should not be left alone. In that case, it's possible to strongly suggest making a crisis call from the massage office and to sit with the client while he or she gets help. A client who talks of suicide, even idly, should be taken seriously. There is no single, perfect, or foolproof way to respond, but concerned, reflective listening can help you maintain the rapport needed to move the client toward more skilled support. Your compassion and referral skills may make a huge difference.

One easy resource to remember in the United States, United Kingdom, and many other countries is the Samaritans. They have local phone numbers and provide help 24 hours a day. Additional 24-hour help is available at the U.S. National Suicide Hotline US at 1–800-SUICIDE. In most places, help is available in some form—by e-mail or face-to-face as well as phone—24 hours a day.

If you get good help for yourself, you are in a better position to help the client. It is vital for you to get skilled support, because it can be difficult, frightening, traumatic, and burdensome to know about someone's suicide wishes. You can get help while guarding the client's confidentiality. This is not the time to try and be a client's sole resource. Suicide is more than an individual problem, and it takes more than an individual to solve it.

MASSAGE RESEARCH

At the time of this writing, the research literature is short on massage and clinical depression. In massage research, depressed mood is often examined in different populations, such as people with cancer or heart disease. However, only rarely is clinical depression the sole focus of a massage study. In a large ($n = 252$) RCT of adults undergoing cardiac surgery, investigators looked at mood, depression, anxiety, pain, and other variables (Albert et al., 2009). They found no differences between groups that would suggest therapeutic benefit from massage. A Cochrane review of non-pharmacological interventions for prenatal depression found the evidence to be inconclusive for massage therapy (Dennis and Allen, 2008). A review of the literature on massage in people with bipolar disorder noted that the research was lacking on this population (Andreescu et al., 2008).

On the other hand, a meta-analysis of massage therapy studies, published several years ago, looked at the massage research literature as a whole, rather than massage for a single population (Moyer et al., 2004). The reviewers looked at effects of massage on many different populations, and the evidence at the time suggested that, for depression and anxiety, a course of massage therapy treatment was comparable to psychotherapy in effectiveness. This is an interesting observation and invites further research in this area.

POSSIBLE MASSAGE BENEFITS

Mood disorders have unfortunately been misunderstood and mistaken for an absence of will or deficit in character. Depression is a very real condition with complex, poorly understood mechanisms. Because it is on the rise in the western world, its sheer prevalence may come to convince communities that it is a community problem, in need of close attention and compassion from the communities of those who suffer so profoundly. Massage therapists can be part of those communities.

As stated above, as a massage therapist, you can also be the source of a good referral. In cases where depression produces physical symptoms, massage therapy may help with symptom relief. Moreover, depression can be a profoundly isolating experience. Like no other illness, it can make a person feel alone and without peer. As a sensitive, fully present massage therapist, you have the potential to reach into that isolation and provide company. This can be a balm for someone who feels judged by others, or suffers from feelings of helplessness and low self-worth. People who are depressed feel a lot of pressure to be well ("Cheer up," "Get over it," etc.). Pressure comes from those around them and from within themselves. Shun the outdated but still prevailing belief that if someone wanted to "get over" the condition, they could. Whenever people are fully seen, felt, and heard as they are, without the expectation that they be better, different, or well, the interaction can be healing. Therapist's Journal 10-3 describes the power of simply bearing witness to another person's pain.

Peripheral Neuropathy

Peripheral neuropathy is a disturbance in the function of one or more peripheral nerves, causing sensory or motor changes. The term usually describes an injury or a disease of one or more spinal nerves supplying skin or muscle, most often in the hands, feet, or both. It can affect nerves of the special senses (e.g., vision or hearing), or internal organs (autonomic neuropathy). Peripheral neuropathy is often called *neuropathy*, for short. **Polyneuropathy** describes neuropathy occurring at more than one site; it is generally due to a systemic condition.

● BACKGROUND

Peripheral neuropathy is typically a complication of another condition, such as HIV infection (*HIV sensory neuropathy*) or diabetes (*diabetic neuropathy*). It can also be caused by strong medical treatment, such as chemotherapy, or drugs used in managing AIDS. Peripheral nerves can be damaged by excessive alcohol use, toxic exposure, and various inflammatory conditions and infectious diseases. Some people have an inherited predisposition. When neuropathy is caused by chemotherapy, it often subsides after treatment is finished and the medication leaves the body, but in some people it persists indefinitely.

When peripheral nerve function is impaired by pressure against it from surrounding tissues, it is called *compression neuropathy*. Carpal tunnel syndrome is an example of this type of neuropathy (see Conditions in Brief, this chapter).

Signs and Symptoms

Symptoms of neuropathy often occur in the hands, feet, or both, but may in severe cases involve larger areas of the upper or lower extremities. The classic symptoms are neuropathic pain and paresthesia. The pain often has a burning quality, and worsens at night. Mild cases may feature only slight pins-and-needles sensation or slight pain; in severe cases, there is significant sensation loss or burning, disabling pain. People with neuropathy often describe the sensation loss as feeling like thin gloves or socks are over the hands or feet. Peripheral neuropathy can also cause motor weakness in the affected area.

Complications

Peripheral neuropathy pain can restrict movement, and this complication can significantly impair a person's quality of life. When it causes numbness, individuals may become injured without knowing it. A pebble in a shoe, or a small wrinkle in a sock can abrade the skin without being noticed. Skin lesions can then put the individual at risk of infection.

Treatment

The first approach to treating peripheral neuropathy is to address the cause, where possible. Examples are tighter control of blood sugar in diabetes, or changing a medication, if that is a factor.

If control of the cause is not an option, or is ineffective, various medications are used to treat the condition. Topical capsaicin (see "Osteoarthritis," Chapter 9) may be used at the affected area, in the form of a cream. A transdermal patch, an adhesive pad pre-treated with a medication, can release the substance through the skin in a timed-release fashion to the local tissues, or to the bloodstream for a systemic effect. In the case of neuropathy, a local effect is preferred, and the patch may contain capsaicin, or an anesthetic, *lidocaine*. There are few side effects of this approach, beyond slight irritation of the skin at the site of the patch.

Low-dose TCAs such as amitriptyline are used for neuropathy. Low-dose antiseizure medications such as gabapentin (Neurontin), pregabalin (Lyrica), and carbamazepine (Tegretol) are also used. See Table 10-1 for side effects of these medications and massage adjustments. If neuropathy causes severe pain, it may be treated with opioid analgesics (see Chapter 21).

● INTERVIEW QUESTIONS

1. Where do you experience your neuropathy?
2. In general, how does it affect you? How is it affecting you today?
3. How is the condition of your skin in the area?
4. What is the cause of the neuropathy?
5. How is it treated? How does treatment affect you?

● MASSAGE THERAPY GUIDELINES

Once you've established the location and the symptoms of the neuropathy, begin gently with pressure and joint movement at the site. A gentle approach is best for pain or sensation loss, and in some severe cases, any touch will be intolerable. If there is sensation loss, recall the Sensation Principle—that proper perception and pain feedback from the client is used to avoid injuring the area with massage.

> *The Sensation Principle.* **In an area of impaired or absent sensation, use caution with pressure and joint movement.**

The Sensation Principle is based on the client's inability to perceive and give feedback about pain, and it is important to respect it. Yet, bearing this principle in mind, it may be possible to depart from it in small increments, with therapeutic benefit. Most massage therapists are aware of the pressures required to avoid bruising or damaging tissues, even without client feedback. For delicate tissues, levels 1 and 2 are usually appropriate. In an ambulatory person, broad strokes

---

THERAPIST'S JOURNAL 10-4 *Stretching the Rules for Neuropathy*

I am an affiliate at the Shepherd Wellness Community, a nonprofit organization in Pittsburgh. We provide education, social services, meals, fun activities, transportation, and wellness services for people affected by HIV and AIDS. I provide half-hour massage sessions for members.

One complication of HIV infection and some of the medications is peripheral neuropathy, involving the feet. Foot problems affect joints, posture, and social activities when a person is disabled by pain. Many neuropathy sufferers are taking medications and have to deal with unpleasant side effects. In addition, pain and numbness affect people profoundly. We often refer them to a podiatrist for help with their feet.

I am providing massage to people with neuropathy, often accompanied by other issues. In some cases, the interviewing is tricky—I can't be sure I am getting reliable health information 100% of the time. Without complete information, I have to work carefully.

In massage therapy school, I was taught to avoid using pressure on areas of peripheral neuropathy. I agreed with this in principle, because the client's ability to give feedback about your pressure is affected, and you could cause injury. But in reality, my clients were standing and walking a lot; many of them take public transportation, which requires plenty of walking. Also, neuropathy isn't the only foot problem: People have sore and injured feet for other reasons, too.

Faced with this population, the reality of their foot problems, and the knowledge that my massage pressure wasn't nearly as much as their feet withstood by daily pounding the pavement, I began using some pressure on their feet. I still worked conservatively, but it also seemed a good idea to go outside the limits of what I was taught in massage school about neuropathy.

This was some time ago, and one of my first clients with neuropathy was a gentleman with a 20-year HIV-positive history. We started with his low back, using Swedish techniques, light at first, then deeper. I next worked his hips, and did basic leg work—jostling, petrissage, effleurage. I did basic foot massage: kneading, stroking, some thumb work, and focused pressure. We did ROM and traction of all toes. ROM at the ankles, getting in between the bones, some gentle twisting. I mixed in some broad, sweeping work. My techniques were nothing fancy or unusual.

The client was thrilled afterward because he could put his shoes on and walk without pain for the first time in a long time. He started telling other members. People coming for massage began asking specifically for footwork to help with peripheral neuropathy.

I went to the director of the center and said, "I think we have something here." People were telling me they could walk more easily after foot massage. You don't get that kind of reaction all the time from clients. They were so happy. They weren't just saying "Oh, this is so nice." They were getting significant relief. It was very exciting.

We began a Foot for Thought program, with weekly meetings for 5–6 weeks. It includes foot massage, a "foot spa," soaking feet, guided imagery, and progressive muscle relaxation for helping with stress and education. I plan to add warm-up and movement to the program. People who are HIV-positive are often told to reduce the stress in their lives. In these sessions, we actually provide tools for stress reduction, and practice them. We laugh and share a lot, which in and of itself reduces stress.

I'm glad to be able to provide these amazing people with massage, and I'm glad we have the Foot for Thought program for them, too. It's good to give their feet some attention. They walk around on their feet all day, carrying a heavy load.

Valerie Vogel
Pittsburgh, PA

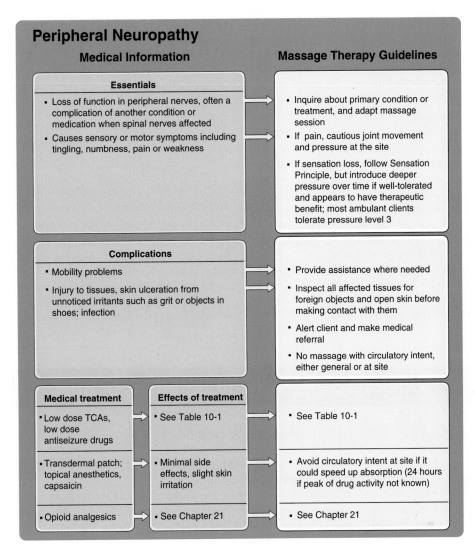

FIGURE 10-11. A Decision Tree for peripheral neuropathy.

on the feet at pressure level 3 are usually well tolerated, appreciated, and do not cause injury (see "Customizing a Massage by Modifying or Overruling a Principle," Chapter 3). Think of the client's daily activities, such as walking with considerable pressure on the feet, or gripping with the hands. If these activities do not cause them pain or injury, you may be able to calibrate the appropriate pressures from there. Also, note that pressures that are too light can be unpleasant when there is sensation loss. One therapist found her way to the right pressure with neuropathy: not too gentle, but not too deep, described in Therapist's Journal 10-4. Although you may end up working at medium pressure over a course of massage therapy, it is usually best to *start* at gentler pressure levels. For the health of the tissues involved, small increments of pressure increase are essential, with careful monitoring over time.

Question 3 points to a common problem in neuropathy: the potential for tissues to become injured by foreign bodies in the shoes, or ill-fitting clothing. Always inspect the tissues for open skin before making contact with them, to avoid introducing infection through contact or lubricant. Look for grit or other foreign material embedded in the tissues that might remain unnoticed due to lack of sensation. By drawing the client's

attention to his or her extremities, you can heighten his or her awareness of the skin health in the area.

> *The Sensation Loss, Injury Prone Principle. If a client has lost sensation in an area, inspect the tissues carefully for injury before beginning the massage.*

Question 4 about the cause of the neuropathy may bring other important medical conditions to light. Contributing conditions such as HIV disease (Chapter 13), diabetes (Chapter 17), and chemotherapy treatment (Chapter 20) should be explored in the interview for any additional massage adjustments.

The last question about neuropathy treatment might raise side effects of antiseizure medications or other drugs. Adaptations for these are straightforward (see Table 10-1). Other guidelines are shown on the Decision Tree (see Figure 10-11).

● MASSAGE RESEARCH

As of this writing, there are no randomized, controlled trials, published in the English language, on peripheral neuropathy and massage indexed in PubMed or the Massage Therapy Foundation Research Database. The NIH RePORTER tool lists no active, federally funded research projects on this topic in the United States. No active projects are listed on the clinicaltrials.gov database (see Chapter 6).

There is a small case series of five patients with HIV/AIDS-related peripheral neuropathy, whose symptom relief was associated with regular massage by an occupational therapist (Acosta et al., 1998).

Even without support from RCTs, there is some evidence that suggests massage and self-massage are being used by people to manage symptoms of peripheral neuropathy: a survey of 1,217 people with HIV/AIDS was conducted in several U.S. cities, Taiwan, and Colombia (Nicholas et al., 2007). Of the respondents, 450 had neuropathy, and about a third of these (156) reported the use of massage.

Growing numbers of massage therapists choose to specialize in work with people with diabetes, HIV/AIDS, and people in cancer treatment. These therapists have a keen interest in helping their clients with peripheral neuropathy. The work of these therapists, together with the compelling need for symptom relief, is likely to inspire more research on this topic. (C. Versagi, personal communication, 2007).

● POSSIBLE MASSAGE BENEFITS

A client with impaired sensation may respond favorably to the pressure, movement, and circulatory intent of massage therapy; there are countless anecdotal reports of this response (see Therapist's Journal 10-4). With neuropathic pain, thoughtful massage work or energy-based therapies may be helpful and are certainly worth trying. Relaxation and stress reduction help everyone; relaxation massage, along with focused massage of affected areas, may prove beneficial to people with peripheral neuropathy. Sleep is disrupted by neuropathic pain, which often worsens at night. Massage may help clients get better sleep.

In general, approach areas of neuropathy with respect, but be willing to try different techniques and document the results. Share your findings with other therapists.

Other Nervous System Conditions in Brief

ANXIETY DISORDER

Background

- Chronic, pervasive, overwhelming, and possibly disabling feeling of being unsafe, with irrational or extreme dread of everyday situations.
- Symptoms are nervousness, fear, terror, restlessness, irritability, feelings of being "on edge," impatience, difficulty concentrating. Physical symptoms include a lump in the throat, teeth grinding, jaw tension, shortness of breath, sweating, headache, GI upset, diarrhea. Insomnia, fatigue, generalized muscle tension are common.
- Generalized anxiety disorder: 6-month interval of at least three of above symptoms; chronic worry, catastrophic thinking, apprehensiveness. Some experience significant interference with daily, normal situations, others avoid them, still others do not experience difficulty with normal situations.
- Post-traumatic stress disorder: anxiety triggered by traumatic event (war, torture, physical or sexual assault, accident, natural disaster). Feelings include fear, horror, helplessness. Reliving trauma through intrusive memories, nightmares, flashbacks. Emotional effects are shame, guilt, anger, numbness, memory problems, sleep difficulties, trouble with memory and concentration, difficulty in relationships. Self-destructive behavior may occur.
- Panic disorder: frequent, sudden, extreme panic attacks (racing heart, shortness of breath, flushed skin, nausea, dizziness). Feelings of doom, terror, fear of dying. Often feels like a heart attack; panic disorder plays a role in many emergency room visits.
- Obsessive-compulsive disorder: recurrent, obsessive, unwanted thoughts and feelings drive individuals to repetitive, ritualized, irresistible actions (e.g., hand washing, counting, cleaning, hoarding, neatness) in order to neutralize the thoughts and feelings. Excessive focus on religious, moral, violent, or sexually explicit images may occur.
- Phobia: major, irrational fear of a trigger that may or may not cause an actual threat. Common triggers are heights, tunnels, blood, animals, closed-in places, crowds, air travel, water. Social phobia (social anxiety disorder) is fear of social scrutiny, public humiliation (e.g., fear of public speaking).
- Complications of anxiety disorders include depression, substance abuse, eating disorders, insomnia, jaw tension and pain, problems with digestion or elimination, headache. Anxiety can contribute to hypertension. Social isolation may result, with avoidance or curtailment of activities. Problems in relationship, work, finances. Quality of life suffers. Suicide may result.

- Drug treatment includes buspirones (Buspar), benzodiazepines (Ativan, Xanax, Valium), β-blockers (see Chapter 11), antidepressants (see "Depression," this chapter). Common side effects of buspirone, benzodiazepines include dizziness, fatigue, dizziness, light-headedness, hypotension, insomnia, headache, weight gain. Psychotherapy includes cognitive behavior therapy, with new coping methods, breathing, and relaxation techniques, gradual exposure to feared objects or experiences. Hypnotherapy and imagery may be used.

Interview Questions	• Is there a specific name for the kind of anxiety you experience? • How does it affect you? • Any complications or physical symptoms resulting from it? • Has your condition been diagnosed? • Can you anticipate anything in the massage setting that might aggravate or provoke your anxiety? • Do you feel tension in your muscles as a result? Would you like me to focus on these areas? If so, how and when? • Treatment? Effects of treatment?
Massage Therapy Guidelines	• Medical referral (possibly to psychotherapy or support resources) if undiagnosed or poorly managed. • Adjust massage and environment to avoid known triggers (including temperature, drape, face cradle, client position, therapist position, music). Consider modifying a spa wrap to be less confining. Follow the Previous Massage Principle. • Approach client with clear communication, clear expectations, compassion and nonjudgment. Begin course of treatment with slow speeds, even rhythms, predictable routines, gentle pressure and joint movement. Increase pressure to tolerance after monitoring client's responses over time. Approach areas of muscle tension, including jaw, with respect and sensitivity; do not try to eliminate tension all at once. • Alter amount of lubricant used if sweating occurs. Be alert for open skin if OCD compulsions include excessive handwashing, scrubbing, or self-injuries; avoid contact, lubricant at open lesions. • For cardiovascular complications, including hypertension, see Chapter 11. For GI symptoms, see Chapter 15. • For fatigue, provide gentle overall session at first. If insomnia present, consider scheduling session late in the day, massage with sedating intent; early in the day with energizing/stimulating intent. • Adjust massage to effects of buspirone, benzodiazepines: see Table 21-1 for massage therapy guidelines. See "Depression," this chapter, for effects of antidepressants; see Table 11-3 for effects of β-blockers. • Offer even rhythms, gentle pressure if medications cause rapid heart rate.

ADDICTION (CHEMICAL DEPENDENCY)

Background	• General signs and symptoms include decline in school or work performance, needing the substance regularly (sometimes many times each day), failing in repeated attempts to stop using, placing self and others at risk to obtain the drug, or under the influence of it; other signs, symptoms specific to the drug. • Often caused by undiagnosed depression, bipolar disorder, other mood disorder or mental illness. • Treated with inpatient or outpatient withdrawal/detoxification therapy (detox), possible substitution substance such as methadone, counseling; side effects of withdrawal depend on the drug, but can be severe.
Interview Questions	• What is the status of your detox program or drug dependence? Any side effects or symptoms of withdrawal? • Any effects on your vital organs from use of the substance? Any tendency to bruise or bleed? • Are you taking any medications during detox program? Effects of medication?
Massage Therapy Guidelines	• Working as part of an integrated medical team is advised; adapt massage to effects of withdrawal, complications of long-term use. • If liver, heart, lung, kidney, CNS function compromised, or if client's body is still detoxifying, follow Vital Organ Principle; if heightened bruising or bleeding, use gentle pressure overall (2 or 3 maximum). • Adjust massage to any side effects of detoxification drugs such as sedatives.

ALCOHOL INTOXICATION

Background	• Altered physiological state produced when consumption exceeds tolerance, impairing both mental function and physical abilities, such as coordination.
Interview Questions	• Ask about recent drinking; observe for slurred speech, poor coordination, impaired attention; ask about headache, nausea, abdominal pain, weakness, and fatigue.
Massage Therapy Guidelines	• Massage not advised during intoxication, since client perception and communication are impaired, security and safety of client or therapist may be at risk. • If you are massaging someone with mild signs of intoxication, pressure and joint movement should be gentle due to altered perception and feedback; avoid general circulatory intent. • In the most conservative approach, avoid general circulatory intent for anyone who has had a drink of alcohol in the last few hours.

BELL PALSY

Background	• Impairment of facial nerve on one side of face, producing flaccid paralysis: drooping, difficulty eating and drinking, and closing eye. • Cause unclear; may be due to viral infection, trauma to face. • Usually resolves without treatment, often improving in days, weeks, or several months (2 weeks to resolution is common). • May be treated with antiviral medication (acyclovir), corticosteroids. • Surgery releases pressure from the nerve when it does not resolve on its own.
Interview Questions	• When did it start? How would it feel to have the area massaged? • Treatment? Effects of treatment?
Massage Therapy Guidelines	• Use gentle pressure (2 max) in affected area. • Adapt to effects of antiviral drugs (see Table 21-1), corticosteroids (see Chapter 21).

BRAIN TUMOR (PRIMARY); METASTATIC BRAIN DISEASE (SECONDARY)

Background	• Primary tumors, beginning in the brain (e.g., glioma, meningioma, and neuroblastoma), are less common than secondary tumors that begin in other tissues and metastasize to brain (e.g., breast cancer, melanoma). • Primary and metastatic conditions cause similar symptoms; most common are headaches (including new headaches or changes in previous headache pattern) and seizures. • Can cause hearing or vision problems, gradual loss of sensation or motor function in arm or leg, speech or balance difficulties, nausea and vomiting, confusion, changes in behavior, mood, or personality. • Symptoms managed with corticosteroids and diuretics for swelling, antiseizure medications for seizures, analgesics for pain. • Disease treatment with surgery, radiation therapy, radiosurgery, chemotherapy, and targeted therapies. Numerous, strong side effects of treatments may occur (see Chapter 20).
Interview Questions	• Where is it in your body? Did it begin in your brain or elsewhere? Does it affect any other tissues or organs? • How does it affect you? Signs or symptoms? Any headache or seizures? • Does it affect your balance, hearing, or vision? • Does it affect your thinking, memory, or mood? Does it affect sensation in any part of your body, or result in weakness? Does it affect your balance or movement? • Treatment? Effects of treatment?
Massage Therapy Guidelines	• Review "Cancer," Chapter 20, for massage therapy guidelines for cancer and cancer treatment. • In general: if brain function is impaired, follow Vital Organ Principle. • If sensation is impaired, follow Sensation Principle. • If motor function is affected, use cautious joint movement; if balance problems, slowly rise from table, provide assistance if needed. Adapt communication to hearing, vision, and any cognitive problems.

- Pay extra attention to possible headache (use massage adaptations similar to those for migraine; see Headache, Migraine, this chapter), seizures (see Conditions in Brief), balance (be mindful of fall risk), cognition, side effects of strong treatments.
- Adjust massage to effects of medication for symptom control, such as antiseizure medications (see Table 10-1), analgesics (see Chapter 21).
- Medical consultation, communication with other health providers strongly advised for safe, coordinated care.

CARPAL TUNNEL SYNDROME

Background	• Compression neuropathy of median nerve where it passes through the carpal tunnel of the wrist; can be caused by overuse, swelling (as in pregnancy), arthritis, and other conditions. • Early symptoms are changes in sensation; later symptoms include motor changes. • Causes pain, tingling, numbness, weakness in thumb, second and third finger, thumb side of fourth finger; also causes pain in wrist, weakening of grip strength, and pain in arm, extending to shoulder in severe cases. • Treatment of root cause, self-care measures help; other conservative measures include splinting, NSAIDs, corticosteroid injections at site. • Surgery may be tried, to sever ligament and decompress tunnel if conservative measures fail.
Interview Questions	• When did symptoms start? When was it diagnosed, and by whom? • What are your symptoms? Where, exactly, are your symptoms? What position would be comfortable for your wrist on the massage table? • Treatment? Effects of treatment?
Massage Therapy Guidelines	• Many people self-diagnose; medical referral if symptoms are unreported to physician. • Avoid pressure or joint movement if symptoms aggravated; position for comfort with wrist in neutral position, well supported. • Focus on easing tension in forearm flexors and other muscles of upper extremity; adapt massage to effects of NSAIDs, corticosteroids, surgery (see Chapter 21)

DEMENTIA/ALZHEIMER DISEASE

Background	• A group of symptoms impairing intellect and social abilities enough to interfere with daily functioning. Problems with at least two brain functions qualify as diagnosis of dementia. • Symptoms/signs include loss of memory, cognition, language; personality change; disorientation. Behavior and mood changes include wandering, sleeplessness, anxiety, depression, agitation. • Coping skills are impaired, and ability to perform self-care, activities of daily living. Difficulty coping with disruptions in routine. • Causes include infection, HIV disease, malnutrition, brain tumor, heart and lung disease, repeated trauma to the head. • Alzheimer disease is one type of progressive, degenerative brain disease causing dementia; others are Lewy body dementia, vascular dementia (may follow stroke). • If cause is reversible, treatment addresses cause (e.g., improvement in nutrition, treatment of infection). • Alzheimer disease and other progressive conditions may be treated with medications to slow cognitive decline: cholinesterase inhibitors, including donepezil hydrochloride (Aricept), rivastigmine (Exelon), galantamine (Razadyne). Side effects include nausea, vomiting, diarrhea. • Memantine (Namenda) prescribed for moderate to severe stages; may cause dizziness, delusional behavior, agitation.
Interview Questions	(Question client or caregiver, depending on disease stage) • How does it affect you? Are there good and bad times of day? • Communication styles and needs? Verbal or nonverbal cues to look for? • Touch and position preferences? • Treatment? Effects of treatment? • Other medical conditions, treatments, and effects?

| Massage Therapy Guidelines | • Depending on severity of symptoms, follow the lead of client and caregivers in learning client's preferences, verbal and nonverbal communication cues, medical issues, daily routine.
• Introduce massage gently, gradually, perhaps beginning with hands or feet; use gentle pressure, joint movement to start; be alert for nonverbal signs of relaxation or tension in breathing, muscle tone.
• Client may be taking multiple medications to manage symptoms; adapt to side effects of medications (see Table 21-1).
• Consider age and other health conditions; if limited mobility, follow DVT Risk Principles (see Chapter 11).
• Refer to massage literature on working with elders, dementia (Nelson, 2006; Rose, 2009, Puszko, 2010) |

ENCEPHALITIS

Background	• Brain infection and inflammation, usually caused by a virus (e.g., herpes simplex, West Nile, Eastern equine encephalitis virus). • Symptoms of mild cases are sudden fever, headache, irritability, lethargy; additional symptoms in severe cases include light sensitivity, nausea, vomiting, confusion, memory loss, seizures, mood changes, and altered personality (rare). • Acute phase lasts 1–2 weeks, neurological symptoms may take several months for full recovery. Permanent neurological impairments in memory, sensation, speech, and motor functions are rare but can occur in severe cases. • Treated with rest, liquids, NSAIDs, antiseizure medications for seizures; antiviral medications (acyclovir, ganciclovir) used, depending on causative virus.
Interview Questions	• When were you diagnosed? Has infection resolved completely? What is the status? • Any current or lasting neurological changes resulting from encephalitis? • Any current treatments for encephalitis symptoms? Effects of treatment?
Massage Therapy Guidelines	• In acute phase, no general circulatory intent, gentle pressure overall, limit joint movement; touch stimulation may be poorly tolerated, medical consultation essential. • Adapt to effects of NSAIDs ("Analgesics," Chapter 21), antiseizure medications (see Table 10-1), antiviral drugs (see Table 21-1) • In severe cases, causing lasting impairment, medical consultation and working as part of an integrated team are strongly advised.

HEADACHE, CLUSTER

Background	• Rapidly developing, moderate to severe throbbing, piercing head pain, typically focused around one eye, lasting 45–90 minutes; on side of pain, flushed cheek, watery eye, swelling under eye, runny nose. Not typically aggravated by same stimuli as migraines. • Occurs once daily or more frequently in clusters of several weeks or months, often with long remission periods (months or years) between clusters. Treatment of acute headache includes breathing pure oxygen, triptans, ergotamine, octreotide, anesthetic nasal spray. • Prevention with calcium channel blockers, low-dose lithium (side effects include tremor, increased urination, diarrhea); corticosteroids for brief cluster periods.
Interview Questions	• Symptoms? Currently or recently in a cluster? Any identified triggers? • If you have ever had massage during a cluster headache or cluster period, how did you respond? Describe the massage. • Treatment for acute episode? Preventive treatment? Effects of treatment?
Massage Therapy Guidelines	• Most clients will avoid massage during acute headache, but headaches are often short-lived, and unlikely to interfere with scheduling. • Position for comfort, especially prone; consider inclined table or propping; general circulatory intent likely to be poorly tolerated when acute, well tolerated at other times. • Use the client's massage history to guide the best pressure, timing, other massage elements. • If the client is not currently having a cluster headache, and historically responds well to massage, attempt to replicate previous successful massage elements where possible. • Adapt massage elements to treatments (see Headache, Migraine, this chapter; "Corticosteroids," Chapter 21; Table 21-1).

HEADACHE, MIGRAINE

Background	• Moderate, severe, or excruciating pain in head, often throbbing, usually unilateral. Pain aggravated by activity. Duration = 4 hours to 3 days; may include nausea and vomiting, watery eye, runny nose on affected side.
	• Often preceded by "aura," symptoms such as bright spots or flashing lights, numbness or tingling, speech changes, weakness.
	• Triggered by stress, hormonal changes during menstrual cycle, lack of sleep, dehydration, foods with nitrates, chocolate, alcohol.
	• Aggravated by stimuli such as odors, light, sound, physical activity; relieved by rest, darkness, quietness; caused by vasoconstriction and subsequent vasodilation in affected hemisphere of brain.
	• Symptom management includes antiemetics, NSAIDs, combination opioid analgesics.
	• Migraine-specific "abortive treatments," for therapy during headache include triptans (Imitrex, Zomig, Relpax), which cause nausea, dizziness, muscle weakness; ergot alkaloids; numerous strong side effects possible.
	• Medications for migraine prevention include CV drugs (β-blockers, calcium channel blockers, other antihypertensive medications); TCAs, antiseizure drugs.
Interview Questions	• How long have you had them? How often? What are your symptoms?
	• Do you have a headache currently, or did you have one recently that's still resolving? Any identified triggers?
	• Have you ever had massage or touch during a migraine or when it was resolving? What kind of massage? How did your body respond to it?
	• How do you treat it when one happens? Do you take any medications to help prevent a migraine or to stop one in progress? How do these treatments affect you?
Massage Therapy Guidelines	• Most clients will avoid massage during acute migraine, as exertion or stimulation may aggravate it.
	• Position for comfort, especially prone; consider inclined table, side-lying position.
	• Stationary techniques are likely to be preferred instead of dynamic strokes; initial pressure gentle (1–2 maximum); after monitoring over course of treatment during migraine, use pressure to tolerance. General circulatory intent likely to be poorly tolerated when acute.
	• Keep outside stimulation (noise, light, movement, odors) to a minimum; avoid headache triggers in environment.
	• Use client's massage history to guide best pressure, timing, other massage elements; be conservative, take care not to overtreat.
	• If client is not currently experiencing migraine and historically responds well to massage, incorporate previous successful massage elements where possible.
	• Be alert for side effects of headache treatment (see Table 10-1 for TCAs, antiseizure drugs; see Chapter 11 for side effects of CV drugs; see Table 21-1 for other side effects).

HEADACHE, TENSION

Background	• Pressure, tightness, steady mild to moderate pain around head and/or neck; tenderness in muscles of shoulders, neck and head; not usually aggravated by activity, duration = 30 minutes to 1 week.
	• Symptom management with NSAIDs; prevention with muscle relaxants (tizanidine), antiseizure medications (gabapentin, topiramate), TCAs.
Interview Questions	• Do you have them frequently, or is this an isolated episode?
	• Do you have one currently? What are your symptoms?
	• Which positions are comfortable for you? In your past experience of massage for headaches, what relieves/aggravates?
	• Treatment? Effects of treatment?
Massage Therapy Guidelines	• Position for comfort, especially prone; consider inclined position.
	• Pressure to tolerance; avoid overtreating neck with too much pressure, focus, or joint movement; use client's past massage experiences as guidelines to avoid overtreating.

• Adapt massage to side effects of treatment (see "NSAIDs," Chapter 21; see Table 10-1 for muscle relaxants, antiseizure drugs, low-dose TCAs; see Table 21-1 for additional side effects).

MENINGITIS

Background	• Infection and inflammation of the meninges, layers of tissue surrounding brain and spinal cord, usually caused by bacterial or viral infection (viral tends to be less severe).
	• Symptoms can appear suddenly: high fever, severe headache and chills, drowsiness, rash, irritability, joint pain, photosensitivity, pain with neck movement, stiff neck and back; nausea, delirium, seizures, confusion may occur.
	• Lasting damage rare with prompt treatment but may include impaired vision or hearing, or cognitive and motor problems.
	• Viral form treated with rest, fluids, antiviral drugs (for some virus types); bacterial form treated with IV antibiotics; side effects of antibiotics include abdominal pain, nausea, vomiting, diarrhea.
	• Symptom control includes corticosteroids for brain swelling (see "Corticosteroids," Chapter 21), antiseizure drugs for seizures (see Table 10-1).
Interview Questions	• When were you diagnosed? Symptoms?
	• Has infection resolved completely?
	• Status of infection?
	• Any current or lasting neurological changes resulting from meningitis?
	• Treatment? Effects of treatment?
Massage Therapy Guidelines	• If infection is acute or still resolving, avoid general circulatory intent, limit overall pressure to level 2, use gentle joint movement; medical consultation; touch stimulation may be poorly tolerated.
	• Adapt to effects of antiseizure medications (see Table 10-1) antibiotics, steroids, antivirals, or other drugs (see Table 21-1); adjust massage to any lasting impairment.

POLIO, POST-POLIO SYNDROME

Background	• Acute infection extremely unlikely to be encountered in massage practice, since the last reported new infection of polio in Europe was in 1998, and in the Western hemisphere in 1991.
	• Paralytic polio survivors experience lasting paralysis; 25% experience post-polio syndrome (PPS) decades later.
	• PPS characterized by sudden fatigue, muscle weakness, muscle and joint pain, breathing or swallowing problems, sleep-related breathing problems, intolerance of cold, and muscle weakness in muscles originally affected by polio, as well as others.
	• PT, OT, and rest are used; medications for pain (NSAIDs) may be administered; Drugs for fatigue, including pyridostigmine, may cause diarrhea, abdominal pain, frequent urination.
Interview Questions	• How has the condition affected you? Which muscles are involved?
	• Activity level? Energy level?
	• Any history of massage? How does it affect you?
	• If post-polio syndrome: Symptoms? Any pain, weakness? If so, where? Fatigue? Breathing, swallowing affected?
	• What positions are you comfortable in? Best temperature of room?
	• Treatment? Effects of treatment?
Massage Therapy Guidelines	• For survivors of paralytic polio: massage is indicated; target functional muscles and muscles known to be helped by past massage; follow Activity and Energy Principle, Previous Massage Principle; consider DVT Risk Principles if mobility limited (see Chapter 11).
	• For post-polio syndrome: adjust position for comfortable breathing, swallowing; consider inclined, seated, side-lying; schedule sessions at client's preference for optimal energy; evening massage may aid sleep.
	• Adjust ambient temperature and draping for cold intolerance.
	• Adapt to side effects of medications (see "NSAIDs," Chapter 21, Table 21-1).

REFLEX SYMPATHETIC DYSTROPHY (COMPLEX REGIONAL PAIN SYNDROME)

Background	• Poorly understood pain syndrome, extreme response of the body to an external stimulus. Sympathetic nervous system activity implicated in creating severe burning pain, inflammation, vasospasm, muscle spasm, sweating, and sleep problems; pain is followed by sympathetic activity, which then worsens pain, perpetuating a pain cycle. • Often follows trauma, commonly involves extremities. Pain is disproportionate to original event, and does not follow known anatomy; frequently extends to other areas of the body. • Localized changes in soft tissue, skin, joints, nerves, blood vessels. • Complications include muscle atrophy, contractures, poor sleep, impaired movement, and self-care. • Pain treated with NSAIDs, TCAs, antiseizure drugs (Neurontin), corticosteroids, topical capsaicin, opioids; nerve blocks (injected anesthetic), transcutaneous electrical nerve stimulation (TENS), delivery of pain medication through intrathecal pump (see "Cerebral Palsy," online), spinal cord stimulation. Numerous strong side effects possible.
Interview Questions	• Where is it? How long have you had it? • Which stimuli can you tolerate in the area, or overall; which stimuli are more/less tolerable: touch, pressure, drape against the skin? • Comfortable and uncomfortable positions? What is your history of massage, and what might be helpful? • Treatment? Effects of treatment?
Massage Therapy Guidelines	• Serious, unpredictable condition; touch, pressure, joint movement may be unwelcome or intolerable at the site. Massage elsewhere could be beneficial if it does not aggravate. • Be extremely cautious with pressure, joint movement. Start very conservatively. Use past massage history, if any, to gauge tolerance, best pressure levels, etc. • Be conscious of stimuli in the massage environment: drape that is too heavy, or air flow from a fan near affected area may cause severe pain. • Adjust massage elements to effects of medications (see Table 10-1 for TCAs, antiseizure drugs; see Table 21-1 for other side effects). • If massage helps anxiety, breathing, depression, it could potentially ease pain. • Encourage medical referral if symptoms are not reported, diagnosed, or treated.

SEIZURES; SEIZURE DISORDERS

Background	• Disturbances in electrical brain activity, resulting in temporary brain dysfunction; history of two or more unprovoked (not caused by known agent) seizures classified as epilepsy. • Caused by fever, injury, tumor, infection, use or withdrawal from drugs, low blood sugar or electrolytes, other stimuli; often, cause is unknown. • May be preceded by "aura," such as unusual taste, smell, or sense of déjà vu. • Symptoms depend on part of the brain affected, but can include violent muscle contractions, numbness or tingling, loss of conscious activity, confusion, and other symptoms. • Absence seizure (*petit mal*) characterized by brief loss of conscious activity, staring into space; Tonic-clonic seizure (*grand mal*) features whole body convulsions, loss of consciousness. • *Status epilepticus* is severe episode: the seizure is prolonged and can be life threatening; medical emergency. • Treated with antiseizure medications, including gabapentin, pregabalin, topiramate, carbamazepine, phenytoin, valproic acid; for side effects, see Table 10-1.
Interview Questions	• How do the seizures affect you? How often do they occur, and when was the last one? • What are the signs? How and when should I respond if one occurs during the massage? How do people keep you safe during a seizure? • How long do they last? At what point should I call emergency services? • Treatment? Effects of treatment?

Massage Therapy Guidelines	• For risk of seizure or seizure occurring during a session: follow Emergency Protocol Principle; watch clock if seizure occurs during a session and time it; call emergency services as specified by client in interview.
	• If seizure lasts more than 5 minutes, or if seizure occurs in a client who has not identified himself/herself as having a seizure disorder, call emergency services.
	• Call emergency medical services immediately if client appears hurt, is pregnant, has diabetes, or is having difficulty breathing.
	• Do not put anything in client's mouth during seizure. Move objects out of the way, try to keep client safe.
	• For frequent or recent seizures: massage can help ease muscle pain, soreness.
	• Adjust massage to antiseizure medications and side effects (see Table 10-1).

SPINA BIFIDA

Background	• During embryonic development, spine fails to cover and protect meninges and spinal cord.
	• Ranges from mild, asymptomatic spina bifida occulta to severe form, in which spinal cord or parts of cauda equina protrude through opening, forming external sac at lumbar spine; many cases include hydrocephalus (buildup of cerebrospinal fluid in brain).
	• Consequences of severe form include lower extremity paralysis, spasticity, loss of sensation, seizures, severe scoliosis, bowel and bladder problems, learning disabilities, skin problems, and urinary tract infections; latex allergies are common.
	• Mild forms require no treatment; more severe forms require surgery, usually in infancy, placement of shunt for hydrocephalus, medications for symptom management.
	• PT, OT used to develop and maintain muscle strength, train in use of assistive devices.
Interview Questions	• How does the condition affect you? Is it mild? Severe? Any areas of reduced sensation, or increased muscle tension?
	• How is the condition of your skin?
	• Any history of seizures, paralysis, bowel or bladder problems?
	• Activity level? Medical restrictions on activity or positions? What positions are comfortable for you?
	• Have you had massage before? How did it affect you?
	• Treatment? Medications or surgery? Effects of treatment?
Massage Therapy Guidelines	• Adapt massage therapy to signs, symptoms, complications; overall, be gentle with joint movement and pressure to start, work in communication with medical team.
	• If mobility is affected, be alert for skin problems (see "Pressure Sores," Chapter 7); consider DVT Risk Principles (see Chapter 11)
	• Latex glove use is contraindicated.
	• If sensation loss, follow Sensation Principle. If spasticity, adapt pressure and joint movement (see "Multiple Sclerosis," this chapter); gentle pressure overall due to susceptibility to fractures.
	• If seizures occur, see "Conditions in Brief," this chapter.
	• Draw on massage history or physician advice to determine pressure and movement in lumbar area; avoid pressure or joint movement that could disturb shunt tubing, extra care at neck and abdomen.
	• Adapt to side effects of treatment (see Table 21-1).

SPINAL CORD INJURY

Background	• Trauma or compression of spinal cord impairs nerve transmission, affecting sensation, voluntary movement, and autonomic functions.
	• Higher levels of injury cause more profound loss of function (quadriplegia versus paraplegia).
	• Paralysis, pain, loss of bladder or bowel control, loss of sexual function, breathing difficulties.
	• Spasticity, contracture are late complications; immobilization may give rise to DVT, lower respiratory infection, pressure sores.
	• Poor bladder emptying requires catheterization, may lead to urinary tract infection (UTI); orthostatic hypotension may occur.

- Autonomic dysreflexia—exaggerated autonomic reflexes—leads to sudden flushing of skin, sweating, nasal congestion, headache, increased spasticity, dangerous rise in BP, slowed heart rate, and other symptoms in response to uncharacteristic stimuli such as pressure at abdomen, creased clothing or sheets, or full bladder; can be life threatening.
- Chronic pain results from injury and from the use of functioning muscles in new ways, to compensate for impairment.
- Chronic pain and limited ROM from bone spurs and *heterotopic ossification* (*HO*), formation of bone fragments in soft tissue that cause inflammation at site. HO causes inflammation (signs/symptoms similar to DVT) and is common in knees, hips, elbows, shoulders.
- Treated with PT, OT, electrical stimulation of peripheral nerves with implanted/applied electrodes (neurostimulation); education and assistance with bowel, bladder dysfunction, proper skin care, assistive devices; drugs for spasticity and to control other symptoms.

Interview Questions	• When was your spinal cord injured, and where? How does it affect you? • Status of sensation: Full? Partial? Where? • Any areas of high tone/spasticity? Any muscle tension from compensation or overuse? • Any areas of pain? What is the cause of the pain? • What does your doctor say about risk of blood clots? • Condition of skin? Any areas of discomfort or open skin? • Any autonomic dysreflexia? If so, what are triggers for reflexes? How do you recognize it and handle it? How do you know if it is an emergency? • Any sites of heterotopic ossification in muscles or joints? Any swelling or pain at hips, knees, elbows? • Treatment? Effects of treatment?
Massage Therapy Guidelines	• For recent (last few months) SCI in which symptom patterns haven't stabilized, follow the Stabilization of an Acute Condition Principle (see Chapter 3) and work in close communication with medical team. • For areas of spasticity, use cautious, slow joint movements, avoid overstretching, monitor results; try firm pressure (level 3) unless lighter and deeper pressures are well tolerated; use even rhythm, slow speeds. • For areas of impaired sensation, follow the Sensation Principle (see Chapter 3); Also follow the Sensation Loss, Injury Prone Principle, and inspect all tissues for injury or pressure sores before making contact (see "Pressure Sores," Chapter 7). • For areas of pain, learn cause of pain (spasticity? heterotopic ossification? muscle spasm?); work with intent to relieve pain, but with careful pressure, joint movement at first. • Limit pressure (2 max) and avoid circulatory intent at sites of known heterotopic ossification; if signs of inflammation haven't been reported to client's doctor, make an urgent or immediate medical referral. • Record all known symptoms and triggers of autonomic dysreflexia and follow the Emergency Protocol Principle (see Chapter 3); avoid common triggers such as pressure of bolster at waist. • Follow DVT Risk Principles (see Chapter 11). • Adapt massage to effects of medications for spasticity (see Table 10-1), other medications (see Table 21-1). • Consultation with PT and OT advised to provide massage care that is consistent with overall treatment goals. • Aim for pain relief, enhancing work of functioning muscles, relief of spasticity, emotional support.

TRIGEMINAL NEURALGIA (TIC DOLOREUX)

Background	• Severe, "lightning-like" stabbing pain on one side of face, along areas served by trigeminal nerve. • Episodes last few seconds to couple of minutes, and recur several to 100 times each day, can last for weeks or months, then resolve. • Can be primary, in which case cause is unknown, or secondary to structural problem pressing on nerve, such as TMJD (see Chapter 9), tumor, bone spur. • Can progress, and be provoked by even light stimulation of certain facial areas, brushing teeth. • May be treated with antiseizure medication, often carbamazepine (see Table 10-1 for common side effects).

Interview Questions	• Is the cause known? How does it affect you? Has it happened recently?
	• How is it triggered? Would you like massage anywhere on your face or head, and if so, how would you like it massaged?
	• How can we position you so that you're comfortable and unlikely to trigger an episode (e.g., in what position do you sleep?)
	• Treatment? Effects of treatment?
Massage Therapy Guidelines	• Adapt massage to cause, if known; avoid any triggers during the session; avoid contact on face and head if requested; avoid positioning with face cradle if necessary.
	• Adapt to effects of antiseizure drugs (see Table 10-1), other treatments (see Table 21-1).

SELF TEST

1. Describe the causes of pain experienced by people with MS.
2. Name and describe the four patterns of disease progression in MS.
3. Describe Lhermitte sign and how massage should be adjusted for it.
4. How is temperature control important in individuals with MS? How is this considered a factor in massage therapy? In spa treatments?
5. Describe the four major features of Parkinson disease.
6. How and why might you adjust positioning for a client with PD?
7. Describe three other conditions to be alert for in PD, as general health declines.
8. Describe the classic stroke symptoms and how the mnemonic FAST is relevant.
9. Describe the three common categories of stroke and the differences between them.
10. What kinds of pain occur after a stroke? How does each affect the massage plan?
11. Describe the differences between major depression and dysthymic disorder.
12. Describe four common side effects of antidepressant medications and corresponding massage adjustments a massage therapist might need to make.
13. What guidelines do you follow if a client discloses suicidal thoughts?
14. What are three common causes of peripheral neuropathy? Where do signs and symptoms of this condition often occur?
15. Explain the two principles that are important to apply in massage with people with peripheral neuropathy.

 For answers to these questions and to see a bibliography for this chapter, visit http://thePoint. lww.com/Walton.

11 Cardiovascular System Conditions

But the body is deeper than the soul and its secrets inscrutable.

—E.M. FORSTER

Cardiovascular conditions are prevalent, and massage therapists encounter them frequently in practice. These diseases affect the heart and blood vessels, at the core and surface of the body. Distributed within and between the layers of tissue, the cardiovascular system supplies each organ and tissue with essential water, nutrients, and oxygen. Cardiovascular disorders will eventually be felt in other parts of the body, but the CV system is so adaptable to adverse internal conditions that things can go wrong for a long time before they become noticeable. Because cardiovascular disease can go unnoticed for so long, it often is not diagnosed until serious complications produce the first signs and symptoms.

In addition to the hidden nature of CV conditions, they do not often appear in isolation. Instead, they tend to occur as comorbidities—two or more diseases appearing simultaneously. Many conditions contribute to others, and some share risk factors. Figure 11-1 shows the web of CV conditions addressed in this chapter, with arrows suggesting some of the contributing or causal relationships. This web suggests that anytime a single cardiovascular condition is identified, there may be multiple conditions, and some of them may be clinically silent.

Although the web of cardiovascular conditions is complex, massage therapists can manage these conditions with ease. Using targeted interview questions, making a couple of assumptions about possible hidden conditions, and following several principles, therapists can make good, safe decisions for their clients.

In this chapter, five common cardiovascular conditions are given full discussion with Decision Trees. The conditions are:

- Deep vein thrombosis
- Atherosclerosis
- Hypertension

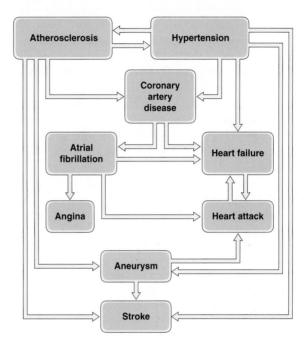

FIGURE 11-1. The web of cardiovascular conditions. Arrows suggest some of the contributing or causal relationships between conditions.

- Heart disease (Coronary artery disease) and heart attack
- Atrial fibrillation

Conditions in Brief addressed in this chapter are aneurysm, angina pectoris, arrhythmia, congestive heart failure, heart murmur, pericarditis, peripheral vascular disease/peripheral artery disease, Raynaud syndrome, and varicose veins.

Stroke is addressed peripherally in this chapter, and full discussion of stroke is in Chapter 10.

General Principles

Several basic principles from Chapter 3 are commonly used with cardiovascular conditions: The Activity and Energy Principle; Filter and Pump Principle; and the Medically Restricted Activity Principle are especially useful when planning massage for a person with a heart condition, and the Core Temperature Principle guides the use of some spa treatments.

Many cardiovascular conditions require a therapist to give time and thought in order to sort out the massage issues. The Massage Setting/Continuity of Care Principle is a reminder

that, in settings without these structures in place, extra caution is advised.

Several new principles are introduced and used in this chapter:

1. The CV Conditions Often "Run in Packs" Principle. *If one cardiovascular condition is present, be alert for others.*

   Because CV conditions have multidimensional relationships, some contributing to others or sharing risk factors, it's important to consider several conditions when one is diagnosed (see Figure 11-1). Therefore, when presented with one identified CV condition, therapists ask about others. In some cases, no matter what the client answers, the therapist assumes others are present, and practices accordingly.

2. The DVT Risk Principle I. *If there is an elevated risk of thrombosis, such as in the lower or upper extremities, use extremely cautious pressure (level 1 or 2 maximum) on areas of risk and avoid joint movement in these areas.*

This principle is usually followed in the lower extremities, the most common site of deep vein thrombosis (DVT), the area of highest risk, and the focus of this chapter. The therapist applies this principle even when there are no symptoms of DVT, just elevated risk. The DVT Risk Principle I specifies the following area of caution: *both* thighs, *both* lower legs, and the dorsal surfaces of *both* feet. In any at risk area, pressure should be limited to 1 or 2, depending on the situation; joint movement at the hips, knees, ankles, and feet should left out of the session. There is one small exception to this: In an ambulatory client, it is likely that massage with pressure level 3 may safely be used on the plantar surfaces of the feet since they sustain comparable pressure through walking. However, if the client is not ambulatory, limit pressure to 2.

If DVT risk is elevated in the upper extremities, or anywhere else in the venous system, then the area of pressure and joint movement caution includes both upper extremities and both lower extremities.

3. The DVT Risk Principle II. *Continue to follow DVT Risk Principle I until the client's physician has assessed the client's risk of DVT, understands the potential for pressure or joint movement to disturb a blood clot at the site, speaks directly to these massage concerns, and approves the use of added pressure and joint movement in the area.*

This principle specifies how long to follow DVT Risk Principle I. It suggests that several key factors—medical assessment, understanding, and agreement about the impact of massage—are vital in therapist-physician communication. If any of one of these factors is missing, then the communication is considered incomplete, and the therapist should continue to follow DVT Risk Principle I.

4. The Suspected DVT Principle. *If DVT is suspected, make an urgent or immediate medical referral.*

This principle is applied when the there are troublesome symptoms or signs of DVT. In such cases, the therapist should not try to determine a massage plan. Instead, the therapist should encourage the client to call his or her physician's office, explain the symptoms, and ask how to proceed. If the client cannot reach his or her physician or nurse, it is time to seek urgent or emergency care.

5. The Plaque Problem Principle. *If atherosclerosis is identified, or is likely to be present, use cautious pressure and joint movement at all arterial pulse points. In particular, limit pressure to level 1 at or near the carotid arteries.*

This principle is designed to adjust to the possibility of atherosclerotic plaque in superficial arteries, accessible to the therapist's hands, and to avoid disturbing clots that can form at sites of plaque.

These five principles are applied across multiple cardiovascular conditions in this chapter. The two DVT Risk Principles appear in other chapters in this book, as well, when medical conditions in other systems contribute to the risk of blood clots.

Deep Vein Thrombosis

The formation of a blood clot, or thrombus, inside a deep vein is called deep vein thrombosis (DVT).

● BACKGROUND

Although blood clotting is a normal physiological function, abnormal ("rogue") blood clots can form inside vessels, as part of a disease process. A thrombus can develop in any vein, but appears most often in the iliac veins and in the veins of the lower extremities. Of these, the femoral, popliteal, and posterior tibial veins in the lower leg are commonly affected. Less commonly, DVT can occur in veins of the upper extremities.

It is estimated that one in twenty individuals will develop DVT over the course of a lifetime; however, most of the time it resolves spontaneously without treatment. DVT is responsible for about 600,000 U.S. hospitalizations per year. The discussion here is focused on DVT in the veins of the lower limbs.

Sometimes a clot appears in a superficial vein and is called superficial venous thrombosis (SVT). If it is associated with inflammation of the vein in either of these areas, it is called thrombophlebitis. Simple inflammation of a vein, without clot formation, is called phlebitis. Thrombophlebitis tends to occur more often in superficial veins, and simple thrombosis in deep veins.

Conditions Favoring DVT

DVT occurs when one of three general conditions is present:

1. *Vessel change.* Injury to the inside of a vein, due to trauma, surgery, or other condition.
2. *Hypercoagulability.* A tendency (often inherited) for the blood to clot more easily than usual.
3. *Abnormal blood flow.* Pooling of blood, intermittent flow, and partial or complete disruption of flow contribute to formation of a blood clot. This is commonly called *venous stasis.*

DVT Risk Factors

These three general conditions that favor DVT translate to numerous risk factors. A risk factor is something that is associated with a higher likelihood of disease or injury. Medical knowledge of DVT risk factors changes, and sources do not always agree on risk factors, so massage therapists do well to stay up to date on DVT information. Some of the recognized risk factors for DVT are:

- Major surgery in the previous 12 weeks (especially abdominal/pelvic, orthopedic, knee/hip replacement, heart surgery)
- Trauma (especially multiple trauma, burns, injury to brain or spinal cord, fracture of hip, thigh, lower leg)

- Prolonged (>72 hours) bed rest or immobility, as in injury or illness
- Paralysis
- History of DVT or thrombophlebitis
- Age 65 or older
- Prolonged sitting, as in long plane or car trip (4+ hours) in the previous 4 weeks
- Cancer (especially advanced cancer, or primary cancers of the breast, prostate, ovary, lung, pancreas, and GI tract)
- Cancer treatment (ongoing or in previous 6 months)
- Congestive heart failure
- Heart attack
- Atrial fibrillation
- Stroke
- Atherosclerosis
- Varicose veins
- Family history of DVT or pulmonary embolism (PE)
- Inherited blood clotting disorders (including *Factor V Leiden*)
- Central venous catheters (port, central line)
- Pregnancy and recent childbirth (previous 6–8 weeks)
- Obesity
- Oral contraceptives
- Estrogen replacement therapy, some hormone therapies in cancer treatment
- Disseminated intravascular coagulation (DIC), a complication of severe infection or organ failure
- Other medical conditions including nephrotic syndrome, ulcerative colitis, systemic lupus erythematosis
- Sepsis
- Cigarette smoking
- High altitude (>14,000 ft)
- IV drug use

Not all of the above risk factors are equal; some are more likely than others to contribute to DVT. Although there is no perfect ranking system, the first five factors on the list are among the greatest risks. Major surgery and trauma both lead to vessel injury and activation of the body's clotting mechanisms. Several other risk factors are notable: Prolonged bed rest, immobility, and paralysis all cause blood pooling, which favors clot formation. DVT in passengers following air travel has underscored the importance of moving around during flights to prevent blood pooling. Previous thrombosis is a major risk factor, and cancer and cancer treatment are closely associated with DVT formation. In particular, the presence of a central venous catheter (such as a *port* or peripheral line) can lead to clot formation in the port or in an upper extremity.

Common CV conditions appear on the list: congestive heart failure (CHF), heart attack, atrial fibrillation, stroke, varicose veins, and atherosclerosis. Their association with DVT supports the CV Conditions often "Run in Packs" Principle. Older adults are more at risk, and age 65 is shown, but it is not an automatic cut-off point: some sources list age 60 instead of 65, and DVT risk begins increasing at age 40. Some clotting disorders are inherited, such as *Factor V Leiden*, which predisposes an individual to clots.

A person is considered to have an average risk of DVT if he or she is active, under 40, with no history of DVT in his or her immediate family, and none of the conditions or illnesses that heighten risk. Having an average risk profile does not shield a person from DVT; it only means the risk is no higher than normal. Although DVT risk assessment is not within the

massage therapy scope of practice, an awareness of DVT risk factors can help in the design of a massage plan.

Signs and Symptoms

About 30–50% of DVT cases are clinically silent, producing no signs or symptoms. When DVT does produce signs and symptoms, they tend to be unilateral (Figure 11-2). Symptoms and signs of DVT include:

- Gradual onset of pain, which can be nonspecific and not localized; it can feel like a deep ache, and is often worse when standing or walking
- Tenderness to touch or pressure, usually in the calf muscles or medial thigh
- Discoloration in skin or nail beds: cyanosis (blue skin, suggestion poor oxygenation), reddish blue color, pallor
- Swelling, often worse when standing or walking
- Warmth
- Redness
- Palpable thrombus (cord-like structure)
- Superficial venous dilation (widened appearance)
- Low-grade fever

Unfortunately, many of these signs and symptoms are not highly specific to DVT, and could signal other conditions. DVT diagnosis can be difficult, because there is no single symptom or combination of symptoms that reliably points to DVT. For example, tenderness to touch or pressure is present in 75% of DVT cases, but it is also common in people without the condition. In DVT, the tenderness is usually, but not always, in the muscles of the calf or medial thigh.

Some sources say the most specific symptom to DVT is swelling, and unilateral swelling is a strong red flag (see Figure 11-2). Yet other conditions, such as achilles tendon injury, cellulitis, and Baker cyst, can also cause swelling. Still other sources state that superficial venous dilation, in which the superficial veins of the leg have a widened appearance, is fairly specific to DVT.

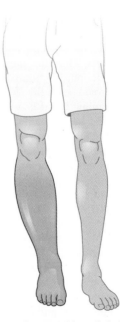

FIGURE 11-2. Signs of DVT. Although half of DVT cases are asymptomatic, signs of DVT tend to be unilateral when they occur. In this figure, swelling is evident in the affected lower leg.

Homans sign, an old test for DVT, is discomfort in the calf upon passive dorsiflexion with the knee extended or flexed 30 degrees. This test produces pain in the calf in about 30% of patients with DVT, but also produces pain in about 50% of people *without* DVT. Because it is not a specific or sensitive test, it is falling out of use in medicine, nursing, and physical therapy, and should not be used in massage therapy.

Blood clots in the veins are diagnosed using several imaging tools: ultrasound, computerized tomography (CT) scan, and magnetic resonance imaging (MRI). *Venography*, an X-ray of the area, is a more invasive test because it follows an injection of a contrast dye in the veins. Although it has been considered the gold standard in DVT diagnosis, the use of the venogram is decreasing because often less invasive images can confirm the diagnosis. A blood test called a D-dimer test is also used, but it is not conclusive.

Complications

A blood clot that remains attached to the inner walls of the vessel may cause little or no damage if it remains small, and often blood clots resolve spontaneously because they are dissolved by the body's normal processes. If the clot enlarges or *propagates* at the site, extending lengthwise through the vein and up the thigh, it is called *proximal DVT*. A propagating clot can cause problems in the area, by blocking the vessel, stretching and injuring the vein, and leading to **chronic venous insufficiency (CVI)**. Formerly called *post-thrombotic syndrome*, CVI is a condition in which veins in the legs become less capable of returning blood to the heart. People with CVI experience lower extremity swelling, pain, and ulceration.

PULMONARY EMBOLISM

A dangerous complication of DVT can occur when a clot detaches from the inner walls of a vessel. Freed from the vessel wall, it travels through the bloodstream as an **embolus**, or moving clot (Figure 11-3). In this process, the clot moves through larger and larger vessels on its return to the heart. It tends to travel easily, because these vessels are wider than the vessel of its origin. The clot usually clears the right heart chambers and valves, entering the main pulmonary artery.

Serious trouble starts when the moving clot enters the pulmonary artery, which branches to smaller arteries and arterioles in the lungs. At some point, the clot becomes stuck, and **occludes** a vessel, stopping blood flow through it. It cannot pass through the smaller vessels and capillaries to the larger pulmonary vein, so it remains in the pulmonary circulation. When a clot from the veins ends up in the pulmonary circulation, it is called **pulmonary embolism (PE)**. The pathway of this process is shown in Figure 11-4.

Once the clot is stuck, blood behind it cannot pass through to be oxygenated; the larger the vessel blocked, the larger the effect. A tiny clot may go unnoticed, and then be dissolved by the body, but larger clots have systemic effects. All of the body's tissues and organs need oxygenated blood to function. Depending on the size of the blockage, systemic tissue death may occur.

Symptoms of PE include shortness of breath, a cough with bloody sputum, rapid heart rate and breathing, and chest pain. An individual with PE commonly feels restless or anxious, with a feeling of impending doom. Fainting and unconsciousness can result. In many cases, PE is fatal, often swiftly so.

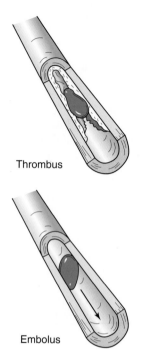

FIGURE 11-3. Thrombus and embolus. A thrombus is a stationary clot. An embolus is a clot that has detached from the wall of a vessel and is moving through the bloodstream.

LEVELS OF THREAT

Not all clots present the same level of threat. Small clots in the lower leg are rarely associated with PE, although they can propagate and become large enough to do more damage when they detach. Larger clots in the thigh or iliac vessels are more often associated with PE symptoms. Without treatment, DVT of the lower extremity has a 3% risk of fatal PE. Death from PE due to upper extremity DVT is very rare.

Emboli from the deep veins are more dangerous than those that occur in the superficial veins. Superficial clots, described previously, tend to dissolve easily; they do not readily dislodge, appearing to be held in place by inflammation. When superficial clots embolize, they tend to do less damage when traveling than deep ones. However, superficial thrombophlebitis appears *alongside* DVT often enough that any client with a superficial inflamed vein should be treated as though DVT could also be present.

VENOUS CLOTS AND STROKE

Although it is a subject of controversy in medicine, another potential complication of a detached venous clot is a stroke in some individuals. Venous clots do not have immediate access to the arteries of the brain, because they are too large to pass through the pulmonary capillary beds and continue to the systemic circulation. However, because many strokes are *cryptogenic*, with unknown cause, attention has turned to the possible role of **patent foramen ovale (PFO)**, a congenital condition featuring a hole between the two atria of the heart, which theoretically allows an embolus from a vein to cross to the left heart, then be pumped to an artery of the brain. PFO occurs in about 20% of individuals. Stroke, which is omitted from the Decision Tree for DVT is addressed in Chapter 10.

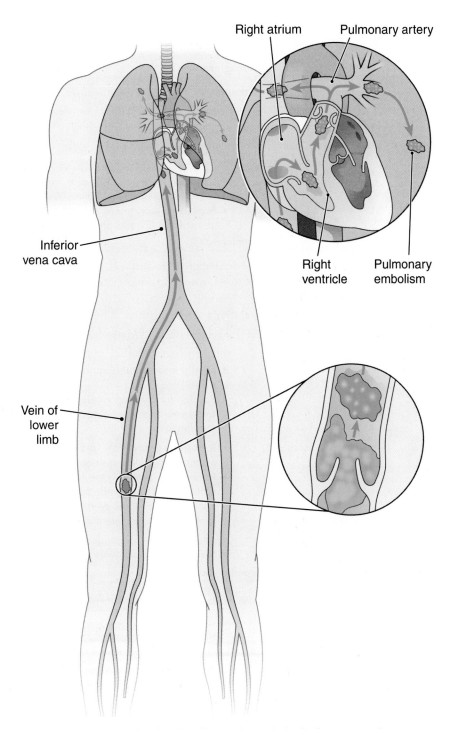

Right atrium Pulmonary artery

Inferior vena cava

Right ventricle Pulmonary embolism

Vein of lower limb

FIGURE 11-4. Pulmonary embolism (PE). A clot detaches from a deep vein in the lower extremity, moves up the inferior vena cava, through the chambers of the right heart, to arteries and arterioles in the pulmonary circulation.

Treatment

Drug treatments are aimed at preventing clot formation, or dissolving clots that have already formed. These treatments are summarized in Table 11-1. A blood clot is treated with blood thinners, also called **anticoagulants**. These drugs include oral anticoagulants such as warfarin (Coumadin), and various forms of heparin. Fast-acting, injectable heparin and low molecular weight heparin (LMWH) are used.

One of the heparins is used to treat acute DVT, during a hospital admission, or on an outpatient basis. A transition is then made to the oral anticoagulant, warfarin. If DVT is attributed to a one-time risk factor that passes, warfarin will be used in a maintenance dose for several months, then discontinued. If a clear DVT cause cannot be found, or the risk persists, then warfarin is prescribed indefinitely. In an effort to be sure the blood is sufficiently thinned, anticoagulants are often given in slightly excessive doses, which can make the individual prone to bruising and bleeding.

Aspirin, an *antiplatelet* medication, may also be used for maintenance. Antiplatelets can help prevent clot formation, but their action is weaker than oral and injectable anticoagulants. Antiplatelets raise the risk of bruising and bleeding, as well, but to a much lesser extent than anticoagulants.

TABLE 11-1.	**MEDICATIONS USED TO TREAT OR PREVENT THROMBOSIS**[a]

	Anticoagulants	
Uses	Prevention or treatment of thrombosis, heart attack, stroke; used in individuals with thrombosis history, atrial fibrillation, phlebitis, CHF	
How They Work	Prevent formation of clots; prevent existing clots from enlarging	
Selected Generic (Trade) Names	Oral warfarin (Coumadin, Warfilone); injected heparin (Hepalean, Uniparin); injected LMWH: enoxaparin (Lovenox) dalteparin (Fragmin), ardeparin (Normiflo)	
Selected Side Effects, Massage Therapy Guidelines	• Easy bruising, bleeding	• Gentle pressure overall (level 1–2 maximum); with physician approval, can use pressure level 3 overall • Avoid circulatory intent at injection sites until drug has been absorbed (4–5 hours after injection)

	Antiplatelets	
Uses	Prevention of arterial thromboembolism in patients with history of atherosclerosis, angina, heart attack, thrombotic stroke; ease symptoms of intermittent claudication by vasodilating, especially in femoral vasculature	
How They Work	Prevent platelets from aggregating and forming clots	
Selected Generic (Trade) Names	Salicylate (Emprin, Bufferin, Aspirin), cilostazol (Pletal), clopidogrel (Plavix)	
Selected Side Effects, Massage Therapy Guidelines	• Slight increase in bruising/bleeding • Nausea	• *Slight* pressure modification overall (usually level 1–3, possibly 4) • Position for comfort, gentle session overall; pressure to tolerance, slow speeds; no uneven rhythms or strong joint movement
	• Dizziness, weakness	• Reposition gently, slow speed and even rhythm, slow rise from table, gentle transition at end of session
	• Headache	• Position for comfort, especially prone; consider inclined table or propping; gentle session overall; pressure to tolerance; slow speed and even rhythm; avoid headache trigger; general circulatory intent may be poorly tolerated
	• Stomach upset/heartburn • Flushing	• Adjust position for comfort; use gentle pressure at site • No massage adjustments

	Thrombolytics	
Uses	Emergency treatment of thrombosis or PE	
How They Work	Dissolve blood clots	
Selected Generic (Trade) Names	Alteplase (Activase, TPA), urokinase (Abbokinase), streptokinase (Streptase, Kabikinase)	
Selected Side Effects, Massage Therapy Guidelines	• Serious, uncontrollable bleeding • Numerous, strong side effects can occur	• Treatment in acute setting; work closely with client's physician and nursing staff and limit overall pressure to level 1

[a]Not all medications are included in this table, nor all side effects of each.

If DVT is serious, or other medications haven't worked, stronger medications called thrombolytics are used to break down clots. These medications are commonly called *clotbusters*. Thrombolytic medications are part of emergency care for PE, followed by a hospitalization of several days, with IV heparin. Because thrombolytics can cause serious bleeding, a patient is carefully monitored (see Table 11-1). Thrombectomy, the surgical removal of a clot, may be performed in some cases, but it is rare.

Compression stockings are routinely worn on the lower legs to prevent swelling from DVT and reduce blood pooling. These apply a pressure gradient to the lower extremities, facilitating venous return.

A permanent metal vena cava filter, commonly called an *umbrella filter* because of its shape, is inserted into the vena cava in some situations. This device, shown in Figure 11-5, can catch emboli and prevent them from reaching the lungs. The use of umbrella filters prevents about 95% of PE complications, leaving 5% of individuals at continued risk of PE. However, the presence of the device itself is thought to add to the ongoing risk of DVT.

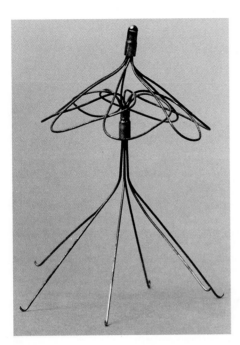

FIGURE 11-5. Vena cava filter. The "umbrella filter" is designed to trap venous thromboemboli before they reach the pulmonary circulation.

● INTERVIEW QUESTIONS

Although interview questions are essential to clinical decision making, there is no single list of interview questions to address the range of DVT scenarios that appear in massage therapy. Instead, interview questions for four different scenarios are listed in the Massage Therapy Guidelines section, below, along with guidelines for each scenario. The Decision Tree for DVT (Figure 11-6) summarizes these guidelines.

● MASSAGE THERAPY GUIDELINES

Massage therapists share the medical concern about DVT: the life-threatening scenario of PE. As of this writing, there are no statistics suggesting that misapplied massage has dislodged venous clots. However, it stands to reason that massage might loosen one, and there are parallel concerns in medicine: a patient with an identified clot may be placed on a movement restriction so the clot stays in place, and there is concern that even performing the Homans sign test—passive dorsiflexion—could dislodge a clot (see "Signs and Symptoms," above).

Many physicians have reinforced this reasoning, that mechanical disturbance should be avoided in the area. Because of this shared concern, DVT has been presented as an absolute "hands-off" massage contraindication.

But this contraindication has been poorly described and understood, and refers only to *diagnosed* DVT, which is a small number of cases. The clinical reality in massage therapy is much larger than this, because massage therapists must also contend with possible *un*diagnosed DVT, as well as other conditions that cause the same signs and symptoms as DVT. In order to practice safely with the range of DVT presentations, more finely tuned guidelines are introduced here, in three areas: *how* to adjust massage, *where* to apply the adjustments, and *when* massage adjustments are necessary:

1. *How to adjust massage: pressure and joint movement.* Pressure at levels 3 and above, or joint movement that

places pressure on involved areas, could conceivably dislodge a stationary thrombus in a deep vein. With this in mind, pressure should be cautious, and joint movement should be limited or avoided entirely in an area where DVT is likely.

What is cautious pressure? On involved areas, a pressure level 2 is probably safe in most cases since heavy lotioning is common in nursing practice, but the safest, most conservative approach is to limit pressure to level 1 (light lotioning). Therapists who are unsure about the five pressure levels, and those who tend to be heavy handed, should aim for level 1 in order to avoid delivering pressure that is too deep. Because of the potential for serious consequences in DVT, this cautious approach is repeated throughout this book.

In massage therapy literature and training, management of DVT has not always been clear. Most therapists are warned away from all contact with someone with DVT. Others are told to avoid circulatory techniques. But the real issue is pressure and joint movement, no matter which strokes or techniques are used. By limiting these elements, you limit mechanical disturbance in the area. (There are certain cases in which to avoid contact, as well, but this is explained below.)

2. *Where to adjust massage: areas of DVT risk.* Because DVT often occurs in the lower extremities, these are usually the areas of cautious pressure and joint movement. About 70–80% of lower extremity clots occur in the popliteal and femoral veins; the remaining 20–30% occurs in the lower leg (the anterior tibial vein, peroneal vein, and posterior tibial vein). In the safest approach, massage therapists avoid disturbing the thighs, lower legs, and dorsal surfaces of the feet. The plantar feet are not usually a concern in an ambulatory client because the action of walking already presses on those surfaces. However, a conservative approach would include the plantar feet, as well.

Because clotting factors are often elevated throughout the body in DVT, both lower extremities are considered at risk. *If there is a DVT concern in one limb, always exercise cautious pressure and joint movement in both.* It is essential to keep this perspective in mind. Even if symptoms appear in just one limb, or DVT is clearly diagnosed there, clots can be present in both limbs, and PE can arise from a clot in the asymptomatic limb. Here is another way to state this important point: Even if there seems to be a risk in just one limb, such as a leg with a previous DVT history, fracture, or trauma, both lower limbs may be at risk.

Figure 11-7 shows the areas that are commonly at risk. These areas are described in the DVT Risk Principles that are repeated throughout this chapter and others. In some cases, these areas should be extended further: iliac vessels should be a concern for bodyworkers who do deeper work at those sites. Also, in the rare event of a clot history or elevated risk in an upper extremity, consider all four extremities to be at risk.

3. *When to adjust massage: a range of clinical scenarios.*
In the realm of DVT, there are four main scenarios to prepare for:

- *Scenario 1:* Diagnosed DVT
- *Scenario 2:* Pulmonary embolism
- *Scenario 3:* Signs and symptoms of DVT
- *Scenario 4:* Elevated DVT risk, with no symptoms

Each of these circumstances is addressed below, with a separate set of interview questions and massage therapy guidelines.

Deep vein thrombosis (DVT)

Medical Information   **Massage Therapy Guidelines**

Essentials

- Formation of an abnormal blood clot within a vein, usually in a lower extremity

  - Diagnosed by ultrasound, d-dimer tests, clinical presentation

  - Signs, symptoms typically unilateral, lower extremity

  - Palpable thrombus, discoloration (pallor, blue or blue-red tinge to skin), superficial venous dilation

  - Signs of inflammation (swelling, warmth, redness)

  - Pain, tenderness to touch

  - Asymptomatic in 30-50% of cases

- Risk factors include recent major surgery, trauma, prolonged bedrest (> 72 hrs), paralysis, DVT or thrombophlebitis history, advanced age (60 or 65+), prolonged sitting (> 4 hrs car or plane trip), cancer/cancer treatment, other cardiovascular conditions, obesity; see text for complete list

- **Diagnosed DVT (Scenario 1 in text):**
  Avoid all contact at diagnosed sites and all sites of DVT risk

- **Signs and symptoms of DVT (Scenario 3 in text):**
  For undiagnosed, nonspecific symptoms (could be DVT or something else), assess whether to use Suspected DVT Principle, DVT Risk Principle I, both DVT Risk Principles, or some combination (see text); consider site of signs or symptoms; consider number of signs, symptoms, risk factors

  - Follow DVT Risk Principle I; avoid contact on symptomatic extremity; strongly urge medical referral for diagnosis

  - As with any undiagnosed inflammation, avoid aggravating it and make medical referral for diagnosis; follow DVT Risk Principle I (pressure level 1, or even no contact); be mindful that swelling is a strong indicator of DVT (most highly specific)

  - If pain is unexplained, worsens with standing or walking, or if accompanied by other signs/symptoms/risk factors, make medical referral and follow DVT Risk Principle I; do not aggravate tenderness (maximum pressure = level 1)

  - Consider risk factors, below

- **Elevated DVT risk with no symptoms (Scenario 4 in text):**
  Follow DVT Risk Principle I and II (especially with single, strong risk factor, or multiple risk factors)

Complications

- Pulmonary embolism (PE) (shortness of breath, chest pain, cough, bloody sputum, rapid heart rate, rapid breathing, anxiety, restlessness, feeling of doom, fainting, loss of consciousness)

- Chronic venous insufficiency (CVI), edema, ulceration, increased DVT risk

- **Pulmonary embolism (Scenario 2 in text):**
  If signs/symptoms, immediate medical referral: contact emergency medical services
  If history of PE, follow DVT Risk Principle I indefinitely

- Avoid circulatory intent at site of edema; inspect skin and avoid contact at ulceration; continue DVT Risk Principles

Medical treatment	Effects of treatment	
- Anticoagulants	- Easy bruising or bleeding	- Use gentle joint movement overall, cautious pressure overall (level 1-2 max); with physician approval, can use pressure level 3 overall
		- If injected, avoid circulatory intent at injection site until medication absorbed (usually 4-5 hours)
- Antiplatelets	- Slightly elevated risk of bruising/bleeding	- Slight pressure adjustment overall (pressure level 3 max; level 4 may be possible)
- Thrombolytics	- Unstable tissues; high risk of hemorrhage	- Work closely with client's physician and nursing staff; limit overall pressure to level 1
- Thrombectomy (surgical removal - rare)	- See Surgery, Chapter 21, for side effects, complications	- Follow the Procedure Principle; see Surgery, Chapter 21
- Compression stockings (routine)	- Can be warm, uncomfortable, difficult to pull on	- Avoid lubricant on stockings; lubricant on skin can make it more difficult to pull on
- Vena cava filter	- DVT risk may continue or increase; is not fully effective against PE	- Avoid deep pressure at abdomen; continue DVT Risk Principle I indefinitely

FIGURE 11-6. A Decision Tree for DVT. See text for further discussion of the four clinical DVT scenarios shown on the tree.

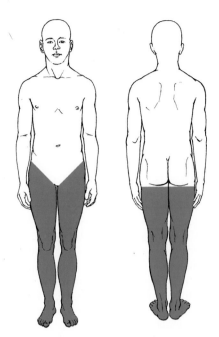

FIGURE 11-7. Areas of DVT Risk. Veins of the lower extremities are common sites of thrombus formation. DVT Risk Principle I covers both lower extremities, as shown by the shaded areas. (Less commonly, upper extremity DVT develops; if this is the case, consider all four limbs at risk.)

DVT Scenarios

Using principles introduced at the beginning of this chapter, sometimes in combination, massage therapists can find their way with each DVT scenario.

SCENARIO 1: DIAGNOSED DVT

Suppose your client tells you that he or she was recently diagnosed with a blood clot or had a blood clot a long time ago. Use the questions in Box 11-1 to learn more about the condition, and develop a massage plan.

Questions 1–4 provide important background on the condition, and possible complications to accommodate. If a client was recently diagnosed with DVT, be cautious with all diagnosed sites and all sites at risk of clot formation. This means

using DVT Risk Principle I, but an even more cautious application of it, limiting pressure to a 1 in the specified areas.

In reality, holding the legs with soft, still hands (without stroking), at a pressure level 1 or less is probably safe. Within that, there is an argument for no *contact* on the diagnosed area until it is clear the condition has resolved. However, the most conservative approach, and the one to follow as a liability precaution, is to avoid contact altogether.

Your caution is justified, even though medications are probably already at work, dissolving the clot and preventing future clot formation. Medications do not eliminate the risk entirely, and some individuals develop DVT while on anticoagulant therapy.

If DVT has resolved, use Question 2 and the client's doctor to find out whether the risk of DVT is fleeting, expected to pass at some point. If the condition resolves and anticoagulant therapy is discontinued, this typically reflects the physician's optimism that an identified, transient risk factor has passed. This will typically be several months later. If the DVT is attributed to a transient factor, such as a medication, recent surgery, or pregnancy, then less caution may be advised when the risk passes. But it is still a good idea to have the physician weigh in on the advisability of heavier pressure in the lower extremities for the near and far future (see Scenario 4 for elevated risk).

On the other hand, if DVT is attributed to a chronic condition that is not expected to go away, it is reasonable to follow DVT Risk Principle I indefinitely, without seeking medical consultation.

If the client's DVT has left CVI in its wake, you may encounter edema in the limb, or ulceration. Avoid circulatory intent at the site of edema. Avoid contact, as always, at an area of open skin, and inspect the skin in the area at each session. Finally, as above, continue the DVT Risk Principles, as CVI may place the area at increased risk.

Questions 5–7 about treatment will likely bring up anticoagulant therapy. This treatment almost always causes easy bruising and bleeding, especially at first. This requires gentle pressure overall, typically level 2 maximum (while continuing to observe any more stringent pressure limits on the DVT risk areas). Use cautious movement at all joints, avoiding strong stretches. As the anticoagulant dose is adjusted over time, an overall pressure level of 3 may be appropriate, but make sure the physician concurs before attempting this. If the client uses injected heparin, avoid circulatory intent at the site of the injection until the drug has been absorbed—typically 4–5

BOX 11-1   QUESTIONS FOR A CLIENT WITH DIAGNOSED DVT

1. Where is or was the clot? When did it occur?
2. Did your doctor state any other areas that are at risk of blood clot? Were there any clear causes or risk factors, and, if so, has it resolved or is it an ongoing concern?
3. Were there any complications, such as embolism, swelling, or skin problems?
4. When and how did the condition resolve? Did it leave any lasting effect, that you know of?
5. How was the condition treated? Is it still being treated, or is treatment planned indefinitely? How does treatment affect you?
6. Do you inject any medications for it? If so, where and when?
7. Do any of your medications cause easy bruising or bleeding? Is it mild, moderate, or severe? Have you and your doctor settled on the correct dose?

BOX 11-2 QUESTIONS FOR A CLIENT WITH A HISTORY OF PE

1. When did you have the blood clot? How serious was the PE?
2. Where did the clot originate?
3. How was it treated? How did (or does) treatment affect you?

hours. If antiplatelet drugs are being used, a slight adjustment in overall pressure may be in order, but these drugs do not heighten bruising or bleeding as much as anticoagulants.

If thrombolytic drugs were administered, it means the client had a difficult case of DVT, or developed PE. For a time, these drugs can leave the tissues especially unstable (prone to bleeding), and the client is or was being treated in the hospital until the condition stabilizes. In this case, work as part of a medical team and limit pressure to level 1 initially. Do not advance the overall pressure without the approval of the client's physician.

If a vena cava filter was inserted, anticoagulants are often discontinued, and overall pressure may not need to be so gentle. However, since filters do not provide a guaranteed safety net, and may even add to the risk of DVT, it is still wise to follow DVT Risk Principle I indefinitely, and avoid sending a clot into the filter. Also, be cautious with pressure at the abdomen.

Always adapt to any known DVT cause or ongoing risk factor (see "DVT Risk Factors," above), and any swelling or vein problems left behind by the clot (see Decision Tree, Figure 11-6).

SCENARIO 2: PULMONARY EMBOLISM

If the client reports symptoms of PE, or you notice signs of PE, call emergency medical services immediately. Review signs and symptoms of PE, above. If client tells you he or she had a PE in the past, ask the questions in Box 11-2.

If a client presents with a history of PE, his or her risk of DVT is likely to be elevated, and this status may be lifelong. The safest approach is to follow DVT Risk Principle I indefinitely. Adapt massage to the likely scenario of lifelong anticoagulant therapy.

SCENARIO 3: SIGNS AND SYMPTOMS OF DVT

Suppose your client shows one or more signs or symptoms of DVT, but has not seen a doctor about it, or has no clear diagnosis. The signs or symptoms could be due to a blood clot, or to something else. In this scenario, your task is much less straightforward than for the client with a DVT diagnosis. Here, you assess the situation and choose one or more of the following actions:

- Make an urgent or immediate medical referral, effectively ending or canceling the session (The Suspected DVT Principle);
- Proceed with a modified session, limiting pressure and joint movement on the at-risk areas (DVT Risk Principle I), until the client's physician can be involved in the massage plan (DVT Risk Principle II);
- Move ahead with the session without modifying the massage plan.

These three responses reflect a wide range of concern and caution. In some cases the first approach would be too alarmist, and in other cases, the last approach would be far too casual. How do you know which response to use, when? For example,

what do you do if a client mentions a sign or symptom, such as swelling or tenderness in a lower extremity, and you know it to be a possible sign or symptom of DVT?

DVT symptoms are *nonspecific*, caused by other conditions that mimic DVT, making it notoriously difficult for physicians to diagnose. Moreover, symptoms are prevalent in the general population. This prevalence, along with multiple other explanations for symptoms, and the complexity of DVT, means there is no clear formula for the massage therapist to follow, and most decisions will be based on a judgment call, rather than an obvious directive.

Use the questions in Box 11-3 to gather signs, symptoms, and risk factors. Along with the history or known cause of the symptoms, these can help you assess the situation, and arrive at massage adjustments, a medical referral, or both.

If the clinical picture is complicated, with signs, symptoms, or risk factors for DVT, then a safe, easy-to-follow approach is to use the DVT Risk Principle I for that session (and, if it is a repeat client, DVT Risk Principle II for subsequent sessions). Principle I (see Figure 11-7) is an invaluable fallback plan because even without much information from the client, and no access to the physician, the principle allows you to safely move forward with the session at hand. No matter what is going on, you can be sure that massage does not worsen the situation. You can also urge the client to see a physician for the signs or symptoms, so that he or she has more information before seeking massage again.

> *The DVT Risk Principle I. If there is an elevated risk of thrombosis, such as in the lower or upper extremities, use extremely cautious pressure (level 1 or 2 maximum) on areas of risk and avoid joint movement in these areas.*

If you have a very strong concern, you can end or cancel the session, with a recommendation for the client to see his or her physician as soon as possible to have it seen. In this case, you are following the Suspected DVT Principle.

> *The Suspected DVT Principle. If DVT is suspected, make an urgent or immediate medical referral.*

In deciding between whether to modify massage, urge a medical referral, or both, consider the following:

1. *The site of signs or symptoms.* DVT typically appears in the lower extremities, although upper extremity DVT is possible. Unilateral symptoms and signs are much more of a concern than bilateral signs and symptoms as DVT signs and symptoms tend to be on one side. (Even though DVT *risk* is often bilateral, the clot itself is usually on one side.)

BOX 11-3 QUESTIONS FOR A CLIENT WITH SIGNS OR SYMPTOMS OF DVT

1. What are your symptoms? Where do you experience them?
2. Have you experienced them before? If so, was the problem diagnosed at the time?
3. Have you seen a doctor for these symptoms? Did you receive a diagnosis? Did the diagnosis seem clear, or was there any uncertainty? Do you know what causes the symptoms?
4. Have any of your current or past health care providers ever said you might be at risk for blood clots? Have you ever been instructed to contact your doctor about any of these symptoms?
5. May I look at it?
6. Do you have any pain in the area? Is it tender to the touch? Any swelling, warmth, or redness in the area?
7. Is there any discoloration of your skin in the area: bluish color or lack of color (pallor)?
8. Any protruding, prominent, or wider looking veins?
9. Do you have any fever, even a low-grade one?
10. Are any of the following true for you? (List risk factors; some may be noted from the client's completed form or interview.)
11. Have you been treating this symptom? Has treatment helped? How has it affected you?

2. *The number of signs, symptoms, and risk factors*. In general, be concerned when more than one sign or symptom is present, or when a single sign or symptom appears along with a risk factor. If a sign or symptom is combined with two risk factors, or a single risk factor that is especially strong, raise your concern higher. If three risk factors are present along with a sign or symptom, an immediate or urgent medical referral is likely in order.

3. *Other DVT signs, such as a palpable cord-like structure, discoloration, or superficial venous dilation*. Any of these is a cause for strong concern and an urgent referral. Any time there is an unfamiliar density in the tissue, it is important to bring it to the client's attention, but if the density is cord-like, an urgent or immediate medical referral is a good idea. And superficial venous dilation is a strong predictor of DVT, according to some of the research. A blue tinge to the skin suggests a vascular problem, in need of medical attention. At minimum, follow DVT Risk Principle I, and raise the issue with the client. Also avoid all contact on the symptomatic extremity.

4. *Signs of inflammation*. Three of the DVT signs—swelling, warmth, and redness—are also signs of inflammation. Irrespective of the cause of inflammation, massage therapists are taught not to aggravate inflammation by pressing on it, and to make a medical referral for undiagnosed or unexplained inflammation. The cause may turn out to be minor—not DVT at all—but other serious causes of inflammation, such as cellulitis or anterior compartment syndrome, should also be seen by a physician.

Unexplained inflammation in a lower extremity calls for DVT Risk Principle I, with the most cautious application (pressure level 1, or even no contact). Of all the DVT symptoms, swelling is the most highly specific to DVT. Undiagnosed, unexplained swelling is a strong argument for an urgent or immediate medical referral.

5. *Pain or tenderness*. Many people have undiagnosed pain or discomfort in one or both lower extremities, and it is not specific to DVT. A host of conditions cause lower limb pain, including claudication, CVI, varicose veins, neuropathy, cellulitis, arthritis, tendinitis, shin splints, a ruptured Baker cyst, or a stress fracture. Note that most of these conditions also contraindicate medium and heavy pressure at the site, and

this is built into DVT Risk Principle I. Moreover, if one of these conditions is causing the problem, it needs to be diagnosed and treated, so that a medical referral may be in order.

Minor pain with a clear cause—"I started a dance class this week," or "I hiked a lot on Sunday"—is less likely to raise concern than unexplained pain. Finding out the history of a certain pain, how familiar it is to the client, and any known alternative causes can help you determine whether or not to suspect DVT. If the client's only complaint is pain or soreness, it doesn't worsen with standing or walking, and there are no other signs, symptoms, or risk factors, you might decide to move forward with a massage plan, with no modifications on the legs. Muscle strain and muscle spasm *indicate* pressure level 3, and they are both common causes of lower extremity pain (see Chapter 8).

On the other hand, if pain is unexplained, worsens with standing or walking, or appears with other symptoms, signs, or risk factors, follow DVT Risk Principle I with pressure level 1, or no contact, and make an urgent medical referral. If there is *tenderness*, pain produced by touch or pressure, use cautious pressure (level 1) or avoid contact at tender sites. In addition to the heightened DVT concern, you do not want to aggravate tenderness.

From the above list, a take home message emerges: if in doubt, follow DVT Risk Principle I for the current session. If in doubt, also avoid contact and any pressure on the symptomatic area. Refer the client for medical care soon, and refer right away if you have a deep concern. If the client's only symptom is pain, your task is made much more difficult, but your concern escalates when there is no explanation or history to the pain.

Avoid the temptation to test the area using the Homans sign. Recall that the test is considered to be of no value in testing for DVT, and the use of it can lead to a false sense of security and to unsafe massage pressure.

The DVT Risk Principle I. If there is an elevated risk of thrombosis, such as in the lower or upper extremities, use extremely cautious pressure (level 1 or 2 maximum) on areas of risk and avoid joint movement in these areas.

After reviewing these factors and making a decision, it is important to convey it to the client. If you decide to follow DVT Risk Principle I, here is one way to communicate your plan:

> Because you have [symptom/sign] in the area, and your health history includes some risk factors for blood clots, I am going to avoid pressure on your legs today. Also, I think it's a good idea for you to bring this [symptom/sign] to your doctor's attention as soon as possible. It could be something minor or something more serious, but your doctor is the best one to say either way.

If you have serious concerns, the *Suspected DVT Principle* is appropriate. Encourage your client to contact his or her doctor immediately, preferably from your office. On the other end of the phone, the nurse, nurse practitioner, or physician assistant will ask questions and recommend how to proceed. If the client cannot reach someone by phone at his or her doctor's office, or does not have a primary care physician, he or she should seek emergency medical care.

> *The Suspected DVT Principle. If DVT is suspected, make an urgent or immediate medical referral.*

If you follow the Suspected DVT Principle, here is one example of how to present your concern to your client:

> Because of the pain in your calf, the swelling, and the protrusion of this vein, I am concerned about that area. It could be caused by something minor, or it could be something very serious like a blood clot in one of the veins. I'm not qualified to diagnose the problem or say for sure. But because it could be serious, I recommend we call your doctor's office and talk with someone there, ask them what to do. Instead of going ahead with the massage, we need to make that call right now because I think you need to have your leg looked at by your doctor. Do you have the phone number of your doctor's office?

Although you communicate your concern calmly, information about DVT is inherently alarming, and the client may or may not respond positively. Therapist's Journal 11-1 tells a story of a client's resistance to a massage therapy student's concern, and how the student managed to work safely and make a good referral.

Symptoms and signs of DVT require your best judgment and effort. It would be convenient, although unrealistic, for every client to arrive with recent test results ruling out DVT. Without this, a certain amount of assessment falls to the therapist. Since assessment is subjective territory, some therapists are more likely to be alarmed than others and more likely to make a medical referral for a minor problem. This is to be expected. The best thing you can do is to learn all you can about DVT symptoms, and talk to health care providers about it. Make conscious, thoughtful decisions, and when in doubt, proceed cautiously.

SCENARIO 4: ELEVATED RISK OF DVT WITH NO SYMPTOMS

Suppose your client has no symptoms but has enough risk factors (or a single strong risk factor) to give you concern about the potential for asymptomatic DVT. Perhaps you see a lot of clients who tend to be at increased risk of DVT, such as older adults (over 60), or people with cancer. Or perhaps a first time client comes in after a long haul airline flight, or a long period of bed rest. In cases like these, one or both DVT Risk Principles are appropriate.

> *The DVT Risk Principle I. If there is an elevated risk of thrombosis, such as in the lower or upper extremities, use extremely cautious pressure (level 1 or 2 maximum) on areas of risk and avoid joint movement in these areas.*

> *The DVT Risk Principle II. Continue to follow DVT Risk Principle I until the client's physician has assessed the client's risk of DVT, understands the potential for pressure or joint movement to disturb a blood clot at the site, speaks directly to these massage concerns, and approves the use of added pressure and joint movement in the area.*

There is no absolute guideline of when to apply these principles, but the questions in Box 11-4 can help you judge whether to use them.

It is usually best to apply the DVT Risk Principles in these cases: (1) If the client has a single strong risk factor, or (2) the client has a medical condition/risk factor that does not go away, such as heart failure. Typically, two risk factors raise the level of concern, and three risk factors argue very strongly for the DVT Risk Principles. If the client is moderately active, it does not completely cancel out other risk factors, but it may reduce the client's DVT risk.

The first DVT Risk Principle specifies the adjustments to make, and the second describes the physician communication required in order to discontinue the first. The form of medical consultation may vary according to the treatment setting or practice. In a medical facility, massage of the lower extremities may be part of physician orders in the patient's chart. If so, check with the patient's nurse about his or her DVT concern before you begin the session. Also, ask about any recent changes to the patient's risk level.

In other settings such as private practice, use the communication steps described in Chapter 5. Recall that it can be ideal to go through the physician's nurse. For something as serious and uncertain as DVT, written communication is strongly advised. Here are some situations in which therapists have successfully used one or both DVT Risk Principles:

- A 68-year-old client who had a recent fall with no fracture but significant bruising at the ankle
- A 64-year-old female with stage 1 hypertension
- A client who gave birth 3 weeks ago
- A client recovering from a spinal cord injury
- A client taking estrogen replacement therapy
- A client who smokes and takes oral contraceptives
- A client with advanced diabetes mellitus

If a single alarm appears in the health history, you have doubts, or there is no time to learn enough about the client's condition to make an educated decision, the DVT Risk Principles provide a safe, default approach. You may also decide to routinely follow the two principles if you work with a special population or client profile that includes elevated DVT risk, such as pregnant women, people with cardiovascular conditions, or people with cancer.

THERAPIST'S JOURNAL 11-1   *Leap of Faith: Pain, Redness, Swelling... Referral!*

In a practice session during my massage training, several red flags arose with my 36-year-old female client: She wore support hose occasionally for severe, painful varicose veins; was active in a profession that required long periods of standing; showed edema in her ankles; and was still carrying 40 extra pounds gained during her pregnancy a year before.

By themselves, the varicose veins and the weight issue were risk factors for DVT—good reasons to communicate with her doctor before I used any pressure on her legs. But she also mentioned her painful lower left leg, which was red, swollen, warm, and tender.

This client wanted deep pressure in the affected area. I knew she was at risk of DVT, and I didn't know why there was inflammation. I took a breath, sat down with her, and told her that we needed to talk, first. First, whatever was going on in her leg, I wasn't qualified to diagnose it; she needed to see her doctor as soon as possible. Second, I would have to hear back from her physician before I used pressure in the area. Finally, I told her my game plan for the day's session, a Reiki session and some careful bolstering for deep relaxation.

Upon hearing the game plan, she was surprised, a little defensive, and not entirely thrilled with me or the treatment plan. I apologized for the conservative treatment, but told her I felt it was in her best interest. In the end, she agreed to the session and was far happier with it than she'd expected. I sent her home with a Release of Medical Records form so that I could communicate with her doctor before her next session.

When I called a day later to follow up, she let me know that her doctor had diagnosed phlebitis. She had started anticoagulant therapy immediately to prevent thrombosis. She was very grateful to me for "sticking up for her" despite her resistance, and for urging her to see her doctor. Her doctor agreed, saying that the client "could have been in a lot of trouble," and my referral was fortunate and extremely timely. The client and physician both said how critical it was for a massage therapist to be aware both of this condition and its risks.

While the client's phlebitis resolved in several weeks, she remains at risk for recurrence and for DVT, and she's still taking anticoagulants. Although she now wears her stockings more consistently, new varicose veins have appeared, and other factors—her weight, her job, and her ankle swelling—remain unchanged. Since graduating from massage school, I have continued to treat her, so I've needed ongoing help from her doctor. My treatment plan excludes pressure on her thighs, lower legs, and tops of her feet, but includes pressure on the plantar surfaces, since she's on her feet so much. Over time, I've been able to adjust massage pressure on her upper body from light to moderate pressure without the risk of bruising. Her physician provides whole-hearted support of the massage plan for her patient's well-being.

From that first session, I remember strongly how challenging it was, as a student, speaking from a position of urgent persuasion and credibility to my client. I kept hearing my massage instructors in my head, reminding me that an occasional treatment decision might not be popular with my client, but I would need to stand by it to be an ethical, responsible professional. Sometimes a "feel good massage" isn't in the client's best interest, but a trip to the doctor is.

When this happened several years ago, my response to the client was considered appropriately cautious. Experience has convinced me that clear guidelines for suspected DVT support immediate physician referral rather than waiting overnight or providing any massage in the moment. Still, I know that I responded proactively, thoughtfully, and with all of my resources at the time, and that my response may very well have saved the client's life.

Elizabeth Terhune
Westboro, MA

Here is one way to communicate the massage plan to the client:

There are some things in your health history that can increase the risk of blood clot formation in the legs. In massage therapy, we avoid disturbing the area until a client's doctor can advise us on that, even if there are no symptoms. For that reason, today I am going to avoid significant pressure and movement of your legs, and focus instead on the rest of your body, from your hips upward. It's a pretty cautious approach, but we find it's the best one. If you would like me to work some pressure back into the massage of your legs, I can tell you how we can include your doctor's input. Your doctor is the best one to look closely at your health history and answer my questions about blood clot risk, then advise us about massage. Today, one place we *can* use more pressure is the bottoms of

your feet, which are getting "massaged" as you walk. Would you like me to do that?

Most of the time, it is not possible to initiate a meaningful exchange about DVT before a client's first massage session—instead, a risk factor comes up during the interview, or later in the session. If this is the case, incorporate DVT Principle I into the massage plan for that session, or for the remaining time left in the session. If subsequent sessions are in the picture, you can initiate some form of medical consultation before the next one.

Because this is a one time session while you're here on vacation, I need to work gently in this area. If you were scheduled for a course of massage treatment, we could bring your doctor into the conversation. Right now, the goal should be to help you feel better, not worse. Today I should focus my pressure on some other areas, such as your shoulders, neck, and back, instead. How does that sound?

BOX 11-4 QUESTIONS ABOUT DVT RISK

1. Have any of your past or current health care providers expressed concern about your risk of blood clots? If so, what did they say?
2. Are any of the following things true for you (list risk factors)?
3. What is your age?
4. Do you have any cardiovascular conditions, or are you on any blood pressure or heart medications?
5. Do you have any of the following symptoms (list signs and symptoms of DVT)?
6. What is your activity level, day to day, or week to week?

If there is no mechanism for physician communication in your massage setting, DVT Principle I is a reasonable precaution, for the purpose of liability as well as safety. In many cases, this plan is well received because many people prefer attention to the back, shoulders, and neck area. If a client is disappointed in the massage plan defined by DVT Principle I, then he or she can take steps to include his or her physician's input in subsequent sessions.

Likewise, if a medical consultation about DVT does not produce the necessary level of communication, you can continue to follow DVT Principle I indefinitely. In "When My DVT Concern is Heard," online, a therapist tells about two cases of DVT risk, with different physician's responses, and differences in the resulting massage plans (See http://thePoint.lww.com/Walton).

There are medical situations that call for *indefinite* use of DVT Principle I, without attempting a medical consultation. If the client's risk of DVT seems significant, you can choose this cautious approach, regardless of input from the client's doctor. Examples include chronic immobility, a DVT history, CHF, or any other client presentation that poses a high risk, or a risk that does not go away. In this case, communicate your concern to the client, and develop creative, nonmechanical ways to address issues in the lower limbs: Gentle touch, energy techniques, and reflexive techniques may be welcome and appropriate.

The Massage Therapist's Role

Management of the various DVT presentations can be intimidating. The chance of provoking injury is small, but the grave consequences cause anxiety among massage therapists and students. You may feel uneasy, asking alarming medical questions and listing off risk factors to a client. It is natural to be concerned about overreacting to a client's symptom, then having it turn out to be something minor.

Keep in mind that it is not your responsibility, your set of skills, or your scope of practice to diagnose DVT correctly; it is only your responsibility to notice and respond to red flags, and figure out how and when to involve the client's doctor. Your task is similar to flagging a change in a skin lesion, one that could signal skin cancer. Massage therapists are not experts on skin cancer, or DVT. But each time you bring a possible health issue to your client's attention, you provide an important service, whether or not your concern is confirmed by later test results.

As described in "Inflammation, DVT, and Massage," online, many massage therapists have at least one story of a client referral that ended in the client receiving essential medical care. Even one DVT "pickup" story is worth a handful of false alarms.

The principles in this chapter share the common purpose of engaging the help of the client's physician, *placing the task of DVT assessment on the physician, not the massage therapist.* Help can come from the doctor or nurse in several forms: a medical workup, diagnosis and treatment, or a response to your concern about pressure in the area.

DVT is poorly understood and notoriously difficult to diagnose. In medicine, physicians use scoring systems of signs, symptoms, and risk factors to predict the likelihood of DVT in patients, and decide when to follow up with invasive, expensive tests and treatment (Scarvelis and Wells, 2006). There, too, practitioners do their best even though no set of guidelines or predictors is reliable (Oudega et al., 2005). In the end, a successful DVT diagnosis is a result of skill, experience, and sometimes good luck. Often, on the basis of a history and a physical examination, DVT is suspected, tests are ordered, and come back negative. In many of those cases, the cause of the symptoms is finally identified as muscle tension.

Clearly, current knowledge about DVT limits the ability of physicians to follow up, and better tools are needed for the day-to-day clinical scenarios they face. Massage therapists, with much less education and no reliable tools to guide referral, can be at a loss for what to do. But even without a perfect guideline for what to do, it is important to do *something.* Massage therapists bring several assets to the problem of undiagnosed DVT: prolonged contact with clients' tissues, hands that are sensitive to tissue changes, good referral skills, and intuition. Therapist's Journal 11-2 tells a story of a therapist's recognition of DVT symptoms, and her good judgment and intuition. Watch for red flags, ask questions, avoid high-risk areas when there is uncertainty, and work hard for a medical consultation or referral. If you are ever unsure of what to do, act conservatively.

The Shred of Doubt Principle. If there is a shred of doubt about whether a massage element is safe, it is contraindicated until its safety is established. When in doubt, don't.

● MASSAGE RESEARCH

As of this writing, there are no randomized, controlled trials, published in the English language, on DVT and massage indexed in PubMed or the Massage Therapy Foundation Research Database. The NIH RePORTER tool lists no active, federally funded research projects on this topic in the United States. No active projects are listed on the clinicaltrials.gov database (see Chapter 6).

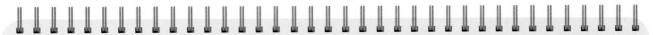

I've been a massage therapist for 13 years. For my first job after massage school, I worked in a chiropractic office, providing brief, focused massage to prepare patients for their chiropractic treatments. I worked for someone who supported massage therapy but did not fully understand the modality. (I have since worked in similar settings, but with more positive experiences.)

I had only been working for a few months when a 65-year-old man came in for help with his lower back and legs. When he got on the table, I noticed that one lower leg was swollen, there was some protrusion, and it was discolored. My boss instructed me to work very deeply on the area, telling me it was necessary to help the area heal. In general, that was often his approach to use with swelling, to order the massage therapist to use deep pressure and "flush it through." Yet, as I looked at this man's leg, every fiber of my being told me this could be a blood clot. I raised this concern to the client and to my boss, but both of them insisted I work the area using deep pressure. I was new to the work, and felt I had to do what I was told. My compromise was to massage the area, but at much gentler pressure than I was instructed to use.

I followed this approach for a few sessions, while continuing to urge the client to see his doctor. The condition persisted and he finally complied. Afterward he told me, "I did have a blood clot, and my doctor told me no way should I have had massage on it." The clot never came loose. He was treated successfully with blood thinners and continued to see me. Because of the blood thinners, I modified my overall pressure for his sessions, but I never used pressure on his legs again.

Do I have any advice for others? Intuition is one of our most important tools. If your intuition tells you something isn't quite right, be open to it and listen.

Seraphina Ashe
Corona, CA

● POSSIBLE MASSAGE BENEFITS

DVT is a stressful, frightening condition, and someone with a recent or past history of DVT can benefit from skilled touch. The focus of this chapter is on the potential harm of massage to someone with DVT. However, as already discussed, the more likely outcome is a referral for needed medical care.

Atherosclerosis

Atherosclerosis is a common condition of the arteries involving deposits of fatty plaque on the linings of the artery walls. These deposits are called **atherosclerotic plaque**.

● BACKGROUND

Atherosclerosis is the most common type of **arteriosclerosis**, a group of diseases characterized by thickening and loss of elasticity in artery walls. The terms atherosclerosis and arteriosclerosis are often used interchangeably. Deposits of plaque combine with other substances, such as cholesterol, cellular waste products, and calcium, thickening of the artery wall, and narrowing of the opening of the artery (Figure 11-8).

Signs and Symptoms

Atherosclerosis can be clinically silent for decades. Signs and symptoms do not usually become noticeable until there are complications.

Complications

There are three main complications of atherosclerosis:

1. *Stenosis.* When plaques partially or completely block an artery, the narrowing is known as **stenosis**. Significant stenosis results in ischemia and symptoms in the area. If the artery is fully occluded, tissue death can result from oxygen starvation. System-wide narrowing of vessels contributes to hypertension (this chapter).

2. *Thrombosis.* If a plaque ruptures, it can lead to rapid thrombus formation in the artery, or **arterial thrombosis**. Large clots can obstruct blood flow, producing ischemia. Like venous clots, detached clots can also do damage, but not specifically in the lungs. In a process called **arterial thromboembolism**, the thrombus detaches from where it formed, then moves downstream through smaller arteries and arterioles, eventually blocking a smaller vessel and causing ischemia in the tissues supplied by that vessel. Figure 11-9 shows where arterial clots can travel and occlude vessels, after being dislodged from an artery, or even from the heart.

3. *Aneurysm.* Atherosclerosis weakens arteries over time. A weak spot in an artery wall can bulge outward in an **aneurysm** (see Conditions in Brief, this chapter). The bulge can rupture, causing bleeding into the surrounding tissue. Even if it doesn't rupture, an aneurysm can cause problems. An intact aneurysm is a site of blood pooling, and sluggish blood flow in the pocket of pooled blood can give rise to arterial clots, which can embolize.

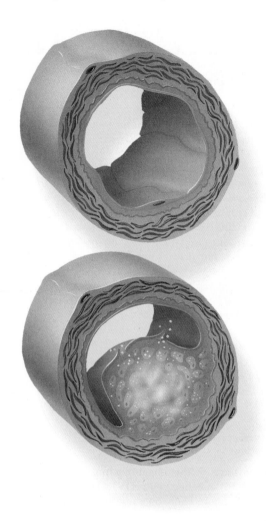

FIGURE 11-8. Atherosclerosis. The vessel above is normal; the vessel below shows formation of atherosclerotic plaque.

Wherever atherosclerosis forms, stenosis, thrombosis, and aneurysm can develop. Complications of these three factors play out in these areas of the body:

- *Cerebral artery disease.* In the arteries of the brain, atherosclerosis can lead to a stroke (see Chapter 10).
- *Heart disease.* In the arteries of the heart, atherosclerosis can cause a heart attack, or a less severe condition called angina (see "Heart Disease [Coronary Artery Disease]"; see Angina pectoris, Conditions in Brief).
- *Atherosclerotic renal artery disease.* In the kidneys, atherosclerosis can narrow arteries and occlude blood flow, impairing kidney function (see "Chronic Kidney Failure," Chapter 18).
- *Intestinal ischemic syndrome.* In the mesenteric arteries, atherosclerosis can occlude blood flow to the intestines and lead to tissue death.
- *Peripheral artery disease.* In the arteries of the extremities, atherosclerosis can cause aneurysm, often in the popliteal or iliofemoral artery. If deposits occlude vessels in the lower limbs, it can lead to **claudication**, or pain when walking, as well as other problems (see Peripheral Vascular Disease, Conditions in Brief).
- *Aortic aneurysm.* Atherosclerosis can weaken the walls of the abdominal or thoracic aorta, causing aneurysms to form (see Aneurysm, Conditions in Brief).

Treatment

Many early cases of atherosclerosis are *subclinical*, meaning they do not produce symptoms. There is no obvious reason to start treatment at that point. Once complications arise, the emphasis of treatment is on managing the complications.

Atherosclerosis is difficult to reverse; however, some treatments are focused on slowing its progression. Dietary changes and increased exercise can help. So can cholesterol-lowering drugs, BP medications, and antiplatelet medications such as aspirin.

Cholesterol-lowering drugs called **statins** are most commonly prescribed if lifestyle changes don't succeed in lowering cholesterol to healthy levels. Statins do not usually have strong side effects, although some can cause constipation (Wible, 2005). Antiplatelet drugs and blood pressure medications are used, with a range of side effects (see Tables 11-1 and 11-3).

One treatment for a narrowed vessel is **angioplasty**, the insertion of a balloon into the vessel. The balloon is inflated and the vessel is stretched. Angioplasty may be followed by the insertion of a **stent**, a metal spring or mesh-like tube that holds open a vessel so that blood can pass through freely. The stent may be coated with medication that prevents scar tissue from forming at the site. Another surgical procedure is **endarterectomy**, in which plaques are shaved off, collected, and removed. **Bypass surgery** may be done, in which another vessel is grafted in to allow blood to bypass the blocked artery. These procedures have a high success rate, but complications of some procedures include re-stenosis (narrowing) of the vessels, arterial thrombosis, and stroke.

● INTERVIEW QUESTIONS

1. How and when was atherosclerosis diagnosed?
2. Have there been any complications? Are there any effects on your heart, brain, kidneys, digestion, or legs?
3. Do you have any history of heart attack or stroke?
4. Do you have any history of blood clots?
5. How is your atherosclerosis being treated? Have there been any changes in diet, activity, medications, or surgery?
6. How does treatment affect you?

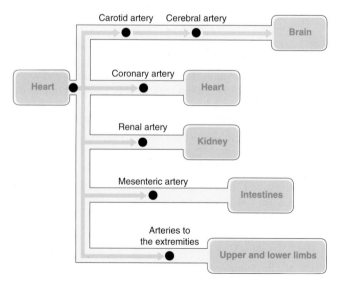

FIGURE 11-9. Organs and tissues affected in arterial thromboembolism.

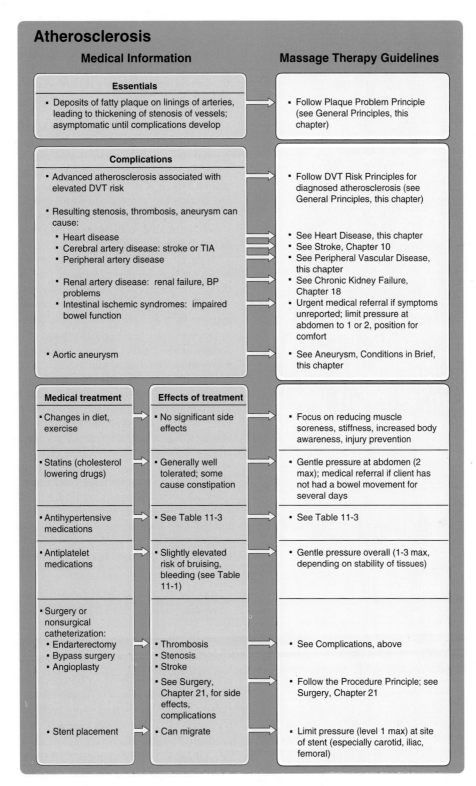

FIGURE 11-10. A Decision Tree for atherosclerosis.

● MASSAGE THERAPY GUIDELINES

Because atherosclerosis can create an environment for blood clots, there are massage adjustments to be aware of, but the issues are slightly different from venous clots. First, massage therapists take care to avoid rupturing atherosclerotic plaques so that they do not create a favorable environment for throm-

bus formation. Second, therapists avoid undue pressure on any accessible arteries in case clots have already formed there.

Most arterial plaques are too deep for the massage therapist to reach, but some may occur in superficial arteries. For this reason, limit pressure to level 1 or 2 on **arterial pulse points**, where the arterial pulse can be felt (Figure 11-11). In massage therapy, these are considered *vascular endangerment sites*,

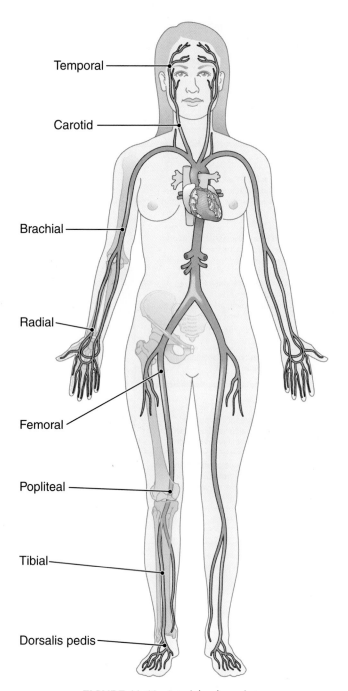

Temporal

Carotid

Brachial

Radial

Femoral

Popliteal

Tibial

Dorsalis pedis

FIGURE 11-11. Arterial pulse points.

where arteries are accessible to massage pressure. Too much focused pressure, especially while pinning the tissues to the surrounding bone, could injure plaques at these sites. Or, if a clot is already present in a carotid or femoral artery, the mechanical stress placed on the structure could dislodge it. Even a clot formed in an abdominal aortic aneurysm is theoretically accessible to direct pressure, and invasive massage techniques are contraindicated. This is the Plaque Problem Principle.

The Plaque Problem Principle. If atherosclerosis is identified, or is likely to be present, use cautious pressure and joint movement at all arterial pulse points. In particular, limit pressure to level 1 at or near the carotid arteries.

This principle is based on theory, not research evidence. Still, it is an easy enough principle to follow, and should be observed for all clients with atherosclerosis, regardless of their answers to the interview questions. It highlights the hazard at the carotid artery, where a dislodged clot could continue on to cause a stroke. Most massage techniques are designed to avoid these hazards.

At the time of this writing, there is little information in the medical literature about the ability of massage to dislodge an arterial clot. One physician, reassuring a concerned consumer, stated that neck massage is unlikely to move or injure arterial plaque, which is strongly attached (Lee, 2008). However, the article failed to address clot formation at the site of a plaque. A clot formed at such a site can be much less stable, and caution is warranted until more information about risk emerges in the literature.

If the client's doctor agrees that deeper pressure is safe at the neck, you may be able to increase the pressure to level 3, but do not use focused, fingertip pressure, and do not linger. Neck work should be gentle at this site, anyway, because of reflex changes in blood pressure that can occur when the **carotid sinus**, located at the branching point of each carotid artery, is pressed. Pressure that is too deep can bring about a drop in BP, followed by dizziness or fainting. For all of these reasons, pressure should be cautious at the lateral/anterior neck.

Another massage adjustment may be broadly applied in atherosclerosis: the DVT Risk Principles. Even though arterial clots and venous clots are in separate vessels, research has emerged that shows an association between atherosclerosis and formation of clots in the veins (Prandoni et al., 2003). Whether one problem contributes to the other, or whether they merely share risk factors, is unclear. Although diagnosed atherosclerosis argues for the DVT Risk Principles, if the client has made reasonable lifestyle changes resulting in limited need for atherosclerosis medications, it may be safe to resume pressure and joint movement on the lower extremities. On this point, guidance is needed from the client's doctor.

The CV Conditions Often "Run in Packs" Principle. If one cardiovascular condition is present, be alert for others.

Questions 1–4 help you evaluate how strong the effects of atherosclerosis have been in the client, and whether there are other CV conditions to be concerned about. Usually by the time atherosclerosis is diagnosed, there is something else present, because atherosclerosis is clinically silent until complications make themselves known. If heart or kidney function is affected by atherosclerosis, follow the Vital Organ Principle (see Chapter 3). See Chapter 10 if the client has a stroke or TIA history. For blood clots or a heart attack history, refer to the relevant sections in this chapter ("Deep Vein Thrombosis," "Heart Disease [Coronary Artery Disease]"). If the intestines are affected, the client could be experiencing nausea, vomiting, acute abdominal pain (worse after eating), weight loss, and blood in the stool. If these symptoms have not been reported to the physician, an immediate medical referral is in order. If you see a client who has been treated and is stabilizing, limit pressure at the abdomen to levels 1 and 2. Position for client comfort; the prone position is likely to be uncomfortable. If the client's atherosclerosis affects blood flow to the lower

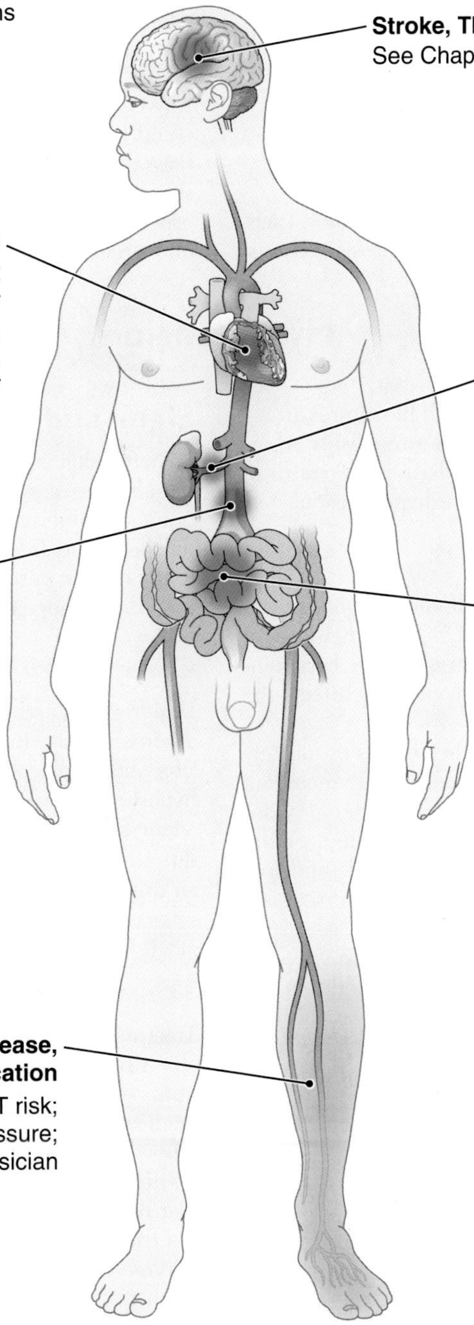

For all atherosclerosis
Follow Plaque Problem Principle; consider DVT Risk Principles; adapt to antihypertensives, cholesterol lowering drugs, antiplatelet or anticoagulant medications

Stroke, TIA
See Chapter 10

Heart disease
Adjust intent; consult physician; consider DVT risk, also see Angina, Congestive heart failure, this chapter

Renal artery stenosis
Adjust intent (see Chronic Kidney Failure, Chapter 18)

Aortic aneurysm
Adjust pressure at site; cautious use of abdominal supports

Intestinal ischemic disease
Possible medical referral; adjust position and pressure

Peripheral artery disease, intermittent claudication
Consider DVT risk; adjust pressure; consult physician

FIGURE 11-12. Atherosclerosis: Selected clinical features and massage adjustments to consider. Specific instructions and additional massage therapy guidelines are in Decision Tree and text.

extremities, you may need to modify pressure there, and communicate with the client's doctor. The DVT Principle I is advised, indefinitely (see Peripheral vascular disease, Conditions in Brief). Complications of atherosclerosis, along with massage therapy guidelines, are summarized in Figure 11-12.

Adjust massage to any medications: if there is easy bruising or bleeding, overall pressure should be in the 1–3 range, and is dependent on tissue stability. Usually aspirin is not much cause

for concern, but anticoagulants are. Side effects of medications used against blood clots are shown in Table 11-1.

For any recent surgical procedure, see "Surgery," Chapter 21. Adapt to any complications of surgical procedures, which in this case, are complications of atherosclerosis, itself (thrombosis, stenosis, and stroke). The various surgical procedures, from stretching of vessels to removal of plaque, provide management but not cure. Because surgical treatments do not change the underlying systemic condition, massage adjustments for the atherosclerosis are still in force. If a stent was inserted, find out where it is. Most stents are not easily disturbed by massage therapy because they are placed in deep vessels, but find out about any superficial or accessible stents in the iliac, femoral, or carotid arteries. Avoid any pressure that could displace these stents from their sites: level 1 is safest. There is at least one account in the medical literature that attributes stent migration to deep tissue massage (Haskal, 2008).

● MASSAGE RESEARCH

As of this writing, there are no randomized, controlled trials, published in the English language, on atherosclerosis and mas-

sage indexed in PubMed or the Massage Therapy Foundation Research Database. The NIH RePORTER tool lists no active, federally funded research projects on this topic in the United States. No active projects are listed on the clinicaltrials.gov database (see Chapter 6).

● POSSIBLE MASSAGE BENEFITS

Any complication of atherosclerosis is stressful, and massage could help manage that stress. By relaxing skeletal muscles, massage may also support movement and exercise, which is strongly encouraged for those who are able. Massage could be especially helpful to a client who wants to add more movement or exercise to a regular routine.

Hypertension

Hypertension is persistent, sustained high blood pressure—above-normal pressure of the blood against artery walls. A systolic blood pressure of 140 mm Hg, a diastolic pressure of 90 mm Hg or more, or both is classified as hypertension.

● BACKGROUND

In hypertension, excessive pressure results from a greater volume of blood pushing through the vessels, from the tightness of the vessel walls, or from both. Although pulmonary hypertension can also occur, hypertension more commonly affects the systemic arteries.

The regulation of blood pressure in the body is exquisitely refined. The body has several ways of raising BP, including increased frequency of cardiac contractions, arterial vasoconstriction, emptying blood from the venous system or the spleen into the systemic circulation, or decreased fluid loss from the blood from filtration by the kidneys. In reverse, each of these mechanisms can lower the BP.

About 10–15% of people with hypertension have **secondary hypertension**, which is caused by another condition. Of those, most have a problem with kidney function, as the kidneys are pivotal in regulating blood pressure. About 85%, have **essential hypertension**, for which there is no identifiable cause. This section will focus on the most common condition, essential hypertension.

Three levels of hypertension are classified according to blood pressure readings: pre-hypertension, stage 1, and stage 2. These categories are shown in Table 11-2.

The specific causes of hypertension are still being studied, but there are clear risk factors, such as a high-fat and high-salt diet, smoking, obesity, lack of exercise, stress, age, and family history, that play a role. Some of these risk factors, such as smoking, exercise, and diet, are *modifiable risk factors*. Others, such as age and family history, are not modifiable.

Atherosclerosis is a risk factor for hypertension because partially hardened arteries have lost elasticity and cannot adequately dilate when blood presses against the walls. This absence of "give" in the vessels increases the blood pressure. (Note that atherosclerosis seems to be both a cause and an effect of hypertension, supporting the principle that cardiovascular conditions often "run in packs.") Hypertension is a more serious concern when other conditions are present, such as diabetes, kidney problems, or peripheral vascular disease.

Signs and Symptoms

Hypertension is sometimes called the "silent killer" because of the absence of symptoms until complications affect the heart, brain, or kidneys. A few symptoms of hypertension—dizziness, dull headache, frequent nosebleeds—may appear in early stages of the disease in some people, but in most people, these symptoms do not appear until the disease is considerably advanced.

Complications

Hypertension stresses arterial walls over time, increasing atherosclerosis. In arteries supplying organs, both hypertension and atherosclerosis place stress on these organs. In fact, hypertension can cause heart failure or heart attack, stroke, aneurysm, and kidney damage. Even vision can be affected due to **retinopathy**, changes in the retina of the eye. Once an organ is damaged by hypertension, the situation is hard to reverse.

Treatment

Treatments for hypertension include modifying the modifiable risk factors, and taking blood pressure-lowering medications, called **antihypertensives**. Many people take multiple medications for blood pressure. **Diuretics**, also called "water pills," help the body shed excess fluid through the urine, and **β-blockers** inhibit impulses in the sympathetic nervous system that raise BP. If these drugs are not effective enough, others are tried, including **ACE inhibitors** (angiotensin-converting enzyme inhibitors), **angiotensin II receptor blockers, calcium channel blockers,** and **vasodilators**. Through different mechanisms, these drugs cause blood vessels to relax and lower BP. ACE inhibitors and angiotensin II receptor blockers are often used to control BP in people with heart disease, heart failure, and kidney failure. Calcium channel blockers decrease cardiac output and relax blood vessels. Table 11-3 summarizes these medications: the mechanisms of action, selected side effects, and massage therapy guidelines.

● INTERVIEW QUESTIONS

1. When were you diagnosed with high blood pressure?
2. What is your usual blood pressure reading?
3. Is your blood pressure stable and well controlled, or do you have trouble controlling it?

TABLE 11-2.	CLASSIFICATION OF BLOOD PRESSURE LEVELS[a]		
Classification	Systolic	Diastolic	Usual medical follow-up and management
Normal	<120	<80	None. Recheck every 2 years
Prehypertension	120–139	80–89	Lifestyle advice provided, recheck BP in a year
Stage 1 (Mild)	140–159	90–99	Recheck in 1 month to confirm, lifestyle advice provided; if BP levels do not drop after 6 months, low doses of antihypertensive medication prescribed, usually beginning with diuretic.
Stage 2 (Moderate To Severe)	160+	100+	Reevaluate within 1 month and refer for care; two drugs usually used, such as diuretic combined with a β-blocker, ACE inhibitor, or angiotensin II receptor blocker; a calcium channel blocker may be combined with an ACE inhibitor or angiotensin II receptor blocker.

[a]Severe high blood pressure is classified as anything over 180/110.

4. How often do you see your doctor about it? How recently?
5. Do you have any complications of hypertension, such as effects on your heart?
6. Do you have a history of stroke or "mini-stroke" (TIA, or transient ischemic attack)?
7. Do you have any swelling?
8. Do you ever experience headaches, vision changes, or fainting? If so, are these thought to be related to hypertension?
9. Have you had any other CV conditions such as varicose veins, blood clots, peripheral vascular disease, or atherosclerosis?
10. Any other conditions such as diabetes or kidney problems?
11. Do you take medication for it? What is the name?
12. How does the BP medication affect you?

● MASSAGE THERAPY GUIDELINES

In any case of hypertension, medium or deep pressure (level 3 or above) is contraindicated in the abdomen, to avoid triggering the vasovagal reaction, a reflexive slowing of the heart rate (bradycardia) and dilation of vessels in the legs. The reflex can be elicited in some individuals by direct pressure in the abdomen, a full bowel, straining in the bathroom, or even by a restrictive waistband. The resulting drop in blood available to the brain, dizziness, and faintness can lead to vasovagal syncope, a fainting episode. Direct work on the psoas muscles at these pressure levels is contraindicated in clients with hypertension, even if there is good BP control. You might want to reconsider bolstering the abdomen when the client is prone.

Because atherosclerosis is likely to be part of the picture along with hypertension, a universal massage guideline for hypertension is to follow the Plaque Problem Principle. Avoid pressure on arterial pulse points, especially the carotid arteries.

The first interview question tells you how long the client has known he or she has high BP, and therefore how familiar he or she might be with the condition and its treatment. Refer to Table 11-2 to consider the client's usual BP readings. If his hypertension is classified as stage 1 or 2, a certain amount of atherosclerosis is also likely; review the corresponding massage therapy guidelines (see "Atherosclerosis," this chapter).

A client whose BP is well monitored, stable, and controlled by medication is more tolerant of massage stimulation than a client whose BP is poorly controlled or monitored, or for whom the medicine is not effective. In the latter case, if the client's hypertension is at Stage 1 or 2 levels, slower speeds, even rhythms, and gradual transitions are best, to avoid sympathetic activity and increasing blood pressure.

For pre-hypertension and Stage 1, ask more questions to decide whether to follow the DVT Risk Principles. Ask about other DVT risk factors; note changes in risk factors when working with a client over time. For example, if a client with Stage 1 hypertension presents with an additional DVT risk factor such as smoking, advanced age (over 60), oral contraceptives, or a recent, extended period of bed rest, apply the two DVT Risk Principles.

The DVT risk is more clear-cut in Stage 2 hypertension. The best approach is to follow the DVT Risk Principles universally. This is especially important if there are complications of hypertension, or if the client has coexisting conditions such as diabetes, kidney problems, or peripheral vascular disease (Questions 9 and 10).

The answers to Questions 5–7 indicate whether the client's complications from hypertension are significant. Adapt your massage to the complication. If swelling is a complication of hypertension, avoid general circulatory intent. For coronary artery disease and heart attack history, review the heart disease section in this chapter. For stroke history or threat, see Chapter 10. If the client's kidney function is affected, see "Chronic Kidney Failure," Chapter 18. If the client has had an aneurysm at any site, including the aorta, see Aneurysm, Conditions in Brief.

Question 8 is aimed at any symptoms that suggest it is at dangerous levels or that BP is rising too fast. If these symptoms (headache, vision changes, or fainting) are occurring, even if they have been addressed by a physician, know that they could be a sign of unstable or dangerous hypertension and make an immediate medical referral.

Question 9 is asked to catch any other CV conditions that were missed by earlier questions, and Question 10 looks at other associated conditions. Follow the DVT Risk Principles if any of these emerge. Also refer to the appropriate chapters in this text, or sections in this chapter.

In the absence of clear symptoms, it is hard to guess at the complications of hypertension. It is not always clear whether to assume other things are going wrong, and how conservative your approach should be. This is especially challenging when working in high-volume, fast-turnaround, and low-documentation settings, such as spas and vacation settings. If you work

TABLE 11-3.	DRUGS FOR HYPERTENSION AND RELATED CONDITIONS[a]

β-Blockers

Uses	Hypertension, CHF, arrhythmia, angina, prevention of future heart attack in heart attack patients
How They Work	By blocking the effects of epinephrine (adrenaline), slowing nerve impulses through the heart, relaxing heart muscle
Selected Generic (Trade) Names	Acebutolol (Sectral), atenolol (Tenormin), propanolol (Inderal)

Selected Side Effects, Massage Therapy Guidelines	
• Hypotension, drowsiness, dizziness, weakness, fatigue	• Gentle session overall; reposition gently, slow speed and even rhythm, slow rise from table, gradual transition at end of session
• Depression	• Medical referral if unreported (see "Depression," Chapter 10)
• Insomnia	• When appropriate, use sedative intent at end of day, activating or stimulating intent at beginning
• Cold hands and feet	• No massage adjustments; drape for warmth

Diuretics

Uses	Hypertension, CHF
How They Work	By increasing movement of salt, water from blood to urine
Selected Generic (Trade) Names	furosemide (Lasix), hydrochlorothiazide (Esidrix, Hydrodiuril), amiloride (Midamar), spironolactone (Aldactone)

Selected Side Effects, Massage Therapy Guidelines	
• Dizziness, lightheadedness, weakness	• Reposition gently, slow speed and even rhythm, slow rise from table, gentle transition at end of session
• Urinary frequency	• Easy bathroom access; schedule session away from time of peak effect of medication
• Diarrhea	• Easy bathroom access; gentle session overall; avoid contact or pressure at abdomen that could aggravate
• Muscle cramps	• See "Cramp," Conditions in Brief, Chapter 8

ACE Inhibitors

Uses	Hypertension, CHF, post heart attack to prevent further heart muscle damage
How They Work	Interfere with enzyme responsible for vasoconstriction; lower salt and water content of body
Selected Generic (Trade) Names	Ramipril (Altace), fosinopril (Monopril), quinapril (Accupril), benazepril (Lotensin)

Selected Side Effects, Massage Therapy Guidelines	
• Dizziness, lightheadedness, fainting, fatigue, orthostatic hypotension	• Reposition gently, slow speed and even rhythm, slow rise from table, gentle transition at end of session
• Numbness, tingling in hands, feet	• Lighter pressure and joint movement at site, depending on significance of sensation loss (usually mild), keep hand contact full and firm
• Dry cough	• No massage adjustments
• Joint pain	• Position for comfort, limit joint movement

Angiotensin II Receptor Blockers

Uses	Hypertension
How They Work	Block the action of an enzyme (angiotensin II), a natural chemical that constricts vessels.
Selected Generic (Trade) Names	Candesartan (Atacand), valsartan (Diovan), irbesartan (Avapro), telmisartan (Micardis)

Selected Side Efects, Massage Therapy Guidelines	
• Orthostatic hypotension, dizziness	• Reposition gently, slow speed and even rhythm, slow rise from table, gentle transition at end of session
• Headache	• Position for comfort, especially prone; consider inclined table or propping; gentle session overall; pressure to tolerance; slow speed and even rhythm; general circulatory intent may be poorly tolerated

(continued)

TABLE 11-3.	DRUGS FOR HYPERTENSION AND RELATED CONDITIONS*a* (Continued)
	• Stomach upset, heartburn	• Adjust position for comfort; use gentle pressure at site
	• Diarrhea	• Easy bathroom access; gentle session overall; avoid contact or pressure at abdomen that could aggravate
	• Back pain, leg pain	• No massage adjustments
	• Nasal congestion	• Position for comfort

Calcium Channel Blockers

Uses	Hypertension, angina, arrhythmia
How They Work	Slow rate of calcium flow into vessel walls, heart muscle, relaxing vessels
Selected Generic (Trade) Names	diltiazem (Cardizem, Dilacor XR, Syn-Diltiazem, Tiazac), amlodipine (Norvasc), nifedipine (Procardia), nicardipine (Cardene), verapimil (Isoptin)
Selected Side Effects, Massage Therapy Guidelines	• Orthostatic hypotension, dizziness, fatigue — • Reposition gently, slow speed and even rhythm, slow rise from table, gentle transition at end of session
	• Headache — • Position for comfort, especially prone; consider inclined table or propping; gentle session overall; pressure to tolerance; slow speed and even rhythm; general circulatory intent may be poorly tolerated
	• Swelling of abdomen, ankles, feet — • Avoid circulatory intent at site; avoid general circulatory intent
	• Heartburn — • Adjust position for comfort; use gentle pressure at site
	• Flushing — • No massage adjustment

Vasodilators

Uses	Hypertension
How They Work	Dilate vessels
Selected Generic (Trade) Names	Hydralazine (Apresoline), minoxidil (Loniten)
Selected Side Effects, Massage Therapy Guidelines	• Headache — • Position for comfort, especially prone; consider inclined table or propping; gentle session overall; pressure to tolerance; slow speed and even rhythm; avoid headache trigger; general circulatory intent may be poorly tolerated
	• Fluid retention — • Avoid circulatory intent at site; avoid general circulatory intent
	• Joint pain — • Limit joint movement
	• Rapid heartbeat — • See "Arrhythmia," this chapter

aNot all medications are included in this table, nor all side effects of each. Not all drugs in a class cause all side effects.

in such a setting, you will want to practice more conservatively than if you can document, ask lots of questions, and consult the client's physician. Without the time to investigate and document, it's safest to plan as though additional issues are present, and implement the Plaque Problem Principle and the two DVT Risk Principles. This extra level of caution is appropriate where follow-up and continuity of care are not possible.

The Massage Setting/Continuity of Care Principle. In massage settings favoring single-time rather than repeat clients, lacking continuity of care, or using little or no documentation, therapists should take a cautious approach to medical conditions.

Questions 11 and 12 probe for side effects of antihypertensive drugs, since these medications can have strong effects

on the body (see Table 11-3). In fact, many BP medications "overcorrect," producing *hypo*tension. If the client experiences low blood pressure in general, or while standing up, called orthostatic hypotension, then symptoms of dizziness and faintness may result, and there is a risk of falling. This problem can be averted in two ways: by ending the session with slightly more stimulating speeds and rhythms, to prepare the client for activity (Wible, 2005), or by facilitating a gradual rise from the table, including sitting for several minutes. This approach is also a good idea for clients complaining of dizziness, weakness, and fatigue.

If the client is taking a diuretic, frequent and urgent urination can be an issue. Easy bathroom access and sensible scheduling of the massage, after the peak effect of the medication, can help prevent interruptions. If swelling is a side effect, as in calcium channel blockers, then avoid circulatory intent at the site of swelling, and avoid general circulatory intent.

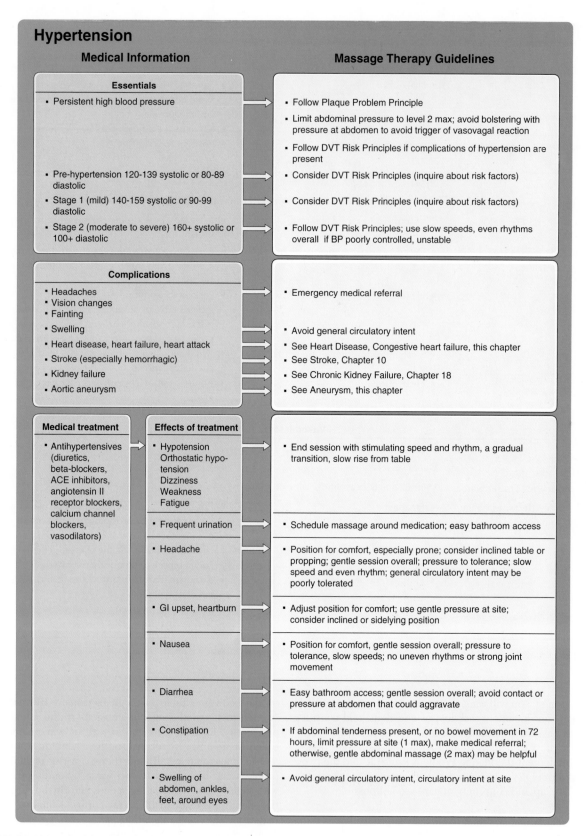

FIGURE 11-13. A Decision Tree for hypertension. Selected side effects of antihypertensives are shown; not all medications and side effects are included. Not all antihypertensive medications cause all side effects.

You may need to work around other side effects, such as headache or GI problems (nausea, diarrhea, constipation). See the Decision Tree (Figure 11-13) for additional selected side effects, and Table 11-3. If the client is experiencing side effects that are not mentioned in this chapter, see Table 21-1.

● MASSAGE RESEARCH

Blood pressure is one indicator of stress, and it is measured in a range of client populations in massage research. Drops in blood pressure are frequently claimed as benefits of massage; however, the evidence on massage and blood pressure is mixed. Even if massage causes a brief drop in BP, the effect does not necessarily translate to a sustained effect in people with hypertension.

In a large study of 263 volunteers with muscle spasm and muscle strain, researchers looked at BP and heart rate (Kaye et al., 2008). This study included subjects with normal BP as well as hypertension. The study suggested that deep tissue massage lowered BP and heart rate. Although the sample size is impressive, there was no control group, so it is impossible to tell whether the outcomes were a true effect of massage.

Other small pilot studies have looked at BP in hypertensive subjects (Olney, 2005) and in healthy volunteers (Ejindu, 2007). Both found some reductions in BP associated with massage, but the studies are too small to provide firm conclusions. In a larger study of aromatherapy massage in 58 menopausal women, the active treatment was associated with declines in blood pressure (Hur et al., 2007). But in another RCT, with 60 nurses serving as subjects, 15 minutes of back massage each week for 5 weeks failed to result in a drop in blood pressure (Bost and Wallis, 2006).

Two other studies have compared different massage protocols and blood pressure. In one, authors reported that massage of the back, neck, and chest might be more effective at reducing BP than massage of the extremities and face (Aourell et al., 2005). And in a large study of 150 clients at a student clinic, researchers reported small reductions in blood pressure after massage, using pre-post measurements (Cambron et al., 2006). In the student clinic study, there was no link found between BP change and massage duration, pressure used, sites massaged, or the experience level of the student therapist. Researchers saw little change when Swedish, deep tissue, myofascial release techniques, or cranial-sacral techniques were used. However, they did find that trigger point and sports massage techniques were associated with a BP *increase*.

The study of massage and blood pressure is still in its early stages. Even though BP reduction is a frequently claimed benefit of massage, there is not yet a foundation of research evidence in support of it.

● POSSIBLE MASSAGE BENEFITS

Individuals with hypertension are often instructed to work with modifiable risk factors in order to lower blood pressure. These include weight loss and increased exercise. If massage therapy reduces muscle tension and enhances body awareness, clients might benefit from fewer injuries and be able to maintain a consistent exercise program. Massage may also provide emotional support for the endeavor.

The overall relaxation provided by massage is well-recognized, and the potential for massage to relieve stress may have an effect on blood pressure. Time (and more research) will tell.

Heart Disease (Coronary Artery Disease)

Heart disease is an umbrella term that includes any disease of the heart walls, valves, muscle, or conduction system. Heart disease takes many forms and has many causes, but the most common is **Coronary artery disease (CAD)**, also known as *Coronary heart disease*. This form of heart disease is the focus of this section.

● BACKGROUND

CAD is the presence of atherosclerosis in the arteries that supply the heart (see "Atherosclerosis," this chapter). In CAD, changes to the vessel walls over time compromise the coronary arteries, occluding them and rendering them vulnerable to clot formation, or, less commonly, to aneurysm. Hypertension puts additional stress on the heart, forcing it to work harder against the resistance of peripheral vessels. Hypertension also narrows vessels to the heart itself.

Signs and Symptoms

Like many other cardiovascular conditions, CAD is often clinically silent until it is far enough along to produce complications. It is usually diagnosed when the symptoms of complications are present and is difficult to diagnose otherwise. Routine screening for heart disease is limited to looking for risk factors such as family history, smoking, poor diet, excess

weight, alcohol intake, and inactivity. It also includes blood tests for cholesterol and diabetes.

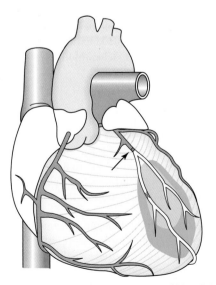

FIGURE 11-14. Heart attack. Interruption of blood flow to cardiac muscle leads to ischemia and death of cardiac muscle tissue (shaded area).

Complications

Complications of CAD include angina (see Conditions in Brief) and heart attack, in which parts of the heart muscle become ischemic, then die from lack of oxygen (Figure 11-14). The medical name for a heart attack is myocardial infarction: the heart muscle sustains an infarct, or death of tissue due to a sudden, acute interruption in blood flow.

Pain in the chest is considered the classic symptom of heart attack, but this pain can also extend to the jaw, back, abdomen, shoulder, and arm. In fact, if pain in the upper abdomen is prolonged, it can signal a heart attack; unfortunately, if it is burning pain, it can easily be mistaken for indigestion, especially in older individuals. A heart attack can also be felt as crushing pressure, squeezing, or feeling of fullness in the chest. Women are slightly more likely than men to experience other symptoms, such as nausea, jaw pain, or back pain.

Other general symptoms of a heart attack are shortness of breath, palpitations, lightheadedness, weakness, confusion, and nausea and vomiting. Some individuals feel a sense of doom; some faint and become unconscious. Many heart attacks occur within a few hours after rising in the morning, although they can occur at any time of day or night.

Sometimes a heart attack is asymptomatic, and goes unnoticed. Approximately 25% of heart attack cases present this way, and these are particularly common in individuals who also have diabetes mellitus.

The severity of a heart attack depends on the amount of damage to the heart muscle, walls, valves, and conduction system. Irregular heartbeat, or arrhythmia, can develop if so much muscle tissue dies that the electrical conduction system "short-circuits." One common arrhythmia that can accompany a heart attack is ventricular fibrillation, in which the contractions of the ventricles become uncoordinated. This common complication can compromise blood flow to the brain, causing death from a heart attack when the individual cannot make it to a hospital in time for treatment.

In severe heart attacks, heart walls and valves may be damaged. In general, an aneurysm in the heart walls, rupture of the heart walls, or damage to the tissues supporting the heart valves are serious complications, compromising its function of pumping blood. These conditions can be severely debilitating or fatal. Heart failure is tissue damage that makes it impossible for the heart to pump blood to meet the body's demands. It can develop into congestive heart failure (see Conditions in Brief, this chapter).

Treatment

Because atherosclerosis has affected the coronary arteries, a person with CAD is treated for atherosclerosis. Various methods of slowing the progression of atherosclerosis, changing lifestyle risk factors that contribute to it, medications to lower cholesterol and widen the arteries (see Table 11-3), and medications to reduce clot formation in the arteries are involved (see Table 11-1).

Often, before treatment begins, an important diagnostic test is performed via cardiac catheterization. In this procedure, a thin catheter is inserted, usually through a small incision in the groin, up through the aorta to the point where the coronary arteries branch. A dye is injected at that point, and its progression through the coronary arteries is followed via X-ray, a process called coronary angiography or *coronary arteriography*. In this procedure, it is possible to see if vessels are occluded, and it takes 1–2 hours to perform.

If this test suggests a problem, or the person has had a heart attack, *coronary artery angioplasty* may be performed. This may be done at the time of the catheterization. The angioplasty procedure is called percutaneous transluminal coronary angioplasty (PTCA). In PTCA, the insertion of a catheter through a vein in the groin or arm, and dye injection is followed by the insertion of a balloon to widen the blocked vessel. A stent may be placed to keep the vessel open.

Some individuals undergo a more invasive procedure, *coronary artery bypass surgery*, in which surgeons use a vein from another part of the body to fashion a vessel that substitutes for the diseased coronary artery. The vessel graft usually comes from a saphenous vein, a mammary artery, or even a radial artery. This is major surgery, which requires an inpatient stay in intensive care.

Emergency treatment for a heart attack includes administering aspirin to prevent blood clot formation, oxygen, pain medications, β-blockers to diminish the sympathetic nervous system's tendency to raise blood pressure, and possibly nitroglycerin, a drug used to quickly dilate the blood vessels. Long-term treatment of heart attacks focuses on eliminating arterial clots, widening arteries to the heart, lowering blood pressure so that the heart doesn't have to work as hard, and making it pump more efficiently. To these ends, anticoagulants, antiplatelet drugs, and antihypertensive medications are used (see Tables 11-1 and 11-3).

The primary treatment goal is restoring blood flow to the heart. This can be done chemically, with medications such as thrombolytics, or mechanically, with angioplasty.

A program of cardiac rehabilitation consists of education, emotional support, ongoing medications, and support for lifestyle changes. To the extent possible, cardiovascular exercise and strengthening exercises are carried out in a supervised setting; the heart is healed and strengthened so that the patient can be as active as possible. The first phase of cardiac rehabilitation typically begins in the hospital, and a second phase of classes continues, with careful monitoring, for 12 weeks after discharge. A third phase, a maintenance program, is designed for those who are stable and independent after completing the second phase.

● INTERVIEW QUESTIONS

1. When were you diagnosed with heart disease? What prompted the diagnosis?
2. Have there been any complications, such as angina or heart attack?
3. If you have experienced a heart attack, please tell me more about it:

   - When did it occur? How severe was it?
   - Were there any complications, such as effects on other organs or tissues, heart failure, or other functions?
   - How was it treated? Have you gone through a cardiac rehabilitation program? If so, please describe it.

4. Do you have any other cardiovascular conditions?
5. Are your doctors concerned about how well your heart pumps?
6. Are there any medical restrictions on your activity?
7. What is your activity level, day to day or week to week?

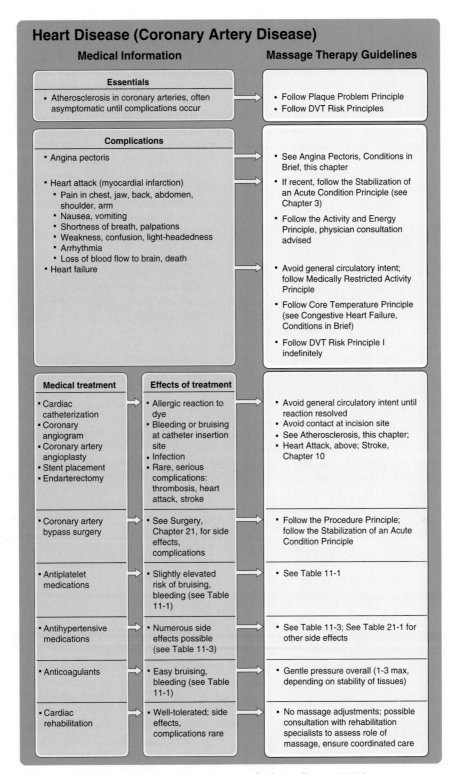

FIGURE 11-15. A Decision Tree for heart disease (CAD).

8. How are you being treated? Are you taking any medications?
9. How does treatment affect you?

● MASSAGE THERAPY GUIDELINES

For anyone with diagnosed CAD, with or without a heart attack history, follow the Plaque Problem Principle and the DVT Risk Principles.

Question 1 will lead into Questions 2–4, about complications, because in most cases heart disease is not diagnosed until it has caused a problem such as angina or a heart attack. Complications and related conditions will complete the CV picture, as you learn about varicose veins, or coexisting effects of atherosclerosis on the kidneys, brain, or other tissues. Adapt the massage accordingly to any of these (see Kidney Failure, Chapter 18; "Stroke" or TIA, Chapter 10; Angina Pectoris or Peripheral Vascular Disease, Conditions in Brief, this chapter).

If the client has experienced a heart attack, listen closely to the client's answers to your follow-up questions about it. Some clients have experienced more than one heart attack and should be asked about the most recent one. Multiple heart attacks should be treated with more cautious massage than a single incident.

If the heart attack was recent, follow up with "Has your heart stabilized since then?" If there is a sense that it is still stabilizing, and medications are still being adjusted, then apply the Stabilization of an Acute Condition Principle (see Chapter 3). The stabilization period is likely to last for around 12 weeks after the heart attack.

> *The Stabilization of an Acute Condition Principle.* Until an acute medical condition has stabilized, massage should be conservative.

Along with the question about stabilization, establish how severe the heart attack was. Clinical presentations after a heart attack can range widely. One client with a mild heart attack could have used the episode as a "wake up call" that allowed him to make significant lifestyle changes that increased his general health: running or other aerobic exercise, eating well, losing weight, quitting smoking. Another could be so debilitated by the heart attack that she is left with significant heart failure, and a low level of function, able to complete only the most basic activities of daily living. Your compassion and support are necessary in both scenarios, but the massage plan is very different. Questions 5–7, discussed below, help determine where the client is on the function spectrum; a client who has been through cardiac rehabilitation will have a good sense of how strong his heart is.

Stabilization after angioplasty and stent placement also takes around 12 weeks; stabilization after bypass surgery takes several additional weeks. During this time, the client may have completed the pivotal second phase of cardiac rehabilitation. This is a good time to communicate with the client's doctor and nurse because the client has been carefully monitored during exercise, and there is a clear understanding of how strong the heart is.

With or without feedback from a cardiac rehabilitation program, your client's answers to Questions 5–7 are pivotal to the massage plan. If the client is relatively active, with no activity restrictions, and doctors are unconcerned about the risk of exercise and the heart's ability to pump, then massage with general circulatory intent is likely to be well tolerated.

> *The Activity and Energy Principle.* A client who enjoys regular, moderate physical activity or a good overall energy level is better able to tolerate strong massage elements—including circulatory intent—than one whose activity or energy level is low.

Even if the client is active, do not extend circulatory intent to the entire body if you are also following the Plaque Problem Principle and DVT Risk Principles; limit circulatory intent to the remaining areas of the body, such as the back and shoulders. However, for an active client, the client's doctor is likely to speak favorably to your question about DVT risk so that massage with pressure and joint movement can eventually be resumed on the lower extremities.

If the client is left with significant impairment in heart function, with little improvement in the risk profile for a subsequent heart attack, then exclude general circulatory intent from the massage plan, to avoid further strain on the heart. In this case, a client's daily activities may be limited to minimal self-care, and the physician may have advised restrictions on activity to avoid strain on the heart. In keeping with these restrictions, follow the Medically Restricted Activity Principle. Also, because of the poor cardiovascular environment, the DVT Risk Principle I stays in place indefinitely.

The client's doctor may also have discouraged exertion or overheating in saunas or hot tubs because the client's heart cannot withstand any increased strain. If this is the case, avoid spa treatments such as steam wraps, which increase core temperature (see Congestive Heart Failure, this chapter).

> *The Core Temperature Principle.* Avoid spa treatments that raise the core temperature if a client's cardiovascular system, respiratory system, skin, or other tissue or system might be overly challenged by heat, or if there are comparable medical restrictions.

The treatments for CAD and heart attack may include several procedures and many medications. For common procedures including cardiac catheterization, coronary angiogram, angioplasty, stent placement, and coronary endarterectomy, side effects are likely to be limited to tenderness or bruising at the site of the catheter insertion. Allergic reaction to the dye used is managed with medication, but in the event it occurs, avoid general circulatory intent after the procedure. If rare complications occur, such as thrombosis, stroke, or heart attack, refer to the relevant sections in this chapter. For stroke, see Chapter 10.

Although pressure is contraindicated at the site of a stent, this is not relevant in the case of a coronary artery, which is obviously inaccessible to massage pressure.

If the client has had coronary bypass surgery, see "Surgery," Chapter 21, and follow the Stabilization of an Acute Condition Principle. Be mindful of any incision used to remove the graft used in the bypass, and avoid pressure at the incision site—usually the lower or upper extremity. Again, in the event of serious complications, refer to relevant sections elsewhere in this text.

For medications, ask the four medication questions (see Chapter 4) about each drug the client is taking, and adapt accordingly. You will likely need to adjust to the effects of antiplatelet medication, anticoagulants, and antihypertensive drugs. Most of these are addressed in Tables 11-1 and 11-3. If you encounter any unfamiliar side effects not mentioned here, see Table 21-1 for a general list of drug side effects and massage therapy guidelines. Finally, if the client is in cardiac rehabilitation, it is a good idea to consult with the specialist to share the massage plan and align it with the goals of rehabilitation.

● MASSAGE RESEARCH

There is little available research data on massage for people with CAD or heart attack history. However, in two studies, massage was tested on patients before cardiac catheterization, widely recognized as a stressful procedure. In one RCT (Okvat et al., 2002), patients provided with a 10-minute massage were compared to those receiving 10 minutes of quiet time with a massage therapist. Seventy-eight patients were in the sample. The group concluded that, while it was feasible to incorporate massage therapy into the wait time before cardiac catheterization, the active treatment (massage) did not produce significant improvement in discomfort or anxiety before the procedure. In another RCT of 46 patients awaiting cardiac catheterization (McNamara et al., 2003), a 20-minute back massage was compared to usual care. The investigators found a reduction in systolic BP in the massage group. These data are not large enough to be conclusive.

As the body of massage therapy research grows, it is likely that more investigators will focus on massage for people with CAD and heart attack histories. Because stress is thought to be a risk factor in heart disease, the effect of massage therapy on this parameter is a natural area of further study.

● POSSIBLE MASSAGE BENEFITS

Most people with CAD know their diagnosis because they have experienced a heart attack or angina, and these are obviously stressful. Depression and anxiety are common in this population.

Relaxation massage therapy, by reducing stress, may play an important role in recovery, or in the management of these conditions. Massage may also support body awareness as well as the health and flexibility of skeletal muscles; each of these is in the service of cardiac rehabilitation. No matter what a client's level of function, massage may help body image and support psychological as well as physical healing.

Atrial Fibrillation

Atrial fibrillation is one of the most common types of **arrhythmia**, or irregular heart rhythm, the interruption of the smooth conduction of electrical impulses controlling contractions of the heart. In **atrial fibrillation**, electrical discharges that control the contraction of the atria occur very rapidly, resulting in rapid, chaotic rhythm. Because the ventricles cannot keep up with the pace set by the atria, the atria empty incompletely.

● BACKGROUND

Atrial fibrillation can be caused by disorders in the valves, congenital heart defects, rheumatic fever, hypertension, CAD, hyperthyroidism, chronic lung disease, and binge alcohol drinking. These conditions make the heart work harder and enlarge; enlarged atria are more likely to develop atrial fibrillation.

Signs and Symptoms

Atrial fibrillation is often asymptomatic, but in many cases it causes **palpitations**—a heightened awareness of an irregular or fast heartbeat—as well as weakness, chest discomfort, mild shortness of breath and fatigue, dizziness, and lightheadedness. In more severe cases, people experience more pronounced chest discomfort, fainting, confusion, and worsening shortness of breath. These symptoms occur because of reduced blood flow and hypotension. Acute episodes last for less than a few days. In *paroxysmal atrial fibrillation*, symptoms come and go suddenly. In *chronic atrial fibrillation*, the disrupted heart rhythm is enduring. Symptoms of atrial fibrillation can be aggravated by exertion and stress.

Complications

Complications occur when blood is pumped inefficiently, including a drop in blood pressure. If the BP drop is precipitous, especially in older adults, the shock can be life threatening. Also, when atrial fibrillation occurs for more than a day or two, blood pooling in the atria can form clots. If pieces of these clots detach, they embolize on the arterial side and can block an artery in almost any location, including the extremities, the kidney, GI tract, or the eye. Emboli may lodge in other organs such as the brain, or the heart itself. In the brain or heart, the blockage can produce stroke or heart attack (see "Stroke [Cerebrovascular Accident]," Chapter 10; "Heart Disease," this chapter). If atrial fibrillation is allowed to go on for several

months, the rapid heart rate can weaken the heart muscle, causing heart failure.

Treatment

Treatments are aimed at slowing the heart rate, restoring normal rhythm, and preventing thromboembolism. Often people with atrial fibrillation can tolerate the uneven heart rate as long as it is slowed down. Medications used to slow the rate include β-blockers and calcium channel blockers (see "Hypertension," this chapter). A digitalis preparation, **digoxin** (Lanoxin), may be used to slow the heart rate. Among other side effects, it can cause mild nausea and diarrhea. Evening out the heart rhythm is a greater challenge: Antiarrhythmic drugs such as amiodarone (Cordarone, Pacerone), propafenone (Rythmol), and dofetilide (Tikosyn) are administered. These can produce strong side effects, including nausea, dizziness, and fatigue. Instead of long-term treatment with these drugs, some people are given the "pill in the pocket" approach: an oral dose to take when arrhythmia recurs. This typically relieves symptoms and reduces emergency room visits.

Because of the concern about stroke, aspirin use is necessary to prevent thromboembolism. In people at increased risk of stroke, such as those over 60, stronger anticoagulation with warfarin is necessary.

A procedure known as **cardioversion** is the delivery of a controlled electrical shock to the chest, designed to normalize the heart rhythm. It is a brief procedure, typically performed under general anesthesia. It can be used on an emergency basis to stop severe symptoms such as fainting, or it can be administered on a voluntary basis when an individual has chronic, milder symptoms. Cardioversion often offers only short-term relief, and atrial fibrillation recurs in many people. The procedure increases the risk of thrombus formation in the heart, and can cause thromboembolism, with stroke being the chief concern. A person choosing voluntary cardioversion may be prescribed warfarin for several weeks before the procedure, and warfarin is taken for 3–4 weeks afterward.

Ablation is the destruction of the heart's malfunctioning pacemaker tissue. This can be done through a catheter, using a tiny device that emits radio waves, or it can be done surgically by making incisions in the tissue, blocking the faulty electrical impulses. Some surgical approaches are more invasive than others, requiring hospitalization and longer recovery times.

In some cases, an artificial pacemaker must be implanted to regulate rhythm.

● INTERVIEW QUESTIONS

1. What are the symptoms and signs of your atrial fibrillation? Are the symptoms mild, moderate, or severe?
2. Are your symptoms constant, or intermittent? Have you had them recently, or currently?
3. Do you feel dizzy or light-headed when it happens? Are you at risk of fainting or falling when you have symptoms?
4. What does your doctor tell you to do when you have symptoms? How could I assist you if so?
5. How does atrial fibrillation affect your activities? (See "Follow-Up Questions About Activity and Energy," Chapter 4)
6. What is the cause, if known?
7. Do you have any complications of atrial fibrillation? Has the condition ever given you problems with very low blood pressure, heart problems, or blood clots forming in your heart?
8. Do you have other cardiovascular conditions such as high blood pressure, a heart condition, varicose veins, atherosclerosis, or a risk of forming blood clots in your legs?
9. How has your condition been treated? How long have you been in treatment? Is cardioversion among your treatments?
10. How do the treatments affect you?

● MASSAGE THERAPY GUIDELINES

Most of the time, a person with diagnosed atrial fibrillation has a mild or moderate condition, is followed closely by his doctor, and is being treated with rate-slowing medications and anticoagulants. Severe, unstable symptoms are less common, and a person with a stubborn case of atrial fibrillation is likely to also have other cardiac conditions that call for a gentle massage approach. In all cases, if severe symptoms appear, producing visible discomfort, or making it hard for the client to talk, call emergency services.

Questions 1–7 are for determining how stable or severe the client's condition is. Follow the Emergency Protocol Principle (see Chapter 3), listening carefully to the client's answers to Questions 3 and 4, and get a clear understanding of how to proceed if symptoms suddenly appear or worsen during a session.

Because atrial fibrillation can range from a "nuisance" condition to one, which creates additional, serious heart problems, massage should be adapted to the severity. The Activity and Energy Questions are essential when questioning a client with atrial fibrillation (see Chapter 4). Some clients will require a gentle overall session, and others can tolerate stronger work, with general circulatory intent. Use the Activity and Energy Principle, the Medically Restricted Activity Principle, and, if necessary, the client's doctor to determine how gently to work. In most cases, physicians support a moderate to high level of activity. Sometimes, a limit on exertion is imposed to prevent further damage to the heart from atrial fibrillation; in these cases, general circulatory intent is not the best plan for the session.

> *The Medically Restricted Activity Principle.* **If there are any medical restrictions on a client's activities, explore and apply any equivalent massage contraindications.**

Follow any other medical concerns: for example, do not raise the client's core temperature if it could aggravate symptoms. In all cases, encourage the client to rise slowly from the table, and if dizziness is an issue, be prepared to assist the client.

From questions 6-8, adapt to any known causes or complications of the condition, such as hypertension, hypotension, hyperthyroidism (see Chapter 17), heart disease or heart failure, and refer to sections in this chapter or others, when appropriate. If other CV disease is present, the Plaque Problem Principle and DVT Risk Principles should be considered. For dizziness, faintness, or weakness, a gradual rise from the table is indicated at the end of the session. In particular, be alert for signs of stroke (see Chapter 10) if the client has undergone cardioversion, or has other risk factors for stroke.

Question 8 is a standard question for any cardiovascular condition. Observe the CV Conditions Often "Run in Packs" Principle. For any yes answers, consult the appropriate section, or the Conditions Brief table at the end of this chapter.

Questions 9 and 10, about treatments for atrial fibrillation, can cue you to any side effects of medications, such as nausea, diarrhea, dizziness, and fatigue. Massage adaptations appear in the Decision Tree (see Figure 11-16). Gentle pressure overall, in the 1–3 range, is likely to be necessary for long-term anticoagulant therapy such as warfarin; for aspirin, pressure does not usually need to be as cautious. Adjust the session to antihypertensives (see Table 11-3, this chapter). If a client has undergone cardioversion, note that stroke risk is elevated in the 4 weeks after the procedure, and be alert for signs of stroke (see Chapter 10). Anticoagulant therapy may be in place in preparation for cardioversion, or following it, so adjust the pressure. If surgery was performed, even if minimally invasive techniques were used, refer to "Surgery," Chapter 21.

● MASSAGE RESEARCH

As of this writing, there are no randomized, controlled trials, published in the English language, on atrial fibrillation and massage therapy indexed in PubMed or the Massage Therapy Foundation Research Database. The NIH RePORTER tool lists no active, federally funded research projects on this topic in the United States. No active projects are listed on the clinicaltrials.gov database (see Chapter 6). There is one story in the nursing literature that describes the use of massage in a patient with atrial fibrillation (Curtis, 1994). It appeared that massage was associated with the restoration of the patient's heart rhythm. Although this is a single story does not demonstrate a clear massage benefit, it does invite systematic research on the topic.

● POSSIBLE MASSAGE BENEFITS

Stress is one of the many triggers for atrial fibrillation, and atrial fibrillation episodes can be very frightening, especially when an individual is new to the experience. Stress management can go a long way. As with many other CV conditions, relaxation massage therapy has a place in stress reduction.

Atrial Fibrillation

Medical Information	Massage Therapy Guidelines

Essentials

- Arrhythmia involving rapid, chaotic contractions of atria, uncoordinated with ventricular contractions; incomplete emptying of atria cause poor blood flow:
- Shortness of breath (mild to severe)
- Weakness, fatigue
- Dizziness, light-headedness, faintness
- Palpitations
- Chest discomfort
- Fainting
- Confusion

- Gentle session overall, depending on activity level; follow Activity and Energy Principle, Medically Restricted Activity Principle
- Reposition gently, slow speed and even rhythm, slow rise from table, gentle transition at end of session
- Follow Core Temperature Principle if heat aggravates symptoms
- For unstable, poorly controlled symptoms, follow Emergency Protocol Principle (see Chapter 3)
- If symptoms severe, produce visible discomfort, or make it difficult for client to talk, call emergency medical services

- Causes include rheumatic fever, congenital heart and valve defects, hypertension, hyperthyroidism, binge alcohol drinking

- Inquire and adapt massage to cause where necessary

Complications

- Thrombosis in atria, arterial thromboembolism

- Hypotension, shock
- Heart failure

- Be alert for signs of stroke (see Chapter 10)
- Emergency medical referral
- See Congestive heart failure, this chapter

Medical treatment	Effects of treatment	
- Beta blockers, calcium channel blockers	- See Table 11-3, this chapter	- See Table 11-3, this chapter
- Digoxin	- Mild nausea	- Position for comfort, gentle session overall; pressure to tolerance, slow speeds; no uneven rhythms or strong joint movement
	- Diarrhea	- Easy bathroom access; gentle session overall; avoid contact or pressure at abdomen that could aggravate
- Antiarrhythmic drugs (amiodarone, propafenone, dofetilide)	- Nausea - Dizziness	- See Nausea, above - Reposition gently, slow speed and even rhythm, slow rise from table, gentle transition at end of session
	- Fatigue	- Gentle session overall
- Aspirin, anticoagulants	- Easy bruising, bleeding	- See Table 11-1
- Cardioversion	- Increased risk of thromboembolism, 3-4 weeks after procedure	- Be alert for signs of stroke
- Ablation, pacemaker placement	- See Surgery, Chapter 21 for side effects, complications	- Follow the Procedure Principle; see Surgery, Chapter 21

FIGURE 11-16. A Decision Tree for atrial fibrillation.

Other Cardiovascular Conditions in Brief

ANEURYSM

Background

- Bulging of weakened arterial wall, due to atherosclerosis, injury, congenital weakness, some types of infection; common in abdominal aorta, thoracic aorta; also occurs in femoral, popliteal, carotid, cerebral, and coronary arteries.
- Often asymptomatic, late symptom is nonspecific pain; most likely to rupture if >2.5″ wide, located in aortic area.
- Rupture results in uncontrolled bleeding, blood loss, hypoxic injury to tissues downstream; aortic aneurysms often fatal.
- Thrombi can form in pooling blood inside bulge; can dislodge and occlude arteries downstream.
- For aortic aneurysm, if <5 cm; may be treated as stable, monitored every 6–12 months; if aneurysm approaches 4 cm, may be monitored every 3 months; if >5 cm, usually treated surgically.
- Surgical repair involves insertion of a synthetic graft with stent to strengthen vessel; may include minimally invasive insertion of a column through a femoral artery, with ring at each end to anchor graft.

Interview Questions

- Where was/is it? When was it diagnosed? Cause?
- Is it considered current? Stable? Resolved? Monitored?
- Complications? Any pressure of aneurysm on nerves? Any rupture or formation/migration of blood clots? Any pain or loss of function? Other CV conditions such as heart disease, atherosclerosis?
- Activity level? Medical restrictions on activity?
- How are you monitored or checked, how often? Treatment performed or planned? Effects of treatment?

Massage Therapy Guidelines

- Avoid excessive pressure at site of aneurysm (relevant for abdominal, carotid, femoral, popliteal area); limit to level 1 maximum at carotid, femoral, popliteal (2 max for abdominal); avoid joint movement at superficial aneurysm site (especially relevant for popliteal).
- Use same precautions for repaired aneurysm, with or without hardware.
- Adjust massage to atherosclerosis; follow Plaque Problem Principle; consider DVT Risk Principles; use slow speeds, even rhythms, gradual transitions to avoid increasing BP.
- Adapt massage plan to complications of aneurysm, usually related to arterial thromboembolism.
- If signs of rupture, including severe or sudden pain (headache, backache), blurred vision, loss of motor function, contact emergency medical services.

ANGINA PECTORIS

Background

- Brief periods of chest pain, discomfort, sensation of heaviness; pain may extend into jaw, shoulder, arm, throat, back; may also experience dizziness, nausea, sweating, shortness of breath, anxiety.
- Caused by CAD, significant occlusion of artery, limiting blood available to heart; triggered by exertion, stress, meals, cold weather, smoking; in stable or chronic condition, symptoms relieved by rest; episodes last 15 minutes or less.
- Unstable angina features change in symptom patterns—different triggers, more easily triggered, increase in symptom intensity, longer episodes, more frequent attacks—can signal heart attack, is a medical emergency.
- Stable or chronic form relieved by rest; unstable angina not relieved by rest.
- Nitrates such as nitroglycerin used in short-acting forms to dilate coronary arteries, relieve episodes within minutes; longer-acting forms used to prevent episodes; aspirin to prevent arterial clots.

- Treatment with cardiac catheterization, angioplasty, stent placement, coronary artery bypass surgery.
- Lifestyle changes include modifying risk factors: weight loss, exercise, smoking cessation, stress reduction.

Interview Questions	• How long since your diagnosis of angina? Is it considered stable? • What triggers an episode? What are your symptoms? How long does it last? What relieves it? • Have there been any changes in your angina episodes recently or are they about the same? • Any other complications of atherosclerosis such as vision or kidney problems? History of heart attack or stroke? High blood pressure? • Treatment? Effects of treatment? • If you have any medication to use for an episode, where do you keep it?
Massage Therapy Guidelines	• General circulatory intent contraindicated in most cases; for mild angina with reasonable activity level, good activity tolerance, no medical restrictions on activity, general circulatory intent may be okay with input from physician. • Follow Plaque Problem Principle; apply DVT Risk Principles (may follow DVT Risk Principle 1 indefinitely). • If client shows signs/symptoms of unstable angina, emergency medical referral. • Determine how to access rescue medication (nitroglycerin) quickly in order to hand it to client in case it is needed during session (do not administer medication). • Adapt to medications, procedures for associated conditions and treatment (see "Hypertension," "Heart Disease [Coronary Artery Disease]," this chapter).

ARRHYTHMIA

Background	• Umbrella term for abnormal heart rhythms, taking several forms: too fast (tachycardia), too slow (bradycardia), uneven (various). Range from mild (such as premature atrial contractions) to life threatening (such as ventricular fibrillation). See "Atrial Fibrillation," this chapter. • Treated with anti-arrhythmic medications, β-blockers, anticoagulants, antiplatelets; nonpharmacological treatments include defibrillation, pacemaker implantation, ablation, surgery.
Interview Questions	• Type of arrhythmia? Symptoms? Mild, moderate, or severe? • Is it stable, well controlled? • Any effects on heart function? Any associated heart disease, blood pressure problem, or atherosclerosis? Known cause? • Activity level? Any medical restrictions on activity? • Treatments? Effects of treatment?
Massage Therapy Guidelines	• Limit pressure (2 max) on abdomen to avoid stimulating vasovagal reaction (see "Hypertension," this chapter). • If additional CV disease, consider Plaque Problem Principle, DVT Risk Principles. • Follow Activity and Energy Principle, Medically Restricted Activity Principle (see Chapter 3); if heart function compromised, avoid general circulatory intent. • If atrial fibrillation present, see Decision Tree (Figure 11-16). • Adjust position if implanted device (usually below clavicle) causes discomfort). • Adapt massage plan to any side effects of medications (see Tables 11-1 and 11-3). For surgery, follow the Procedure Principle, see Chapter 21.

CONGESTIVE HEART FAILURE

Background	• Heart is unable to pump sufficient blood for tissue needs; backup of blood leads to congestion in body tissues. • If right heart insufficiency, backup occurs in systemic veins, causing fluid accumulation in liver, extremities, abdomen; if left heart impaired, congestion occurs in lungs. • Signs, symptoms include edema in lower extremities, abdomen, shortness of breath with exertion (or at rest, in advanced cases); weakness, drowsiness, confusion (as blood supply to brain affected).

- Complications include blood clot formation in heart chambers, embolization, stroke, heart attack.
- Treatments are diuretics, antihypertensive drugs, anticoagulants, support stockings to facilitate venous return; angioplasty or surgical correction of faulty heart valve, heart transplant (experimental, used in younger individuals).

Interview Questions	• When were you diagnosed with CHF? Is it considered mild, moderate, or severe? Symptoms? Is left or right side of heart most affected? • How much movement or activity can you tolerate each day? How does it affect you? • Do you have swelling anywhere? How is your breathing? What do you do if your breathing becomes difficult? • Are there any complications of your CHF, does it affect other areas or systems of your body? Are there other cardiovascular conditions that you know of? • What positions are you comfortable in? For example, how do you sleep? • Treatment? Effects of treatment?
Massage Therapy Guidelines	• Avoid general circulatory intent (follow Filter and Pump Principle). Gentle session overall (Vital Organ Principle). • Observe Plaque Problem Principle; follow DVT Risk Principle I indefinitely. • If right heart affected, positioning changes may include elevating extremities, padding around swelling in midsection, or using side-lying position. • If left side of heart involved, adjust position for shortness of breath (side-lying may be welcome, or inclined position). • If both sides involved, elevating lower extremities along with upper body may be necessary. • Support stockings should be left in place unless physician approves removing them for contact with lower extremities; avoid lubricant if it makes it difficult to replace stockings after massage. • Adapt to medications: easy bathroom access or sensitive scheduling for diuretics; effects of anticoagulants, antiplatelets (see Table 11-1), antihypertensives (see Table 11-3). • For surgery, follow Procedure Principle, see Chapter 21.

HEART MURMUR

Background	• Backflow of blood during contraction of a heart chamber, detected by a stethoscope. Includes mitral valve prolapse (MVP), stenosis of aortic or mitral valve, other structural defects in valves or walls. • Caused by rheumatic fever, heart disease, endocarditis (infection of heart). • Most are harmless, but some affect heart function, requiring surgical correction.
Interview Questions	• When was it diagnosed? How does it affect you? Does it give you symptoms, or require treatment? • Does it affect your activities? What is your activity level? Are there any medical restrictions on activities? • Do you have any other cardiovascular conditions such as heart disease? • Treatment? Effects of treatment?
Massage Therapy Guidelines	• Most heart murmurs have no bearing on the massage. However, if condition affects activity level, is due to an underlying heart condition or considered serious, see Decision Tree for heart disease, Figure 11-15, or Congestive heart failure, Conditions in Brief. Follow Filter and Pump Principle, Activity and Energy Principle (see Chapter 3).

PERICARDITIS

Background	• Inflammation of pericardium (membrane surrounding the heart); caused by infection, heart attack, radiation therapy, immunosuppressive therapies, autoimmune conditions. • Chest pain and breathing difficulty when lying down; relieved by sitting and leaning forward, cough, fatigue, fever, anxiety.

- Complications are arrhythmias, cardiac tamponade (emergency condition, too much pressure from fluid interferes with heart pumping), heart failure.
- Treatment depends on cause; antibiotics or antifungal drugs for infection, pain relievers for pain, NSAIDs for inflammation, diuretics for reducing fluid accumulation.
- If severe, pericardiocentesis is performed (fluid aspiration from around heart).
- Usually resolves in several weeks to several months with effective treatment.

Interview Questions	<ul><li>When was it diagnosed? What is the cause? Is it worsening or improving?</li><li>Where are your symptoms? Any dizziness, lightheadedness, faintness, drowsiness? Any swelling anywhere?</li><li>What is your activity level? Any medical restrictions on your activities? Is your doctor concerned about the health of your heart?</li><li>Which positions are you comfortable in?</li></ul>
Massage Therapy Guidelines	<ul><li>Avoid general circulatory intent unless client is closely monitored, improving, with good heart function, increasing activity level, no activity restrictions; medical consultation advised.</li><li>If condition still acute, use gentle pressure overall (level 2 maximum).</li><li>Adapt positioning for client comfort and ease of breathing; consider seated, slight incline, side-lying position.</li><li>Follow DVT Risk Principles for all clients.</li><li>Emergency medical referral for new signs or symptoms (swelling in abdomen or extremities, dizziness, faintness).</li><li>Adjust to treatments, effects of treatments (see Diuretics, Table 11-3; "NSAIDs," Chapter 21; Common Side Effects of Medications, Table 21-1).</li></ul>

PERIPHERAL VASCULAR DISEASE/PERIPHERAL ARTERY DISEASE

Background	<ul><li>Reduced blood flow in peripheral circulation, usually due to atherosclerosis; symptoms occur in extremities, commonly in lower limbs.</li><li>Causes color change, absence of pulse, cold feet, lower legs, hands, muscle pain, numbness.</li><li>Causes intermittent claudication (pain with walking, relieved by rest).</li><li>Treated with vasodilating medications, antiplatelets, statins, angioplasty; intermittent claudication treated with pentoxifylline (Trental), cilostazol (Pletal).</li></ul>
Interview Questions	<ul><li>When was it diagnosed? How does it affect you?</li><li>What is your activity level? Any medical restrictions on activities?</li><li>Any complications of your condition? Any other associated CV conditions such as high BP, atherosclerosis, heart disease?</li><li>Treatments? Effects of treatments?</li></ul>
Massage Therapy Guidelines	<ul><li>Limit pressure at extremities to level 2; if heart disease present, avoid general circulatory intent (see "Heart Disease [Coronary Artery Disease]," this chapter).</li><li>Follow Plaque Problem Principle; follow DVT Risk Principle I indefinitely.</li><li>Adapt to associated CV conditions, complications.</li><li>Adjust massage to effects of medications (Tables 11-1 and 11-3). For angioplasty, see "Atherosclerosis," this chapter.</li><li>If client is taking Trental, limit overall pressure to level 3 because of changes in blood viscosity (Wible, 2009).</li></ul>

RAYNAUD SYNDROME

Background	<ul><li>Spasm of peripheral arteries, often from cold; vasoconstriction leads to numbness, pain, discoloration of hands and/or feet; uncomfortable and painful, but rarely severe.</li><li>Treatments are calcium channel blockers, vasodilators, other medications.</li></ul>
Interview Questions	<ul><li>When was it diagnosed? Triggers? How does it affect you?</li><li>Treatments? Effects of treatments?</li></ul>

Massage Therapy Guidelines	• During Raynaud episode, gentle massage only, as numbness may occur. Although massage seems ideal for increasing circulation, increasing it too quickly can produce throbbing; circulatory intent should be gradually introduced. • Adapt to effects of medications (see calcium channel blockers, vasodilators, Table 11-3; see Table 21-1 for side effects of other medications).

VARICOSE VEINS

Background	• Enlargement of veins, resulting in permanent impairment of one-way valves and development of back pressure in veins; usually appears in lower extremities. • Veins appear large, protruding. In mild cases, veins appear discolored, or spider veins—starburst-shaped red or blue lines—form in superficial tissues. • In severe cases, veins protrude, harden, becoming tortuous (twisted, ropy), and can be surrounded by bruises. • Risk factors include pregnancy, sedentary lifestyle, obesity, family history. • Complications may occur in both mild and severe cases, and include pain and achiness, swelling, dermatitis with itching, ulceration, superficial phlebitis, thrombophlebitis. • Conservative treatments include elevation, compression stockings. • Procedures include sclerotherapy (injection therapy with saline to collapse the diseased vessel); ablation of the diseased vessel with heat, laser treatment; stripping (surgical removal). Treatments are usually well tolerated, with few side effects or complications.
Interview Questions	• Where are the varicose veins? Do they protrude from the skin? • Are they painful, itchy, or ulcerated (open skin)? • Do you ever have any swelling in the area? Any complications such as phlebitis, or an inflamed vein? • Has your doctor ever expressed any concern about your varicose veins, or about anything else developing in the veins of your legs, such as swelling, pain, or blood clot? • Treatment? Effects of treatment?
Massage Therapy Guidelines	• Consider varicose veins to be injured veins, and limit pressure at affected areas. • Most mild varicose veins (spider veins, or larger discolored veins with no protrusion) are safe to massage at level 3, but avoid focused pressure on the injured vessels, and in all cases direct strokes toward the heart in order to avoid aggravating blood backflow. • If moderate or severe veins are present, limit pressure to level 2 or 1, respectively, at site. • If additional signs/symptoms present, such as swelling, itching, pain, follow DVT Risk Principles, and avoid friction in the involved region; if open skin (from scratching, or from poor circulation causing ulceration), contact and lubricant are contraindicated at the site. • If superficial thrombophlebitis is evident, deep vein thrombosis is often present; follow the DVT Risk Principles, urgent medical referral if unreported to physician. • Adapt massage to treatments, such as avoiding lubricant on support stockings. If veins were treated recently with saline, heat, laser, or surgery, continue gentle pressure in affected areas. If the surgery was long ago and incisions are healed, then adjust massage pressure to any current varicose veins or DVT risk.

SELF TEST

1. Explain the CV Conditions often "Run in Packs" Principle. How does it affect the practice of massage?

2. Compare the Plaque Problem Principle and the DVT Risk Principle I. How are they similar? How are they different? In each case, which areas of the body are treated with caution?

3. Describe how DVT Risk Principle II affects DVT Risk Principle I. What are three essential elements of physician communication in DVT Risk Principle II?

4. List eight risk factors for DVT. Of all the DVT risk factors mentioned, what are five of the strongest?

5. Regarding nonspecific DVT symptoms, in order to decide whether to modify massage, urge a medical referral, or both, describe five things to look for, ask about, and consider.

6. Explain why the Homans sign should not be used to test for DVT.

7. Describe how atherosclerosis affects the health of arteries, and the three main complications of atherosclerosis.

8. List six organs or areas of the body that are typically affected by atherosclerosis.

9. What is the difference between stent placement and bypass surgery? Which sites of stent placement should be treated with caution in massage therapy?

10. Explain why it is important for a massage therapist to know pulse points when working with a client with atherosclerosis. How should massage be modified at these sites, and which site requires the most caution?

11. Explain why cautious abdominal pressure is necessary in a client with hypertension, the steps of the reaction that may occur with too much pressure, and the consequences.

12. Explain orthostatic hypotension, why it might be a problem for someone with hypertension, and two ways that massage can be adjusted to accommodate it.

13. Describe the three levels of hypertension. What is the typical medical management in each case?

14. What are three signs/symptoms of dangerously high blood pressure? What should the massage therapist do if the client complains of them?

15. Does research support the claim that massage lowers blood pressure in hypertensive individuals, or in individuals with normal blood pressure? Describe two studies that looked at massage and blood pressure, and what the researchers reported about it.

16. Which two principles should you follow with anyone with diagnosed heart disease, whether or not they have a heart attack history?

17. Which massage principles can help you determine whether a client with heart disease can withstand massage with circulatory intent, or a spa treatment that involves heat treatment? Describe the principles and how to use them.

18. What are the signs and symptoms of a heart attack? Can a person have a heart attack without having any symptoms?

19. Describe three symptoms of atrial fibrillation, and two complications.

20. If a client has atrial fibrillation, what questions should you ask about other cardiovascular conditions that might be present?

 For answers to these questions and to see a bibliography for this chapter, visit http://thePoint. lww.com/Walton.

Chapter

12 Blood Conditions

You have stars in your bones and oceans in blood.

—ALLA RENEE BOZARTH

The body's ocean—the bloodstream—carries out essential functions, serving all of the tissues of the body. The blood delivers nutrients from the digestive system to the tissues, and transports oxygen from the lungs to the tissues. Blood hydrates the body and carries away wastes, delivers hormones from glands to target tissues, and distributes immune factors to fight infection.

Blood is a complex mixture of water, proteins, minerals, nutrients, and hormones. The three types of formed elements—red blood cells, white blood cells, and platelets—are present in varying concentrations, according to conditions in the body. These elements are born in the bone marrow, then transferred to the bloodstream. Health problems arise when there are imbalances in any of these blood components, such as too many white blood cells, or too few platelets. Impairment of bone marrow function can cause reduced populations of blood cells or an overpopulation of immature or incompetent cells that crowd out healthy cells.

The structures that pump and conduct blood—the heart and vessels—are addressed in Chapter 11. This chapter is focused on the blood itself. Three conditions of the blood are addressed with full discussion, with full Decision Trees. They are:

- Anemia
- Thrombocytopenia
- Leukemia

Conditions in Brief are **Hemochromatosis, Hemophilia, Neutropenia** (leukopenia), **Multiple myeloma, Polycythemia vera, Sickle-cell disease, Thrombocythemia,** and **Thrombophilia.**

General Principles

When working with people with blood and bone marrow conditions, therapists can draw on principles introduced in Chapter 3. Massage adjustments depend on the nature of the blood imbalance. For example, if there is an overtendency to clot, from too many platelets, clotting proteins, or otherwise thickened blood, the therapist should involve the physician before using pressure or movement on areas where clots tend to form (see DVT Risk Principles, Chapter 11). If the condition causes inadequate clotting, then easy bruising or bleeding may require lighter pressure. Use the Unstable Tissue Principle (see Chapter 3).

If there is poor immunity, the therapist may need to strengthen infection control, according to instructions from the client's nurse and doctor.

Whenever a component of blood is in excess, it is important to consider whether any of the major blood filters is being worked harder, such as the spleen, liver, or kidney. If this is a possibility, the therapist can avoid any additional stress on these organs by avoiding massage with general circulatory intent. This is in keeping with the Filter and Pump Principle (see Chapter 3).

Anemia

Anemia refers to a deficiency in the number, structure, or hemoglobin makeup of red blood cells.

● BACKGROUND

The primary function of **red blood cells (RBCs)**, also called **erythrocytes**, is to deliver oxygen from the lungs to all the tissues of the body, then carry carbon dioxide back to the lungs where it can be expelled from the body. A deficit in this cell population results in systemic effects, because the body's tissues function poorly with inadequate oxygen (O_2), or excess carbon dioxide (CO_2).

A familiar name for anemia is "tired blood," because of the common symptom of fatigue. The many types of anemia, ranging from mild to severe, have different causes. One common cause of anemia is iron deficiency, because iron is needed in healthy **hemoglobin**, the O_2- and CO_2-carrying molecule that is the major element of RBC. It is crucial for the structure and function of RBCs. Iron deficiency may occur in anyone who is losing blood, such as during heavy menstrual bleeding, or blood loss from the gastrointestinal (GI) tract due to peptic ulcers or colitis. Cancer of the GI tract can also contribute to blood loss and anemia.

Anemia can be due to a deficiency of vitamin B_{12} (called *pernicious anemia*), folic acid, or other vitamin, as some vitamins are especially important in the manufacture of RBCs. Some people get plenty of dietary vitamins but absorb them poorly from the GI tract, a process known as malabsorption.

Anemia is often secondary to other bone marrow diseases, such as leukemia. In one inherited form of anemia, sickle-cell disease, the structure of hemoglobin is compromised by a defective gene, leading to fragile RBCs with a shorter life cycle, and thus an inadequate supply (see Conditions in Brief). Aplastic anemia, a rare and particularly serious form of anemia, occurs when the bone marrow stops producing enough RBCs. Although its cause is uncertain, it has been linked to chemical and radiation exposure, viral exposures, and possible inherited vulnerability. Cancer treatments, such as chemotherapy, or drugs for treating HIV infection, can injure bone marrow in predictable ways, leading to anemia. When administering such medications, physicians anticipate anemia and prevent it with other treatment, if necessary.

Signs and Symptoms

The hallmark of anemia is fatigue—tiring easily, exhaustion, and weakness. Shortness of breath can occur. People with anemia may be intolerant of cold temperatures, or the extremities can be numb or cold. Pallor (paleness) is easiest to recognize in a range of skin tones by observing the nail beds and lips for a lack of the usual pink color. Cognitive problems suggest the brain is getting less oxygen, and dizziness can occur upon rising from lying down. Headache may occur.

In milder forms of anemia, none of these symptoms may occur, and the condition remains unnoticed. In some cases, the individual feels general overall tiredness, but no other symptoms.

Complications

Chronic, unchecked anemia can lead to arrhythmia, either a rapid or irregular heartbeat, as the heart attempts to compensate for the poor quality of blood by pumping it more quickly through the body. In severe cases, or in people with other heart or lung problems, this overwork can lead to congestive heart failure (see chapter 11).

Treatment

Treatment for anemia depends on the cause. If the cause is iron deficiency, it may be addressed by dietary iron supplementation and improved diet. With supplementation, the condition usually improves in about 2 months. If the iron deficiency is itself caused by blood loss other than from menstruation, then the source of the bleeding, such as GI bleeding, needs to be identified and addressed. Iron supplementation cannot maintain adequate iron levels if it is continually depleted through blood loss. If the cause of anemia is B_{12} deficiency, injections of vitamin B_{12} are used, or if folic acid is deficient, supplements are given.

Anemia due to treatments for cancer or HIV infection can be managed by the administration of a colony-stimulating factor (CSF), which stimulates the bone marrow to increase blood cell production. An example of a CSF for RBC production is the drug epoietin alfa (Epogen, Procrit). This approach often resolves the problem quickly, although it can cause pain in the sternum, or in long bones near the joints, due to pressure from the internal increase in marrow production.

If aplastic anemia is present, or if the anemia is acute, the person may require a blood transfusion to replace RBCs. A stem cell transplant, commonly called a bone marrow transplant, may be required to replace diseased marrow (see Chapter 20). In this procedure, healthy stem cells are gathered from the bone marrow or blood, and infused into the recipient.

If sickle-cell disease is present, treatment typically focuses on symptom management (see Sickle-Cell Disease, Conditions in Brief). If anemia is caused by kidney disease, or another bone marrow disease such as leukemia, the anemia resolves when the underlying condition is successfully treated.

● INTERVIEW QUESTIONS

1. What kind of anemia do you have? What is the cause of it?
2. Does your doctor describe it as mild, or serious, or somewhere in between?
3. How does the anemia affect you? (Any fatigue, light-headedness, intolerance of cold, numbness, or cold extremities?)
4. What is your activity level? What are your movement habits, day to day or week to week?
5. Are there any complications of anemia, such as effects on your cardiovascular system or other systems?
6. How is your anemia treated?
7. How does the treatment affect you?

● MASSAGE THERAPY GUIDELINES

The first task is to identify the type of anemia, and whether another health condition is causing it. If your client cannot define it closely, you can get a basic idea of the client's situation from the answers to Question 2 and about severity and Question 6 about treatment. The seriousness of the anemia is often proportional to the aggressiveness of the treatment: from a simple iron or vitamin supplement at the milder end to a stem cell transplant at the most severe end of the spectrum. In any event, if the cause represents another, definable condition, ask more about that condition and adjust the session accordingly. An additional Decision Tree for that condition may be in order.

If blood loss is suspected but the source has not been identified, then massage pressure and the session elements should be gentle overall until the source is determined by the client's physician. If the source of blood loss, such as a peptic ulcer, has been identified, then adapt the session to the causative condition (see Chapter 15).

If cancer and chemotherapy are causing the anemia, then numerous massage adjustments may be necessary (see Chapter 20). If a blood cancer, such as leukemia, is at fault, adjustments may likewise need to be made for effects on other blood cell populations (refer to the section "Leukemia," this chapter). If kidney disease is involved, general circulatory intent is probably contraindicated. Adjust massage for the other effects of kidney disease, complications, and treatments (see Kidney failure, Chapter 18). Kidney disease may be associated with diabetes, which also calls for other adjustments (see Diabetes, Chapter 17).

> The Ask the Cause Principle. Consider the cause of a sign or symptom, as well as the sign or symptom itself, when making a massage therapy plan.

If Question 2 reveals one of the more serious causes of anemia, a medical consultation or more information is likely to be essential to the massage plan. Aplastic anemia will require

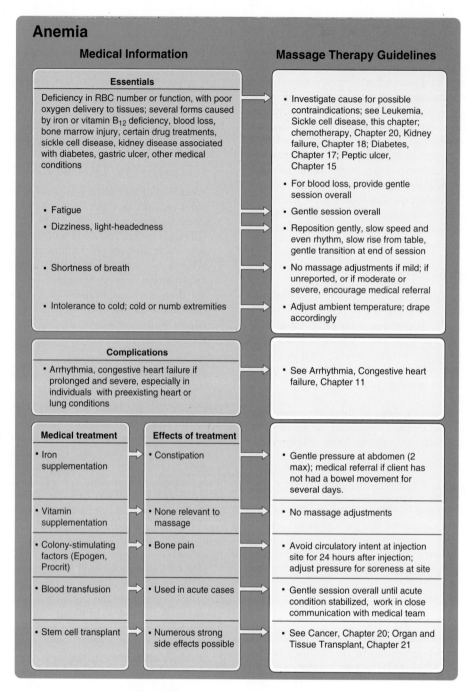

FIGURE 12-1. A Decision Tree for Anemia.

careful questioning and adaptation to the condition itself and to its strong treatments; refer to Chapter 20 for massage guidelines for cancer therapies, which are often used in the treatment of aplastic anemia.

Questions 3–5, about symptoms, activity, and complications, help you determine how strong or gentle to make the session overall. The more fatigued and inactive the client is, the gentler the session should be. In addition, each individual effect of anemia should be considered in the massage plan. If there is dizziness or light-headedness, encourage the client to rise slowly from the table—sit for a while, then stand. If cold extremities are a problem, or intolerance to cold, use an extra drape, or a lightly warmed massage table. Adjust the ambient temperature, as well. Mild shortness of breath does not usually call for

specific massage adjustments, but urge the client to report the symptom to his or her doctor if he or she hasn't already.

The Activity and Energy Principle. A client who enjoys regular, moderate physical activity or a good overall energy level is better able to tolerate strong massage elements—including circulatory intent—than one whose activity or energy level is low.

Most signs and symptoms of anemia require straightforward massage adjustments such as these. Severe or prolonged anemia can cause complications that affect the massage plan. Question 5 will get at this issue. The most common concern is the effect of anemia on heart function over time. If this has occurred, pay specific attention to cardiovascular issues such as arrhythmia or heart failure (see Chapter 11).

Questions 6 and 7 about treatment and its effects could signal a number of massage therapy guidelines, ranging from minor to significant, depending on the strength of the treatment. Iron supplementation is known to help most cases of iron deficiency anemia, but it causes constipation in some people. Appropriate abdominal massage is indicated for constipation, but if the client has not had a bowel movement in several days, advise him or her to report it to the doctor. Use light pressure (levels 1–2) on the abdomen in the meantime. If a colony-stimulating factor such as epoietin has been injected, avoid circulatory intent at the injection site for 24 hours after the injection, to avoid increasing the rate of absorption. The site will often be sore, so pressure there should be gentle. The bone pain that often follows epoietin injection may benefit from gentle touch or energetic techniques at the site of the pain (often in the sternum, hips, or ends of long bones).

When working with a client with aplastic anemia, or with blood loss, the client may require a blood transfusion. In such a situation, work extremely gently until the condition has stabilized. A physician's input is advised, in this case. For symptom management in the case of refer to Sickle-cell disease, Conditions in Brief.

A stem cell transplant brings significant medical concerns, with numerous side effects or complications, and consultation with the client's physician is in order (see "Organ and Tissue Transplant," Chapter 21).

● MASSAGE RESEARCH

As of this writing, there are a limited number of randomized, controlled trials, published in the English language, on anemia and massage indexed in PubMed and the Massage Therapy Foundation Research Database. The NIH RePORTER tool lists no active, federally funded research projects on the topic in the United States. No active projects are listed on the clinicaltrials.gov database (see Chapter 6).

The available research focuses on sickle-cell disease, in which pain management is essential (see Conditions in Brief, this chapter). Only a few research papers are published on the topic, but preliminary reports are optimistic (Lemanek et al., 2009). More research is likely to be forthcoming, as interest grows in massage therapy and other nonpharmacological methods for alleviating pain and other symptoms (Post-White et al., 2009; Sibinga et al., 2006; Yoon and Black, 2006). The pain of sickle-cell disease is notorious, and efforts in complementary and integrative approaches will be welcome if their effectiveness is established.

● POSSIBLE MASSAGE BENEFITS

Severe anemia, with serious illness at the heart of it, is stressful for obvious reasons, but chronic anemia can be demoralizing, too. People have to give up their usual activities, or perform them less well. It is possible that massage therapy could improve sleep and energy levels in some way. If the underlying condition is severe, a client might welcome massage during aggressive medical treatment as part of a combined approach.

Thrombocytopenia

Thrombocytopenia is a condition of reduced **platelets**, also known as **thrombocytes**, the cell fragments in blood that are essential for blood clotting. The low platelet count can be caused by three general conditions: reduced production by the bone marrow, destruction of platelets in circulation, or trapping of platelets in the spleen, making them unavailable to the blood circulation.

● BACKGROUND

Normal platelet counts are between 150,000 and 450,000/µL of blood (referred to as 150 and 450). Although definitions vary, thrombocytopenia is usually established at around 100. At this level, platelets are low, but not dangerously so. At 50, individuals are monitored closely for platelet status and changes. Below 40 is considered *profound thrombocytopenia*, and platelets below 20 are called *acute profound thrombocytopenia*.

Decreased platelet production may result from primary cancers of the bone marrow (see "Leukemia," this chapter), in cancers that spread to the bone marrow, or in aplastic anemia. Hepatitis, HIV, HSV, herpes zoster, and other viral infections may also suppress platelet production. Heavy alcohol use can diminish platelet production, and certain medications, including some chemotherapy drugs, suppress bone marrow activity. High dose chemotherapy is often responsible for severely low platelet counts.

In some cases, platelets are produced in adequate numbers, but they are destroyed more quickly than usual in the bloodstream, spleen, or liver. Examples of this are autoimmune conditions such as rheumatoid arthritis (see Chapter 9), systemic lupus erythematosus (see Chapter 13). An enlarged spleen, known as **splenomegaly**, can cause thrombocytopenia by trapping platelets and sequestering them, preventing their return to the bloodstream.

Signs and Symptoms

If thrombocytopenia is mild, it may be asymptomatic. Depending on the cause of the condition, symptoms may develop slowly or suddenly. Because platelets are essential for normal blood clotting, the markers of thrombocytopenia all suggest easy bruising and bleeding. These signs are nosebleeds, bleeding gums, heavy menstrual bleeding, or **petechiae**, pinpoint-sized, painless red spots that signal superficial bleeding into the skin (Figure 12-2A). Deeper bleeding in the skin is indicated by purple, green, or gold bruises called **ecchymoses** (Figure 12-2B).

Complications

If thrombocytopenia is not treated successfully, complications may include **hemorrhage**, or uncontrolled bleeding. Only minor trauma is needed to cause bleeding when platelets are in the 20–30 range, and spontaneous bleeding can occur without injury when platelets are below 10 or 20. Individuals with platelet counts this low are advised to stay in bed to avoid injury, or are monitored in the hospital.

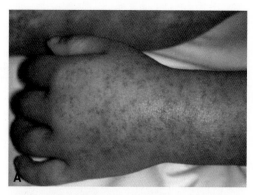

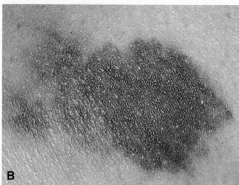

FIGURE 12-2. Petechiae and ecchymosis. (A) In petechiae, small, painless red spots indicate isolated bleeding into the skin. (B) In ecchymosis, the bleeding is deeper and more extensive.

Bleeding in the brain (*intracranial hemorrhage*) amounts to a stroke and can be life threatening (see Chapter 10). GI bleeding can also occur, leading to severe blood loss.

In one common type of thrombocytopenia, *idiopathic thrombocytopenic purpura*, the cause is unknown, and the condition ranges from mild and asymptomatic, to severely symptomatic. The condition can be chronic in young and older adults, and is attributed to an autoimmune process.

In another, rare type of thrombocytopenia, *thrombotic thrombocytopenic purpura*, both bleeding and clotting are problems. Tiny blood clots develop, causing damage to the brain or other vital organs. The prevalence of the clots leads to platelet depletion, and normal clotting is impaired. This condition can be life threatening.

Treatment

Treatment depends on the cause of thrombocytopenia. If it appears to be drug induced, then the drug is usually discontinued, with a range of consequences that depend on the drug, and the availability of a substitute. If thrombocytopenia is due to chemotherapy in cancer treatment, the next chemotherapy session may be delayed until the normal platelet population is restored.

If thrombocytopenia is caused by an autoimmune condition, a corticosteroid may be used to dampen the immune response, or chemotherapy may be started to suppress the bone marrow. If an enlarged spleen is at fault, the spleen can be removed surgically.

If platelets are dangerously low, treatment may include a platelet transfusion from a donor. This approach is used in acute situations in order to stop bleeding or prevent it when the patient is vulnerable. In some cases of platelet transfusion,

reactions occur, including allergy or fever, and allergic reactions can be extreme and even life threatening. Although increasingly strict guidelines are in place to ensure the purity of donated blood, complications can occur whenever blood or blood products are transfused.

Thrombotic thrombocytopenic purpura is treated by **plasmapheresis**, the removal of blood from an individual. This is part of a procedure called **plasma exchange**, in which the individual's blood cells are reconstituted in fresh blood *plasma* (the liquid portion of blood), then returned to the patient.

● INTERVIEW QUESTIONS

1. What is the cause of your thrombocytopenia?
2. Does your doctor describe it as mild, serious, or somewhere in between? Do you know your platelet count?
3. How does the condition affect you? Do you have easy bruising, bleeding, clotting, or skin changes?
4. Do you have any complications? Are there any effects on your cardiovascular system or nervous system? Is your liver, kidney, or spleen affected?
5. Are there any medical restrictions on your activity because of concern about bruising or clotting?
6. What is your activity level? What are your movement habits?
7. How is it treated?
8. How does the treatment affect you?

● MASSAGE THERAPY GUIDELINES

In most cases, the *cause* of the thrombocytopenia, as well as the thrombocytopenia itself, is likely to necessitate massage adjustments. Question 1 could uncover a range of causes, from medication to HIV infection, or another blood disease such as leukemia. Many causes of thrombocytopenia are addressed in other chapters of this book. If the bone marrow is compromised by cancer, see "Leukemia," this chapter, and Chapter 20. If viral infection is the cause, see Herpes, Chapter 7; "HIV", Chapter 13; Hepatitis, Chapter 16.

For chemotherapy-induced thrombocytopenia, refer to "Chemotherapy," Chapter 20. If another drug is causing the condition, ask the four medication questions (see Chapter 4) and follow the Medication Principle.

> *The Medication Principle. Adapt massage to the condition for which the medication is taken or prescribed and to any side effects.*

Spleen enlargement may require a position modification, depending on how severe it is. Consider the side-lying or seated position to gain access to ease pressure on the spleen, while still allowing access to the client's back. For any spleen congestion, avoid general circulatory intent, in keeping with the Filter and Pump Principle.

From Questions 2–5, you can get an idea of how serious the condition is and whether broad adjustments are necessary in massage pressure. If the client is seeing the doctor frequently, or his or her activities are restricted, it is a sign that pressure should be in the 1–2 range.

If you know the current platelet count, you can use it to gauge the best pressure. Most people with platelet counts in the 50–100 range can tolerate pressure levels 2–3, depending on how easily bruising is occurring; but below 50, limit overall

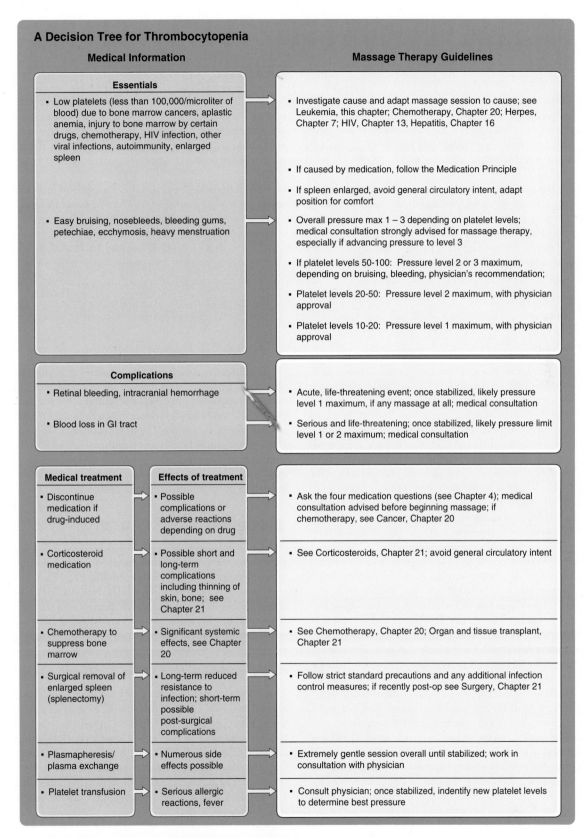

FIGURE 12-3. A Decision Tree for Thrombocytopenia.

pressure to level 2 so that your hands do not go beyond the superficial muscle layers (MacDonald, 2005, 2008). At this level, physician communication and permission to massage are strongly urged. Below 20, pressure level 1 is an absolute maximum. The client's treating physician and nurse should be consulted for permission to work with the client. Discuss any cautions against other activities, such as applying lotion, or pressure from the client's garments or bedding.

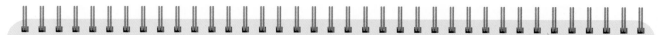

If you do not know the platelet count, and are not sure which pressure to use, stick with level 1, and always initiate a medical consultation before advancing pressure.

Taken together with the client's actual activity level in Question 6, a fairly complete picture should emerge of the client's health and vulnerability, and therefore a guide for overall pressure. If there are cardiovascular or neurological complications, the condition is very serious, and you may need to refer to Chapter 11 or Chapter 10 for more information on a specific condition. If the kidneys are affected by the condition, avoid general circulatory intent, but limiting pressure to 1 or 2 automatically takes care of that precaution. See the Decision Tree (Figure 12-3) for other bleeding complications.

Questions 7 and 8 could yield a range of treatments for thrombocytopenia, depending on the cause of the condition and the form it takes. If a client has had to discontinue a medication, it should cue you to a whole set of questions about what the drug was used for in the first place, and any related massage guidelines. A medical consultation may be necessary before beginning massage.

If the client is receiving corticosteroids, then fluid balance may be affected, and general circulatory intent should be avoided. There are other adjustments for corticosteroid treatment in Chapter 21. If the spleen was removed, see "Surgery," Chapter 21, and follow good infection control measures.

Notice that chemotherapy shows up twice in the Decision Tree: when used to treat cancer, chemotherapy may be a *cause* of thrombocytopenia, or when used to suppress immunity, it may be a *treatment* for an autoimmune condition. In either case, chemotherapy is strong medication with sweeping effects to consider. Consult Chapter 20 where chemotherapy is addressed in detail.

In acute thrombocytopenia, platelet transfusion may be necessary. Be alert for complications of transfusion. Moreover, new platelet levels must be established after transfusion, and potentially new massage pressure guidelines. Once the client has stabilized, determine the new platelet levels to determine the best pressure. If you are planning work with a client post-transfusion, work with the approval of the treating physician, and in communication with the medical team. This is a good guideline for plasmapheresis, as well.

● MASSAGE RESEARCH

As of this writing, there are no randomized, controlled trials, published in the English language, on thrombocytopenia and massage indexed in PubMed or the Massage Therapy Foundation Research Database. The NIH RePORTER tool lists no active, federally funded research projects on the topic in the United States. No active projects are listed on the clinicaltrials.gov database (see Chapter 6).

● POSSIBLE MASSAGE BENEFITS

Thrombocytopenia can be a serious condition, or it can be secondary to a serious condition; it is stressful, in either case. Whether acute or chronic, touch may be welcomed by someone who is concerned about possible complications or strong treatment. Living with such a heightened sense of fragility, knowing that tissues can bleed and bruise easily, a person might appreciate skilled, reassuring touch. Therapist's Journal 12-1 tells a story of massage therapy during a platelet transfusion.

Leukemia

Leukemia is a cancer of blood and bone marrow, affecting the bone marrow, the circulating white blood cells, the spleen, and lymph nodes.

● BACKGROUND

White blood cells (WBCs), or **leukocytes**, function in the body's immunity, fighting infection. There are several types of white blood cells, including *granulocytes, monocytes*, and *lymphocytes*. **Lymphocytes** are responsible for the production of antibodies to microorganisms, and for attacking the body's cells that have been invaded by viruses, destroying them. Of equal importance are **neutrophils**, a type of granulocyte that is on the front line of the immune system, one of the first to travel to a site of infection, attack, and destroy invading microorganisms. Neutrophils serve in the body's defense against bacterial and fungal infections.

In leukemia, immature, poorly functioning blood cells are produced in great number in the bone marrow, eventually spilling into the bloodstream. For this reason, a person with leukemia can have a very high WBC count, but low WBC function. These proliferating cells crowd out the production and distribution of other healthy and mature WBCs, RBCs, and platelets. Depending on the type of leukemia, the effect on healthy cells can be slight or significant; if significant, the condition is life threatening.

These deficiencies in blood cell function are felt throughout the body: both anemia and thrombocytopenia have systemic effects. Defective WBCs, especially neutrophils, lead to poor immunity and leave the body vulnerable to infection (see Neutropenia, Conditions in Brief). Immature cells in the blood can also infiltrate other tissues and organs, such as the joints, brain, liver, spleen, and kidneys. Their presence in these tissues causes pain or swelling, and impairs tissue and organ function.

There are many types of leukemia, typically classified by the cell types affected, and by how quickly the disease develops and progresses. **Lymphocytic** or *lymphoid* leukemia affects lymphocytes, and **myelogenous**, or *myeloid* leukemia affects myeloid cells, the precursors to other blood cell types. **Chronic leukemia** develops and progresses slowly, and individuals with the condition may be on a "watch and wait" monitoring program rather than treatment. In chronic leukemia, there is still room for some mature, healthy blood cells to carry out normal function. **Acute leukemia** develops and progresses rapidly, and blood cell functions are significantly impaired. Medical treatment is generally started as quickly as possible in these cases.

From these classifications, four main types of leukemia emerge. These are:

- Acute Lymphocytic Leukemia (ALL)
- Acute Myelogenous Leukemia (AML)
- Chronic Lymphocytic Leukemia (CLL)
- Chronic Myelogenous Leukemia (CML)

Acute lymphocytic leukemia (ALL) typically affects children and is sometimes called *acute childhood leukemia*. It is also referred to as *acute lymphoblastic leukemia* because the proliferating cells are immature lymphocytes, called lymphoblasts. For a massage therapist's account of her young child's ALL, see Therapist's Journal 12-2.

Acute myelogenous leukemia (AML) is most prevalent in older adults—age 60 and older, and it occurs more often in men than women. Risk factors include previous radiation and chemical exposures, smoking, and previous chemotherapy for another cancer, such as ovarian cancer or ALL.

Chronic lymphocytic leukemia (CLL) tends to affect adults aged 50 and older. There are few known risk factors, although exposure to agricultural chemicals and certain environmental toxins has been implicated. CLL develops gradually, and may go unnoticed until a routine physical examination.

See "My Journey with CLL," online at http://thePoint.lww.com/Walton, for one massage therapist's experience of it.

Chronic myelogenous leukemia (CML) is a rare, poorly understood form of leukemia that occurs in adults, affecting more men than women. It rarely occurs in children. There are few known risk factors. It is not linked to chemical exposure, and few people with CML have a history of exposure to high levels of radiation.

Signs and Symptoms

Although the signs and symptoms of leukemia vary somewhat according to the specific type, the common ones are listed here. For massage therapists, it is essential to learn which symptoms are present in a given client, and the interview questions below are designed accordingly.

Typically leukemia causes anemia, along with fatigue and weakness, susceptibility to infection due to deficient WBC activity, and easy bruising and bleeding when platelet function is compromised. Impaired clotting can produce bleeding gums, nosebleeds, and bleeding into the skin, producing petechiae and ecchymoses (see "Thrombocytopenia," this chapter). Lumps and swelling may form in the lymph nodes, and swelling can occur in the spleen, liver, or thymus. The spleen may become congested and enlarged and extend well beyond its normal borders, as shown in Figure 12-4. The ribs may flare with massive enlargement, which can occur in CML.

As they proliferate, immature blood cells of leukemia infiltrate the joint spaces, giving rise to joint pain. Pain is also felt in the bones, especially in the sternum, ribs, and tibia, because of the space occupied in the marrow by leukemic cells. If cells infiltrate the brain or spinal cord, CNS symptoms can result, such as headache, seizures, nausea and vomiting, vision changes, and dizziness. If the thymus swells (as in ALL), the nearby vasculature may be compressed, producing swelling in the arms and head; this constitutes a medical emergency.

Leukemia symptoms can also include fever, loss of appetite, weight loss, and night sweats. Especially with chronic types, the symptoms may be vague and nonspecific. Leukemia is diagnosed using a combination of physical exam, blood work, and **bone marrow examination**, in which needles are used to aspirate liquid and withdraw marrow from the bone (*bone marrow biopsy*) for examination. The bone marrow is accessed with special needles, often at the iliac crest, shown in Figure 12-5. The area may be extremely tender for several days after the procedure.

Complications

It is difficult to separate the complications of leukemia from the essential signs, symptoms, and problems presented by the disease. The complications listed here will include problems caused by acute, severe, and in some cases later disease.

One of the obvious complications is serious infection, because leukemia involves a deficiency in the immune response: respiratory infections, mouth and throat ulcerations, and urinary tract infections are common. Severe cases can result in pneumonia, or even **sepsis**, a blood infection, usually bacterial, that can lead to the failure of multiple organs. Sepsis is life threatening.

Severe bleeding is another complication of leukemia. Impaired clotting may lead to hemorrhage into the joints, central nervous system, retina, and other vital tissues.

In ALL, one particularly grave complication is **disseminated intravascular coagulation (DIC)**. In this condition, the blood

THERAPIST'S JOURNAL 12-2 *Everyone Has a Story: My Son's Leukemia*

When my first son Michael was 2 years old, he was diagnosed with acute lymphocytic leukemia (ALL). He was very sick at the time: low platelets, low RBCs, and a white count off the charts, but the white cells were immature and not doing their job, so he was vulnerable to infection.

He underwent two phases of chemotherapy. The first, remission induction, lasted 8 weeks. It was very strong chemotherapy. Although it did induce remission, this meant that the leukemia was not detectable; not that it was gone. Then he went through consolidation for 2 years, less intense chemotherapy. During this phase of treatment, he was hospitalized every other weekend for a year for 4 days to receive the medication. At the end of that time, our lives started to return to some type of normal, and because of my experience with Michael and his illness, I was inspired to start massage school at the end of his consolidation treatment.

Eight months later, he was feeling well, but on a routine follow-up visit, he was diagnosed with ALL again. He was treated even more aggressively this time, including a 21-day cycle of radiation to the brain.

It was a long, long haul, but he is now a healthy 15-year-old. He is undergoing growth hormone treatments because the chemotherapy affected his growth, but he is well and full of life.

During his treatments, I massaged him a lot. I remember once, when he was 3 years old, playing in the playroom of the hospital in his little yellow hospital gown—I reached for his shoulders and massaged them. He stopped playing and stood absolutely still, taking it in. I remember needing to massage him, how important it was to be able to offer him soothing human contact, since all the medical tests and treatments were so invasive.

I made massage adjustments according to changes in his condition. His platelets were low, so I used gentle pressure. When his WBC count was low from the chemotherapy, we were careful about infection precautions. We couldn't have visitors in the house, and in terms of massage, I had to be careful, too. If he had an infection, or when he had discomfort or symptoms I didn't fully understand, then I would massage his head carefully. I massaged his feet a lot—it was my interest in reflexology that got me into massage school. I didn't do much in the way of circulatory massage. It was too much for him, and he was too little.

Massage seemed to help Michael. It eased his nausea and pain, and it served as a distraction tool. When he was hurting from injections and blood draws, I would massage his head, arm, or foot to distract him from the needle, and head massage settled him. I felt so helpless, and it was good to offer him comfort, connection, and, when necessary, distraction.

Leukemia turned our world upside down. Having had this experience with Michael and his treatments brought me a broader understanding of my massage clients who are ill. The biggest part is compassion and empathy. I have been through the emotions, so I understand them in others. I have a client with fibromyalgia and she struggles some days. Feelings I've had are similar to what my clients describe. I recognize the emotional piece, and I'm not afraid of it in my clients.

Also, I realized each person has a story. This one happens to be mine: my son had leukemia. The story is behind me, but it's with me still. Everyone has a story. I remind myself of this whenever I'm aggravated because someone is giving me a hard time. She or he has a story, too, a story that's still present, making it difficult for both of us. Remembering that, I remember my compassion.

Kim Bonadio
Waltham, MA

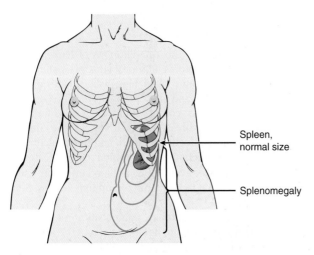

FIGURE 12-4. Enlargement of the spleen (splenomegaly). The spleen extends downward and toward the midline as it expands in size.

Spleen, normal size

Splenomegaly

clots abnormally, resulting in clots throughout peripheral blood vessels. Clotting factors get used up in this extreme process, preventing the normal clotting mechanism when an injury occurs; this leads to uncontrolled bleeding. In DIC, bleeding and clotting occur simultaneously. It is a medical emergency.

Treatment

Although treatment approaches differ, depending on the type of leukemia, it is often treated with chemotherapy, given in stages. The first goal is to bring about remission, especially if there is a crisis of proliferating cells. Chemotherapy often starts with **remission induction therapy**, to destroy the leukemia cells in the bone marrow and blood. **Consolidation therapy** follows; in leukemia, this usually consists of high doses of chemotherapy to continue eliminating residual cells. A course of **maintenance therapy**, with lower doses, may follow over several years to preserve remission.

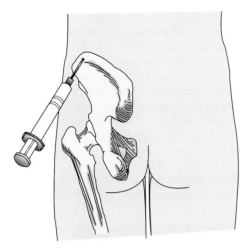

FIGURE 12-5. A bone marrow examination. A needle is used to draw off bone marrow for laboratory testing.

Other anticancer drugs, such as *kinase inhibitors* including imatinib (Gleevec), dasatinib (Sprycell), and nilotinib (Tasigna), may be used in leukemia treatment. These drugs may cause side effects including fever, low blood counts, and edema. Radiation therapy may be used over the whole body, or focused on an area of the body. Biologic therapies (e.g., immunotherapy with interferon) and monoclonal antibodies, large numbers of antibodies to cancer cells, are another type of therapy used in leukemia. A stem cell transplant may be necessary in order to replace the leukemic cells with healthy cells (see Organ and Tissue Transplant, Chapter 21).

Leukemia therapies are strong treatments, with multiple side effects. See Chapter 20, for more discussion of the common side effects of cancer treatments.

● INTERVIEW QUESTIONS

1. What type of leukemia do you have?
2. How does it affect you? Do you have any areas of pain?
3. How are your blood cells affected? Are there any effects on red blood cells or platelets? Are there any effects on white blood cell function?
4. Are any of your organs congested or swollen, such as your liver, spleen, kidney, or thymus?
5. Are any of your lymph nodes swollen?
6. Is there any swelling or risk of swelling anywhere?
7. Does the condition affect your skin? Do you have any bruising or bleeding?
8. Has leukemia affected any vital organs, such as your liver, brain, or kidney?
9. Has your condition led to any acute problems or episodes, requiring emergency medical attention? If so, how recently?
10. How is your energy level? Your activity level?
11. How is it being treated?
12. How does treatment affect you?

● MASSAGE THERAPY GUIDELINES

Question 1 will typically yield one of the four most common types of leukemia. Listen for the word "acute" or "chronic." If it is acute and current, it is much more serious, although chronic leukemia can develop into an acute situation over time. If the leukemia is a type that you don't

recognize, the client may be able to provide helpful information. The remaining questions should deliver the most relevant information for massage, regardless of the type of the leukemia.

Question 2 addresses the general effects of the disease. Answers can range from "not at all," signifying either a resolved condition, to "a lot," signaling widely felt effects on blood cells or organs. Leukemia causes numerous signs and symptoms, and most call for a gentle session overall. Fever is one example of this: Avoid general circulatory intent, in keeping with the Compromised Client Principle.

If the client reports pain in the bones or joints, pressure should be gentle, at level 1–2 for most, and joint movement should be performed well within the client's comfortable range. If a recent bone marrow biopsy was performed, ask the client to point to the area and use either cautious pressure there, or avoid contact entirely. If you do work over areas of pain, try using full hand contact, gentle pressure, and attention over affected areas. Stationary holds may be particularly likely to ease the client's pain.

The answers to Questions 2–12 will help you determine how strong or gentle the massage session should be. Common clinical features of leukemia and appropriate massage therapy adjustments are shown in Figure 12-7. For symptoms that are not flagged by Questions 2–12, or are not addressed here, think through any possible massage adjustments and consult the client's physician.

Question 3 gets at the heart of any problems caused by the condition. In general, since chronic conditions allow room for some mature blood cells to function, massage adjustments in chronic conditions may be only slight. If effects are significant, as in acute conditions, massage adjustments are also significant. If leukemia is crowding out RBCs, use the simple massage adjustments for anemia symptoms in Figure 12-6; see "Anemia," this chapter, for a full discussion. If the client bruises and bleeds easily, general pressure will need adjusting; see "Thrombocytopenia," this chapter, for specific massage therapy guidelines.

For deficiencies in WBC function, follow appropriate infection control precautions dictated by the client's medical team. Monitor your own health carefully, and offer to cancel or reschedule if you are feeling sick or have symptoms that could indicate respiratory, skin, or GI infection. Even a scratchy throat, which could signify allergies, is of interest to someone with impaired immunity, and they should be notified. See Neutropenia, Conditions in Brief, for more discussion of modifying massage in compromised immunity.

Questions 4–6 address swelling in different ways and from different perspectives. In a good interview, there is more than one chance to answer an important question, with several chances to cue the answers. Swelling in leukemia is an important consideration for massage, and so Question 6 can be a "catch-all" for anything not captured in the answers to Questions 4 and 5. If a lymph node is swollen, carefully avoid circulatory intent at and near the site, limiting your pressure to level 1 at the site and the general region drained by the affected node.

If the liver or spleen is congested, avoid massage with general circulatory intent, following the Filter and Pump Principle. If swelling occurs in the face, head, or arms, it is a medical emergency, and do not massage any of the swollen areas with pressure or circulatory intent.

The Filter and Pump Principle. If a filtering organ—liver, spleen, kidney, or lymph node—or a pumping organ—the heart—is functioning poorly or overworking, do not work it harder with massage that is circulatory in intent.

If the spleen is significantly swollen, lying on the table may be uncomfortable for the client. Massive splenomegaly may occur in some types of leukemia, to the point where the spleen visibly expands the ribs and abdomen (see Figure 12-4). See "Positioning for an Enlarged Spleen," online, for a therapist's adaptations to the condition.

Question 7, about skin changes, is an additional catch-all question: another cue for bruising or bleeding, and a cue for any skin reactions to treatment, rashes, itching, or dryness relevant to massage. See "General Principles," Chapter 7, for possible massage concerns when working with skin changes.

If the client responds affirmatively to Question 8 about infiltration of the liver, brain, or kidneys, follow the Vital Organ Principle. Gentle massage elements are appropriate overall, and in the case of liver and kidney impairment, avoid massage with general circulatory intent. Any time a vital organ is affected by leukemia, medical consultation is a good idea.

If the CNS is affected (brain or spinal cord), additional problems may be present, such as seizures or headaches. For

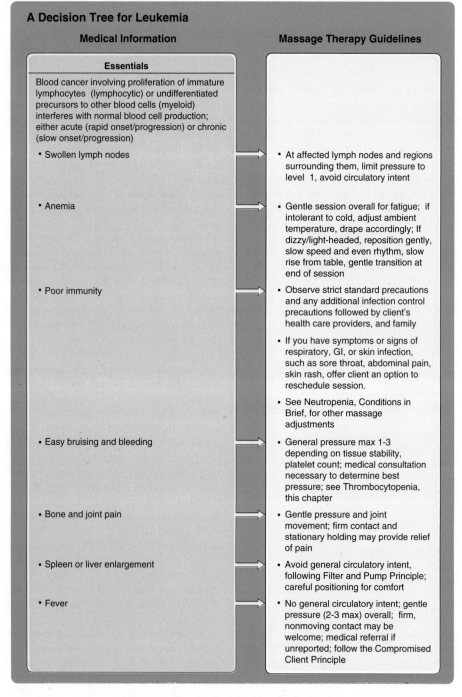

FIGURE 12-6. A Decision Tree for leukemia.

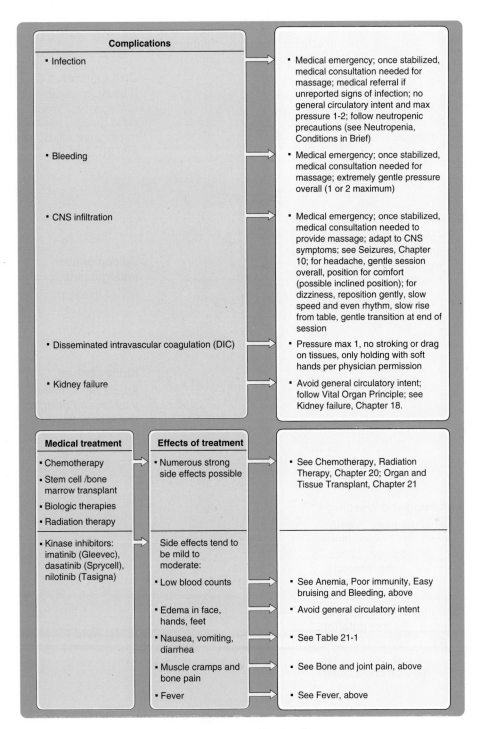

FIGURE 12-6. (*Continued*).

seizures, see Conditions in Brief, Chapter 10. For headaches associated with leukemia, extremely gentle work is indicated, with positioning for comfort, including propping or placing the client in the inclined position. For dizziness, see the Decision Tree (Figure 12-6).

> *The Vital Organ Principle. If a vital organ—heart, lung, kidney, liver, or brain—is compromised in function, use gentle massage elements and adjust them to pose minimal challenge to the client's body.*

Questions 9 and 10 are ways to determine how acute the condition is, or how acute it has recently been. A current or recently acute condition, such as infection, kidney failure, or bleeding, calls for a very gentle session overall; see the Decision Tree for more detail (Figure 12-6). For DIC, the pressure level should be limited to 1, with no drag on the tissues; any massage should be limited to holding with soft hands, and the permission of the physician is advised.

A gentler session is in order for a client with low energy and activity levels, but at the other end of the leukemia spectrum, some people with chronic types of leukemia maintain good activity levels and high function. These clients are better able

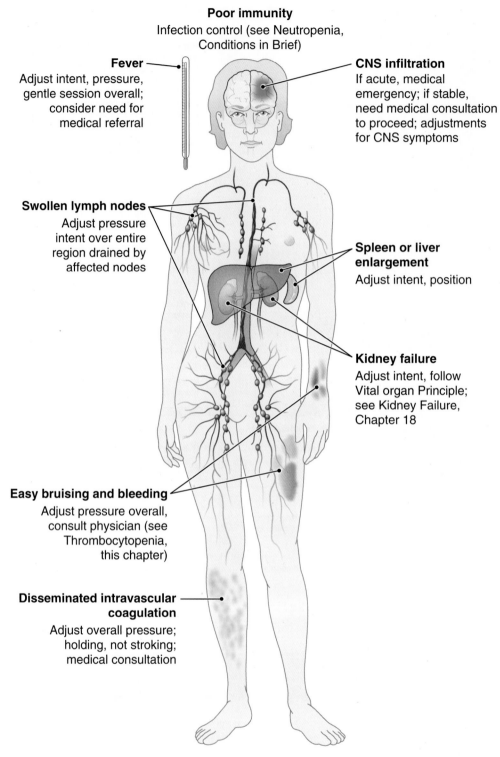

Poor immunity
Infection control (see Neutropenia,
Conditions in Brief)

Fever
Adjust intent, pressure,
gentle session overall;
consider need for
medical referral

CNS infiltration
If acute, medical
emergency; if stable,
need medical consultation
to proceed; adjustments
for CNS symptoms

Swollen lymph nodes
Adjust pressure
intent over entire
region drained by
affected nodes

**Spleen or liver
enlargement**
Adjust intent, position

Kidney failure
Adjust intent, follow
Vital organ Principle;
see Kidney Failure,
Chapter 18

Easy bruising and bleeding
Adjust pressure overall,
consult physician (see
Thrombocytopenia,
this chapter)

**Disseminated intravascular
coagulation**
Adjust overall pressure;
holding, not stroking;
medical consultation

FIGURE 12-7. Leukemia: Selected clinical features and massage adjustments to consider. Specific instructions and additional massage therapy guidelines are in Decision Tree and text.

to tolerate stronger massage elements. The Activity and Energy Principle (see Chapter 3) is useful here.

Questions 11 and 12 are essential if the client is in current treatment, or has recently (in the past year) completed treatment for leukemia. Side effects, such as those caused by kinase inhibitors, are described in the Decision Tree and should be incorporated into the massage session. Treatments for leukemia tend to be strong—chemotherapy, stem cell transplant, radiation

therapy, and biologic therapies. In fact, chemotherapy is carefully calibrated in leukemia patients because it has effects on blood cell populations that are similar to the effects of the leukemia itself. Massage therapy needs to be adjusted to the effects of strong treatment on blood cells, skin, neurological function, and well-being, among other parameters. These issues are handled in detail in Chapter 20 on cancer, and in Chapter 21 on medical treatments.

● MASSAGE RESEARCH

There is little research focused on massage and leukemia. A small RCT of 20 subjects reports that daily, parent-provided massage of children with leukemia improves overall WBC and neutrophil counts (Field et al, 2001); however, re-analysis of the data (Beider and Moyer, 2006) suggested no effect from massage. Even though a "boost" in immunity from massage is a popular claim in massage therapy, there is not yet sufficient research to support it (see "Making Accurate Claims about Massage," Chapter 6).

In another small study, with a sample size of 12, researchers looked at Healing Touch in people with leukemia (Danhauer et al., 2008). Healing Touch is a gentle energy therapy. The authors noticed some improvement in patients after the intervention, but there was no control group in the study, so it was difficult to draw firm conclusions.

Although a solid foundation of research evidence on massage and leukemia has yet to be built, patients with leukemia are often included in studies on massage and cancer (see Chapter 20), and are heavily represented in research on stem cell and bone marrow transplant (see Chapter 21). Research in both of these areas is growing.

● POSSIBLE MASSAGE BENEFITS

Leukemia is a serious disease, and individuals can benefit from the stress relief of skilled massage. Skilled touch may even provide symptom relief for nausea, fatigue, and pain, as these are often aggravated by stress and may be eased by relaxation. Chronic leukemia can be managed and monitored for years, and it can be stressful, even without the acute events characterized by ALL and AML. Individuals experiencing chronic disease can also benefit from the human connection that massage provides.

Other Blood Conditions in Brief

HEMOCHROMATOSIS

Background	• Inherited liver disorder, causing overabsorption of dietary iron and storage of excess in liver, pancreas, and heart; usually diagnosed in midlife. • Signs and symptoms are joint pain (especially in hands), bronze skin pigmentation, fatigue, abdominal pain, hypothyroidism, loss of sex drive, loss of menstrual periods (amenorrhea). • Late complications include cirrhosis, liver failure, liver cancer, arrhythmia, congestive heart failure, diabetes. • Treated by periodic removal of blood (phlebotomy) to reduce iron levels.
Interview Questions	• How does it affect you? Any effects on your joints, or abdomen? • Do you have any complications, such as effects on your liver, pancreas, or heart? Do you have any cirrhosis? Any diabetes? Any heart problems? • Treatment? Effects of treatment?
Massage Therapy Guidelines	• Adjust massage to symptoms; use gentle movement if joint pain present; if hypothyroidism is present, see Chapter 17. • If fatigue, gentle session overall; follow Activity and Energy Principle; abdominal pain may dictate a position change, or no use of prone position. • Address complications affecting major organs; if "Arrhythmia" or "Congestive Heart Failure," see Chapter 11; if "Liver Disease," see Chapter 16; if "Diabetes," see Chapter 17.

HEMOPHILIA

Background	• A group of blood clotting disorders, range in severity depending on which clotting factor is missing. Classified as mild hemophilia A, moderate to severe hemophilia A, hemophilia B, and hemophilia C. • Causes easy bruising and bleeding, tendency to prolonged bleeding; nosebleeds or large bruises may occur. • Complications include bleeding into joints, with joint pain and swelling; blood may appear in urine or stool. • Emergency signs or symptoms include sudden pain in large joints and muscles, with swelling, warmth; persistent or painful headache, neck pain, blurred vision, extreme fatigue, vomiting.

- Significant blood loss or cerebral hemorrhage can be fatal.
- Treatment depends on severity: Injected, infused, or nasal desmopressin (DDAVP), a clotting factor stimulator, is given for mild hemophilia, either in acute bleeding, or prophylactically; side effects are mild headache, nausea, abdominal cramping, flushing.
- Clotting factors are replaced through blood transfusions, genetically engineered clotting factors; may cause nausea, fatigue, fever, chills.

Interview Questions	
	• What type of hemophilia do you have: Is it mild, moderate, or severe? How does it affect you?

- What type of hemophilia do you have: Is it mild, moderate, or severe? How does it affect you?
- How do your tissues respond to various massage pressures, or the pressure of applying lotion?
- Any effects on joints or muscles? Any pain in joints or neck?
- Treatment? Effects of treatment?

Massage Therapy Guidelines

- Reduce overall pressure, depending on severity of condition and stability of tissues; input from physician and thorough client history are needed.
- Perform joint movement with care, especially if joints are stiff or swollen from bleeding into joints.
- Adapt to side effects of medications or clotting factors (see Table 21-1); follow Emergency Protocol Principle for emergency signs or symptoms.

MYELOMA, MULTIPLE MYELOMA

Background

- Cancer of bone marrow, causing plasma cells, a subset of WBC's, to proliferate, diminishing production of other blood cells and antibodies.
- May be slow growing; tumors invade and erode compact bone at multiple sites in the body, weakening bone at lesion sites; substances produced by tumor also cause generalized bone thinning (see "Osteoporosis," Chapter 9).
- Bone breakdown leads to increased blood calcium levels, causing constipation, excessive thirst, increased urination, confusion, nausea, loss of appetite; kidney failure and kidney stones may result.
- Tumors cause pain with invasion of the spine, ribs, and hips; in 70% of cases, bone pain occurs in lumbar area; in 20% of cases, spinal cord compression occurs.
- Complications include anemia (this chapter), frequent infections from poor immunity (often in bladder, kidney, sinuses, lungs), easy bruising and bleeding from low platelets; rarely, blood thickens, impeding flow to skin, fingers, toes, kidneys, brain.
- Treatment may include watch and wait approach if no symptoms are present or diagnosis uncertain; in advanced cases, chemotherapy, radiation therapy, and stem cell transplantation may be used (see Chapter 20).
- Dialysis, pain medications, antibiotics, colony-stimulating factors such as filgrastim, erythropoietin (see "Anemia," this chapter) are used to manage symptoms and complications.

Interview Questions

- How serious is your multiple myeloma considered to be? Are you being treated for it, or just monitored ("watch and wait")?
- Where is it and how does it affect you?
- Any effects of myeloma on your bone or spine stability? Are your doctors or nurses concerned about the stability of your bones, or risk of fracture? Are you monitored for bone stability or risk of fracture?
- What is your activity level? Any medical restrictions on activity?
- Do you have any areas of pain? Any pain in your back? Any areas of new or worsening weakness, numbness, tingling, sharp or radiating pain, or problems with bladder/bowel control?
- Do you have any complications? Any effects on your blood or blood cells, including anemia or fatigue? Is your immune system functioning well? Any current or recent infections?
- Are your platelets affected? Do you have any clotting problems, or easy bruising or bleeding?
- Are there any effects on your kidneys?
- Treatment? Effects of treatment?

Massage Therapy Guidelines

- Review "Cancer," Chapter 20, for massage therapy guidelines for cancer and cancer treatment; no direct massage pressure at/over active tumor site.
- Assess bone stability to determine safe pressure. Be careful with joint movement and pressure at site where bone stability is in question; pressure level 1 or 2 may be maximum, depending on stability; use very cautious pressure for pain unless client has reported to physician, physician has followed up, and approves advancing massage pressure to level 3.
- Use client activity level, medical restrictions on activity, regular checking in about diagnostic tests for bone stability in assessing safest pressure.
- If client reports new pain, urgent medical referral; follow the Waiting for a Diagnosis Principle (see Chapter 3); if client reports new neurologic symptoms such as weakness, numbness, sharp pain, or problems with bladder/bowel control, immediate medical referral.
- Adapt massage to low RBC, WBC, or platelet counts (see "Leukemia," this chapter).
- Adjust massage to complications such as infection (general circulatory intent contraindicated), easy bruising and bleeding (gentle pressure overall). If kidney function affected, follow the Filter and Pump Principle (see Kidney failure, Chapter 18).
- Adapt to treatments (see Chapter 20). If client takes pain medications, use gentle pressure overall and adapt to side effects (see "Analgesics," Chapter 21). If side effects of antibiotics occur, see Table 21-1 for massage guidelines. For colony-stimulating factors, adjust pressure and avoid circulatory intent at the injection site until the medication has absorbed.

NEUTROPENIA, LEUKOPENIA

Background

- Low WBC count (leukopenia); abnormally low blood level of neutrophils (neutropenia), white blood cells that make up 45%–75% of total WBCs in bloodstream under normal conditions.
- Normal neutrophil counts = 1,200–1,500 cells/mm^3 of blood; below 1,000, risk of infection increases; below 500, serious risk of infection; below 200, severe risk of infection.
- Causes include cancer treatments, bone marrow/blood cancers and aplastic anemia, autoimmune diseases, congested spleen, Vitamin B$_{12}$ or folic acid deficiency, drugs and environmental toxins.
- Can be chronic, acute, or cyclical, with intermittent bouts of neutropenia over time; causes fatigue; frequent or unusual infections occur (skin, respiratory), can become uncontrolled, life threatening. Mouth sores (stomatitis) common as immune function declines
- Acute neutropenia (with neutropenic fever) treated with antibiotics, antifungals; colony-stimulating factors used to stimulate WBC include filgrastim (Neupogen), long-acting pegfilgrastim (Neulasta); common side effects include bone or muscle pain, headache, nausea, cough.
- Cause is treated where possible (removal of environmental toxin, stopping immunosuppressive drug treatment, corticosteroids for autoimmune condition).
- Infection prevention through neutropenic precautions such as avoiding crowds, avoiding contact with people who are ill or recently vaccinated, requiring others to glove, mask, or gown; when WBC count below 1,000, avoiding uncooked foods, fresh flowers, soil, dental work.

Interview Questions

- How serious is your neutropenia? Is it acute, chronic, cyclical? What is the cause?
- How does it affect you? How are your WBC counts, and how concerned is your doctor about your counts?
- Any signs or symptoms of infection, such as fever? Any mouth sores?
- Are there any medical restrictions on your activities?
- Describe any steps you are instructed to take for hygiene or infection control. Do the people around you need to take special precautions?
- Treatment? Effects of treatment?

Massage Therapy Guidelines

- Adapt to cause of neutropenia such as cancer treatment (see Chapter 20), blood cancers (see "Leukemia," Multiple Myeloma, this chapter), spleen enlargement (avoid general circulatory intent, adjust position for comfort, and investigate cause), and others.
- Avoid general circulatory intent, use gentle massage overall, even if no infection is present.
- Observe strict standard precautions *and* implement additional infection control precautions as specified by client's physician or nurse, including gloving or masking; scheduling client for low-traffic times, etc.

- If you have symptoms or signs of infection, such as sore throat, abdominal pain, skin rash, then call client with neutropenia (or at risk of neutropenia) and offer option to reschedule session.
- If mouth sores present, avoid pull or pressure at site (on chin, jaw); use alternatives to face cradle to avoid pressure or drag on the face.
- Adjust massage to any side effects of antibiotics (see Table 21-1); if client's spleen was surgically removed, lifelong hygienic precautions are in place.
- Urgent or immediate medical referral if client has fever, unreported to physician.

POLYCYTHEMIA VERA

Background	- Rare, serious increase in RBC's with unknown cause. - Blood thickening causes breathing difficulty when lying down, shortness of breath, spleen congestion, headache, dizziness, itching, reddened skin, thrombosis. - Poor platelet formation can result, causing abnormal bleeding; platelets and WBCs may also be *increased*. - Treatment with phlebotomy (blood removal); low-dose aspirin (see "NSAIDs," Chapter 21) used to prevent blood clots. - Hydroxyurea, anagrelide used to suppress bone marrow; interferon alpha also used; see "Thrombocythemia," this chapter, for side effects.
Interview Questions	- When diagnosed? How does it affect you? Do you have increases in other blood cells (WBC's, platelets) as a result? - Do you have any complications, such as breathing problems, enlarged spleen, headache, or dizziness? Any itching or reddened skin? - Any bruising or bleeding problems? - Have you had any problems with blood clots? What is your doctor's assessment of your blood clot, stroke, or heart attack risk? - Treatment? Effects of treatment?
Massage Therapy Guidelines	- Risk of bleeding and/or clotting is serious; medical consultation strongly recommended for massage, especially if advancing pressure past level 2. - In milder forms, use gentle pressure overall (pr = 2–3 maximum), and follow DVT Risk Principles; in moderate or severe cases, follow DVT Risk Principle I indefinitely (see Chapter 11). - Avoid general circulatory intent; use cautious pressure at arterial pulse points; avoid friction if itching is a problem. - If spleen enlarged, adjust massage position for comfort; consider inclined, side-lying or seated position for breathing difficulties. See "Thrombocythemia," this chapter, and Table 21-1 for massage therapy guidelines for other medication side effects.

SICKLE-CELL DISEASE

Background	- Inherited form of anemia. Altered RBC's form fragile crescent shape, destroyed prematurely; cells block blood flow, causing symptoms; milder form is sickle-cell trait. - Sickle-cell crisis is pain in long bones, spine, abdomen, chest; episodes are mild (a few hours) or severe (lasting days, requiring hospitalization). - Rapid RBC turnover causes jaundice, swollen spleen, frequent infection. Blocked blood flow causes hand-foot syndrome (swollen feet and hands). - Vision problems, stunted and delayed growth in children. - Complications include stroke, vision impairment, ulcerations on legs, gallstones, organ damage. - Acute chest syndrome (chest pain, fever, breathing difficulty), a medical emergency, is caused by blocked vessels in lungs; repeated episodes can lead to lung damage, pulmonary hypertension. - May increase risk of DVT. - Treatments: hydroxyurea (see "Thrombocythemia," this chapter). Pain relief with NSAIDs, opioid analgesics (see Chapter 21). Antibiotics given for acute infection, and prophylactically in children and young adults. - Symptoms result from sickle-cell trait; moderate to severe symptoms result from sickle-cell disease. - In some cases, may be treated with bone marrow transplant (see Chapter 20).

Interview Questions	• What are your symptoms? Are you currently having a sickle-cell crisis? • Do you have frequent pain? For how long? Are you in pain now? If so, where? What are comfortable positions for you? • Effects of the disease on liver function? Kidney function? Lung function/breathing? • Condition of your skin, especially on thighs and lower legs? Any swelling anywhere? • Any complications of the condition? Recent hospitalization for this? When? • Treatment? Effects of treatment?
Massage Therapy Guidelines	• If symptoms are present, avoid general circulatory intent; adapt to pain with positioning changes, gentle pressure (2 max) overall, especially at pain sites. • If chronic breathing difficulty, adjust position for breathing comfort (consider sidelying, seated, semireclining); inquire to be sure it has been reported to physician to rule out acute chest syndrome (medical emergency). • Avoid contact at any ulceration sites; if liver, kidney, or lung function is affected, follow Vital Organ Principle. • Limit pressure to level 1–2 at sites of swelling; avoid circulatory intent at sites of swelling. • Limit joint movement to tolerance at painful joints. • Consider DVT Risk Principles (see Chapter 11)

THROMBOCYTHEMIA

Background	• Excess platelet production, with overtendency to clot and abnormal clotting; resulting platelet shortage can lead to clotting deficiency and hemorrhage. • May be primary, with unknown cause, or secondary to other conditions, such as splenectomy, bleeding, some infections, rheumatoid arthritis. • My be mild or asymptomatic, or include mild bleeding (nosebleeds) or bleeding into GI tract; liver or spleen may enlarge. • Clots form and block blood vessels, can cause tingling in hands and feet, headaches, dizziness, weakness; thrombotic events include stroke, DVT, pulmonary embolism, heart attack. • Treated with hydroxyurea (Droxia, Hydrea), which can cause diarrhea, constipation, nausea, vomiting, drowsiness, rash, itchiness; anagrelide (Agrylin) may cause fluid retention, heart problems, nausea, diarrhea, dizziness, headache. • May be treated with interferon-alpha injections, which can cause flu-like symptoms, nausea, diarrhea, seizures, confusion, sleepiness, depression. • Platelet removal from whole blood (plateletpheresis) used in emergencies.
Interview Questions	• What is the cause, if known? • How does it affect you? What are your symptoms? • Have you had any complications? History of blood clot, stroke, heart problems, other cardiovascular problems? • Treatment? Effects of treatment?
Massage Therapy Guidelines	• If caused by another condition, investigate massage therapy guidelines (see Rheumatoid arthritis, Chapter 9). • If liver, spleen enlarged, avoid general circulatory intent, adjust positioning for comfort (consider sidelying). • If medications cause fluid retention or heart problems, avoid general circulatory intent; avoid circulatory intent at site; see Table 21-1 for other side effects, massage therapy guidelines.

	THROMBOPHILIA
Background	• Increase in tendency to clotting in veins, or in both arteries and veins; due to inherited disorders in clotting proteins (*factor V Leiden*), or to acquired disorders such as lupus or DIC, sometimes associated with cancer. • May be asymptomatic, with no thrombosis, or may cause DVT, superficial venous thrombosis, PE. • For history of a single clot incident, treatment is with anticoagulants during periods of heightened risk, such as prolonged bed rest (see Table 11-1, Chapter 11). • For history of two or more clots, lifelong anticoagulant therapy.
Interview Questions	• When was it diagnosed? What is the cause? How does it affect you? • Have you ever developed a blood clot in the veins or arteries of your arms, legs, or elsewhere? Have there been any complications of the conditions, such as damage to tissues or pulmonary embolism? • Treatment? Effects of treatment?
Massage Therapy Guidelines	• Follow DVT Risk Principles, or DVT Risk Principle I indefinitely. • Anticoagulant therapy requires gentle pressure overall (pr 1–2 maximum), depending on tissue stability. • If DVT or PE history, see "Deep Vein Thrombosis," Chapter 11.

SELF TEST

1. Why is the Filter and Pump Principle used for many blood conditions? Which organs may be affected, and how should massage be adapted?
2. Describe five symptoms and two complications of anemia.
3. Why is it important for you to know the cause of a client's anemia?
4. Explain the massage adaptations that are necessary after a recent injection of a colony-stimulating factor, such as erythropoietin.
5. What are normal platelet levels? Describe the complications that occur at low platelet levels.
6. Describe how and when pressure may need to be modified for a client with thrombocytopenia.
7. Discuss how the Filter and Pump Principle can be an important consideration in working with some clients with low platelets.
8. What are two visible surface signs of thrombocytopenia, signaling a pressure modification?

9. Describe an activity restriction that is advised for an individual with severe thrombocytopenia.
10. Explain why WBC counts are high in leukemia, while resistance to infection may be compromised.
11. What are the four common types of leukemia and how do they differ from one another? Which type of leukemia usually affects children, and which form is common in older adults?
12. How does leukemia affect the function of RBCs and platelets? What are the signs and symptoms that can result?
13. Regarding leukemia, what modifications in massage therapy might be necessary for a client with a heightened vulnerability to infection?
14. List three side effects of kinase inhibitors, given in some cases of leukemia. Do side effects tend to be mild, moderate, or severe? How should massage be modified in each case?
15. Does the research on massage and leukemia support the claim that massage boosts immunity? Why or why not?

 For answers to these questions and to see a bibliography for this chapter, visit http://thePoint. lww.com/Walton.

13 Immune and Lymphatic System Conditions

All interest in disease and death is only another expression of interest in life.

—THOMAS MANN

When the immune and lymphatic systems work properly, they maintain a comfortable and clean internal environment in the blood and tissues. Together with the bone marrow and blood, these systems provide layers of protection against infection and other threats to health. Whenever the immune and lymphatic systems are injured or attacked, it presents a significant challenge to health and life.

White blood cells (WBCs) straddle the immune and lymphatic systems. They originate in the bone marrow, travel in the blood, and then function in the various lymphatic tissues, including the thymus, spleen, and lymph nodes of the lymphatic system. They also work to eradicate infection in any infected tissue of the body. Lymphoma, a disease of WBCs that appears in the lymphatic system, is addressed in this chapter, while leukemia, a WBC defined by its origin in bone marrow, is discussed in Chapter 12.

The lymphatic system is more anatomically distinct than the immune system. It is made up of a network of vessels and filters that drain the tissues. It concentrates immune activity in its various filters, including clusters of lymph nodes located in key regions of the body and in the spleen, the largest lymphoid organ. Tissues are cleansed of waste products,

excess plasma proteins left behind by the blood, and foreign substances. These materials are filtered and neutralized in the lymph nodes, and the filtered fluid is returned to the bloodstream. Immune system cells, and the substances they produce to neutralize foreign invaders, are scattered throughout the body, but they are concentrated most highly in tissues near the body's surface, at openings in the body, and wherever infection is likely to occur.

Immunodeficiency describes a medical condition or state in which some part of the immune system is inadequate, resulting in reduced resistance to infection. AIDS is an example of immunodeficiency. **Autoimmunity** is the tendency of the immune system to mount a defense against the body's own tissues as if they were foreign. Systemic lupus erythematosus, rheumatoid arthritis, and Crohn disease are autoimmune conditions.

This chapter addresses the following conditions at length, with full Decision Trees:

- HIV Disease
- Non-Hodgkin Lymphoma
- Lymphedema

Conditions in Brief included in this chapter are **allergy** (allergic reaction, hypersensitivity reaction), **autoimmunity**, **edema**, **Hodgkin lymphoma** (Hodgkin disease), **inflammation**, **lymphangitis and lymphadenitis**, and **systemic lupus erythematosus (SLE)**.

General Principles

Several principles from Chapter 3 can be applied to massage with clients who have immune and lymphatic conditions. In addition, two new principles are:

1. The Swelling Principle. *Adjust massage to the cause of swelling as well as the swelling itself. Swelling that appears suddenly, has no identified cause, is widespread, or is severe, persistent, or shiny, calls for an urgent medical referral; avoid general circulatory intent and circulatory intent at the site.*

   Because swelling can indicate a minor condition or a serious one, there is no single approach to swelling. Rather than applying massage indiscriminately, with the intent of alleviating it, find out the cause. Widespread swelling, such as in the face or the abdomen, can be very serious. Swelling in the ankles can be mild, from premenstrual syndrome, or it can indicate serious disease, such as heart failure. Because of this range, look for a diagnosis, or at least a clear

cause, such as an injury. Then adapt massage to the cause. If the advisability of circulatory intent is in question, then avoid it.

2. The Quadrant Principle for Lymphedema History. *In an area of lymphedema history, as well as the associated trunk quadrant, use extreme caution to avoid aggravating lymphedema. In these areas, follow any precautions specified by the client's lymphedema therapist and health care team, limit pressure to level 1, and avoid reddening the tissues. Also avoid circulatory intent, friction, joint movement, and excessive focus on the area, and any client positions known to compromise lymph flow.*

   This principle is used with any client who currently has, or has had, lymphedema—a type of swelling caused by an inherited or acquired structural problem in the lymphatic system. This principle is a refinement of the "Filter and Pump Principle" (see Chapter 3). It reflects the therapist's response to injury, deficiency, or disease in the lymphatic system. These conditions are explained further in the lymphedema section of this chapter. Because lymphedema most often occurs as a result of certain cancer treatments, this principle may be applied in many cases of cancer represented in this book.

HIV Disease

HIV disease is a broad term for the chronic disease resulting from infection with the **human immunodeficiency virus (HIV)**. HIV disease includes an asymptomatic phase, progressive impairment of the immune system, and AIDS. **Acquired immune deficiency syndrome (AIDS)** is the advanced form of the disease, in which the immune system is severely compromised and the individual is profoundly vulnerable to infection.

● BACKGROUND

HIV is spread through certain body fluids: blood, semen, breast milk, and vaginal secretions. HIV is transmitted by the passing of an infected fluid into the bloodstream of another person. Transmission occurs through sexual contact involving oral, vaginal, or anal penetration, by intravenous needle sharing, via the transfusion of blood or blood products, and from mother to child during pregnancy, birth, or breast-feeding.

A **T cell** or *T lymphocyte* is a type of white blood cell that matures in the thymus, and then plays a central role in the immune response, regulating the body's response to infection. One type of T cell, called a **CD4 lymphocyte** or *T helper cell*, is largely responsible for coordinating the immune response. HIV targets and damages CD4 cells, and the CD4 count is a measurement of how far HIV infection has progressed. Physicians also pay attention to the *viral load*, the number of HIV particles in the blood, to assess the infection status.

A person can live with HIV asymptomatically for many years. When an individual's CD4 marker, or *CD4 lymphocyte counts* drop to the 200–500 range (normal values are between 600 and 1,000), the risk of certain infections increases. HIV infection is officially called AIDS when an individual has a positive HIV test, plus either the development of one opportunistic infection or a CD4 lymphocyte count of 200 or less. A diagnosis of AIDS generally occurs 10 or more years after the initial infection.

Signs and Symptoms

The signs and symptoms of HIV infection vary depending on the progression of the disease, an individual's level of resistance, and treatment. During early infection, most people do not experience any distinct symptoms. Nonspecific flu-like symptoms, such as fatigue, fever, sore throat, and swollen lymph nodes, may occur a few weeks after HIV infection and may last several weeks. However, because of the nonspecific nature of these symptoms, and because they often subside, a person might not be prompted to seek medical attention and receive an HIV test. Thus, it is possible to be infected and to transmit HIV to others unknowingly. In fact, a person can be HIV-positive and not have symptoms for 8 or 9 years or more.

As immune system impairment progresses, the nonspecific symptoms of earlier infection tend to reappear. In addition, individuals experience mouth sores, muscle aches, cough, diarrhea, weight loss, shortness of breath, rash, and frequent, stubborn vaginal yeast infections.

Complications

Complications of HIV disease can be debilitating and even fatal. They tend to occur in later stages of infection. When the immune system is compromised, **opportunistic infections (OIs)** can develop. These are infections that would not take hold as easily in a person with a healthy immune system, but in the absence of a strong immune defense, they have the opportunity to thrive.

Opportunistic infections often cause serious illness in people with HIV disease. When CD4 counts drop to 200–500, the risk of OIs such as shingles and other skin infections increases, and thrush, upper respiratory and pulmonary infections can appear. Tuberculosis is also a risk at this level. When CD4 cells drop below 200, the risk of OI increases even more, and infections such as PCP and MAC appear with greater frequency.

The symptoms and signs of OI complications include high fever that lasts several weeks, chronic swollen lymph nodes, soaking night sweats, chills, persistent headaches, chronic diarrhea, debilitating fatigue, weight loss, and vision changes. Many of these symptoms occur even without an opportunistic infection and are due to HIV infection itself. Common OIs are:

- Bacterial infections: bacterial pneumonia; *mycobacterium avium complex (MAC)*, which affects the respiratory tract and other organs including bone marrow, liver, and spleen; tuberculosis (TB) (see Chapter 14); salmonella; *bacillary angiomatosis*, which produces skin lesions and spreads to liver and spleen.
- Viral infections: *cytomegalovirus (CMV)*, which causes damage to lungs, GI tract, and retina; viral hepatitis (see Chapter 16); herpes simplex virus (see Chapter 7); *human papillomavirus (HPV)*, which causes genital warts and increased risk of cervical cancer; *progressive multifocal leukoencephalopathy (PML)*, a serious CNS infection, which affects brain function.
- Fungal infections: candidiasis, which affects the oral cavity (thrush), esophagus, and vagina; *cryptococcal meningitis*, which can produce severe CNS complications.
- Parasitic infections: *pneumocystis pneumonia (PCP)*, which produces respiratory/pulmonary symptoms; *toxoplasmosis*, which can spread to all organs, especially the heart, lungs, eyes, and brain; *cryptosporidiosis*, which infects the intestines and bile duct.

Nausea, vomiting, and diarrhea occur in people with advanced disease, and AIDS can produce a **wasting syndrome**, or rapid loss of 10% or more of body weight. Treatments can help prevent this condition, and it is less common than it was in the early years of the disease. One neurological complication is **AIDS dementia complex**, a loss of cognitive function due to direct impact of HIV on the brain. Another neurological complication is peripheral neuropathy, which is not limited to the hands and feet as it often is in other conditions (see Chapter 10). In AIDS, peripheral neuropathy can also occur in other areas, including the face, and impair the function of autonomic nerves as well as somatic nerves.

Certain types of cancer are associated with HIV infection, such as non-Hodgkin lymphoma (this chapter). **Kaposi sarcoma (KS)**, a tumor of the blood vessels, appears at skin surfaces and the mouth as black or dark brown lesions in darker-skinned individuals, or purple, red, or pink lesions in lighter-skinned individuals (Figure 13-1). In addition women with HIV are at much higher risk of developing cervical cancer than women without HIV.

Treatment

Three general types of treatment are discussed here and on the Decision Tree: treatment that acts directly on HIV, treatment for opportunistic infections, and cancer treatment.

Treatment for HIV is often in the form of **highly active antiretroviral therapy (HAART)**, also called combination therapy, or the **cocktail**. HAART is a group of medications that attack the ability of the virus to replicate. The drugs include **protease inhibitors**, **entry inhibitors**, and **reverse transcriptase inhibitors**. Each of these inhibitors works against a different step in the process of viral replication. The drugs are very expensive and are used primarily in developed countries. Since the advent of HAART in 1996, death rates from HIV disease have dropped dramatically in countries with access to it.

The drugs in the HAART cocktail are very strong, and they affect different people differently. Fewer studies have been done on how they affect women than men, so some side effects in women are only beginning to be recognized and understood. Nausea, vomiting, and diarrhea are common side effects of starting or changing the medications, but in some people these pass after a few weeks of adjustment. Others who are on HAART therapies continue to struggle with chronic side effects and must continue to organize their lives around where the nearest bathroom is.

Fatigue can be a chronic side effect, some of it due to anemia. Women are more prone to anemia from HIV drugs than men, and it is important for anemia to be treated because untreated anemia is associated with HIV disease progression.

Other common side effects of HAART include headache; neurological symptoms such as tingling, pain, dizziness, and neuropathy; and rash. Neuropathy is a particularly troubling side effect, since it is also a complication of HIV, and can be difficult to treat. More common in women than men, a rash is a common response to HIV drugs. In rare cases, the rash can be severe and even life threatening.

Some changes in the shape and distribution of fat tissue, called **lipodystrophy**, can occur as a side effect of HIV drugs. Loss of fat from the face and extremities occurs, and fat can accumulate in the abdomen and at the back of the neck.

Over time, the drugs put women at risk for excessive menstrual bleeding and osteoporosis. Anemia in women may be due, at least in part, to excessive menstrual bleeding that can occur with HAART.

HAART dosage must be closely monitored by a physician, and careful planning is needed to sequence the drugs over time. HIV can develop a resistance to certain drugs, and in some cases, HIV can become resistant to an *entire class* of drugs in response to exposure to just *one* drug in that class. Specific sequencing of drugs can prevent this resistance, thereby continuing the effectiveness of the cocktail. It is not necessarily the massage therapist's role to memorize all the HIV/AIDS drugs and their possible side effects, but to stay on top of the individual client's condition. Ask about side effects and also ask if there are any additional signs or symptoms not listed here.

Treatments for complications, such as opportunistic infections and HIV-related cancers, involve other kinds of drugs. Antibacterial, antifungal, antiviral, and antiparasitic drugs are given for OIs. Side effects are similar to those of the cocktail, and some are similar to HIV itself: fever, headache, nausea, vomiting, and rash. Altered taste sensation, chills, and reduced appetite may also occur, as can neuropathy, abdominal pain, and muscle pain.

Standard cancer treatments are administered for HIV-related cancers. Because medications such as chemotherapy are immunosuppressive, and people in later stages of HIV disease already have weakened immune systems, the chemotherapy doses may be lower than usual. See Chapter 20 for discussion of standard cancer treatments.

With people living longer with HIV due to HAART therapy, management of chronic symptoms can be challenging. Medications are used to treat neuropathy (see "Peripheral Neuropathy," Chapter 10), control pain (see "Analgesics," Chapter 21), and ease fatigue and nausea, as well as other conditions.

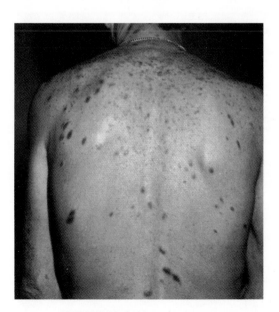

FIGURE 13-1. Kaposi sarcoma.

● INTERVIEW QUESTIONS

1. How has HIV infection affected you?
2. Would you describe your condition as mild, moderate, or severe? Do your blood counts leave you vulnerable to infection?
3. What are your symptoms, if any?
4. Have you had any opportunistic infections or other complications?
5. How is your condition being treated? Are you taking medications for HIV itself, to prevent other infections, or treat any complications?
6. How do your treatments affect you? Any side effects or complications of treatment?

7. Does the condition or the treatment affect your skin?
8. Does the condition or the treatment cause any sensation changes such as numbness or pain?

● MASSAGE THERAPY GUIDELINES

It can be difficult to tell whether a certain sign or symptom is due to HIV disease itself, or to the treatments, and in some cases, it is impossible to know. For example, neuropathy occurs with HIV disease, but it also is a side effect of the cocktail. Fatigue and nausea may be from the disease or from treatments, and additional drugs, with additional side effects, may be used to treat these symptoms. For HIV disease, it may not be possible to determine where every sign or symptom goes on the Decision Tree, with 100% accuracy. However, you can find out as much as you can about the person's condition in order to make a massage plan.

HIV Disease

Medical Information	Massage Therapy Guidelines
Essentials	
• Initial HIV infection causes mild flu-like symptoms, may be asymptomatic	• If known, avoid general circulatory intent, overall pressure 3 max depending on symptoms; no significant massage adjustments if asymptomatic
• Rash	• See General Principles, Chapter 7
• Mouth sores	• Avoid pressure or drag at jaw, chin; avoid face cradle if aggravates
• Muscle aches	• Begin with limited pressure (pr = max 1-2 for most), increase pressure to tolerance slowly over course of massage treatment; monitor response
• Shortness of breath	• If mild, no massage adjustment; for moderate or severe, adjust position (consider sidelying, seated, inclined positions)
• Vulnerability to infection	• Observe additional infection control measures recommended by client's physician or requested by client, including offering to reschedule if you have symptoms of infection (skin, GI, respiratory)
• AIDS (CD4 count below 200 or history of one opportunistic infection)	• Follow Activity and Energy Principle (see Chapter 3)
Complications	
• Opportunistic infections (OIs), causing fever, swollen lymph nodes, sweats, chills, headaches, fatigue, diarrhea, vision changes	• Avoid general circulatory intent; overall pressure 1-3 max depending on symptoms and tolerance; no direct pressure on or near swollen lymph nodes • Adapt to effects of pathogen, individual symptoms, such as sweating, chills, fever; use proper precautions if communicable
• Skin lesions (including herpes simplex, herpes zoster)	• See General Principles, Chapter 7; see Herpes simplex, Shingles, Chapter 7
• Nausea, vomiting, diarrhea	• Easy bathroom access; position for comfort (flat prone or supine position may be poorly tolerated; side-lying may be preferred); gentle session overall; pressure to tolerance (typically 3 max), but with full, reassuring contact; slow speeds; no uneven rhythms or strong joint movement; avoid scents in lubricant and odors in environment; avoid contact or pressure at abdomen that could aggravate
• Wasting syndrome	• Use gentle pressure (level 1-2 max) overall; use cautious joint movement ; be sensitive to possible poor body image; position for comfort
• Neuropathy	• Follow Sensation Principle, Sensation Loss, Injury Prone Principle; see Peripheral Neuropathy, Chapter 10, for adaptations to symptoms and treatment
• Dementia	• Simplify communication; establish clear consent; observe for nonverbal cues of comfort, discomfort
• Kaposi sarcoma (KS)	• No pressure (level 1 max) or drag at site; avoid contact at site if KS lesion open
• Lymphoma, cervical cancer	• See Hodgkin lymphoma, Non-Hodgkin lymphoma, this chapter; see Cervical cancer, Chapter 19; see Cancer, Chapter 20

FIGURE 13-2. A Decision Tree for HIV disease.

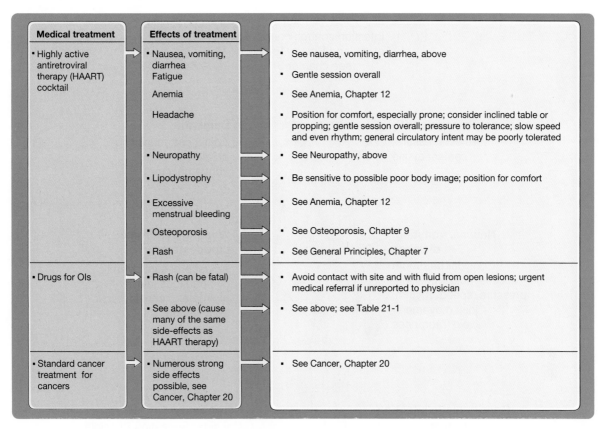

Medical treatment	Effects of treatment	
• Highly active antiretroviral therapy (HAART) cocktail	• Nausea, vomiting, diarrhea Fatigue Anemia Headache	• See nausea, vomiting, diarrhea, above • Gentle session overall • See Anemia, Chapter 12 • Position for comfort, especially prone; consider inclined table or propping; gentle session overall; pressure to tolerance; slow speed and even rhythm; general circulatory intent may be poorly tolerated
	• Neuropathy	• See Neuropathy, above
	• Lipodystrophy	• Be sensitive to possible poor body image; position for comfort
	• Excessive menstrual bleeding	• See Anemia, Chapter 12
	• Osteoporosis	• See Osteoporosis, Chapter 9
	• Rash	• See General Principles, Chapter 7
• Drugs for OIs	• Rash (can be fatal)	• Avoid contact with site and with fluid from open lesions; urgent medical referral if unreported to physician
	• See above (cause many of the same side-effects as HAART therapy)	• See above; see Table 21-1
• Standard cancer treatment for cancers	• Numerous strong side effects possible, see Cancer, Chapter 20	• See Cancer, Chapter 20

FIGURE 13-2. (*Continued*)

In many cases, tolerance to massage elements, such as pressure, is individualized rather than linked to a certain drug. As always, during a course of massage treatment, you can monitor an individual's massage tolerance over time, but for one-time clients, it is harder. Remember to begin conservatively, especially if the person's disease is advanced. Follow the Activity and Energy Principle (see Chapter 3), and investigate each sign, symptom, complication, and infection carefully. See the Decision Tree in Figure 13-2 for additional massage guidelines for the condition.

The answers to Questions 1–4 establish background on the client's HIV experience, including whether the disease has advanced to AIDS and whether the client is vulnerable to infection, or has experienced any OIs. Although there is a wide range in OI pathogens and scenarios, massage adjustments are pretty uniform across the range: avoid general circulatory intent, limit overall pressure to level 1–2 for most people, up to level 3 for those who tolerate it well, and do not press on swollen lymph nodes. In addition, take extra care with infections that cause skin lesions (such as HSV, or shingles), reviewing "General Principles" in Chapter 7.

Common symptoms of progressing infection are mouth sores, muscle aches, and shortness of breath. If mouth sores are present, pressure and drag at the jaw and chin are ill-advised. You may need to avoid the face cradle, or adjust the client's position in it so that the tissues of the chin and cheek are comfortable. If the client has muscle aches, begin with limited pressure at first; if more pressure is preferred, increase it in small increments, to tolerance, over time. With moderate or severe shortness of breath, adjust the client's position for breathing comfort. The side-lying, seated, and inclined positions may work best.

If the client's CD4 count leaves him or her vulnerable to infection, or he or she expresses concern about it, it's important to go beyond standard precautions and include any additional infection control precautions requested by the client, or recommended by the client's doctor. At minimum, this includes notifying the client if you are sick, or if you have signs or symptoms that could indicate infection, but you are planning to work. Offer the client a chance to reschedule. With ongoing clients, it's a good idea to establish a plan in such an event, and respect the client's wishes.

If the client reports nausea, vomiting, or diarrhea, easy access to a bathroom from the massage room is important, even if it means the client has to wrap up in the drape and move quickly. Provide a gentle session overall (see Decision Tree, Figure 13-2). Pressure on the abdomen is usually unwelcome with these symptoms. If the client has experienced wasting syndrome, limit overall pressure to level 1–2. Because muscle mass is lost in wasting syndrome, muscles are less able to stabilize the joints, so use gentle joint movement, as well. Position for comfort, with plenty of padding. Wasting syndrome calls for extra compassion as the signs of AIDS are more obvious. With more pronounced signs, an individual can feel acutely self-conscious.

Neuropathy, a common clinical feature of HIV disease, may cause absence of sensation, or painful burning or tingling. Here, the Sensation Principle (see Chapter 3) is in force. See "Peripheral Neuropathy," Chapter 10, for massage adaptations for neuropathy and several types of neuropathy treatment.

Dementia calls for a gentle overall session, clear consent, and attentiveness to nonverbal signs of discomfort and comfort. Simplify and streamline communication to offer one choice at a time, for example: "Would you like this lotion

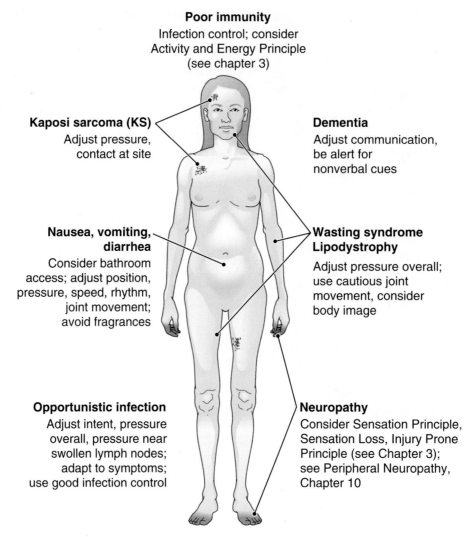

Poor immunity
Infection control; consider
Activity and Energy Principle
(see chapter 3)

Kaposi sarcoma (KS)
Adjust pressure,
contact at site

Dementia
Adjust communication,
be alert for
nonverbal cues

Nausea, vomiting, diarrhea
Consider bathroom
access; adjust position,
pressure, speed, rhythm,
joint movement;
avoid fragrances

Wasting syndrome Lipodystrophy
Adjust pressure overall;
use cautious joint
movement, consider
body image

Opportunistic infection
Adjust intent, pressure
overall, pressure near
swollen lymph nodes;
adapt to symptoms;
use good infection control

Neuropathy
Consider Sensation Principle,
Sensation Loss, Injury Prone
Principle (see Chapter 3);
see Peripheral Neuropathy,
Chapter 10

FIGURE 13-3. Acquired immune deficiency syndrome: selected clinical features and massage therapy guidelines.

here?" rather than "Would you like lotion or oil on your hands and feet?" The client's caregivers can provide guidance for communication and massage.

If HIV disease has led to a cancer diagnosis, such as Kaposi sarcoma, lymphoma, or cervical cancer, review cancer and cancer treatment in Chapter 20. Adapt to Kaposi sarcoma by avoiding too much pressure and drag at the site, and avoid contact with lesions and any fluid draining from open lesions. For other cancers, see "Hodgkin Lymphoma," "Non-Hodgkin Lymphoma," this chapter, and "Cervical Cancer," Chapter 19.

A client's answers to Questions 6–8 may be lengthy if the client is receiving HAART therapy. If the client experiences fatigue or anemia in response to medications, provide a gentle session overall, and see "Anemia," Chapter 12. Recall that excessive menstrual bleeding may cause anemia in women. If headache is a problem, position for comfort, and avoid general circulatory intent at first; start with gentle pressure, and then monitor over time whether specific focused areas of pressure or treatment tend to help or aggravate the headache.

If lipodystrophy is a problem, be sensitive to the poor body image that can result. Be prepared for position changes: if a large fat pad behind the neck causes pain, you may need to skip the supine position. Loss of fat tissue in the extremities or buttocks may require extra soft bolstering. As more becomes known about lipodystrophy and the effects on metabolism,

such as associated metabolic syndrome (see Conditions in Brief, Chapter 17), massage adjustments may continue to evolve.

If the client mentions a rash, or you notice one during the session, give this issue extra attention. A rash can be a mild or moderate reaction to a drug; it often appears in the first few weeks of starting or changing medications and resolves after a few weeks. Rashes occur more in women than men. Some rashes are associated with medications, and can result in serious and even fatal complications. Treat a rash as you normally would, asking about the cause, avoiding contact and lubricant at the site and with any fluids coming from the lesions, and even avoiding contact altogether until the cause of the rash is known. If it seems associated with medication, be sure to ask whether the client has reported it to his or her doctor and urge the client to report it right away if he or she has not. The medication causing the reaction may need to be changed, or the client may need to be treated with antihistamines, or even hospitalized and treated with anti-inflammatories.

Complications of HIV disease, due either to the condition or the treatment, are complex, and a conservative approach is warranted at first, for a variety of reasons. Clinical features and massage adaptations for AIDS are shown in Figure 13-3.

Finally, be aware that not everyone with HIV is comfortable disclosing his or her HIV status. Even though HIV is not transmitted by touch or other casual contact, people with HIV live each day with others' fear, judgment, prejudice, and outright discrimination. In this environment, extra sensitivity is in order. In the massage setting, real issues stem from OIs, skin health, general health, and effects of medication, but not usually from the virus itself. Standard precautions, practiced with every client, prevent transmission of HIV and many other pathogens. With a good medical history, you can cover all the bases, whether or not the client knows or reports his or her HIV status. Many people with HIV, including massage therapists, receive and give massage. Obviously, massage can safely be exchanged between persons who are HIV-positive and HIV-negative.

● MASSAGE RESEARCH

Massage therapy and HIV disease is a growing area of research, but available evidence falls short of conclusive benefit from massage. There is some interest in massage and immune function, especially in terms of CD4 counts, given the role that CD4 lymphocytes play in HIV disease. In one RCT, investigators provided weekly massage alone, and in combination with other stress management interventions, to 42 HIV positive subjects (Birk et al., 2000), but massage did not appear to improve CD4 counts. The researchers did find that combining stress management-biofeedback with massage was associated with some improved quality of life (QOL) measures.

Two other small RCTs reported improvement in immune function following massage, one in adolescents with HIV disease (Diego et al., 2001) and another in younger children (Shor-Posner et al., 2004), however, re-analysis of the data from these studies (Beider & Moyer, 2006) suggested no effect on immunity from massage. As of this writing, the question of whether massage boosts immune function in HIV disease remains open, and it is too early to claim that benefit for people with HIV.

THERAPIST'S JOURNAL 13-1 *Massage, Stress, and HIV*

I began providing volunteer massage services at the Whitman-Walker Clinic in Washington, DC, 10 years ago. The clinic is a nonprofit, community-based organization whose mission statement includes the goal of "ending suffering of all those infected and affected by HIV/AIDS." Over my years working in the community, I have seen the U.S. demographics for HIV change. It used to affect primarily men who have sex with men, but now it affects heterosexuals, people sharing needles, women, and children. HIV has a particularly strong effect on poor populations. I notice that the disease affects people differently depending on their access to care, but all are affected by stress. I have continued to offer free massage sessions in my office to some of my clients from the Whitman-Walker Clinic and have grown to know them well over the years.

One HIV-positive client, a homemaker and mother of two children, has been coming to me monthly for five years. She learned of her HIV status eleven years ago during a pregnancy. She has neuralgia in her hip that causes her a fair amount of intermittent pain, but it doesn't manifest on the skin. Her doctors have suggested she visit a pain clinic and take medications for it but she doesn't want to, perhaps because she is already taking so many drugs for HIV.

Over the course of our time and many conversations together, she's realized that the pain comes and goes depending on her stress level. If a financial or family stress enters the picture, she will start to hurt. When the stress subsides and she feels good again, the pain subsides. Pain is a perfect barometer for her stress level.

Once the pattern became clear, this client worked hard to keep her stress down and avoid having to take more medications. She adopted several approaches to managing and minimizing stress. She gets regular exercise, swimming with her son at a municipal pool a few times a week. This allows them family time together and helps keep her healthy. I also see her limiting her time and interactions with difficult people who cause her stress, and making other conscious choices to keep her stress down. My client is well connected in her community, with the clinic, with her children's school, and to services available to her family. I think all of these keep her stress as low as possible. Finally, she gets monthly massage to help her with her stress level and feels strongly that this makes the difference in her pain.

Her viral load, a measure of HIV in the blood, is undetectable, and her CD4 count hovers around 400. She's had no opportunistic infections. She is taking several different drugs, a cocktail designed to inhibit the replication of HIV. They have strong side effects, one of which is making her anemic. So she struggles with low energy. Perhaps because of this, my massage sessions include an overall pressure of just 2 or 3. At first when I used pressures of 3–4, she left the sessions seeming "drugged," because the pressure was too much for her.

I have met her husband and children, and they are wonderful people. She talks a lot about what great kids she has and what an inspiration they are to her. They give her so many reasons to stay healthy, to lower her stress so that she can live as well as possible and be there for her children. We talk about making sure she lives until they've reached 18, at least. It's inspiring to see her and to be so directly involved in her health, with such palpable results.

From this client, I have learned that several things are part of surviving and thriving with HIV. Perseverance is one; she works hard to locate good programs and resources for herself and her family. Another is the commitment to stay healthy and be available to loved ones. And a third one is finding joy in simple things. She is an amazing person. I feel lucky to know her and to be one of her resources.

David Cockrell
Silver Spring, MD

Another RCT suggested that twice-weekly massage helped reduce anxious and depressed behaviors and negative thoughts in HIV-positive children. In this study of HIV-positive Dominican children who were not receiving HAART therapy, massage was also associated with enhanced communication and self-help skills (Hernandez-Reif et al., 2008). This study raised questions about the value of touch in populations where resources do not exist for HAART and other expensive therapies.

In an interesting paper on massage therapy and meditation, researchers measured spiritual quality of life (QOL) in 58 people with late-stage AIDS. The authors noted the relative absence of spiritual quality of life care in the delivery of end of life care in the United States. They compared a massage therapy intervention, a Metta "loving-kindness" meditation intervention, and a combination of the two with a standard care control. They found spiritual QOL improvement associated with each individual intervention, but the improvement was not statistically significant. However, the combination of massage *and* meditation was much more favorable: *the apparent effect was greater than the sum of the two separate interventions*. This synergistic phenomenon points to the need for more research. If convincing data emerge in favor of massage, then massage could have a significant role in HIV care.

● POSSIBLE MASSAGE BENEFITS

Many people with HIV disease report stress as an important factor in their symptoms, well-being, and tolerance of medications. As described in Therapist's Journal 13-1, massage therapy can be an integral part of health care for HIV-positive individuals, targeted at stress relief. See also Therapist's Journal 10-4, which suggests that carefully performed foot massage can help neuropathic pain in people with HIV. Finally, massage therapy has the potential to help with anxiety and depression. Both are serious concerns with HIV disease (Fulk et al., 2004).

Non-Hodgkin Lymphoma

Non-Hodgkin lymphoma (NHL) is a group of more than thirty types of cancer that occurs in the lymphatic system. NHL is formed from an abnormal B cell, a type of WBC, usually beginning in a lymph node. B cells or *B lymphocytes* secrete antibodies to foreign substances. Although all white blood cells are born in the bone marrow, B cells become distinct from T cells, in that they go on to mature in the bone marrow rather than the thymus.

● BACKGROUND

Non-Hodgkin lymphoma is most common in older adults, and it has been rapidly increasing in incidence in the United States and Canada. One type of NHL, Burkitt lymphoma, is common in Africa and is associated with infection by a virus called Epstein-Barr virus.

NHL shares similarities with *Hodgkin lymphoma* (Hodgkin disease), so some of the information here is useful for working with someone with Hodgkin; however, there are some differences in medical treatment between the types of lymphoma. Hodgkin lymphoma is covered in the Conditions in Brief table at the end of this chapter.

NHL may be indolent, which means slow growing or low grade; in other cases, it is rapidly growing, also called *aggressive* or *highly malignant*. Risk factors for some types of lymphoma include organ transplants and other conditions in which the immune system is not working effectively, such as HIV disease.

Signs and Symptoms

Many symptoms may occur with non-Hodgkin lymphoma, including one or more swollen lymph nodes in which abnormal cells form a mass. These tend to be painless and show up in the neck, axilla (armpit), or inguinal (groin) areas. Sometimes swollen lymph nodes are the only early sign of NHL. As the condition advances, it may cause fatigue as well as fever, unexplained weight loss, itchiness, and night sweats. If these generalized symptoms are present at diagnosis, they are associated with a poorer prognosis, signifying aggressive lymphoma growth.

Complications

Complications of NHL depend on its location, and whether the function of an organ or tissue is affected by a mass. Swollen lymph nodes can press against surrounding organs and tissues, causing swelling in those tissues, impairing function, and causing discomfort. Lymph nodes can swell in the GI tract, causing difficulties in digestion and elimination, as well as injury to GI structures. Signs and symptoms include abdominal pain, constipation, loss of appetite, nausea, and vomiting. Tearing of tissues can cause blood loss.

Enlarged lymph nodes in the chest can press against the airways, causing cough and difficulty breathing. Heart function can be affected if advanced NHL causes pericardial effusion, a buildup of fluid surrounding the heart, or if spread to the heart tissue causes arrhythmia. When NHL spreads to the spleen and liver, the organs become congested; enlargement is called splenomegaly (see Figure 12-4) and hepatomegaly, respectively.

If lymph nodes deep in the abdomen are swollen, they can obstruct circulation, producing swelling in the lower limbs. In some cases, tumors can also grow massive enough to press on the superior vena cava, causing back pressure and swelling in the head, face, and arms. This condition, called vena cava syndrome (VCS), is a medical emergency. Although there are some treatment measures for VCS, it appears in the late stage of the disease, and treatment for it is palliative at that point.

If NHL affects the bone marrow, it can cause pain and various cytopenias (reductions in blood cell counts), such as anemia, thrombocytopenia, or leukopenia, a reduced WBC count (see Chapter 12). NHL can spread to the outer structure of the bone itself. Although it is not a true metastatic process, the effects are similar, and it can compromise compact bone and cause pathologic fracture, as some other cancers do. This is especially serious if fracture occurs in a vertebra, causing spinal cord compression; bone fragments and displacement injure the spinal cord, causing pain, sensory loss, and paralysis.

In some cases, the primary lymphoma forms in the brain, causing headaches, cognitive and motor problems, and seizures. If the skin is affected, red or purple nodules or lumps form under the skin, and they may itch.

Treatment

If the NHL is slow growing and in its earlier stages, it is often treated with radiation at the site of the mass. If it is early but aggressive, chemotherapy is the likely treatment, along with local radiation therapy (see Chapter 20). If it is in later stages and is slow growing, a **watch and wait** approach may be adopted in which no treatment is provided but the condition is closely monitored to see if it grows more rapidly. If it progresses, treatment often includes chemotherapy and radiation therapy. A *stem cell transplant* (see Chapter 20) may be needed in order to allow high-dose chemotherapy. Newer treatments include vaccines and biologic therapies. Side effects of cancer therapies are summarized in Chapter 20 on cancer.

● INTERVIEW QUESTIONS

1. What kind of lymphoma do you have?
2. Where is it concentrated in your body? Is it considered to be slow growing, or rapidly growing?
3. How does it affect you? Does it affect any body functions?
4. Have you had any complications from the lymphoma? Are there any effects on your bones, bone stability, bone marrow, or blood cells?
5. Has lymphoma had any effect on your liver, spleen, breathing, digestion, or heart function?
6. Do you have any swelling or congestion anywhere?
7. Do you have any areas of pain or discomfort?
8. How is it treated?
9. How do the treatments affect you?

● MASSAGE THERAPY GUIDELINES

Questions 1 and 2 provide general background. The second question about lymphoma site is critical for determining where to avoid pressure. If it is rapidly growing or aggressive, prepare to ask these interview questions periodically and frequently over time, since medical presentations can change quickly. Recall that in the early stages of NHL, the physician may adopt a watch and wait approach to see if things change.

From Questions 3–5 and specific follow-up, you can determine how gentle you need to be. If the client reports any general symptoms such as night sweats, weight loss, or fatigue, these all call for gentle massage overall. (The disease is likely to be fairly advanced.) Sweating may require a mid-session "mop up" with a towel in order to resume the session and restore glide to the lotion or oil used. The client may also become chilled after a soaking sweat, requiring additional draping. Itching calls for firm holds, providing distraction, rather than stroking or friction; the lubricant may need to be carefully chosen to avoid aggravating itching.

Follow-up questions about specific organ involvement or complications will also point to specific massage adaptations. If the client reports that his or her spleen or liver function is affected, avoid general circulatory intent, follow the Vital Organ Principle if liver function is impaired, and adjust massage position for any distended organs. If lymphoma or its effects are in the GI tract or abdomen, avoid abdominal massage with pressure in the area. Even if the client is constipated, refrain from using strokes with pressure. Limit any contact at the abdomen to pressure level 1 or 2, depending on the advice of the client's physician; recall that NHL can cause serious symptoms, such as bowel blockage or bleeding in the area.

If the heart or lungs are affected, observe the Vital Organ Principle (see Chapter 3). Adjust the client's position to facilitate breathing; an inclined or side-lying position is usually best, or the client may need to be seated for the session. If heart function is affected, refer to Arrhythmia and other appropriate sections in Chapter 11.

> *The Vital Organ Principle. If a vital organ—heart, lung, kidney, liver, or brain—is compromised in function, use gentle massage elements and adjust them to pose minimal challenge to the client's body.*

In the event that Questions 1–5 do not bring up any swelling, Question 6 provides an additional layer of inquiry. It may identify vital organ involvement, uncomfortable pressure or positions, as above, or superior vena cava syndrome (VCS), which can be chronic in the end stages of lymphoma. In any of these cases, avoid general circulatory intent. Also avoid circulatory intent at the site of swelling. Do not attempt to use massage to treat swelling, and use extremely gentle pressure at the site, maximum level 1. If the client has developed new swelling, but has not reported it to his or her doctor, urge him or her to do so; if the swelling has suddenly appeared in the face, head, neck, or arms, an emergency medical referral is in order, as this can signal life-threatening VCS. In most cases, if you are seeing someone with VCS, it is in a palliative care setting.

Question 4 may reveal additional massage adjustments: if blood cell counts are affected, find out which blood cell population is low, the extent of the problem, and adapt accordingly (see "Anemia," "Thrombocytopenia," "Neutropenia/Leukopenia," Chapter 12). If bone structure is compromised, adjustments in joint movement and pressure may be in order. In this case, ask *very* pointed follow-up questions to determine how stable the bones are. Even though bone involvement in NHL is not a true metastatic process, the same principles apply. See "Bone Metastasis," Chapter 20.

Question 7 about pain is another layered question. Pain in NHL can signal various serious issues: bone involvement with spinal cord compression, swelling that presses on nearby structures, congested organs, or even bone marrow problems. Even back pain, which often responds well to massage, can be a sign of some of the serious complications mentioned above. For this reason refrain from pressing or moving an area of pain until its cause is clear, the client's physician feels it's safe to do so, and it won't injure tissues. Using pressure level 1 to hold or stroke an area of pain should be okay in most cases.

Questions 8 and 9 about treatment may reveal effects of treatment similar to the effects of NHL itself. For example, chemotherapy can cause various cytopenias, although they tend to be treated quickly once identified. Whether complications are from treatment or from the NHL itself has little bearing on the massage; the adjustments are made in either case. Aggressive cancer treatments, including radiation, chemotherapy, stem cell transplant, and biologic therapies may be being used, with strong effects on the body. See Chapter 20 for proper interview questions relating to these therapies, side effects, and appropriate massage therapy adjustments.

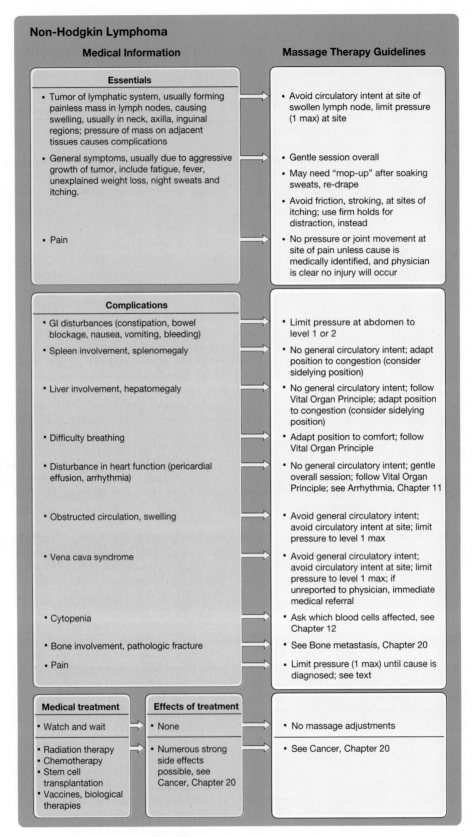

FIGURE 13-4. A Decision Tree for non-Hodgkin lymphoma.

On the other hand, an individual with NHL maybe in a watch and wait mode to see whether the lymphoma progresses rapidly or not. In this event, massage adjustments for medical treatment are unlikely to be necessary.

● MASSAGE RESEARCH

As of this writing, there are no randomized, controlled trials, published in the English language, on non-Hodgkin lymphoma and massage indexed in PubMed or the Massage Therapy

Foundation Research Database. The NIH RePORTER tool lists no active, federally funded research projects on the topic in the United States. No active projects are listed on the clinicaltrials.gov database (see Chapter 6). However, many massage research projects focus on people with cancer, and presumably some of these include patients with lymphoma in the study sample.

● POSSIBLE MASSAGE BENEFITS

Lymphoma is a stressful diagnosis, regardless of whether the individual is in a watch and wait period, or in strong treatment. The effects across organ systems of advanced NHL can be frightening. Massage makes sense for people with lymphoma, as it does for anyone with cancer. Massage may support people through treatments, during watch and wait, at the end of life, or during survivorship. Massage may help manage symptoms of the disease, or side effects of treatment.

Lymphedema

Lymphedema is an accumulation of fluid, or swelling, in the tissues. Unlike other forms of edema, caused by inflammation or poor blood circulation, lymphedema is caused by faulty drainage through the lymphatic system. The fluid backup is perpetuated by fluid stagnation and increasing concentrations of protein in the fluid over time.

There are several causes of lymphedema. In developed countries, lymphedema is most often caused by surgery or radiation for cancer, in which lymph nodes are removed or injured. The discussion in this chapter focuses on lymphedema from cancer treatment.

Other causes of lymphedema include a congenital structural deficiency in the lymphatic system, which usually produces lymphedema in the legs. More often, however, lymphedema is acquired later in life. A local obstruction in the lymphatic system can occur when a solid tumor forms in an area, causing lymphedema in the region drained by the affected network. Trauma, in which lymphatic structures are injured, can produce lymphedema. Widespread scarring of lymphatic structures, as in *filiariasis*, a tropical parasitic infection, can produce a profound form of lymphedema known as *elephantiasis*.

Lymphedema usually occurs in a limb, although it can also occur in the face, neck, or trunk. Lymphedema in a limb is most evident when compared to the non-affected side. Figure 13-5 shows lymphedema in the upper and lower extremities.

● BACKGROUND

Standard cancer treatment for a solid tumor includes a **lymph node dissection (LND)**, the removal of nearby lymph nodes for diagnostic and therapeutic purposes. As a diagnostic step, the lymph nodes are removed in order to check for the presence of cancer and to help stage the disease. As a therapeutic step, removal of nodes with tumor cells can help arrest the further spread of those cells.

Lymph node dissection, also called *lymphadenectomy*, can aid in cancer diagnosis and treatment, but it can also result in lymphedema. Lymph node dissection and other risk factors for lymphedema are described in Chapter 20 on cancer. There, massage guidelines are presented for clients *at risk* of lymphedema. In this chapter, massage guidelines are discussed for clients *who have already developed* chronic lymphedema, either currently or in the past. It is essential to understand this distinction, between lymphedema risk and lymphedema history.

Many people have lymph nodes removed or irradiated during cancer treatment. It is not known why this leads to lymphedema in some people but not in others. In some people, nearby collateral

lymphatic vessels may function indefinitely, substituting for the missing or damaged structures. In others, collateral structures may function for a short while, until the delicate balance of fluid and

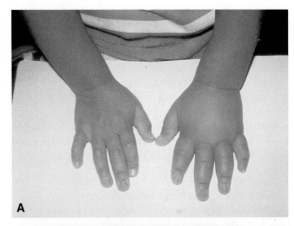

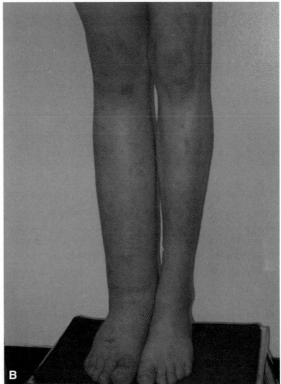

FIGURE 13-5. Lymphedema of the upper and lower extremities.

lymphatic capacity is upset by a stressful event, such as an injury, excessive heat, or inflammation.

At that point, the lymphatic system is overwhelmed by the increased demand on it, and becomes unable to keep up. Even a small inflammatory event can lead to a first episode of lymphedema, which can become chronic and lifelong. See "Surgery," Chapter 20, for further discussion of the events leading to lymphedema.

During normal circulation, blood plasma proteins are pushed from the blood capillaries out to the tissues under high pressure; however, these proteins are too large to re-enter the blood capillaries. Instead, they are transported through lymphatic vessels and returned to the bloodstream at the subclavian veins. In lymphedema, when lymphatic flow is impaired, plasma proteins and cellular debris accumulate in the tissues, and they attract water, which produces further swelling and stagnation. Lymphedema is sometimes called *protein-rich edema* because of this chemical composition of tissue fluid. The combination of structural problems in the lymphatic system and chemical factors in the tissue makes lymphedema very difficult to treat. The swelling can become chronic. It ranges from a mild feeling of fullness or puffiness, to severe disfigurement, in which an extremity expands to several times its normal size.

In the United States, most lymphedema is caused by breast cancer surgery, involving the removal of lymph nodes from under the arm (see "Breast Cancer," Chapter 19). This sets up the structural deficiency in the lymphatic system. Lymphedema risk increases when breast cancer surgery is followed by radiation therapy, which injures the remaining structures.

Less is known about lymphedema risk with nodes removed from other areas, or with a radiation field, such as:

- Inguinal nodes, as in anal and genital cancers
- Cervical nodes, as in head and neck cancers
- Pelvic nodes, as in prostate, bladder, and gynecological cancers

Any of these nodes may be removed in melanoma (see Chapter 7; see Figure 20-2), depending on its location. Not all patients with a given cancer type will have lymph nodes removed from the same places.

Signs and Symptoms

Lymphedema is classified in terms of severity, when its size is compared to the unaffected limb, or to its previous size. It is described as mild if the limb has increased in volume by less than 20%, moderate if it is a 20–40% increase, and severe if it shows a 40% or more increase in volume.

The progression of lymphedema is divided into three stages. In stage I, called the *reversible stage*, the swelling is *pitting*, which means that, after pressed with a fingertip, an indentation remains for a time. The swelling is relieved by elevation, and often disappears overnight, or within a few days, and is therefore reversible. In Stage II lymphedema, also called *spontaneously irreversible lymphedema*, the swelling is no longer pitting. Instead, the tissue feels spongy. In this stage, fibrosis has begun in the affected tissues, and the limb begins to harden and may increase in size. The swelling is not relieved by elevation and does not reverse. This stage can persist for anywhere from weeks to years, and it may increase or decrease in size but it does not tend to go away. In Stage III lymphedema, also called *lymphostatic elephantiasis*, the tissue is very hard, and the limb can be very large. Complications are most likely in this stage.

Complications

With severe or persistent cases of lymphedema, skin changes occur over time—it thickens and becomes rough. Wound healing becomes poor. In the worst cases, skin breaks down and leaks lymph, putting the person at an increased risk of infection.

Infection is a great concern in lymphedema, occurring as cellulitis (see Chapter 7) or lymphangitis (see Conditions in Brief, this chapter). Fungal infections may also appear. Because lymphatic flow is slowed or stopped in places, it becomes more difficult for the body to fight infection in the area. When infection appears, individuals need immediate treatment because infection can aggravate lymphedema or, if the pathogen passes to the blood circulation, it can become life threatening.

Pain and functional impairment can develop when lymphedema is severe; the limb is so heavy with water weight that it becomes hard to use. The pressure of the fluid causes stiffness, achiness, and pain. Disfigurement can have a negative effect on self-esteem and body image, and in some cases can contribute to depression. Lymphedema is isolating: people with the condition often feel conspicuous in public, and some curtail their activities as a result.

Treatment

There is no cure for lymphedema, and complications are serious, so lymphedema patients are instructed to take excellent care of the skin and deeper tissues in the area to avoid aggravating the condition. Traditionally, exercise of the limb has been discouraged, because the increased circulation in muscles and skin places too large a load on the struggling lymphatic system. This view has been challenged in recent years (Schmitz, 2009), and dialogue about the role of exercise in lymphedema is likely to continue.

Patients are encouraged to seek medical care right away for any sign of infection, so that the lymphedema is not aggravated by the infection. In addition, careful compression of the affected limb is advised. Compression bandaging and compression sleeves are customized to the individual's lymphedema and size. Compression is graduated—stronger distally, less strong proximally, to encourage the return of lymph to the trunk (see Figure 13-6).

One of the few effective therapies for lymphedema management is specialized manual work, which bears little resemblance to classical massage. Various lymph drainage therapies are used, some under the umbrella term *manual lymph drainage*. These approaches increase circulation, but in a more methodical, purposeful, and directed way than classical massage. Instead, precise choreography is used, often with extremely gentle pressures, to move excess lymph along "detours," bypassing damaged structures, to other healthy, intact lymphatic vessels for return to the blood. There are several methods of lymph drainage, and intensive, often daily, treatments are needed at first. These manual sessions are usually combined with precise bandaging to bring down the size of the limb. Once this is achieved, a maintenance program includes the use of a custom-fitted sleeve. Often patients are instructed in simple drainage techniques to perform at home.

Elevation is often encouraged to treat lymphedema, as are sequential exercises that help pump lymph in a proximal direction. Sometimes mechanized pneumatic pumps provide the sequential compression from distal to proximal. There is some controversy over the use of these machines, and they are

Elements of the Quadrant Principle for Lymphedema History

Your client may have many lymph nodes left in the area, just a few, or none at all. Because lymph nodes, the filters, have been removed or injured, the Filter and Pump Principle applies (see Chapter 3). This principle, refined for this special, vulnerable condition, is called the Quadrant Principle for Lymphedema History.

> *The Quadrant Principle for Lymphedema History.* **In an area of lymphedema history, as well as the associated trunk quadrant, use extreme caution to avoid aggravating lymphedema. In these areas, follow any precautions specified by the client's lymphedema therapist and health care team, limit pressure to level 1, and avoid reddening the tissues. Also avoid circulatory intent, friction, joint movement, and excessive focus on the area, and any client positions known to compromise lymph flow.**

The Quadrant Principle for Lymphedema History is designed to avoid bringing additional fluid into the area. In these individuals, lymphatic flow is already backed up. Any small increase in circulation, or small inflammation due to injury in the area, can overwhelm the remaining lymphatic structures further, and worsen lymphedema. Therefore, avoid reddening the skin, which is a sure sign of increased circulation (Zuther, 2001, MacDonald, 2008).

In contrast to the finely tuned, carefully organized movements of lymph drainage therapies, the crude circulatory intent of deeper effleurage and petrissage may actually make the situation worse. Likewise, heat applications and cold treatments are obvious elements to avoid in the region. Also avoid introducing any other factor that could stress or slightly injure the area, such as pressure above level 1, and joint movement, which should be done only by a trained lymphedema therapist. Limit any stroking on the area to a minute or two in most cases.

If the client is not already receiving manual treatment for lymphedema, a good referral is in order. If the client is already receiving manual care for her or his lymphedema, follow the lymphedema therapist's lead on any additional precautions. Lymphedema therapists often caution massage therapists to be careful with the *direction* and *placement* of superficial effleurage, with the strokes being directed toward intact lymphatic structures in other quadrants (MacDonald, 2008). By limiting your time and pressure in the area, you can mitigate the movement of fluid in the wrong direction. Gentle (pressure level 1) stationary holds can be done in any sequence or placement.

The massage restrictions in this principle mirror the medically restricted activities for people with lymphedema: exercise, injury, and exposure to heat and cold. Both the massage and medical restrictions are designed to avoid increasing circulation and an increased load on the lymphatic system.

Areas Defined by the Quadrant Principle for Lymphedema History

The Quadrant Principle applies, not only to the swollen limb (or neck/face, in the case of cervical lymph node removal), but also to the trunk quadrant that borders it. The adjacent

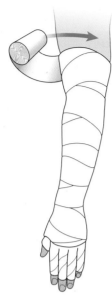

FIGURE 13-6. Graduated pressure bandaging in lymphedema. The pressure gradient is precise, requiring a trained lymphedema therapist to apply it.

criticized for providing pressure that is so strong that it injures tissues and makes the situation even worse.

In some countries, medications called benzopyrones are prescribed for lymphedema. They act on the proteins trapped in the tissues, provoking the immune system to destroy them, and facilitating their removal from the tissues. Results from studies on these drugs are mixed, and liver damage is a concern; as of this writing, these drugs are not approved in the United States or Canada for use with lymphedema. Although there are several surgical procedures in use for lymphedema when it does not respond to more conservative therapy, these procedures are also controversial, and have limited success. Lymphedema is a difficult medical problem to treat.

● INTERVIEW QUESTIONS

1. What is (or was) the cause of your lymphedema? How long have you had it?
2. How does it affect you? Would you call it mild, moderate, or severe?
3. What positions are you comfortable in? Which ones do not aggravate your lymphedema?
4. How is the condition of your skin in the area?
5. What is your expectation of massage in the region? Would you like the body area included in the session, for example, if I simply hold the area or gently rest my hands on the tissues there?
6. What kinds of precautions or restrictions do you observe in light of the lymphedema?
7. How do you treat it? How does treatment affect you?

● MASSAGE THERAPY GUIDELINES

When a client has lymphedema, your primary concern is to not aggravate it. Before turning to the client's answers to interview questions, it is important to understand the general principle that governs massage and lymphedema, and when to apply it. This is the Quadrant Principle for Lymphedema History, introduced at the beginning of this chapter.

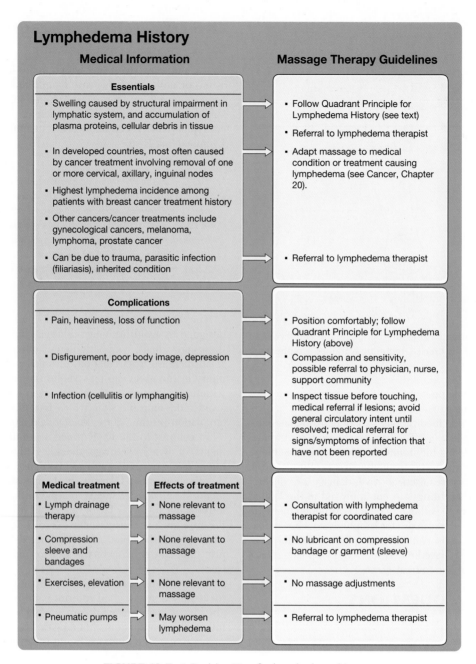

FIGURE 13-7. A Decision Tree for lymphedema history.

trunk area is also served by the missing or damaged lymphatic structures—thus the word "quadrant." Areas defined by the Quadrant Principle are shown in Figure 13-8. They include:

- *Cervical lymph node removal (lymphedema in head, face, or neck).* The front, back, and side of the head and neck, over to the midline and down to the level of the clavicle.
- *Axillary lymph node removal (lymphedema in the upper extremity).* The upper extremity and the bordering trunk quadrant. The quadrant is defined by the midline, the lowest rib, and the clavicle on the front, and the midline, lowest rib, and the level of the clavicle on the back.
- *Inguinal node removal (lymphedema in a lower extremity).* The lower extremity and the bordering trunk quadrant. The quadrant is defined by the midline and the lowest rib, front and back.

When to Use the Quadrant Principle for Lymphedema History

In medicine, a patient presenting with a condition is considered to have a *history* of that condition, even if presenting with the condition for the first time; as any new symptom that day becomes part of the medical history. Thus, this principle applies to any client who presents with current lymphedema, and to anyone with a history of it, as in Grade I lymphedema that has resolved, but can reappear at any time.

A referral to a lymphedema clinic can be very helpful to a client with a lymphedema history. Physical therapists, nurses, occupational therapists, and massage therapists with advanced training in lymphedema treatment have provided hope and relief for people with lymphedema, through detailed assessment and thorough treatment.

Anterior view **Posterior view**

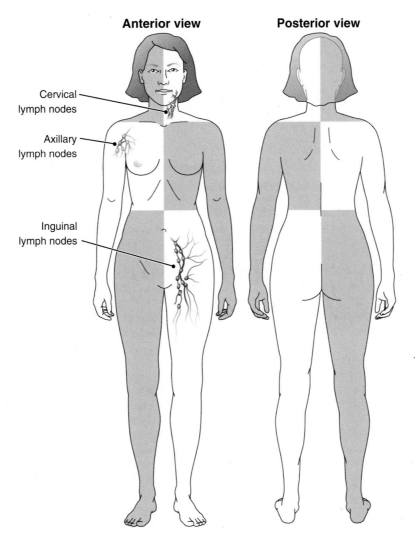

Cervical lymph nodes

Axillary lymph nodes

Inguinal lymph nodes

FIGURE 13-8. Areas defined by the Quadrant Principle for Lymphedema History. The unshaded quadrants show the area of massage caution corresponding to the lymphatic structures in each case.

In Chapter 20 on cancer, the Quadrant Principle for Lymphedema *Risk* is explained, for those who have not developed the condition. Note similarities and differences between the two principles: both include the trunk quadrant as well as an extremity. Both have the same borders at the midline, clavicle, and lowest ribs. Both are conservative approaches, yet slightly more caution is in order for clients with a history of lymphedema than for clients who have not developed it, but who are at risk. The interview questions and massage guidelines in this chapter are aimed at those *who have already experienced lymphedema*.

Question 1 is important to ask if the client has not brought it up already, just in case the cause of the lymphedema presents additional massage concerns. Recall that a common cause of lymphedema is surgery and radiation therapy for cancer, usually breast cancer. The Decision Tree in Figure 13-7 is oriented to this common occurrence. If the cause is lymphatic obstruction due to another type of tumor, review massage precautions for the type of cancer itself, as well as the interview questions and guidelines in Chapter 20. If the cause is filarial infection and the initial infection is resolved, the lymphedema may be especially pronounced. In such

cases, the prohibitions in the Quadrant Principle, above, should be applied over the whole body, but contact without pressure would not be contraindicated, and would likely be welcome.

The Ask the Cause Principle. **Consider the cause of a sign or symptom, as well as the sign or symptom itself, when making a massage plan.**

Question 2 should prompt some background on the condition. The client might be experiencing pain, heaviness, and loss of function from lymphedema. Although it might be tempting to use strokes with circulatory intent to alleviate the symptoms, only therapists with specialized training in lymphatic drainage techniques, with specific attention to lymphedema treatment, are qualified to use this approach. Others should follow the Quadrant Principle. In North America, referral for lymphedema care may be found at the National Lymphedema Network and several schools of lymphatic drainage help patients to locate trained lymphedema therapists (see Bibliography).

For a client with pain or discomfort, you might find that general relaxation massage or reflexive techniques that are not focused directly on the area of caution can provide symptom relief, or at least comfort. Remember that disfiguring lymphedema can affect body image. Compassion, sensitivity, a willingness to make contact with the area, and safely including it in the session could help a client accept the injured area, thereby supporting a more positive body image. Encourage your client to seek help for depression and body image difficulties, by seeking out her or his doctor or nurse, oncology social worker, or support communities.

Answers to Question 3 help you determine how to position the client on the table. In general, it's important not to let the affected limb hang down or sustain focused pressure, as an upper arm might while hanging off the table in the prone position. Some sort of elevation is preferable. Take the client's lead on proper positioning, and offer bolsters that support the limb (e.g., in the supine position, pillows from knee to ankle for a lower extremity, or a soft, folded towel that slightly elevates the arm).

Question 4 refers to the risk that lymphedema poses over time to the health of the skin. Infection is possible, and other conditions may cause skin lesions. While you will not be spending time stroking the skin or "working the tissues," even making simple contact with the skin requires an initial, quick inspection. Avoid contact with any lesions, and bring them to the client's attention. If an infection has not resolved, avoid general circulatory intent and pressure everywhere else on the body, as well as the affected region.

Question 5 sets the stage for open dialogue about the area, to reinforce the Quadrant Principle for Lymphedema History, but to include the area somehow in the treatment. Since you will follow the principle if you do not have advanced training in lymphedema treatment, it is especially important to clarify your expectations and possibly adjust those of your client, if necessary. Most people with lymphedema histories know that too much pressure, improper movement, or a circulatory session can aggravate lymphedema. Others may ask you to give the area a good deal of pressure, or to try to move fluid along. Even if a client wants deep work in the area, observe the guidelines here.

If there is any discrepancy in what the client wants and the Quadrant Principle, Question 6 should help. Lymphedema patients are almost always given specific activity precautions to manage the condition, including avoiding blood pressure cuffs, heat applications, and restrictive clothing (except for custom-made sleeves). Even people who choose not to follow precautions have typically been made aware of them. The Quadrant Principle mirrors these other medical precautions. By describing your massage adjustments and telling the client that they are in line with the standard approach to lymphedema management, you can make your reasoning clear.

If the client is undergoing lymph drainage therapy, a consultation with the therapist is advised for coordinated care; explain the Quadrant Principle that you follow, and ask if there is anything else that you can do to support the lymph drainage therapist's work. If the client is wearing a sleeve, or bandages, avoid getting lubricant on the garments.

● MASSAGE RESEARCH

As of this writing, there is little research published in the English language, on classical massage therapy and lymphedema. Although the term "massage" is sometimes used in the medical literature to describe manual therapies for lymphedema, a closer look at the available research reveals that lymph drainage therapies were studied, not massage. In these papers, there are some small studies, but the results of lymph drainage are mixed, and the various forms of therapy make it difficult to pool the data (Preston et al., 2004).

Lymphedema is poorly understood, but our understanding will evolve as more research is devoted to the subject. This is true in medicine and physical therapy as well as massage therapy. As mentioned before, lymphedema patients are often warned not to exercise the affected arm, to avoid aggravating the condition. Recent research in *The New England Journal of Medicine* has begun to challenge that notion (Schmitz et al., 2009). Women with stable lymphedema were divided into a weight-lifting group and a control group. Those who engaged in twice-weekly progressive weight lifting experienced greater improvements in lymphedema symptoms and fewer exacerbations at the one-year mark.

If, one day, exercise restrictions are lifted for the lymphedema population, then parallel massage restrictions might follow, but a greater understanding of lymphedema and massage dynamics is needed first. For now, a cautious approach is thoughtful, justified, and unlikely to do harm.

● POSSIBLE MASSAGE BENEFITS

While focused, specialized manual techniques to reduce lymphedema may be helpful, basic massage techniques are unlikely to be helpful and may injure the area further. The benefit of massage therapy is to the person with lymphedema, not the lymphedema itself. General relaxation-oriented massage may reduce isolation and even depression. Acceptance of the body without judgment may support the client's own acceptance of his or her body, and this can be healing in and of itself.

Other Immune and Lymphatic Conditions in Brief

ALLERGY (ALLERGIC REACTION, HYPERSENSITIVITY REACTION)

Background

- Immune system response to foreign substance (allergen); can result in congestion, itching, rash, hives, swelling.
- In severe cases, life-threatening anaphylaxis occurs: acute, systemic reaction causing rapid heart rate, difficulty breathing, widespread edema, lightheadedness, loss of consciousness.
- Treated with antihistamines, decongestants, corticosteroids (see Chapter 21), leukotriene modifiers, mast cell stabilizers; widely ranging side effects, depending on medication, dose, and individual tolerance.

Interview Questions	• What are you allergic to? Have you had a reaction recently? How strong was/is it? • How did/does it affect you? Any effects on your skin? • Do you have any allergies to the ingredients in my oil/cream? (List ingredients.) To latex, vinyl, or nitrile? (If you are gloving for any reason.) • Treatment? Effects of treatment?
Massage Therapy Guidelines	• Recent allergic reaction is cause for more investigation. If swelling remains in large area, or over more than one area, avoid general circulatory intent, pressure, and contact at site(s) of swelling. • If current, chronic allergy with rash or hives, avoid general circulatory intent; avoid pressure, friction or lubricant at sites; any hint of anaphylaxis requires emergency medical referral. (Mild seasonal allergies with nasal congestion are an exception, and do not require these modifications.) • In massage environment, avoid use of scented oils and creams; nut oils in lubricant (especially peanut); latex gloves; fabric softener, strong or scented detergents in linens. • Avoid personal use of scented hair products, soaps, or body lotions; avoid perfume, cologne, aftershave; avoid laundering own clothing in fabric softener, strong or scented detergents. • Adapt to any effects of treatment, such as drowsiness; follow Medication Principle, see Table 21-1 for common side effects of drugs and massage therapy guidelines.

AUTOIMMUNITY

Background	• Impairment in immune system function, immune response mounted to body's own tissues; causes inflammation, loss of function in affected tissues and organs. • Mechanism in many diseases, including multiple sclerosis, rheumatoid arthritis, diabetes mellitus type 1, systemic lupus erythematosus, Addison disease.
Interview Questions	• What is the name of the condition? Is it considered mild, moderate, or severe? • Are you currently in a flare-up of the condition? • How does it affect you (signs, symptoms, complications)? • Which tissues or organs are affected? Are any tissues or organs affected by past flare-ups? • Is your skin affected? • Are blood cells affected in your condition? Is blood clotting affected? If so, how is it affected? • Are any lymph nodes enlarged, or is your spleen enlarged? • Any problems with your heart, lung, liver, or kidney function? • Any effects on your nervous system—brain, spinal cord, or nerves? • Do you have any areas of pain and inflammation? Is sensation affected? • What is your activity level, and activity tolerance? • Have you ever received massage therapy during flare-ups, or between flare-ups? Did you tolerate it well? Can you describe the massage used? • Treatment? Effects of treatment?
Massage Therapy Guidelines	• Massage plan depends on client presentation (if disease is active, or if not in flare-up), severity and stability of condition, whether tissues within reach of hands (such as skin, muscles, joints) are inflamed or unstable, and whether organ function is impaired; combine Stabilization of an Acute Condition Principle, Unstable Tissue Principle, where relevant to client presentation (see Chapter 3). • To help determine best overall massage strength, especially between flare-ups, use Activity and Energy Principle, Previous Massage Principle (see Chapter 3). • If disease is active (flare-up), follow Inflammation Principle; if blood cell populations compromised, see Chapter 12. • Follow Vital Organ Principle where appropriate; follow Filter and Pump Principle if liver, spleen, kidney, or heart function affected; adapt positioning to any enlarged or congested organs. • If client is taking strong medications, such as corticosteroids or other immunosuppressants, use gentle pressure overall, avoid general circulatory intent; ask the four medication questions (see Chapter 4), follow Medication Principle. • For specific autoimmune conditions, review sections of this book: multiple sclerosis (see Chapter 10); rheumatoid arthritis (see Chapter 9); systemic lupus erythematosus (see Conditions in Brief, this chapter); Crohn disease (see Chapter 15), diabetes mellitus type I (see Chapter 17).

EDEMA

Background	• Swelling; accumulation of fluid in tissue, in interstitial spaces between cells. May be present in the abdomen (ascites), in swelling or puffiness of skin and/or extremities (peripheral edema), or in lungs (pulmonary edema).
	• Causes include inflammation, infection, and injury; premenstrual syndrome; pregnancy; venous insufficiency; side effects of medication; organ failure (heart, liver, kidney); obstruction due to tumor, blood clot, or obesity.
	• Treatment aimed at reversing underlying cause where possible; can also include restriction of dietary sodium to reduce fluid retention, diuretics (see Table 11-3), paracentesis (see "Liver Failure," Chapter 16), leg elevation, compression garments.
Interview Questions	• Where is it? What is the cause? Has it been seen by your doctor and diagnosed?
	• How long have you had it? Is it new, unfamiliar, or worsening? Was the onset sudden or gradual? How does it affect you?
Massage Therapy Guidelines	• Cause of edema is more important than edema itself in determining appropriate massage adjustments.
	• Undiagnosed edema requires medical referral, especially if sudden onset, severe, worsening, or occurring on face (in this case, it is an urgent or immediate referral). Follow the Swelling Principle. Follow Vital Organ Principle if heart, liver, or kidney function compromised; follow Filter and Pump Principle if lymphatic flow is compromised.
	• If due to obstruction, avoid circulatory intent and limit pressure to level 1 at site. If edema is due to lymphatic obstruction or impairment, see Lymphedema, this chapter. If due to pregnancy, follow pregnancy massage guidelines (Osborne, 2011; Stager, 2009).
	• If lower extremities are involved, follow DVT Risk Principles (see Chapter 11), unless cause is a minor blow, or premenstrual syndrome (presenting as bilateral ankle swelling).
	• If edema is due to a minor injury to soft tissue, circulatory intent at the site may be safe and indicated, depending on your skill level and other client medical conditions.

HODGKIN LYMPHOMA (HODGKIN DISEASE)

Background	• Lymphatic system cancer, malignant WBCs present in cells in lymph nodes, often presenting in upper body (neck, chest, axilla) or groin; advanced disease typically found in liver, lungs, bone marrow.
	• Less common than NHL (this chapter). Hodgkin accounts for 1% of all cancers in United States); tends to occur in young people (most common age range 20–30), and in people over 55. Incidence of Hodgkin lymphoma is declining in United States.
	• Signs and symptoms: painless lymph node enlargement, fever, chills, night sweats, fatigue, itching, loss of appetite, weight loss, cough or shortness of breath, abdominal pain.
	• May also cause cytopenias, hepatomegaly, or splenomegaly.
	• Treatment includes chemotherapy, radiation, combined chemotherapy and radiation, stem cell transplant. Surgery less common.
Interview Questions	• Where is it in your body?
	• How does it affect you? Any complications? Any areas of swelling, pain, or discomfort? Does it affect any body functions?
	• Do you have any liver or spleen involvement or congestion?
	• What are comfortable positions for you?
	• Are blood cell counts affected in your condition? Is your skin affected? If so, how?
	• Treatment? Effects of treatment?
Massage Therapy Guidelines	• Use gentle pressure (level 1 max) at affected lymph nodes or any site of swelling; avoid circulatory intent at sites of swelling.
	• No general circulatory intent if hepatomegaly or splenomegaly; gentle session overall if fever present.
	• Follow Vital Organ Principle if lungs or liver involved. Adapt position to comfort and reduce pressure on congested areas. Adapt to low blood cell counts (see Chapter 12).

- Extremely gentle session overall if profound weight loss.
- See Chapter 20 for descriptions, effects, and massage therapy guidelines for cancer, cancer treatment.

INFLAMMATION

Background	• Body's response to internal tissue damage and invasion by outside substances. Prevents further invasion, begins removal of cellular debris, and prepares tissues for healing. Edema accompanying inflammation also serves to "splint" or immobilize injured area, preventing reinjury during healing. • Can accompany injury, toxicity, infection, autoimmune process, or presence of foreign object.
Interview Questions	• What symptoms do you have: pain, swelling, redness, warmth? Loss of function? • How does it affect you? Which tissues are involved? • What is the cause? Has your doctor diagnosed it? • Is it a new, unfamiliar, or worsening condition, or one you've managed over time or experienced in the past?
Massage Therapy Guidelines	• Learn everything possible about condition, cause, diagnosis. Cause is as important as inflammation itself, and may require massage adjustments in its own right. • Follow Inflammation Principle (see Chapter 3). If inflammation is mild (as in minor insect sting, minor injury), it is probably okay to use general circulatory intent, limiting pressure (max = 1 or 2) and circulatory intent at site. If more serious, consider medical referral, avoid general circulatory intent, circulatory intent at site, friction at site, and limit pressure. • Undiagnosed, especially if new, unfamiliar, or worsening, is cause for concern and urgent medical referral. Follow the Pain, Injury, and Inflammation Principles (see Chapter 3).

LYMPHANGITIS AND LYMPHADENITIS

Background	• Infection and inflammation in the lymphatic capillaries (lymphangitis) or lymph nodes (lymphadenitis), from normal skin flora. • Characterized by acute inflammation, often with red "tracks" of infection heading from infection port of entry (cut, hangnail, other lesion). • Can progress over hours to include lymph nodes, fever, malaise, and septicemia (blood poisoning), which can be fatal; emergency treatment with antibiotics.
Interview Questions	• If client has diagnosed lymphangitis/lymphadenitis, ask: When was it, and where? How did it affect you? Any complications? How treated? Has it resolved? • If signs are evident, but no diagnosis made, ask: How long has it been going on? Have you reported it to a doctor?
Massage Therapy Guidelines	• If condition is diagnosed and resolved, no massage adjustments; if the client is still recovering from recent episode, provide gentle overall massage; avoid general circulatory intent and limit pressure in region until infection resolved. • If you notice symptoms or any undiagnosed acute inflammation, with or without the "tracks," immediate medical referral; massage is not needed, but proper diagnosis and emergency antibiotics are needed without delay.

SYSTEMIC LUPUS ERYTHEMATOSUS (SLE)

Background	• Chronic, inflammatory autoimmune condition affecting connective tissue; can affect mucous membranes, joints, blood vessels, organs. • Symptoms: fever, malaise, joint pain and inflammation, hair loss, petechiae, enlarged lymph nodes, splenomegaly, headaches, and skin rash, including a mask-like pattern across nose and cheeks. • Pulmonary and cardiovascular complications: pleurisy, pleural effusion, pulmonary embolism, pericarditis, angina, heart failure.

- Blood complications: cytopenias, thrombosis.
- Kidney complications: nephritis.
- Nervous system complications: headaches, cognitive impairment, personality changes, stroke, seizure disorders, others.
- GI complications: abdominal pain, blockages, tears in tissue, liver damage, or pancreatitis.
- Mild cases treated with NSAIDs, severe cases treated with corticosteroids (see Chapter 21), other immunosuppressing drugs (azathioprine, cyclophosphamide, mycophenolate mofetil).

Interview Questions	• How does it affect you (signs, symptoms, complications)? Is it considered mild, moderate, or severe? Are you currently in a flare-up? • Which tissues or organs are affected? Are any tissues or organs affected by past flare-ups? • Is your skin affected? If so, how and where? • Are blood cells affected? Is blood clotting affected? If so, how is it affected? • Are any lymph nodes enlarged, or is your spleen enlarged? • Any problems with your heart, lung, liver, or kidney function? • Any effects on your nervous system—brain, spinal cord, or nerves? • Any areas of pain and inflammation? Is sensation affected? • Treatment? Effects of treatment?
Massage Therapy Guidelines	• Avoid circulatory intent at sites of unstable or inflamed tissues, and adjust massage pressure and joint movement at these sites, especially skin, joints; pressure maximum 2–3 in most cases. • If lung, heart, kidney, liver, or CNS affected, observe Vital Organ Principle; see Angina, Congestive heart failure, Pericarditis, Chapter 11. • Position for comfort to accommodate abdominal pain, hepatomegaly, splenomegaly, breathing problems. • Adapt to cytopenias (see Chapter 12); if risk of thrombosis elevated, follow DVT Risk Principles, Chapter 11. • For CNS conditions, see "Headache," "Seizure disorders," "Stroke (Cerebrovascular Accident)," (Chapter 10). • See "NSAIDs," "Corticosteroids," Chapter 21 for side effects and massage guidelines. See Table 21-1 for other side effects.

SELF TEST

1. Describe the difference between autoimmunity and immunodeficiency, and give one example of each.
2. Define opportunistic infection. Describe the four common types of opportunistic infections, and list two examples of each.
3. What is the significance of CD4 cell count for someone with HIV?
4. Describe lipodystrophy, and explain why it appears in HIV disease. Explain how the massage session might need to be adjusted for a client with lipodystrophy.
5. How should you adjust massage positioning for a client with HIV who presents with mouth sores or shortness of breath?
6. Does research show that massage improves immune function in people with HIV? Describe the evidence about massage and CD4 counts.
7. Why do you need to know the locations of any masses in a client with non-Hodgkin lymphoma? What are the massage therapy guidelines for common lymphoma sites?

8. How can non-Hodgkin lymphoma affect the spleen and liver? Explain the massage therapy guidelines in each case.
9. Why might the Vital Organ Principle be important in working with a client who has non-Hodgkin lymphoma?
10. How is bone structure affected in advanced cases of non-Hodgkin lymphoma? How is bone marrow affected? What are the complications of each of these scenarios?
11. Define lymphedema. What distinguishes it from other forms of edema?
12. How is each stage of lymphedema characterized? How are mild, moderate, and severe lymphedema characterized?
13. Describe the areas of massage caution in upper extremity lymphedema and lower extremity lymphedema. What is the trunk quadrant bordered by, in each case?
14. How do you adjust massage for a client with lymphedema? Explain the massage guidelines in detail.
15. Can conventional massage be used to reduce lymphedema? Explain why or why not.

 For answers to these questions and to see a bibliography for this chapter, visit http://thePoint. lww.com/Walton.

14 Respiratory System Conditions

A human being is only breath and shadow.

—SOPHOCLES

The breath defines life to the same degree as the pulse does. In respiratory health, the breath gives oxygen a clear gateway to the blood, and carbon dioxide an escape from the body. Breathing is something we take for granted until it becomes a health issue. In respiratory disease, the body's airways are partially blocked or irritated, or the lung tissue itself is compromised. When breathing is obstructed, a terror like no other overcomes an individual, and even the fear of that fear can be profound. Massage therapy can reach gently inside the isolation created by that experience and help ease its legacy of muscle tension. To that end, massage therapists should be encouraged to work with people with respiratory conditions.

This chapter addresses the following conditions at length, with full Decision Trees:

- The Common cold
- Asthma
- Emphysema

Conditions in Brief included in this chapter are **acute bronchitis, chronic bronchitis, cystic fibrosis, influenza (flu), lung cancer, pneumonia, pulmonary edema, sinusitis,** and **tuberculosis (TB)**.

General Principles

This chapter addresses three common respiratory conditions in depth, and in most of them, breathing difficulty, also called **dyspnea**, is a factor.

Using simple principles from Chapter 3, therapists can reason their way through most respiratory conditions and arrive at a massage plan. However, since some respiratory and pulmonary conditions are contagious, therapists should consider their own health and the health of their clients whenever contagion is an issue. Following standard precautions will protect against transmission in most cases, but viruses and other pathogens can be transmitted through coughing and sneezing as well as contact. In each situation, assess whether you or the client are at risk; if the client's friends, family, or health care providers are instructed to follow special infection control precautions, then bring your massage practices in line with these medical concerns.

The Common Cold

The common cold, also known as an upper respiratory tract infection (URI), or *viral rhinitis*, is caused by a virus.

● BACKGROUND

There are at least 200 different types of viruses that attack the tissues of the upper respiratory tract (the nasal passages and throat). After transmission, it usually takes 2–3 days to develop symptoms, and during this period, a person can be highly contagious. Most colds last a week or two, with the highest risk of contagion in the first 2–3 days. Although technically one is contagious as long as one has symptoms, colds are much less contagious by days 7–10.

Signs and Symptoms

The familiar symptoms of a cold are sneezing, a runny nose, sinus congestion nasal congestion, cough, sore throat, headache, and a mild fever. Adults and older children tend to have no fever or a low one. Young children often have a fever of 100 –102°F (37.8 –38.9°C). A sore throat is often the first symptom to appear, sometimes as early as 10 hours after infection.

Complications

Sometimes a cold leaves a person vulnerable to a bacterial infection, causing sinusitis, laryngitis, a middle ear infection, acute bronchitis, or pneumonia.

Treatment

Because there is no cure for the common cold, colds are primarily treated with rest and drinking fluids. Gargling and steam inhalation may provide symptom relief. Many people use vitamin C, Echinacea, and zinc supplements for a cold. OTC medications treat symptoms but do not eradicate the infection. These medications include pain relievers for sore throat and headache, cough syrups, and decongestants. Some medications can be drying, or can cause drowsiness, but overall, there are few side effects.

Although people are often tempted to ask a physician for antibiotics when they have a cold, antibiotics fight bacteria, not viruses, and will not cure a cold. Concern is growing in medicine and public health about excessive prescriptions of antibiotics. Frequent use of antibiotics has the unfortunate effect of building bacterial resistance to the drugs, thus making bacterial infections harder to treat when they do occur.

● INTERVIEW QUESTIONS

1. What are your cold symptoms?
2. How long have you had the cold?
3. Are you getting worse, or getting better?
4. Have you had a fever? Has it subsided?
5. Are there any complications, such as sinusitis, ear infection, or bronchitis?
6. How have you treated it? How has treatment affected you?

● MASSAGE THERAPY GUIDELINES

Always practice good infection control in the massage setting, to prevent contracting a cold from a client, spreading a cold from one client to others that day, or giving a cold to a client. Cold viruses can generally remain viable outside the body on a surface, such as a doorknob or massage table, for several hours. Every surface in contact with a client, including the

table, your hands, and the oil or lotion bottle, should be freshly cleaned for each client.

It is worthwhile to consider the ethics of working when you have a cold. Given the prolonged contact with a client's skin and the shared air, should you cancel at the first sign of cold symptoms? In a related context, most health care workers are required to report to work with a cold if they are able, but they are also required to practice excellent standard precautions to avoid spreading it. Typically, health care workers with symptoms will avoid contact with vulnerable clients, such as those with neutropenia (see Chapter 12). If you have a cold, consider your clients for the day: if there are individual preferences or vulnerabilities to respect, then offer the chance for clients to cancel if they wish. A scratchy throat could mean a mild allergy or it could be a forerunner of a full-blown cold. This practice is hard to make perfect, but you should be able to make your best judgment.

In massage training and literature, the common cold is listed as a massage contraindication, possibly because cold symptoms seem to worsen after massage. The popular explanation is that circulatory massage "pushes the virus through the body before the immune system can mount a response," but there are no data to support this hypothesis. Rather than try to explain the worsening symptoms, which would be tough to establish scientifically, consider the Compromised Client Principle. While the body is fighting infection, provide

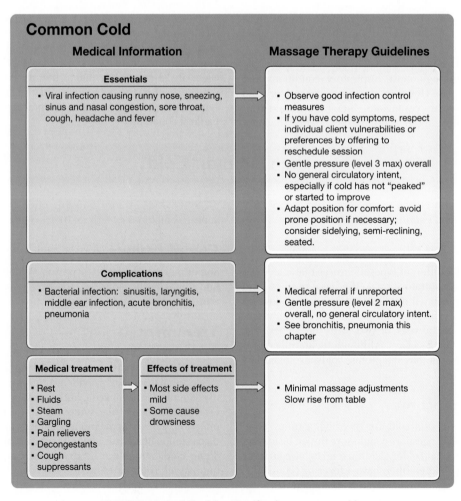

FIGURE 14-1. A Decision Tree for the common cold.

gentle massage. Instead of asking the body to integrate another strong stimulus, respect the body's natural healing processes.

> *The Compromised Client Principle. If a client is not feeling well, be gentle; even if you cannot explain the mechanism behind a contraindication, follow it anyway.*

Questions 1–4 should yield a basic history and status of the client's cold. The course of the infection is important in planning the strength of the massage. As stated before, the best approach, especially while the cold is still worsening, is to use gentle pressure and avoid general circulatory intent. This is true during any infection. However, if Questions 3 and 4 may suggest that the client is improving, not worsening, and the cold seems to have already "peaked." In this case, a slightly stronger session might be well tolerated. Be careful, though, because the client's body is still recovering from the infection. The idea is to give the body support, rather than further challenge.

The flat prone or supine position may be uncomfortable, increasing headache or congestion. The semi-reclining, side-lying, or seated position might provide relief from this discomfort.

Question 5 addresses any secondary bacterial infection. If a client reports severe or worsening symptoms, painful sinuses, loss of voice, pain in one or both ears, body aches, persistent coughing, or trouble breathing, the client is not the best candidate for massage. Instead, a medical referral is a good idea. If they have received a diagnosis and treatment for a complication and have been improving for several days, they might be able to tolerate gentle work, but be cautious: limit the overall pressure to level 2, and continue to avoid general circulatory intent.

The last question, about the effects of treatment, is unlikely to bring out significant massage adjustments. At most, drowsiness from cold remedies suggests a gentle session and a slow transition at the end.

● MASSAGE RESEARCH

As of this writing, there is just one randomized, controlled trial, published in the English language, on the common cold and massage indexed in PubMed and the Massage Therapy Foundation databases. The single listing of research on massage and the common cold, published in the *Journal of Traditional Chinese Medicine* (Zhu et al., 1998), reported on an RCT of massage of specific acupoints to strengthen the constitution of children and prevent respiratory tract infection. The NIH RePORTER tool lists no active, federally funded research projects on this topic in the United States. No active projects are listed on the clinicaltrials.gov database (see Chapter 6).

● POSSIBLE MASSAGE BENEFITS

A popular belief in the massage world is that working with clients after a cold has peaked will "get them better faster," but possibly make their symptoms worse for a day or so. There are no data to support this claim, and there's no way to draw this conclusion from clinical practice, without a control condition. If slow improvement in cold symptoms seems to turn to rapid improvement after a vigorous massage, you cannot tell whether this would have happened in the absence of the massage, with another explanation for the improvement. In other words, the sample size for the study is just 1, and there's no control group to compare it to.

Rather than claim massage will help a cold go away faster, emphasize the health benefits of regular massage. Steer clear of claiming a clear "boost in immunity" from massage, as this is unproven (see Table 6-1). However, it *is* fair to suggest that stress relief may help prevent some diseases, by supporting the body's defenses. Massage may facilitate sleep, which in turn facilitates healing. Perhaps one day we'll find that massage helps prevent the common cold, or even that it helps treat it, but we're nowhere near that claim yet.

Asthma

Asthma is a narrowing of the airways, or bronchial tubes, which is usually reversible. It features inflammation, then **bronchospasm** (constriction of the bronchi and bronchioles) and the production of excess mucus, or mucus plugs. These factors narrow the space through which air can travel during inhalation and exhalation, as shown in Figure 14-2.

● BACKGROUND

Although it usually develops in childhood, some adults can also develop asthma. Asthma attacks can last from a few minutes to several days, and can range from mild to severe. In severe cases, asthma can be life threatening.

Asthma is a common disorder, and it is on the rise in the United States, Canada, England, Australia, and New Zealand. In the United States alone, both the prevalence and the death rate from the condition have dramatically increased over the last three decades. Although the reasons are not conclusively known, theories include (1) an increase in allergens, such as dust mites and cockroaches, in indoor environments, due to

tighter insulation in buildings, and (2) the use of vaccines and antibiotics in children, causing a shift in the immune response toward allergies rather than fighting infection. Allergens such as molds, animal dander, and pollen are known triggers for asthma. Other asthma triggers include exercise; breathing cold, dry air; inhaling smoke or chemical fumes; taking certain medications; emotional stress; and a cold or the flu. There is also an association between gastroesophageal reflux disease (see Conditions in Brief, Chapter 15) and asthma, although the nature of the association is not well understood. Unfortunately, in some people who have severe asthma, the triggers remain unidentified.

Signs and Symptoms

Asthma manifests as attacks of wheezing and coughing, a feeling of tightness in the chest, and shortness of breath. Increased sputum production and reduced exercise tolerance are other signs. During an attack, the individual may feel better sitting up. In severe episodes, a fast pulse, sweating, **cyanosis**— bluish discoloration of lips, nailbeds, and skin—can occur.

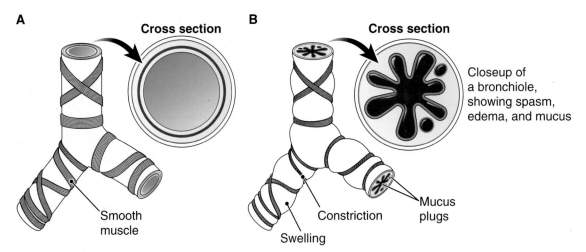

FIGURE 14-2. Asthma: normal bronchiole (A) and bronchiole during asthma episode (B). (From Willis MC. *Medical Terminology: A Programmed Learning Approach to the Language of Health Care*, 2nd ed. Philadelphia: Lippincott Williams & Wilkins, 2008.)

Over time, asthma can produce a "barrel chest" configuration, with chronically overinflated lungs (Figure 14-3).

Complications

Complications of asthma can include pneumonia, respiratory fatigue, and respiratory failure, which can be fatal. In especially severe cases, the alveoli can rupture, allowing air into the pleural space and collapsing the lungs. This rare complication is called **pneumothorax** and requires a chest tube to draw off the air and restore the lung to its expanded form.

Treatment

Conventional asthma treatments fall into three groups: long-term control to prevent attacks, rescue medications for immediate relief from an attack, and long-term allergy shots for allergic asthma.

Long-term prevention medications include corticosteroids, which may be inhaled (Pulmicort, Flovent) or oral (Decadron). Prevention is also achieved with long-acting **bronchodilators** (Serevent, Foradil, Oxeze), which open up the airways slowly and keep them open, usually over a 12-hour period. Increasingly, combination therapies such as Symbicort and Advair are used; these preparations are a blend of corticosteroid and bronchodilating medicines. Theophylline, another bronchodilator in the form of a daily pill, is used for severe cases, or in the evening if asthma disturbs sleep. It can cause GI upset, headache, nervousness, confusion, and rapid heartbeat.

Inhaled corticosteroids cause minimal side effects—just a cough or huskiness for a few minutes. However, if the medication remains in the mouth, it can cause a fungal infection of the mouth and throat called **thrush**, so patients are advised to rinse with water after taking it. Oral corticosteroids also have side effects, so prolonged use is discouraged (see "Corticosteroids," Chapter 21). Bronchodilators may cause headache, nervousness, rapid heartbeat, insomnia, and dizziness, among other effects.

Other asthma prevention medications are *leukotriene receptor antagonists*, such as Singulair or Accolate. These have rare side effects, including headache, dizziness, GI upset, and fatigue. Some patients with mild or moderate allergic asthma are prescribed *mast cell stabilizers*, such as cromolyn and nedocromil (Tilade), which dampen allergic reactions. They have few side effects, most commonly throat irritation, nausea, heartburn, or abdominal pain.

Rescue medications are usually inhaled, as in short-acting bronchodilators such as albuterol or ipratropium (Atrovent). These take effect within minutes and last 4–6 hours. Short-acting bronchodilators can cause nervousness, dizziness, insomnia, trembling, and increased heart rate. Individuals taking strong asthma medication are monitored closely for the correct dosage in order to minimize side effects.

If the asthma seems to be triggered by allergens, the individual may undergo **desensitization therapy**, also called *allergy shots*. This approach involves injecting allergenic substances in increasing amounts in order to desensitize the immune system, thereby discouraging an allergic reaction. Another immune system approach is called **anti-IgE monoclonal antibody therapy** or *antibody-blocking therapy* (Xolair). This newer therapy blocks the action of the antibodies involved in the allergic response. In both of these immune system approaches, serious allergic reactions are possible, and patients are carefully monitored.

A severe asthma attack is treated in the emergency department of a hospital. There, oxygen and IV equipment are available for rapid delivery of medicine, and, in some instances, an *endotracheal tube* or breathing tube is needed.

● INTERVIEW QUESTIONS

1. How long have you had asthma?
2. How often do you have trouble breathing? When was the last episode?
3. How does an episode affect you?
4. Is your asthma well controlled?
5. What are the identified triggers? Do you have any sensitivity to lotions or oils?
6. How do you manage an attack when it occurs?
7. Where can I find your inhaler, in case you want me to locate it for you while you are here?
8. How do you treat the asthma?
9. How do the treatments affect you?
10. Do you notice muscle tension anywhere caused by your breathing? Have you had massage therapy on those muscles before? If so, what worked and what didn't work?

● MASSAGE THERAPY GUIDELINES

Massage during an acute asthma attack is obviously not appropriate. Most massage adjustments are for a history of asthma.

The answers to Questions 1–4 establish important history: in particular, if the last episode was recent, the client might welcome massage therapy to relax fatigued muscles of breathing. Work these muscles gently and increase pressure gradually over a course of treatment, avoiding sudden changes in direction, rhythm, and rapid speeds so as not to aggravate tension.

Listen carefully to answers to Question 5 because it is important to eliminate or at least minimize triggers in the massage environment. In all cases, avoid using linens that have been washed in scented detergents or fabric softener, especially near the client's face. Avoid using shampoos, lotions, or other personal care products that contain fragrances. Ask about the client's sensitivity to plants in your office. Show the client the ingredients of lotions or oils you plan to use in the massage. It may be necessary to provide a massage with no lubricant, or to have the client bring his or her own, time-tested lotion or oil to the session, just to be safe. All of this depends on how well the client knows the asthma triggers and how strongly he or she reacts to them.

Keep these things in mind if you are working with a client whose asthma is poorly controlled: how to respond if an asthma attack occurs during the session (Questions 6 and 7); any complications (see Decision Tree); and the possible side effects from medication (Question 9). Observing the Emergency Protocol Principle, identify what to do if the client has an episode during the session, such as the best position for the client, locating the rescue medicine, and how to know whether to summon emergency services.

> *The Emergency Protocol Principle. **If a client has a condition with rapid or unpredictable changes in symptoms, ask about any warning signs and appropriate responses in case they occur during a massage.***

In regard to side effects of medication, the common concern for people on long-term oral corticosteroids is the thinning effect on bone and skin. There may also be effects on blood pressure and immunity (see "Corticosteroids," Chapter 21). Inhaled steroids cause fewer problems because the medicine is directed to the target area, and less goes into the bloodstream. In the rare event that an inhaled steroid leads to thrush, use gentler pressure overall and avoid general circulatory intent until it resolves.

There are no significant massage adjustments for nervousness, trembling, or increased heart rate, but it may take longer for the relaxing effect of massage to occur in these cases, and ultimately massage may help ease these symptoms (Wible, 2008). See the Decision Tree (Figure 14-4) for massage therapy guidelines for other bronchodilator side effects, such as dizziness, headache, and insomnia.

Side effects of leukotriene receptor antagonists are rare, and those of mast cell stabilizers are mild. If you identify side effects from these drugs in the interview, follow the Medication Principle, locate the side effect in Table 21-1, and follow the corresponding massage guidelines. Although severe reactions to desensitization therapy or antibody-blocking therapy are possible, patients are carefully monitored, and you are unlikely to encounter an acute reaction in the massage setting.

The answer to Question 10 will help you focus on specific skeletal muscles used in breathing, such as the intercostals, the sternocleidomastoids, and other muscles of ventilation. In particular, the SCMs can be prominent. Go in gently and gradually, and give these areas some time and attention during the session.

● MASSAGE RESEARCH

As of this writing, there are several studies of CAM use among children and adults with asthma (Braganza et al., 2003), and interest in massage is notable. However, there are few RCTs specific to massage therapy. In an updated Cochrane review of manual therapies for asthma (Hondras et al., 2005), authors surveyed the massage research and concluded that there was not enough evidence to support the use of manual therapies with asthma, finding just one RCT on the subject. In that study (Field et al., 1998), authors randomized 32 children with asthma to a daily massage from a parent or to a relaxation therapy group. Although this study reported improvement in the massaged children, the sample size is too small to claim clear benefit.

In an RCT comparing reflexology with sham control sessions (Brygge et al., 2001), authors observed little difference between the two procedures in effects on asthma symptoms. The NIH RePORTER tool lists no active, federally funded research projects on this topic in the United States. No active projects are listed on the clinicaltrials.gov database (see Chapter 6). Clearly, there is not an evidence base for the claim that massage can ease asthma symptoms, although further research is warranted.

● POSSIBLE MASSAGE BENEFITS

Depending on the individual, asthma may have a stress component, and massage therapy can be a beneficial component in a stress management program. Therapist's Journal 14-1 tells about the value of relaxation to a person with asthma.

Breathing difficulties require extra effort from the muscles of breathing. Even other muscles, when tense, can make it more difficult to breathe. Massage therapy, focused on specific muscles wrapping the rib cage, may turn out to be an important support for a person with asthma.

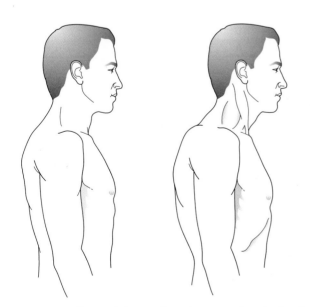

FIGURE 14-3. Postural changes in asthma over time. In the picture at right, note the "barrel chest" development, neck muscle tension, and forward head posture.

Asthma

Medical Information	Massage Therapy Guidelines

Essentials

- Narrowing of bronchial tubes caused by inflammation, bronchospasm and mucus production
- Causes shortness of breath, wheezing, coughing and chest tightness
- In severe episodes, rapid heart rate, sweating, cyanosis
- May be triggered by allergens

→

- No massage during acute attack
- Follow Emergency Protocol Principle if attack occurs during session; locate rescue medication

- Ask about triggers; avoid common triggers in massage lubricants, linens and environment

Complications

- Pneumonia
- Pneumothorax (rare)
- Respiratory fatigue, respiratory failure

→

- See "Pneumonia," this chapter
- Medical emergency; massage generally in inpatient setting with physician consultation, extremely gentle session overall

Medical treatment	Effects of treatment	
Oral corticosteroids	Long-term use thins bone and skin, increases BP, weakens immunity; see Corticosteroids, Chapter 21	See Corticosteroids, Chapter 21 Gentle pressure for thinned bone and skin See Hypertension, Chapter 11
Inhaled corticosteroids	Thrush (oral fungal infection)	No general circulatory intent, lighter pressure and gentler session overall
Inhaled bronchodilators	Possible strong side effects (usually well monitored)	Be able to locate inhaler if needed
	Nervousness, trembling, increased heart rate	Allow longer for relaxation effect of massage to occur
	Dizziness	Reposition gently, slow speed and even rhythm, slow rise from table, gentle transition at end of session
	Headache	Position for comfort, especially prone; consider inclined table or propping; gentle session overall; pressure to tolerance; slow speed and even rhythm; general circulatory intent may be poorly tolerated
	Insomnia	When appropriate, use sedative intent at end of day, activating/stimulating intent at beginning
Leukotriene receptor antagonists	Rare side effects (see text)	Follow Medication Principle; see Table 21-1 for massage therapy guidelines
Mast cell stabilizers	Some mild side effects possible (see text)	Follow Medication Principle; see Table 21-1 for massage therapy guidelines
Desensitization therapy and antibody-blocking therapy	Severe allergic reactions possible; patients well monitored	Medical emergency. Follow Medication Principle; see Table 21-1 for massage therapy guidelines

FIGURE 14-4. A Decision Tree for asthma.

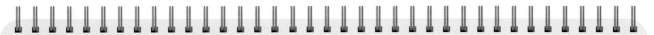

A man in his mid-thirties came to me for massage therapy and, during the interview, told me about his asthma. He was taking several medications, and used an inhaler, and he was a regular visitor to the ER. He had a great doctor who was supportive of massage therapy.

My initial contract with him was for weekly massage, 1-hour sessions. I gave a whole-body session but focused my work on his neck, shoulders, chest, and back—the whole thorax where his muscles were tight.

Sometime in the 1st year, though, I was inspired to ask him if he'd like to try a simple meditation during the session, focusing on his breath—noticing it but not judging it—and adding in a short mantra. I can't remember the exact words that he chose for his mantra, but I remember his spirituality figured into it. That can be the best kind of mantra: personal, brief, meaningful. I would never tell him to meditate instead of using his prescribed medication, but I suggested he add this awareness and focus to the massage, and even to his tool kit in dealing with asthma.

He really took to it. Somehow practicing meditation during the relaxation session of a massage emboldened him to try it elsewhere, too. He began using the meditation and the breath focus outside of the session to great effect. Because he practiced it in a setting where he was relaxed, it seemed like he took that relaxed sense with him whenever he did the exercise. He also began learning yoga, and after trying a few different teachers and schedules, he settled on a yoga teacher. He had encouragement from me and from his doctor.

After a year or so of these measures, he began noticing gradual changes in his asthma control. When he felt an impending attack, he would practice focusing on his breath and using the mantra before he reached for his inhaler. He knew he could use the inhaler or go to the ER if he had to, but he would try this first. It helped; his inhaler use and ER visits became less frequent. And he felt that his other meds were working better to prevent an attack. He was much less anxious and less controlled by the asthma.

Some asthma is life threatening, but even if it isn't, it's quality of life- threatening. Asthma really robs people, making them feel frightened and very out of control. They don't always feel like they can draw on their own resources— they have to reach for rescue medications or practitioners. Any measure that gives back some control is a grand thing.

I saw my client becoming more empowered. He had more self-confidence, more inner resources, and therefore more hope. I continued to see him for several more years, until he relocated and now sees another massage therapist. We still keep in touch, though, and he continues to do well.

Barbara Coughlin-Martin
Dennis, MA

Emphysema

Along with chronic bronchitis, **emphysema** is one of a group of conditions called **chronic obstructive pulmonary disease (COPD)**, in which the flow of air through the airways is persistently and irreversibly obstructed.

● BACKGROUND

In emphysema, the alveoli of the lungs are damaged, impairing the exchange of oxygen and carbon dioxide across their membranes. Oxygen cannot flow as freely to the bloodstream, and carbon dioxide cannot flow from the blood to the lungs to be exhaled. While cigarette smoking is the most common cause of emphysema, other pollutants can also damage alveoli of the lungs.

Signs and Symptoms

The classic symptom of emphysema is **air hunger**, which is dyspnea accompanied by the constant inability to catch one's breath. This is due to the inability to expel "used air" from the lungs, and CO_2 accumulates in the lungs and blood. In emphysema, chronic cough may also occur. Fatigue is common because of inadequate oxygen supply to the muscles. Cyanosis may be visible in the skin, lips, or nailbeds. For a while, there

may be no symptoms of emphysema, but the course of the disease becomes noticeable when shortness of breath, cough, and wheezing occur, and activity becomes difficult.

At first, a walk might be too fatiguing and cause uncomfortable shortness of breath. Over a period of years, other activities of daily living, such as a short trip across a room, getting out of bed, and even chewing food become difficult. As shown in Figure 14-5, people with emphysema and other forms of COPD will often lean forward and use the accessory muscles of inspiration to breathe. They might prefer loose waistbands, or may even unbutton them in order to reduce constriction at the abdomen and allow the diaphragm more space. As in asthma, an individual with emphysema may develop an enlarged barrel chest (see a side view in Figure 14-3). Because it becomes impossible to exhale completely, residual air becomes trapped in the lungs, and they are chronically overinflated. This sign appears along with *kyphosis* and forward head posture.

Complications

Complications of emphysema are many, as the body struggles to maintain homeostasis with less oxygen available. Hypertension on the pulmonary side may occur, and disease of the right side

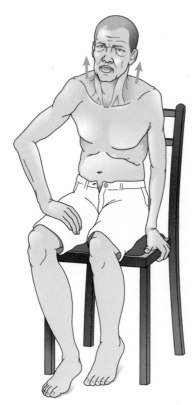

FIGURE 14-5. Common position for breathing in emphysema. People with emphysema often lean forward to more effectively use the accessory muscles of breathing, and loosen waistbands or undo fastenings to reduce constriction at the abdomen. Note tension in the sternocleidomastoid muscles.

of the heart, which results in swelling of the legs and abdomen. The risk of thrombosis is elevated in people with emphysema.

To compensate for poor blood oxygen levels, the red blood cell count may increase to capture as much oxygen as possible from each pass through the pulmonary circulation, a condition called *secondary polycythemia*. Although the disease process is different from polycythemia vera, it causes similar symptoms, such as headache (see Conditions in Brief, Chapter 12). In severe cases, secondary polycythemia causes fatigue, chest and leg pain, ringing in the ears, and burning sensations in the hands and feet. It also increases risk of thrombosis and other cardiovascular problems.

Oxygen delivery to the brain is compromised in advanced emphysema, resulting in confusion. Because breathlessness can make eating difficult, unintentional weight loss may occur, and malnourishment can contribute to an overall decline in health. People with emphysema are particularly vulnerable to recurrent respiratory infections. Chronic bacterial infection of the lower airways may occur, aggravating symptoms. Pneumonia can be a factor in causing death.

Claustrophobia is a problem, and people with emphysema are sensitive to being overheated. Anxiety, difficulty sleeping, and difficulty concentrating can also occur as emphysema advances.

Treatment

There is no known cure for emphysema, but its effects are managed. Patients with emphysema who smoke are advised to stop in order to stop the progression of the disease. Breathing medications include short- and long-acting bronchodilators,

similar to those used for asthma. Most bronchodilators are inhaled rather taken orally. Corticosteroids may be inhaled as needed, or taken orally if further anti-inflammatory action is required. A common combination therapy is an inhaled corticosteroid (fluticasone) and bronchodilator (salmeterol). See "Asthma," this chapter, for the side effects of bronchodilators and corticosteroids.

Antibiotics are given for chronic and acute respiratory infection. Even if no pneumonia is present, antibiotics can help manage exacerbations of emphysema and improve breathing during respiratory infection. Common side effects of antibiotics are mild nausea and diarrhea.

As the disease advances, low-flow oxygen may be used only at night, during exercise, or continuously. The oxygen may be stored in a large free-standing or lightweight portable tank, or be purified and concentrated from the air in a room, then delivered by a machine called an **oxygen concentrator**. Both of these devices are connected by plastic tubing either to a **nasal cannula** worn under the nostrils, or to a mask. Side effects of supplemental oxygen are minimal, and most patients experience significant relief. Pulmonary rehabilitation, including education and exercise, can help optimize function in people with emphysema.

Some patients may receive a lung transplant. Others may have **lung volume reduction surgery (LVRS)**, in which diseased portions of the lung are removed. This procedure makes room for healthier portions of the lung to expand, thereby improving the oxygenation of the blood. As with any surgery, this procedure can carry a risk of complications (see Chapter 21).

● INTERVIEW QUESTIONS

1. How long has it been since your diagnosis of emphysema?
2. How does it affect you? Is it considered mild, moderate, or severe?
3. Are there any complications of your emphysema?
4. Are there any effects on your heart function? Have your blood counts or blood pressure been affected? Have you experienced any swelling?
5. How do you manage sudden breathing difficulty if it occurs?
6. Where can I find your inhaler, in case you want me to locate it for you during the session?
7. Are there ideal positions for you for coughing or breathing, and what would be ideal positions for your massage?
8. How is it treated? How do treatments affect you?
9. Do you notice muscle tension anywhere caused by your breathing? Have you had massage therapy on those muscles before? If so, what worked and what didn't work?

● MASSAGE THERAPY GUIDELINES

Some of the common clinical features and massage adjustments for emphysema are summarized in Figure 14-7. In general, massage with people who have emphysema or any chronic breathing difficulty should begin gently, with particular attention to slow speeds and even rhythms, and avoiding sudden changes in pressure on the thorax. Positioning should be adapted to optimize breathing. Because a client may be claustrophobic, the drape should not be too constrictive, and a hot, dry massage room may be very uncomfortable. Spa treatments that use heat or body wrapping will likely be poorly tolerated by most clients who have emphysema. Follow the Core Temperature Principle.

THERAPIST'S JOURNAL 14-2 *Emphysema, Equipment, and Massage Therapy*

I've been a hospice volunteer for 12 years. I worked with a 64-year-old client with emphysema. Although she had lung reduction surgery the year before we started, she was quite compromised, and had reached the point where she had no energy to leave her bed. I visited her in her home every week for the last 6 months of her life.

Picture a tiny room, crammed with the furniture and belongings of a full life, a wall with plaques and other accolades for her many years of work with a nonprofit organization. There was a huge hospital bed, and a very small person in the middle of it. The other presence in the room was the oxygen concentrator: a large, noisy machine with tubing connected to a cannula that fed oxygen into her nose. Because her breathing was so labored, the machine was cranked to the maximum setting and gave off a lot of heat. For this reason, the client kept the windows open in winter, so the bedroom was freezing.

The client's skin was gray and her toes bluish from poor oxygenation. She was tired and often dozed off during our sessions. She was not always lucid, I believe because her brain had to work with less oxygen, but for the most part we had good conversations and she gave good feedback during her sessions. I suggested massage might help soften her breathing muscles and perhaps help her get more air.

In terms of massage adjustments, about all she could tolerate was a 20- or 25-minute session. I avoided massage on her thighs and lower legs because she had been in bed for so long and I was concerned about blood clots. All my movements were slow, gentle, rhythmic, and predictable, with pressure at a maximum of 2 or 3. We began her session with her supine, and the head of the bed elevated about 30 degrees. I would work at her sternum and let my fingers "stack" and sink in between her ribs and engage her intercostal muscles. I also worked the lower intercostals, reaching across the bed and using gentle pulling strokes with one finger between each rib, gliding toward her sternum. I used effleurage and petrissage on her feet and hands. Then she would sit up for 10 minutes or so, a position that was good for breathing and for getting at the scalenes, the trapezius muscles, and other muscles of her back. I sat behind her on the bed with a pillow between us to support her for this work, and finished with a bit of tapotement on her upper back. Then she would lie down supine again, and I would finish with work on her scalp, which she loved. To get to her, I had to move some furniture, squeeze behind the bed, fold myself up to get to the head and foot of the bed, and replace everything afterward. I was conscious of my body mechanics, but I also had to respect her belongings and her environment.

Sometimes we would use her oximeter, a device clipped to her finger that measures oxygen saturation. We would check it pre-massage and post-massage, and see improvement over the course of the session. Her readings would often be in the high 80s before the massage, then in the 90s afterward. Perhaps her position changes were partly responsible for the improvement, not the massage. Still, it was interesting to take these measurements and wonder whether massage, by relaxing and deepening breathing, played a role.

This client was rather reserved, and it took a while to establish rapport with her. But she became more comfortable over time. We would chat sometimes, and she reported fingering her own intercostals and scalenes to relax them. We'd sometimes share a chuckle over the goofy positions we found ourselves in as I navigated positioning to give her a massage. I'd like to think the massage therapy was helpful over those last months. Either way, it was an honor to work with her during that time.

Lee Blank
Rockville, MD

The Core Temperature Principle. **Avoid spa treatments that raise the core temperature if a client's cardiovascular system, respiratory system, skin, or other tissue or system might be overly challenged by heat, or if there are comparable medical restrictions.**

Because people with emphysema can suffer aggravated breathing difficulties during a respiratory infection, it is particularly important to practice excellent infection control, and to avoid exposing a client to your own viruses when you are sick. Offer to reschedule a session if you are experiencing cold or flu symptoms.

Without dwelling on your client's condition, your compassion and sensitivity can be particularly welcome, because air hunger is so difficult and frightening. It can be difficult to watch, too. Remember to breathe and settle during the interview and the session.

Questions 1–4 establish basic health information related to the emphysema. Work more cautiously with clients who have advanced disease. Emphysema complications cause people to be medically frail, so your work will be extremely gentle. Follow the Vital Organ Principle. By using gentle pressure overall, avoiding circulatory intent, and modifying other elements of massage, you accommodate most emphysema complications, including problems due to secondary polycythemia (headache, fatigue, pain and cardiovascular complications).

The Vital Organ Principle. **If a Vital Organ—heart, lung, kidney, liver, or brain—is compromised in function, use gentle massage elements and adjust them to pose minimal challenge to the client's body.**

If the client's cognitive function is affected by advanced disease, simplify and streamline your communication, establish clear consent for the massage, and observe for nonverbal signs of discomfort. The client's caregivers can provide additional guidance for communication and massage.

Pulmonary hypertension occurs with emphysema, but it is more localized than general hypertension. If a person has complications of emphysema, it is likely that the heart, at least on the right side, is taxed by the condition. While this contraindicates general circulatory intent, you have already handled this precaution with the Vital Organ Principle. If swelling is present in the lower extremities or abdomen, avoid pressure and circulatory intent at these sites.

Advanced disease raises the risk of thrombosis, and, because emphysema tends to worsen rather than improve, it is best to apply DVT Risk Principle I indefinitely (see Chapter 11). With emphysema, weight loss can be profound, and is another reason to provide a gentle session overall.

Questions 5 and 6 help you plan ahead, in case breathing becomes more difficult and "rescue" measures are necessary. A client may want to change position, reach for the inhaler, or both, so it's good to know where the inhaler is kept.

The questions about positioning will help you plan the session, as well. Inclining the upper body or placing the client in the side-lying position may be best for breathing. Some clients will want to sit up during the session. In Therapist's Journal 14-2, a practitioner describes several positions and adaptations used in sessions with a client with advanced emphysema.

Question 8 might illuminate a variety of medications, some with strong side effects. Selected effects of bronchodilators are described in the Decision Tree along with simple massage therapy adjustments. If the client is taking corticosteroids, adjust to any long-term effects on bone, skin, blood pressure, and immunity, and review "Corticosteroids," Chapter 21. If the client is taking antibiotics, most likely it's for a recent or current aggravation of emphysema symptoms, or recent or current pneumonia. Adjust to any diarrhea or nausea caused by the medications (see Figure 14-6).

If the client uses supplemental oxygen, be careful not to get lubricant on the tubing, especially at the cannula or mask (see Figure 14-7). Some clients choose to remove the cannula for certain activities; they might choose to remove it for brief periods during the massage. Tubing is pretty stiff, and stepping briefly on it will not affect oxygen flow, but prolonged crimping or pressure on it may, so check the tubing after each position change to see that it is free. Also, avoid the use of lighted candles in a room with supplemental oxygen.

If your client has had a lung transplant or LVRS, review massage therapy guidelines for organ transplant and surgery, Chapter 21. With lung transplant, there may be lingering effects from antirejection drugs, which may need to be taken indefinitely.

Question 9 points to the possibility of massage benefit by loosening the muscles of breathing. If possible, use the client's previous experience of massage to inform your massage of the muscles. Move in gently.

● MASSAGE RESEARCH

As of this writing, there are no randomized, controlled trials, published in the English language, on emphysema and massage indexed in PubMed or the Massage Therapy Foundation Research Database. The NIH RePORTER tool lists no active, federally funded research projects on this topic in the United States. No active projects are listed on the clinicaltrials.gov database (see Chapter 6).

● POSSIBLE MASSAGE BENEFITS

As with other conditions characterized by breathing problems, massage therapy can benefit clients with emphysema. While massage should not be initiated with too much pressure, experimenting over time with releasing muscle tension around the thorax, especially in the intercostals and scalenes, may aid breathing and be welcome (see Therapist's Journal 14-2).

Emphysema

Medical Information

Essentials

- Chronic obstructive pulmonary disease reducing gas exchange in alveoli
- Air hunger, cough, wheezing, fatigue, cyanosis
- Overuse and tension in accessory muscles of inspiration, kyphosis, enlarged barrel chest

Complications

- Pulmonary hypertension, right heart failure
- Swelling (lower extremities, abdomen)
- Thrombosis
- Secondary polycythemia: headache, fatigue, chest and leg pain, burning in hands and feet, cardiovascular complications
- Weight loss
- Respiratory infection

- Anxiety, claustrophobia, difficulty with sleep, concentration

Medical treatment

- Bronchodilators

- Corticosteroids

Effects of treatment

- Possible strong side effects (usually well monitored):
- Nervousness, trembling, increased heart rate
- Dizziness
- Headache

- Insomnia

- Long-term use thins bone and skin, increases BP, weakens immunity See Corticosteroids, Chapter 21

Massage Therapy Guidelines

- Follow Vital Organ Principle
- Gentle pressure on thorax, slow speeds, even rhythms, gradual transitions
- Position to facilitate breathing, cough: inclined upper body, seated, sidelying

- No general circulatory intent; gentle session overall
- Avoid general circulatory intent, circulatory intent at site
- Follow DVT Risk Principle I indefinitely (see Chapter 11)
- No general circulatory intent; gentle session overall
- Follow the Compromised Client Principle; see Chapter 11 for cardiovascular conditions such as thrombosis, heart failure
- Gentle session overall
- See Acute Bronchitis and Pneumonia, Conditions in Brief
- Observe strict infection control measures
- Compassion and sensitivity; predictable session, clear communication
- No constricting drape or spa wraps
- Avoid overheating environment, heat therapies

- Be able to locate inhaler if needed

- Allow longer for relaxation effect of massage to occur

- Reposition gently, slow speed and even rhythm, slow rise from table, gentle transition at end of session
- Position for comfort, especially prone; consider inclined table or propping; gentle session overall; pressure to tolerance; slow speed and even rhythm; general circulatory intent may be poorly tolerated
- When appropriate, use sedative intent at end of day, activating/stimulating intent at beginning

- See Corticosteroids, Chapter 21 Gentle pressure for thinned bone and skin See Hypertension, Chapter 11

FIGURE 14-6. A Decision Tree for emphysema.

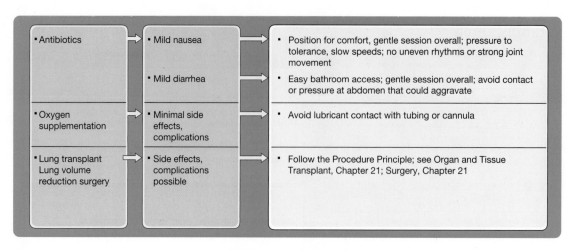

FIGURE 14-6. (*Continued*).

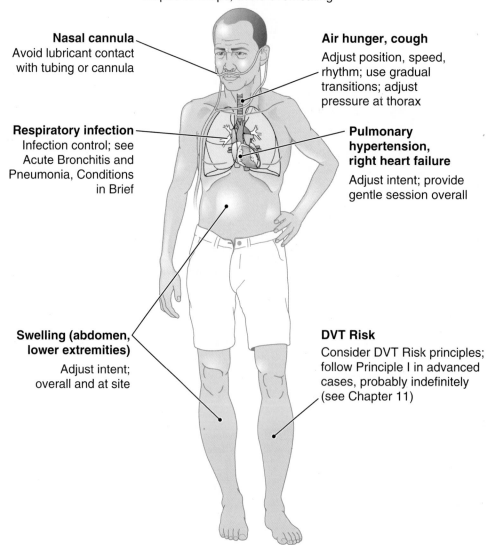

FIGURE 14-7. Emphysema: selected clinical features and massage therapy guidelines. Specific instructions and additional massage therapy guidelines are in Decision Tree and text.

Other Respiratory Conditions in Brief

BRONCHITIS, ACUTE

| Background | • One type of COPD , with infection and irritation of bronchial tubes, often caused by a secondary bacterial infection following the common cold.
• Unlike chronic bronchitis (see Conditions in Brief, this chapter), acute bronchitis does not cause irreversible scarring and narrowing of bronchial tubes.
• Symptoms are sore throat, fever, nasal congestion, fatigue, cough (dry or productive), with clear, discolored, or bloody mucus, wheezing, shortness of breath, chest pain. Pneumonia is a complication (see Conditions in Brief, this chapter).
• Treated with rest, fluids, steam, OTC pain relievers, antibiotics, inhaled corticosteroids; most side effects mild. |
|---|---|
| Interview Questions | • Have you seen your doctor about your symptoms? How long have you had them?
• Are symptoms worsening or improving? How is your cough? Your breathing?
• What is your activity level?
• Which resting or sleeping positions are most comfortable for you?
• Treatment? Effects of treatment? |
| Massage Therapy Guidelines | • If client has symptoms but has not reported it to her doctor, encourage a medical referral.
• Avoid general circulatory intent, limit overall pressure to level 3 until resolved, and individual has resumed normal activities.
• Adjust positioning for breathing comfort, and to minimize coughing: semi-reclining, side-lying, seated.
• Adjust massage to side effects of treatments (usually mild, as in nausea or diarrhea from antibiotics, see Table 21-1 for massage therapy guidelines).
• Focused, gentle work on muscles used in breathing and coughing may provide relief: thoracic, abdominal muscles, especially intercostals and scalenes. |

BRONCHITIS, CHRONIC

| Background | • One type of COPD, with irritation, irreversible scarring, narrowing of bronchial tubes over time.
• Caused by chronic lung irritation from cigarette smoke, pollution.
• Symptoms develop slowly, starting with mild cough; chronic bronchitis is diagnosed when cough occurs on most days for at least 3 months each year for 2 consecutive years.
• Sputum is thick, either clear, white, yellow-gray, green.
• Can complicate to pneumonia (this chapter); progressive damage can be accompanied by emphysema (this chapter). |
|---|---|
| Interview Questions | • How long have you had it, and when was it diagnosed?
• How does it affect you? Any complications?
• Is your doctor concerned about your blood circulation or heart?
• How is your breathing or cough?
• What positions are best for your breathing? Sleeping? How should we position you for massage?
• Treatment? Effects of treatment? |
| Massage Therapy Guidelines | • If advanced, assume cardiovascular strain or consult physician and avoid general circulatory intent.
• Locate inhaler before session.
• Position for breathing comfort, coughing (see Acute Bronchitis, this chapter). |

CYSTIC FIBROSIS

Background	• Genetic disorder affecting exocrine gland function in respiratory, digestive, reproductive, and integumentary systems; primary effects on respiratory system; usually diagnosed around age 3, average lifespan 30 years.

- Membranous secretions become thick and sticky, difficult to clear in respiratory tract, causing dry or productive cough, dyspnea, chest pain, cyanosis, and vulnerability to respiratory infection.
- Digestive function affected by poor secretion of pancreatic enzymes, low production or transfer of bile.
- Complications include pneumothorax, right heart failure, enlarged spleen, duodenal ulcers (see Chapter 15), gallstones, cirrhosis (see Chapter 16); poor absorption of nutrients from digestive tract can lead to osteoporosis; men are usually infertile.
- Skin perspiration is thick and salty, leading to poor thermoregulation.
- Treatment includes mucus-thinning medications that can irritate airway and cause sore throat, bronchodilators (see "Asthma," this chapter), pain relievers (see Chapter 21), antibiotics for infection (with nausea, vomiting, diarrhea as side effects), manual percussion of thorax to drain airways.

Interview Questions	<ul><li>How does it affect you? Which systems or organs are affected?</li><li>Have you had any complications? Any effects on your heart, spleen, liver, or other organs?</li><li>How is your bone stability? Do you have any osteoporosis?</li><li>Any signs or symptoms of infection? Are there any precautions you take to avoid infection?</li><li>How is your breathing? What do you do if you have trouble breathing?</li><li>What are the best positions for you during massage? In which positions do you sleep?</li><li>Treatment? Effects of treatment?</li></ul>
Massage Therapy Guidelines	<ul><li>Maintain comfortable room temperature during warm weather and drape lightly to avoid overheating client.</li><li>Observe excellent infection control measures; offer to reschedule if you feel ill.</li><li>If infection present, or client feels weak, avoid general circulatory intent and limit pressure to level 2, depending on tolerance (Vital Organ Principle).</li><li>Position to optimize breathing/coughing with inclined upper body, seated, possibly side-lying.</li><li>If complications affect spleen or liver, follow Filter and Pump Principle (see Chapter 3).</li><li>If client has osteoporosis, gentle pressure overall, with medical consultation about bone stability.</li><li>Adjust massage to medications and side effects (see Table 21-1).</li></ul>

INFLUENZA (FLU)

Background	<ul><li>Viral infection of respiratory tract, similar to common cold, but with higher fever that lasts 3 days or more.</li><li>Inflamed respiratory tract, headache, dry cough, achy muscles and joints, fever, chills, sore throat, swollen lymph nodes, profound fatigue; may also feature vomiting, diarrhea.</li><li>Continues to be contagious about a week after symptoms develop.</li><li>Complications include sinusitis, ear infections, bronchitis, pneumonia.</li><li>Treated with rest, fluids, pain relievers (see Chapter 21), antivirals (Tamiflu, Relenza) in some cases; antivirals can cause confusion.</li></ul>
Interview Questions	<ul><li>What were your symptoms? How did it affect you?</li><li>When did you develop symptoms, and how long were you sick? When did it resolve? How long have you been feeling better?</li><li>Treatment? Effects of treatment?</li></ul>
Massage Therapy Guidelines	<ul><li>Do not massage a person with flu until symptoms resolve and risk of transmission has passed.</li><li>Because flu is more contagious than common cold, lasts longer, and is spread by inhaling airborne viruses, be careful to avoid contracting or transmitting it; observe good infection control procedures, use well-ventilated room, especially during flu season.</li></ul>

LUNG CANCER

Background	• Primary tumor of the lung, most common cancer type, two principal types: non-small cell lung cancer (NSCLC), small cell lung cancer (SCLC); NSCLC is 75% of lung cancer diagnoses. • SCLC more aggressive, more likely to be inoperable, but more responsive to chemotherapy and radiation than NSCLC. • Symptoms: cough, bloody sputum, difficulty breathing or swallowing, hoarseness, fatigue, weight loss; may be asymptomatic for extended period of time. • Metastasis most often to brain and bone, also to liver and adrenal glands. • Can be difficult to treat; may be inoperable, treated with chemotherapy, radiation therapy (see Chapter 20); palliative care common.
Interview Questions	• Where is it in your body? In lungs, or other places also? • How does it affect you? Is your breathing affected? • Is there any bone involvement? (See "Bone Metastasis," Chapter 20.) Any areas of pain? • What would be the most comfortable position for you during the massage? In what position do you sleep? • Treatment? Effects of Treatment?
Massage Therapy Guidelines	• Review Cancer, Chapter 20, for massage therapy guidelines for cancer and cancer treatment; follow Vital Organ Principle (see Chapter 3) • Adjust massage to sites of cancer spread, such as liver, bone, brain. • If bone involvement, see "Bone Metastasis," Chapter 20; if pain, especially new, unfamiliar, or increasing pain, do not use pressure or joint movement at site until physician verifies that no bone metastasis is present. • If liver function impaired, avoid general circulatory intent, adjust position for liver enlargement; (see "Liver Cancer," Chapter 16). • Adjust massage position for comfort and ease of breathing (consider side-lying, seated, semi-reclining); gentle focus on muscles of breathing may assist respiration. • Adapt to brain involvement (see "Brain Metastasis," Chapter 20). • Follow DVT Risk Principle I indefinitely throughout active lung cancer, advanced lung cancer, treatment; for successful, completed treatment, add DVT Risk Principle II (see Chapter 11).

PNEUMONIA

Background	• Inflammation of lungs, caused by bacterial infection (most common), or by other organisms (viral, fungal, parasitic). • Can be complication of other respiratory infection (bronchitis, common cold); more easily acquired in nursing facilities, in immunocompromised individuals (e.g., people with HIV, in chemotherapy, or on immunosuppressive medications). • May develop when vomit is aspirated, or when food is aspirated in an individual who has difficulty swallowing. • Cough with yellow or green mucus, bloody sputum, fever, chills, chest pain aggravated by inhalation or coughing, breathing difficulty; some forms milder than others ("walking pneumonia"). • Complications include severe breathing difficulty (acute respiratory distress syndrome), bacteria in blood (bacteremia), abscess formation on the lung, fluid accumulation in pleura (pleural effusion) with inflammation (pleurisy) and infection (empyema); DVT and PE can occur, especially with prolonged bedrest. • Treatment includes rest, fluids, productive coughing, OTC pain relievers, cough suppressants. • Oral or IV antibiotics, antivirals, antifungals given depending on pathogen, side effects include nausea, vomiting, diarrhea. • Supplemental oxygen or mechanical ventilation provided for complications in hospitalized patients.

Interview Questions	• How long have you had pneumonia? What is the cause? • How does pneumonia affect you? Are you getting worse or better? • Do you have any cough, or difficulty breathing? • Any complications or worsening of the disease? • What is your activity level? Tolerance of activity? • Which positions are comfortable sleeping positions? What position would you prefer during the massage? • Treatment? Effects of treatment?
Massage Therapy Guidelines	• Follow Vital Organ Principle; avoid general circulatory intent until resolved; limit overall pressure to level 2 until client resumes normal activity and tolerates it well. • In most cases, limit overall pressure to level 1 if complications have developed, work in consultation with client's physician. • Because bedrest may increase DVT risk, follow DVT Risk Principles for at least several weeks after infection resolves and client resumes normal activity. • Adapt position for comfort and ease of breathing; consider side-lying, semi-reclining, seated. • Adjust massage to side effects of medications, including mild nausea or diarrhea from antibiotics, mild, rare side effects of cough suppressants, expectorants (see Table 21-1); see Analgesics Chapter 21.

PULMONARY EDEMA

Background	• Life-threatening condition of fluid accumulation in lungs, caused by blood flow backup in pulmonary circuit, with backpressure in lungs. • Can be caused by heart condition, pneumonia, being at high altitude, some medications. • Symptoms are shortness of breath, cough, sweating, pallor, fluid weight gain; can be first sign of heart condition. • In complicated cases, swelling occurs in lower extremities, abdomen, pleura (pleural effusion). • Oxygen therapy, diuretics to reduce fluid accumulation, other antihypertensives (see Chapter 11).
Interview Questions	• How long have you had it? What is the cause? Is it considered acute? • Signs and symptoms? Did they develop quickly or slowly? • What is your activity level? Are there any medical restrictions on your activities? • Treatment? Effects of treatment?
Massage Therapy Guidelines	• Acute symptoms require immediate medical attention. • Gentle session overall; follow Vital Organ Principle. Refer to Chapter 11 if heart condition involved (most cases); follow DVT Risk Principles (see Chapter 11). • For chronic cases, adapt position for breathing comfort (semi-reclining, side-lying, seated). • Adapt massage to treatments and side effects (see Table 21-1).

SINUSITIS

Background	• Inflammation of sinuses, either acute or chronic (lasting more than 8 weeks); can be caused by infection (viral, bacterial, fungal) or allergy (dust, mold, pollen). • Sinus pressure causes headache, facial pain, aching in jaw, teeth, aggravated by bending down, nasal congestion, thick, yellow or green nasal discharge, cough. • Infectious sinusitis features thick, sticky discolored mucus and cold symptoms, possible fever and chills if bacterial. • Allergic rhinitis features thin, clear mucus without signs of infection. • First-line treatment with fluids, rest, nasal rinse, decongestants, NSAIDs (see Chapter 21), drugs that thin mucus (guaifenesin); if bacterial cause, antibiotics, corticosteroid nasal sprays; antifungal sinusitis treated with IV antifungal drugs, surgical drainage. • Numerous mild side effects possible, drowsiness common.

Interview Questions	• Do you know if it is due to infection or allergy? • Other symptoms? • Treatment? Effects of treatment?
Massage Therapy Guidelines	• If infectious, no general circulatory intent; limit overall pressure to level 2; practice excellent infection control precautions. • Flat supine or prone position in face cradle can aggravate symptoms; consider semi-reclining, seated, or side-lying position for comfort. • Limit pressure at the site of facial pain. • Adapt to effects of treatment (see NSAIDs, corticosteroids, Chapter 21; see Table 21-1).

TUBERCULOSIS

Background	• Bacterial infection of lungs; can be latent (non-contagious, inactive, no symptoms) or active (contagious, symptomatic); active infection can be fatal. About one third of all people in the world are thought to have latent infection; 5–10% of those progress to active TB. • Active TB causes unexplained weight loss, fever, chills, night sweats, chest pain, coughing that persists 3+ weeks, bloody sputum, damage to lung tissue. • Disseminated TB, in which bacteria enter lymphatic system and blood circulation, can cause multiple organ dysfunction, including impairment of kidneys, liver, spleen, pancreas, adrenal glands, bone, and CNS. • Latent TB treated preventively with 9-month course of isoniazid; initial treatment of active TB is with four different antibiotics (isoniazid, rifampin, ethambutol, pyrazinamide); typically 2 weeks of treatment while in isolation (in hospital) renders individual non-contagious, followed by 6+ months of continued treatment with at least two antibiotics. • In 95% of patients, side effects are not serious, but liver toxicity can occur, or numbness in extremities. • Compliance with TB drugs is low because of side effects and prolonged course of treatment; compliance essential to prevent development of drug-resistant strains.
Interview Questions	• Do you have active TB or just a positive TB test? • What are your symptoms? Do you have pain or discomfort anywhere? • Which organs are affected? Has it affected your lung function, or function of your liver, spleen, pancreas, or other organs? • How long have you been treated? Are you being monitored by your doctor? Has he or she established that your TB is no longer communicable and cleared you for contact with others, etc.?
Massage Therapy Guidelines	• If TB symptoms unreported, urgent medical referral. • If latent TB, no massage adjustments. • If active TB, refrain from all contact until physician clears client for contact with others, is unlikely to transmit disease. • If complications have occurred, avoid general circulatory intent, use gentle pressure overall (level 2–3 depending on tolerance and physician consultation). • If disseminated TB has occurred, plan extremely gentle session overall, avoid general circulatory intent, adjust positioning for comfort (liver or spleen enlargement); if infection involves the meninges, see "Meningitis," Chapter 10. • TB medications are notoriously strong and toxic, with low compliance rate; general circulatory intent may be poorly tolerated if client is taking TB drugs; follow the Filter and Pump Principle if impairment of liver function results from medications.

SELF TEST

1. For a cold, why should massage pressure and general circulatory intent be modified?
2. At what point, during the course of the common cold, is the person with the cold most contagious? When does the risk of virus transmission drop?
3. List five signs and symptoms indicating that a secondary bacterial infection, such as bronchitis, may have set in following a common cold.
4. If you have a cold, what factors do you consider when deciding whether to cancel your massage sessions for the day?
5. Is there research supporting the claim that massage, provided after cold symptoms have peaked, will help rapidly resolve the condition? If so, describe the evidence.
6. What are three ways you might have to modify your massage environment for a client with allergic asthma?
7. How does the Emergency Protocol Principle apply to massage with clients who have asthma?

8. List three side effects of bronchodilators, and massage therapy modifications for each.
9. Are claims of massage benefit for people with asthma supported by research? Explain.
10. Describe air hunger in emphysema. What is the cause?
11. How does emphysema change posture and breathing?
12. Describe two cardiovascular complications of emphysema, and explain the corresponding massage guidelines.
13. Name three massage therapy positions that may ease breathing for a client with emphysema.
14. In a client with emphysema, which skeletal muscles may benefit from extra focus in the massage plan?
15. Describe the use of supplemental oxygen and how you might adapt to it during the massage session.

 For answers to these questions and to see a bibliography for this chapter, visit http://thePoint.lww.com/Walton.

15 Gastrointestinal Conditions

Digestion exists for health, and health exists for life, and life exists for the love of music or beautiful things.

—G.K. CHESTERTON

The digestive process consists of the breakdown of food and the absorption of nutrients. Like breathing, these essential functions of the body are taken for granted most of the time, because they are performed without our conscious awareness.

The gastrointestinal (GI) tract is a single, continuous tube running through the body; sections of the tube are cordoned off from each other by sphincter muscles to compartmentalize their functions. The tube varies in width, from the widened stomach to the narrowed small intestine. It begins in the mouth, or oral cavity, continues as the esophagus, the stomach, the small intestine, large intestine or colon, and ends with the rectum and anus.

Along the GI tract, accessory organs assist with digestion. These include the pancreas, which produces pancreatic enzymes used in the breakdown of food, the liver, which produces bile salts for the breakdown of fats, and the gallbladder, which stores the bile. Any of these structures can be affected by inflammation, infection, cancer, or other disease processes that affect function.

This chapter addresses the following conditions at length, with full Decision Trees:

- Constipation
- Peptic ulcer disease
- Ulcerative colitis (UC)

In addition, a full discussion of diverticular disease (diverticulosis and diverticulitis), including a Decision Tree, may be found online at http://thePoint.lww.com/Walton. Conditions in Brief in this chapter include diseases of the GI tract, pancreas, and gallbladder. (Liver conditions are discussed in Chapter 16.) Conditions in Brief included in this chapter are appendicitis, celiac disease, colorectal cancer, Crohn disease, diarrhea, esophageal cancer, gallstones (cholelithiasis), gastroenteritis (food poisoning, "stomach flu"), gastroesophageal reflux disease (GERD), irritable bowel syndrome (IBS), nausea and vomiting, pancreatic cancer, pancreatitis, peritonitis, and stomach cancer (gastric cancer).

General Principles

Many disorders of the GI tract involve inflammation, described with the suffix, -itis. Gastroenteritis is inflammation of the stomach and small intestine, colitis is inflammation of the colon, and so on. Inflammation may be due to viral, bacterial, fungal, or parasitic infection. It may also be caused by food allergy or intolerance, or by imbalances in digestion and absorption. No matter what the cause, the Inflammation Principle (see Chapter 3) is applied in these cases; avoiding pressure on any affected areas within reach. By following this principle, and positioning the client for comfort, the massage therapist can work safely with most conditions.

Classic signs and symptoms of GI problems include nausea, vomiting, diarrhea, constipation, gas, abdominal distension, cramping, and pain in the area. In most massage settings, massage therapists are unlikely to encounter acute symptoms, but chronic, low level GI symptoms are common in the general population. Therapists working with medically compromised clients frequently encounter acute GI symptoms and conditions.

Constipation

A common GI problem, constipation consists of infrequent bowel movements, passing hard and dry stools, and/or straining or discomfort during bowel movements. The medical definition of constipation is a bowel movement frequency of less than three times per week. Although there is a lot of variation in the frequency of normal bowel movements, most adults have them ranging from three times each day to three times a week.

● BACKGROUND

Constipation is not a disease or medical condition by itself; it is a symptom or complication of another condition. Contributing factors can include inadequate dietary fluid or fiber, a sedentary lifestyle, pregnancy and recent childbirth, surgery with anesthesia, aging, thyroid problems, delaying bowel movements, pain, and depression. Some medications, such as opioid analgesics, calcium channel blockers, antidepressants, antiseizure drugs, and diuretics, can cause constipation.

Constipation can be a sign of a serious problem in the bowel, such as a bowel obstruction, inflammatory bowel disease, diverticulitis, or colorectal cancer.

Signs and Symptoms

In constipation, bowel movements are less frequent than the normal range, or stool is difficult to pass because of hardness and/or dryness. Straining and discomfort may accompany symptoms of constipation.

Complications

Frequent straining can cause **hemorrhoids**, itchy or painful swelling of varicose veins around the anus; **abrasions**, the wearing away of the membrane surface; and **fissures**, splits or tears in the anus. Abrasions cause burning pain and fissures cause sharp pain. Chronic constipation can lead to a **bowel impaction**, the formation of a mass of dry, hard stool in the rectum that cannot exit the body. A bowel impaction is a serious situation, and watery stool may move around it, leaking from the anus.

Treatment

Dietary changes that include more fiber and water may help constipation, and fiber supplements are popular. Stool softeners, such as mineral oil or docusate, may help the passage of stool, although long-term use is discouraged. Laxatives may also help, but long-term use is discouraged to avoid dependency. Some laxatives have side effects of fatigue and weakness, as well as gas. People with constipation are encouraged to move around and exercise as much as possible to facilitate movement.

Manual treatment may be necessary for a bowel impaction, in which the physician inserts fingers into the rectum and breaks up the fecal mass so that the smaller pieces may be passed.

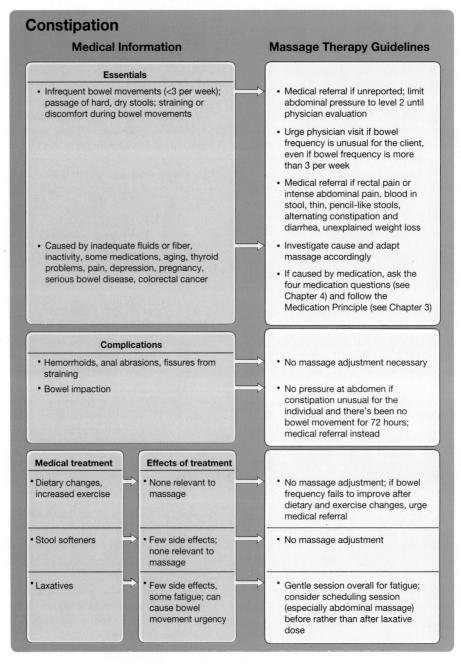

FIGURE 15-1. A Decision Tree for constipation.

● INTERVIEW QUESTIONS

1. How often are you constipated? How long do you go between bowel movements?
2. Is this unusual for you?
3. Do you know the cause?
4. Have you reported it to your doctor?
5. Do you have any abdominal pain or tenderness?
6. Is there any intense pain, bleeding, tearing, or hemorrhoids?
7. How is it being treated?
8. How does the treatment affect you?

● MASSAGE THERAPY GUIDELINES

Although some therapists might be uncomfortable asking certain delicate questions of their clients, and some clients may be shy in answering them, the first six questions determine the advisability of abdominal pressure during the massage, and whether a medical referral is in order. Bowel movement frequency of less than three times per week is low—it is cause for gentler pressure at the abdomen and a strong medical referral. If the client has already seen a doctor about the problem, has made changes in diet and exercise, and the condition persists, refer the client back to his or her doctor and continue to be gentle in the area.

Also, consider what is normal for the person, because any change in bowel habits is cause for concern. For example, if your client reports just four bowel movements per week, compared to his or her normal frequency of two per day, he or she needs medical attention. This also goes for rectal or intense abdominal pain; blood in the stool; thin, pencil-like stools; unexplained weight loss; and alternating constipation and diarrhea.

Supporters of massage therapy report that abdominal massage with some pressure (usually around level 3) can help constipation. In a minor case of constipation and a slight departure from the client's normal frequency, that may be appropriate. However, the safest approach is to stay at pressure level 1 or 2 when the client does not know the cause of the condition, it persists, bowel frequency is less than three times per week, or significantly different from the client's usual habits. In the meantime, you might help the condition without using direct pressure: by placing your hands gently over the abdomen or low back, or by using reflexology or other modalities that are not directed at the site.

To explain your reasoning to the client, you might say something like this: "Because it could be something serious or something minor, getting a doctor's opinion is a good idea. I recommend you see your doctor. In the meantime, I am going to use only the gentlest pressure on your abdomen."

Adapt the massage to any cause of constipation reported in answer to Question 3. Causes such as low fluid or fiber intake don't usually require specific massage adjustments; but review adjustments for more serious causes, such as colorectal cancer and ulcerative colitis (this chapter). If a client's constipation is caused by medication, then you will need to ask the four medication questions (see Chapter 4) and follow the Medication Principle (see Chapter 3).

THERAPIST'S JOURNAL 15-1 *Unexpected Outcomes*

I'm a hair stylist as well as a massage therapist. For a while, I worked in a hair salon and had my own massage business there, too. I learned reflexology in my basic training in school and practice it a lot, although my thumbs are more sensitive than my index finger so I learned to apply the pressure and do the assessment with my thumbs instead.

I've been a massage therapist for many years, and the beauty of massage is in the unexpected results of massage as well as the expected ones. A person comes in thinking, "I'm getting my body worked," or "I'm getting my feet rubbed," that's expected. People who have a massage don't necessarily expect to feel great for a few days or to sleep better. And if they're just one-time clients I only get to know how they feel right after the session—I don't get to find out how the massage affected them the next day.

In this salon, the other employees knew about my massage work and many had experienced it firsthand. One day one of the staff was giving a client a manicure and the client, I'll call her Krista, was complaining of terrible constipation. She was really uncomfortable. The manicurist told her, "You should see Starr for reflexology—that might help. Believe me, I know this from experience!" The client was doubtful, but you could tell she was interested. The manicurist came and got me and I talked with Krista for a few minutes. She told me she hadn't had a bowel movement for nine days. She'd tried everything. I told her reflexology might help. The look on her face was something like, "Yeah…right!" But she said let's give it a shot—we have nothing to lose, and she would try it for a few minutes. I had a long break, so I took her back to the treatment room and she removed her socks.

I started with broad strokes on her feet, which were tender. I followed with gentle work over the colon points, which were very sore, then deeper work over those points. I worked for maybe 10–15 minutes. I told her, "You might have some movement in the next couple of hours." I could tell she wasn't convinced, but she was polite about it. She put on her socks and left.

The next day I arrived at work, and she had sent me flowers. The note said, simply:

Thank you. —Krista.

It gave me a pretty good idea of how things turned out.

Starr Pugh
Lawrence, KS

For complications due to straining, such as abrasions or fissures, there is no massage adjustment required. However, a bowel impaction could be present in prolonged constipation; this is one reason for limiting your pressure at the abdomen if it has been more than 3 days since the last bowel movement.

Although constipation remedies have few side effects that are relevant to massage, some laxatives cause fatigue and weakness, calling for a gentler session. In addition, the client may want to consider the timing of abdominal massage and laxatives, to avoid bathroom interruptions during the session.

● MASSAGE RESEARCH

There are a few studies on massage and constipation. They are too small to be conclusive, but they should inspire further research. In an RCT of 60 subjects with constipation, investigators compared a laxative-only control intervention with laxatives and abdominal massage (Lamas et al., 2009). They found that abdominal massage was associated with more frequent bowel movements and fewer GI symptoms. The investigators concluded that massage might complement laxative treatment but did not suggest that massage replaces it.

In another study of 24 spinal cord injured patients, investigators reported some improvement in constipation after abdominal massage (Ayas et al., 2006). The study was uncontrolled, and too small to yield firm conclusions, but the practice of abdominal massage in this population deserves further

investigation. Meanwhile, case reports suggest a revival of interest in massage for constipation (Preece, 2002), and it can be a part of a patient's self care at home (Harrington and Haskvitz, 2006). More research may support the practice of abdominal massage in such cases.

● POSSIBLE MASSAGE BENEFITS

Massage and bodywork for constipation are based on simple, straightforward approaches. General relaxation massage may be helpful: by enhancing flexibility and body awareness, it may facilitate exercise, which promotes normal bowel function.

Direct massage of the abdomen, with gentle pressure in the direction of intestinal peristaltic flow, may help relieve constipation. The classic protocol addresses each segment of colon, beginning with the most distal: downward strokes at the descending colon, followed by strokes across the transverse colon and then down the descending colon. Finally, strokes go up the ascending colon, across the transverse colon, and down the descending colon. In this last, rounded stroke, you draw a clockwise circle on the client's abdomen.

Whether the strokes actually move the intestinal contents, or simply stimulate normal peristaltic movements that propel the contents is not yet clear. However, people therapists report benefits from this approach and from other common therapies such as acupressure and reflexology. Therapist's Journal 15-1 tells the story of simple reflexology techniques for a client with constipation.

Peptic Ulcer Disease

An **ulcer** is an open sore in skin or mucous membrane. **Peptic ulcer disease** is a collective term for ulcers in the GI tract, from the esophagus to the small intestine (Figure 15-2). An **esophageal ulcer** is an open sore in the lining of the esophagus. A **gastric ulcer**, also known as a *stomach ulcer*, is an open sore in the lining of the stomach. A **duodenal ulcer** is located in the upper part of the small intestine, or *duodenum*.

● BACKGROUND

The condition used to be attributed to lifestyle issues such as poor diet, overindulgence in certain foods, and stress. In the 1980s, researchers discovered that one kind of bacterial infection, from the bacterium *Helicobacter pylori*, is at the root of most ulcers, and that esophageal ulcers may also be due to stomach acid reflux. The regular use of NSAIDs, smoking, excessive alcohol consumption, and unmanaged stress can contribute to ulcer development. These factors can also aggravate ulcers and delay healing. Regardless of the cause, the open sore is aggravated by contact with stomach acid.

Signs and Symptoms

The most common symptom of peptic ulcer disease is burning pain, experienced anywhere from the sternum to the navel. It can last just a few minutes or many hours. The pain is sometimes worse on an empty stomach, and is temporarily relieved by eating. Flare-ups of pain are common at night. Severe signs or symptoms of ulcers include nausea or vomiting, vomiting blood, dark or tarry stool, chest pain, and unexplained weight loss.

Complications

An ulcer that does not heal in response to treatment is called a **refractory ulcer**. If a peptic ulcer is left untreated over time, it can cause internal bleeding, and blood loss over time can cause anemia. It can also produce scarring that obstructs the movement of material through the digestive tract, leading to a feeling of fullness, vomiting, and weight loss. This condition is typically treated surgically.

Another serious complication of peptic ulcer occurs when erosion of the stomach lining leads to **perforation** of the stomach. A tear in the stomach wall allows the movement of contents into the abdominal cavity, causing **peritonitis**, an uncontrolled infection in the abdominal cavity that can be life threatening (see Conditions in Brief, this chapter). With peritonitis, **sepsis** may occur, in which an infection overwhelms the body, a systemic inflammatory response occurs, and multiple organ failure may follow.

Treatments

There are two treatment options for peptic ulcer disease, and they are often used together. One approach is a combination of antibiotics to treat the bacterial infection. Another is the reduction of stomach acid, to relieve pain and promote healing of the ulcer. Drugs that reduce the effects of stomach acid include antacids (Maalox, Mylanta, Amphojel), which neutralize stomach acid, *acid blockers* or *H2 blockers* (such as Tagamet, Pepsid, and Zantac); and proton pump inhibitors (Nexium, Prilosec, Prevacid), which shut down the production of acid. Combination antibiotic therapy can take a while, but

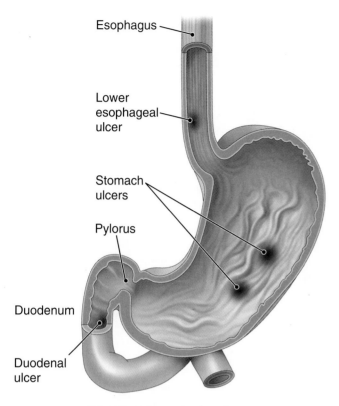

Esophagus

Lower esophageal ulcer

Stomach ulcers

Pylorus

Duodenum

Duodenal ulcer

FIGURE 15-2. Peptic ulcer disease.

once the bacterial infection has been eradicated, it prevents the return of ulcers. Antibiotics for ulcers can cause diarrhea. Some antacids also cause diarrhea, and others cause constipation. H2 blockers have few side effects, but occasionally patients report headache, fatigue, and other problems. Proton pump inhibitors tend to be well tolerated, but side effects can include diarrhea, nausea, vomiting, constipation, headaches, rash, and dizziness.

If the ulcer does not respond to medication, or if complications develop, surgery may be performed. A part of the vagus nerve may be severed (*vagotomy*) to interrupt acid secretion in the stomach, or a part of the stomach may be removed to reduce the secretion of digestive enzymes and acid.

● INTERVIEW QUESTIONS

1. How long have you had the ulcer?
2. Have you reported it to a doctor, and has it been diagnosed?
3. How does it affect you? Do you have any positioning preferences while on the massage table, so that your are comfortable?
4. Are there any complications or long-term effects? Any bleeding or scarring?
5. How was or is it treated?
6. Has it responded to treatment?
7. How does the treatment affect you?

● MASSAGE THERAPY GUIDELINES

Questions 1–4 provide basic background information. Because many people self-diagnose peptic ulcer, Question 2 should be asked as a matter of course. If the client has not seen a physician to evaluate an ulcer, or symptoms of an ulcer, then a medical referral is in order.

If peptic ulcer symptoms still persist, adjust the massage position according to the client's comfort, and avoid any pressure in the painful area. The side-lying position may be the most comfortable. Because symptoms can be worse on an empty stomach, consider suggesting that the client schedule massage after meals.

If the client's ulcer has not responded to treatment over time, it is likely to have caused internal bleeding and scarring. If these complications have not been treated surgically, and the client is still feeling the effects of fullness, vomiting, and weight loss, then a gentle session overall is indicated, and it is wise to schedule the massage session when the pain levels are lowest. For anemia due to blood loss, see Chapter 12. If the client reports any symptoms of complications but has not seen a physician about them, a medical referral is in order. However, in most cases, bleeding or scarring will already have been treated—perhaps with surgery—and and the condition has resolved by the time the individual seeks massage. If the ulcer has led to perforation and peritonitis, it will have been surgically corrected on an emergency basis. Wait until the client's condition has stabilized and he has returned to normal activity before resuming strong massage. If a client with a diagnosed ulcer reports severe abdominal pain, an emergency medical referral is in order.

The questions about treatment may bring up past treatment that resolved the condition, in which case massage adjustments will probably not be necessary. If the client is feeling the side effects of medications, you may need to adjust to diarrhea, constipation, nausea, headache, fatigue, skin rash, or dizziness. These are addressed in the Decision Tree (see Figure 15-3). For recent surgery, see Chapter 21.

● MASSAGE THERAPY RESEARCH

As of this writing, there are no randomized, controlled trials, published in the English language, on peptic ulcer disease and massage indexed in PubMed or the Massage Therapy Foundation Research Database. The NIH RePORTER tool lists no active, federally funded research projects on this topic in the United States. No active projects are listed on the clinicaltrials.gov database (see Chapter 6).

● POSSIBLE MASSAGE BENEFITS

Ulcers usually respond well to medical treatment, so the benefit of massage therapy during such a small window of time would be hard to determine. However, if combination therapy is taking some time, or if a client has refractory ulcers, she or he could use the support and possible stress relief of massage over time. As in the case of many other conditions, a massage therapist can provide gentle encouragement to see a physician for needed medical care.

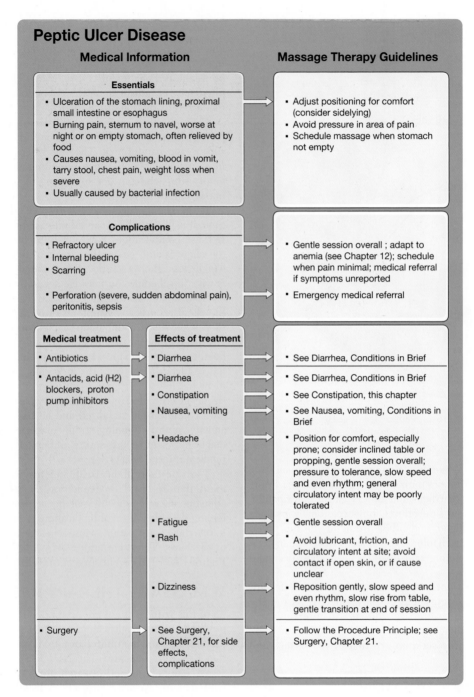

FIGURE 15-3. A Decision Tree for peptic ulcer disease. Not all side effects of medications are shown. Not all medications cause all side effects.

Ulcerative Colitis

Ulcerative colitis (UC) is an inflammation of the lining of the large intestine or rectum, or both. Along with Crohn disease, (see Conditions in Brief), it is one type of **inflammatory bowel disease (IBD)**.

● BACKGROUND

Ulcerative colitis can affect the colon, rectum, and in some cases, part of the ileum. *Proctitis* is rectum involvement only, and *proctosigmoiditis* involves the sigmoid colon and rectum.

Although ulcerative colitis and Crohn disease both involve inflammation and ulceration of the colon (Figure 15-4), Crohn disease is not as isolated in its effect: it can involve any portion of the GI tract, from the mouth to the anus.

Signs and Symptoms

Ulcerative colitis features periods of flare-up and remission. The flare-ups can be mild, moderate, or severe. Symptoms of mild UC include mild diarrhea, mild abdominal cramping, painful straining with bowel movements, periods of constipation, bleeding from the rectum, and discharge of mucus with the stool.

Moderate disease also includes frequent (up to ten per day) loose bloody stools, mild or moderate abdominal pain, mild anemia, and low-grade fever. Severe UC is characterized by more colon involvement, and may involve the entire colon. More than ten loose stools per day, severe abdominal cramping, significant bleeding, and fever are typical.

Complications

Dehydration and rapid weight loss are complications of severe UC, and people with the disease may suffer from malnutrition. In general, people with ulcerative colitis are at increased risk for anemia and blood clots. In fulminant ulcerative colitis, a high WBC count occurs, as well as a loss of appetite and severe abdominal pain. In some cases, the disease progresses to extraintestinal ulcerative colitis, meaning that other structures are affected, in addition to the colon. In extraintestinal disease, inflammation may occur in the large joints, the eyes (*uveitis*), the skin (*erythema nodosum*), and, less frequently, the lungs. Even during a period of remission, ankylosing spondylitis can occur (see Chapter 9). A rare extraintestinal complication of UC is inflammation of the bile ducts and liver disease.

In refractory ulcerative colitis, the disease does not respond well to drug treatment. Stronger medications, such as steroids and immunosuppressants, are required to control their symptoms.

One life-threatening complication of UC and Crohn disease is toxic megacolon, in which the colon dilates with infection or inflammation, growing rapidly within a few days. This can cause intense pain and abdominal distention, fever, weakness, rapid heart rate, dehydration, and shock. If untreated, toxic megacolon can lead to perforation of the colon and peritonitis (see Conditions in Brief). Ulcerative colitis can also increase the risk of colon cancer.

Treatment

There are many different drugs used to treat ulcerative colitis. Anti-inflammatories called *aminosalicylates* are used. These include mesalamine, sulfasalazine, olsalazine, and balsalazide. For proctitis or proctosigmoiditis, topical anti-inflammatory drugs are generally delivered by suppository, foam, or enema. This local treatment can be quite effective.

If the colitis extends above the rectum, sigmoid colon, or splenic flexure, suppositories and enemas cannot reach, so oral medications are necessary. An oral form of mesalamine (Asacol, Canasa) is one of the most common drugs; remission occurs in most people after several weeks of administration. Some side effects of aminosalicylates are headache, nausea, fatigue, and cramping; skin rash and hair loss may also occur.

For moderate to severe symptoms, corticosteroid medication—usually prednisone—is administered orally or in IV form in the hospital. The common side effects of corticosteroids are addressed in Chapter 21. Immunosuppressants such as Imuran, Neoral, Sandimmune, and Remicade may be prescribed. They can have strong side effects, and side effects are well monitored. An obvious side effect is reduced resistance to infection.

Surgery for UC is done to remove the affected segment of colon and splice together the two healthy ends. It may also involve an *ostomy*, a surgical procedure to create an artificial opening or passageway out of the body. In a colostomy, the diseased colon is removed and the healthy portion is attached to the exterior of the abdomen. The opening itself is called a stoma, and the external receptacle is called a colostomy bag (Figure 15-5). The ostomy may be permanent, or it may be temporary, giving the colon a rest for some time before the ends are rejoined surgically. A plastic bag is attached to the stoma, and the site depends on the location of the original bowel disease. A colostomy bag needs emptying about once daily.

● INTERVIEW QUESTIONS

1. Are you having a flare-up of ulcerative colitis right now, or is it in remission?
2. How does it affect you? What are your signs and symptoms?
3. Which structures are affected by it? Is it considered mild, moderate, or severe?
4. Are there any complications of your condition? Any dehydration, weight loss, effects on blood counts?
5. How has it been treated?
6. How has your treatment affected you?
7. How well hydrated do you feel you are?
8. What is your preference for comfortable positions on the table?
9. Are you likely to need access to the bathroom during the session?

● MASSAGE THERAPY GUIDELINES

The most defining information for the massage session is whether or not the client is in a flare-up of UC. If this is the case, observe the Inflammation Principle, with respect to the abdomen. If the client is in remission, the colon should still not be massaged with heavy pressure, although level 2 or 3 will be tolerable for most people.

> The Inflammation Principle. **If an area of tissue is inflamed, don't aggravate it with pressure, friction, or circulatory intent at the site.**

The client's answers to Questions 2–4 will give you an appreciation for the extent and severity of the condition. There is a wide range of disease severity in UC, and massage adjustments can be minimal or multiple in response. Clinical features of ulcerative colitis are shown, along with massage adjustments to consider, in Figure 15-7.

In mild cases of UC, or during remission, only a single massage adjustment may be necessary: limiting abdominal pressure to level 2. However, dehydration is important to consider for all clients with UC. Even with only a few loose, watery stools per day, an individual may struggle to stay hydrated. Use gentle pressure, slow speeds, and even rhythm, and avoid general circulatory intent if the client is mildly dehydrated. If the client is moderately dehydrated, an urgent medical referral is in order. If signs or symptoms of severe dehydration are present, the client needs emergency medical attention. For the signs and symptoms of mild, moderate, and severe dehydration, see Diarrhea, Conditions in Brief.

If the client has experienced ongoing blood loss, leading to anemia, provide a gentle overall session. This is true, too, for anyone with a high WBC count, severe abdominal pain, refractory ulcerative colitis, or rapid weight loss.

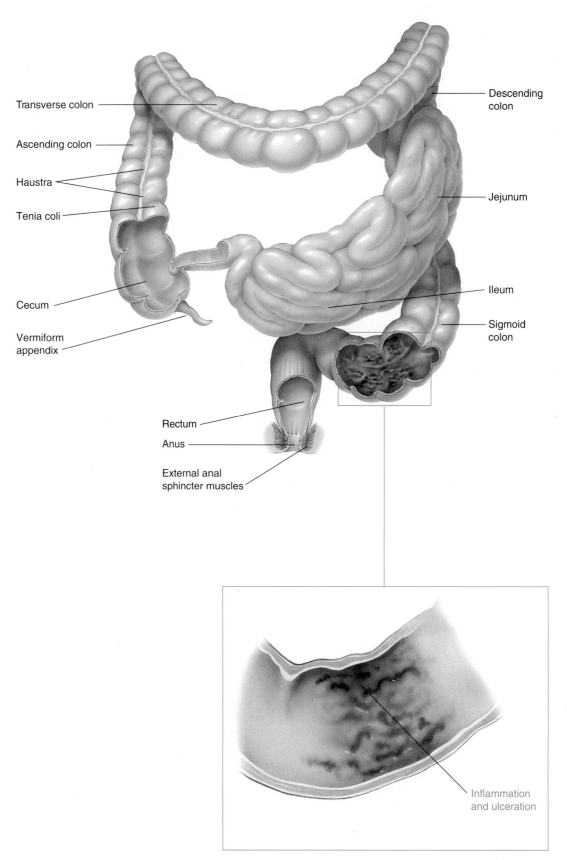

Transverse colon

Ascending colon

Haustra

Tenia coli

Cecum

Vermiform appendix

Rectum

Anus

External anal sphincter muscles

Descending colon

Jejunum

Ileum

Sigmoid colon

Inflammation and ulceration

FIGURE 15-4. Ulcerative colitis.

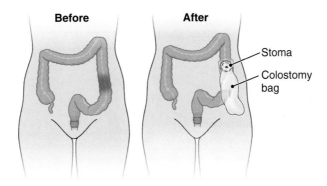

FIGURE 15-5. A colostomy. The colostomy bag is attached to the stoma, an opening in the abdominal wall attached to the surgically created end of the colon.

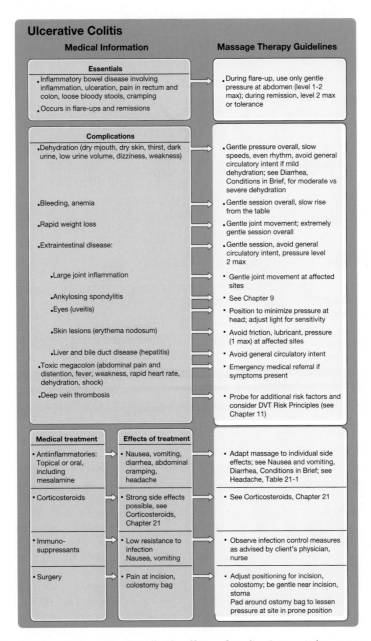

FIGURE 15-6. A Decision Tree for ulcerative colitis. Not all side effects of medications are shown. Not all medications cause all side effects.

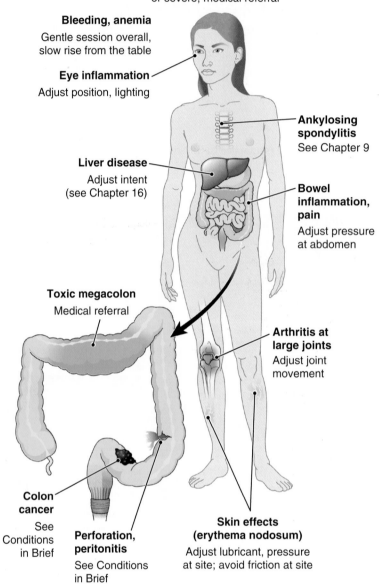

Dehydration
If mild, adjust overall pressure,
speed, rhythm, intent; if moderate
or severe, medical referral

Bleeding, anemia
Gentle session overall,
slow rise from the table

Eye inflammation
Adjust position, lighting

**Ankylosing
spondylitis**
See Chapter 9

Liver disease
Adjust intent
(see Chapter 16)

**Bowel
inflammation,
pain**
Adjust pressure
at abdomen

Toxic megacolon
Medical referral

**Arthritis at
large joints**
Adjust joint
movement

**Colon
cancer**
See
Conditions
in Brief

**Perforation,
peritonitis**
See Conditions
in Brief

**Skin effects
(erythema nodosum)**
Adjust lubricant, pressure
at site; avoid friction at site

FIGURE 15-7. Ulcerative colitis: selected clinical features and massage therapy guidelines. Specific instructions and additional massage therapy guidelines are in Decision Tree and text.

Severe cases with extraintestinal disease also call for gentle work overall (pressure level 2 max, no circulatory intent). Also, use caution near the affected structures: avoid friction, lubricant, and pressure, for example, in areas of erythema nodosum, or avoid contact entirely if the area is tender. Limit joint movement at any large joints affected by the disease. For a client with ankylosing spondylitis, see Chapter 9. If hepatitis is present, avoid general circulatory intent (see Chapter 16). A client with eye involvement may appreciate adjustments in lighting, as well as inclined position to minimize pressure in the head.

Toxic megacolon is a serious complication of ulcerative colitis. If any symptoms are present, such as increasing abdominal pain, rapid abdominal distention over a period

of 1–3 days, fever, weakness, or rapid heart rate, make an emergency medical referral. If peritonitis has occurred, the client will need time to stabilize before stronger massage can be used (see Conditions in Brief).

Ulcerative colitis increases one's risk of DVT, although it's unclear whether that isolated risk factor is enough to warrant following the DVT Risk Principles (see Chapter 11). As a general guideline, increase caution on the lower extremities with multiple risk factors, be mindful of DVT risk, and follow the principles if there is any doubt. If the client has developed cancer of the colon, see Colorectal cancer, Conditions in Brief.

Questions 5 and 6 help determine any massage adjustments that might be necessary due to treatment. UC treatments, ranging from well-tolerated anti-inflammatories such as mesalamine, to strong corticosteroids, to surgery, require various massage adjustments. Although there are no general massage adjustments for local anti-inflammatory preparations such as enemas, suppositories, and foams, abdominal symptoms in those cases will mean pressure is already limited at the abdomen. Aminosalicylates such as oral mesalamine may cause nausea, diarrhea, abdominal cramping, and headache, in which case gentler work overall is indicated, taking particular care over affected areas. See the Decision Tree (Figure 15-6) for specific massage adjustments. In the rare event that skin rash and hair loss are present, lubricant, contact, or pressure may be avoided in the affected areas. More severe side effects of aminosalicylates are rare and should be investigated on a case-by-case basis.

If a client is taking corticosteroid medication, see Chapter 21 for massage therapy guidelines for strong side effects. If other immunosuppressants are being used, such as Imuran, observe strict infection control measures. Be alert for nausea and vomiting and adapt massage accordingly (see Conditions in Brief).

If surgery has been performed and it was recent, see Chapter 21 for massage considerations. If there is any scarring, work gently on the abdomen. Question 8 about positioning could turn up positioning needs for a colostomy bag or simply for abdominal comfort. If the client is having a flare-up, the flat prone position or one with abdominal support may be uncomfortable, in which case proper supports or the side-lying position may be best.

If the client has had a colostomy or ileostomy, be thoughtful about positioning adjustments for the prone position, being careful to avoid putting pressure or drag on the colostomy bag. For a prone client, you might set up gentle padding around the bag, with a depression or "nest" for it to sit in without pressure, to make the client more comfortable. Or place a large, folded towel across the client's abdomen, superior to the ostomy site, and another towel inferior to it. To minimize anxiety about the bag dislodging from the stoma, be sure to avoid putting pressure or drag on the bag by drawing the drape across it, and by following the client's lead in positioning.

Some possible colostomy sites are shown in Figure 15-8. In most cases, the stoma and bag are located in the lower left abdomen, after removal of all or part of the sigmoid or descending colon. If part of the transverse colon is affected, the bag is often attached at the upper right abdomen. Less often, when the ascending colon is affected, the bag is attached at the lower right abdomen. Sometimes an *ileostomy* is performed, in which the last segment of the small intestine, the ileum, is attached directly to a stoma; in that case, the bag will generally be to the right of the navel, just below the waist. A permanent ileostomy is typically performed when the entire colon is diseased.

Question 9 about bathroom access is good to ask up front so that measures can be taken during the session to get the client to the lavatory quickly if necessary.

● MASSAGE RESEARCH

As of this writing, there are no randomized, controlled trials, published in the English language, on ulcerative colitis or inflammatory bowel disease and massage indexed in PubMed

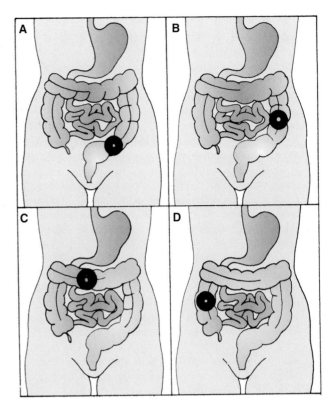

FIGURE 15-8. Colostomy sites. Depending on the area of colon disease, a different area of the colon is removed. Below, in black, stomas are shown in the (A) sigmoid, (B) descending, (C) transverse, and (D) ascending colon. The colostomy bag, attached to the stoma, is attached to the corresponding area of the abdomen.

or the Massage Therapy Foundation Research Database. The NIH RePORTER tool lists no active, federally funded research projects on this topic in the United States. No active projects are listed on the clinicaltrials.gov database (see Chapter 6). The availability of several observational studies on general CAM use among people with IBD (Burgmann et al., 2004; Rawsthorne et al., 1999), suggests that massage therapy research may be warranted.

● POSSIBLE MASSAGE BENEFITS

People with serious diseases, characterized by flare-ups and remission, describe them as "existentially exhausting." Not knowing when the next flare-up is coming, or when the current flare-up will end, makes it hard to plan and enjoy life during the good periods. In addition, any disease that necessitates being near a bathroom at all times obviously has stresses and challenges.

The loss of control one can feel in these circumstances is an indication for massage and bodywork, as it can be an empowering step in self-care. With a caring, sensitive, and fully present massage therapist, an individual with ulcerative colitis may feel less alone on the journey. For an account of ongoing work with a client with IBD in remission, see Therapist's Journal 15-2.

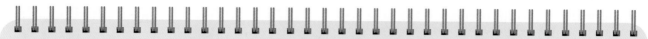

THERAPIST'S JOURNAL 15-2 *A Stretching Partnership with a Client with IBD*

A gentleman in his early forties came to see me a few years ago. At our first session he told me he was taking some pretty serious medications—Imuran and a short course of prednisone—for IBD. He had flare-ups of ulcerative colitis, but at the moment he was feeling pretty good and doing fine.

This client was a musician, but his primary job was in human services and he sat at a desk a lot. His workplace had offered chair massage, and that introduced him to table massage. He had pronounced kyphosis and stiffness—his muscles, especially his hamstrings, were not very flexible. We began with Swedish massage and deep tissue work, mostly effleurage and petrissage. We checked in about medications and effects at each session, and to my knowledge, he didn't have the tissue breakdown, the bone and skin thinning, that can go with prolonged use of corticosteroids, so there wasn't a limitation on massage pressure. He liked abdominal massage, though we kept it gentle and broad, especially near his descending colon where he experienced his bowel trouble. I didn't need to make any position adjustments for his IBD, but I always gave him neck and head support for his kyphosis when he was supine.

Over time he began working with a personal trainer to improve his fitness and flexibility. At that point, I offered him a session of Thai Yoga massage, a modality that involves a lot of stretching on a mat, not a table. After his first session of it, he was hooked! We began very slowly and gently all over. Abdominal work in this modality amounted to palming the abdomen in a circle at first, then specific thumb work in the circular shape, then finishing with the palming. I was careful with the specific work until it was clear he could tolerate it and we weren't aggravating the inflammation. The area would begin gurgling after we worked.

While we adjusted for the IBD, it was really a peripheral issue. Our focus was on his flexibility and overall health, not his abdominal issues. He said that after the Thai Yoga sessions he felt great, with much more flexibility. Plus, he said his energy increased. He loved the stretching in this modality. He would laugh when I pulled his toes, stretching each one. His hamstrings, once so tight, began to loosen so that I could see increased ROM and tolerance of the stretch. He had moved from the massage chair, to the table, to the mat, without looking back! Only occasionally would we do table work after that because he seemed to benefit so much from the stretching.

I saw this client every 3 weeks for a couple of years until he moved to take another job. It was immensely satisfying to work with him. He knew a lot about his health and medical condition, and he gave really good feedback. Looking at his posture at the first session, you would not have thought he would be able to do what we did together. But because he was so open and willing, we were able to set up a dialogue, and his good feedback led us through to the eventual place of increased flexibility. In my notes, I wrote down his comment one day—that the session "was like music." I will always remember that comment, our partnership, and his joyful laugh.

Susan Frikken
Madison, WI

Other Gastrointestinal Conditions in Brief

APPENDICITIS

Background

- Inflamed appendix, fills with pus, causing nausea, vomiting, constipation, diarrhea, abdominal distension, loss of appetite, low-grade fever, pain; usually occurs between ages 10 and 30.
- Pain starts at navel, moves to lower right abdomen, increases over 6–12 hours, can be severe: Sudden, temporary pain relief may appear if rupture occurs, then pain becomes more generalized.
- Rupture can lead to peritonitis, a life-threatening infection of the peritoneal cavity.
- Treated with emergency surgery—appendectomy—to avert perforation and peritonitis; laparoscopic surgery possible, open surgery may be necessary; IV antibiotics administered if peritonitis occurs.

Interview Questions

- Are your symptoms current or recent? Did you see your doctor about them? Did you receive a diagnosis?
- Treatment? When? Effects of treatment?

| Massage Therapy Guidelines | • Acute, diagnosed appendicitis is unlikely to appear in massage practice, as emergency surgery is performed upon diagnosis and the condition resolves. Massage is likely to be unwelcome during acute symptoms.
• If symptoms not reported to physician, immediate medical referral, not massage. See Peritonitis, Conditions in Brief.
• If surgery was recent (last 3 months), see "Surgery," Chapter 21.
• Until client has returned to normal activity, use gentle overall massage. |
|---|---|

CELIAC DISEASE (CELIAC SPRUE, NONTROPICAL SPRUE, GLUTEN-SENSITIVE ENTEROPATHY)

| Background | • Intolerance of gluten protein in wheat, barley, rye, other grains/flours that trigger immune response in small intestine.
• GI symptoms include abdominal pain, bloating, diarrhea; general symptoms are irritability, depression, joint pain, skin rash, mouth sores, neuropathy, anemia, fatigue.
• Disease can emerge after trauma such as injury, infection, stress of pregnancy, surgery.
• Complications include nutrient malabsorption, osteoporosis, lactose intolerance.
• Treated by eliminating dietary gluten. |
|---|---|
| Interview Questions | • Diagnosis?
• Current symptoms?
• Complications such as loss of bone density, neurological effects? |
| Massage Therapy Guidelines | • Adapt massage to symptoms or complications, rather than disease itself.
• Position changes for comfortable abdomen, careful modification of lubricant or contact at site of skin rash.
• Adapt to complications such as osteoporosis (see Chapter 9), neuropathy (see Chapter 10). |

COLORECTAL CANCER

| Background | • Cancer beginning on intestinal or rectal lining, or on a polyp or protrusion of the wall; often advanced before symptoms appear.
• Symptoms include weakness, fatigue, blood in stool, diarrhea, constipation, painful or frequent bowel movements, sensation of incomplete rectal emptying.
• Commonly metastasizes to bones, liver, lungs, ovaries, peritoneum; highly aggressive; prognosis poor when advanced, unless only liver is involved.
• Treated with surgery, including colostomy; also treated with radiation, chemotherapy (see Chapter 20). |
|---|---|
| Interview Questions | • Where is or was the cancer in your body? How does it affect you?
• Have there been any complications of the cancer? Any effects on function of your liver or lungs?
• Is there any bone involvement?
• Treatment? Effects of treatment?
• Do you have any medical devices, such as an ostomy? If so, do you have any positioning preferences that minimize movement or pressure at the device? |
| Massage Therapy Guidelines | • Review Cancer, Chapter 20, for massage therapy guidelines for cancer and cancer treatment; follow Vital Organ Principle (see Chapter 3)
• Limit pressure at abdomen (level 2 max).
• Adapt to symptoms such as constipation, diarrhea, nausea, or vomiting (this chapter), fatigue.
• Adjust massage to sites of cancer spread, such as liver, bone, brain.
• If bone involvement, see "Bone Metastasis," Chapter 20; if pain, especially new, unfamiliar, or increasing pain, do not use pressure or joint movement at site until physician verifies that no bone metastasis is present.
• If liver function impaired, avoid general circulatory intent, adjust position for liver enlargement; (see "Liver Cancer," Chapter 16). Follow DVT Risk Principle I indefinitely throughout active colorectal cancer, advanced colorectal cancer, treatment; for completed treatment and remission, add DVT Risk Principle II (see Chapter 11). |

- Adjust session to effects of cancer treatment (see Chapter 20); if necessary, position carefully for ostomy device (see "Ulcerative Colitis," this Chapter).

CROHN DISEASE

Background	• Together with ulcerative colitis (this chapter), one type of IBD; pathophysiology and symptoms similar to ulcerative colitis.
	• Can occur anywhere in GI tract and affects deeper tissues of GI structures; pain commonly occurs in lower right abdomen; bleeding less common than in UC.
	• Other possible symptoms are from extraintestinal involvement: fever, fatigue, arthritis, eye inflammation, skin problems, liver and bile duct inflammation.
	• Complications include bowel obstruction, open sores along GI tract, *fistula* (formation of tunnel-like connections from bowel to other organs), anal fissure, malnutrition and associated problems (anemia, osteoporosis).
	• Treatments similar to those for UC (anti-inflammatories, immune system suppressors), plus antibiotics (Flagyl, Cipro); side effects of antibiotics include nausea, diarrhea, abdominal pain, headache, dizziness, fatigue.
Interview Questions	• Where does it affect you—which organs and tissues?
	• Symptoms?
	• Complications? Any involvement of skin, joints, liver?
	• Comfortable positions for you?
	• Treatment? Effects of treatment?
Massage Therapy Guidelines	• Follow all applicable precautions for UC (see "Ulcerative Colitis," this chapter) and consider additional tissue involvement; if skin changes present, adapt pressure, lubricant, contact; if joints involved, gentle joint movement only; if liver involved, follow Filter and Pump Principle.
	• Flare-up contraindicates general circulatory intent. Adapt to treatments similar to UC, plus side effects of strong antibiotics (see Table 21-1).

DIARRHEA

Background	• Loose, watery stools, increased volume of stool, urgency, and frequency of bowel movements, often accompanied by abdominal cramping.
	• Causes include viral gastroenteritis, some medications (especially antibiotics), IBS, inflammatory bowel disease (this chapter), celiac disease.
	• Dehydration may occur, can be a serious complication.
	• Mild dehydration: increased thirst, dry mouth, dark yellow urine, reduced urine output.
	• Moderate dehydration: strong thirst, dark amber or brown urine, reduced urine output (half the usual amount in the past 24 hours) lightheadedness (relieved by lying down), irritability, restlessness, muscle cramps, rapid heartbeat, arms/legs feel cool to touch.
	• Severe dehydration (any one of the following): rapid respiration rate, rapid heart rate (weak pulse), faintness unrelieved by lying down, lightheadedness that persists after 2 minutes. standing, behavior changes (confusion, sleepiness, anxiety), skin temperature changes (cold/clammy or hot/dry), little or no urination in last 12 hours.
	• Treatments involve replacement of lost fluids, electrolytes, soft, starchy foods.
	• OTC medications include attapulgite (Kaopectate), bismuth subsalicylate (Pepto-Bismol), few side effects except for constipation.
	• Opioid-related antidiarrheal drugs such as diphenoxylate with atropine (Diphenatol, Lomotil), loperamide (Imodium); side effects include nausea, vomiting, drowsiness, dizziness.
Interview Questions	• How long have you had diarrhea? How severe is it?
	• Do you know the cause? Have you talked to your doctor about it?
	• Any nausea, vomiting, fever, chills? Any chance that you are dehydrated (list symptoms of mild, moderate, severe dehydration, above)?
	• Treatment? Effects of treatment?

Massage Therapy Guidelines	• Adapt to cause of diarrhea (such as IBS, "Ulcerative Colitis," "Celiac Disease," this chapter). If diarrhea has persisted more than 5 days (and pattern is unusual for that person), blood has appeared in stool, or signs/symptoms of moderate/severe dehydration are present, postpone massage session, advise urgent medical referral. • If fever, chills, nausea, vomiting present, advise urgent medical referral, postpone massage session. • If symptoms/signs of mild dehydration, gentle overall session (gentle pressure overall, slow speeds, even rhythm, avoid general circulatory intent); if moderate dehydration, urgent medical referral; if severe dehydration, emergency medical referral. • Adapt to side effects of medication (see Table 21-1). • If diarrhea mild, improving, provide gentle session overall, with careful positioning.

ESOPHAGEAL CANCER

Background	• Cancer of the esophagus, uncommon in United States, but common in Asia and parts of Africa. Poor prognosis, since most cases diagnosed when advanced; early stage may be asymptomatic. • Later stage symptoms include difficulty swallowing, sensation of stuck food in throat or chest; pain in throat, mid chest, or between scapulae; hiccups, vomiting blood, unintentional weight loss. • Complications include severe weight loss, hoarseness, coughing, esophageal bleeding, pain, complete blockage of esophagus, making swallowing impossible. Usually metastasizes to lungs and liver, also spreads to bones, brain, intestines, kidneys. • Treatments aimed at managing symptoms rather than cure: surgical removal of tumor, section of esophagus, upper stomach, reconstruction of esophagus using section of colon; chemotherapy, radiation, combined chemotherapy/radiation (see Chapter 20).
Interview Questions	• Where is or was it in your body? How does it affect you? • Have there been any complications of the cancer? Any effects on function of your liver or lungs? Is there any bone or intestinal involvement? • Any areas of swelling or discomfort? What are comfortable positions for you? • Treatment? Effects of treatment?
Massage Therapy Guidelines	• Review Cancer, Chapter 20, for massage therapy guidelines for cancer and cancer treatment. Avoid pressure at sites of tumor. • Position carefully for difficulty swallowing, minimal pressure on throat, chest, and upper abdomen, effects of radiation on skin. • Gentle overall session if profound weight loss. • Adjust massage to sites of cancer spread; use gentle pressure if bowel involved; follow Vital Organ Principle if liver, kidney, brain involved. • If bone involvement, see "Bone Metastasis," Chapter 20; if pain, especially new, unfamiliar, or increasing pain, do not use pressure or joint movement at site until physician verifies that no bone metastasis is present. • If liver function impaired, avoid general circulatory intent, adjust position for liver enlargement; (see "Liver Cancer," Chapter 16). • Consider DVT Risk Principles; if cancer is advanced, follow DVT Risk Principle I indefinitely (see Chapter 11).

GALLSTONES (CHOLELITHIASIS)

Background	• Solid material forming in gallbladder or bile duct, hardened bile substances including cholesterol, calcium, bile pigments; sizes range from grain of sand to golf ball in diameter. • May be asymptomatic or, when larger than 8 mm, produce symptoms by blocking cystic duct or common bile duct. • Abdominal pain in right or middle upper abdomen, may be sharp, cramping, dull, can radiate to back or right scapula, often appearing several minutes after meal and aggravated by fatty foods; other symptoms are fever, nausea, vomiting, gas.

- Complications include inflammation of gallbladder, pancreatitis, blockage of ducts leading to jaundice, fever, chills.
- Treatment for symptomatic gallstones is usually laparoscopic cholecystectomy (gallbladder removal) or open surgery; sound wave therapy and/or bile salt tablets can break up small stones or small numbers of stones with no strong side effects.

Interview Questions	• Is the condition current or recent? • What are your signs and symptoms? How does it affect you? • Any current areas of pain or discomfort? Any complications of the condition? • Treatment? Effects of treatment?
Massage Therapy Guidelines	• If gallstones were in past and resolved with surgery, massage adjustments are usually unnecessary. • If current pain or discomfort, massage will probably be unwelcome (attacks last a few minutes to 2–3 hours) • Complications include cholecystitis, pancreatitis, or jaundice, avoid general circulatory intent; gentle session overall, position for comfort. • If surgery was recent, see "Surgery," Chapter 21.

GASTROENTERITIS (FOOD POISONING, "STOMACH FLU")

Background	• Inflammation of GI tract caused by viral infection. • Watery diarrhea, abdominal pain, cramping, nausea, vomiting, muscle ache, headache, fever; may last 1–2 days or 10 days in severe cases. • Complications include systemic infection, dehydration; dehydration occurs rapidly in older adults, young children, infants. • No medical treatment available; rest, fluids, gradual advancing of diet as symptoms improve.
Interview Questions	• How does it affect you? Symptoms? • How long have you had it, or did you have it? Any chance that you are dehydrated (list symptoms of mild, moderate, severe dehydration; see Diarrhea, Conditions in Brief)? Have you had any bleeding? • Have you reported it to your doctor?
Massage Therapy Guidelines	• Massage usually too stimulating in acute cases; contact unlikely to be welcome; may be communicable. • If symptoms have persisted more than 5 days, blood has appeared in stool, or signs/symptoms of dehydration are present (see Diarrhea, Conditions in Brief), postpone massage session, advise urgent medical referral. • If milder or improving, very gentle touch with little hand movement, predictable rhythm, slow speed may be tolerated or welcomed. • Observe careful infection control measures. • If diarrhea present, see Conditions in Brief.

GASTROESOPHAGEAL REFLUX DISEASE (GERD)

Background	• Chronic condition, stomach acid, or bile reflux (backflow) into esophagus; acid irritates esophageal lining, causes inflammation. • Symptoms include heartburn and chest pain (both aggravated by lying down), difficulty swallowing, coughing; wheezing, hoarseness, sore throat, regurtitation. • Complications include narrowing and ulceration of esophagus with pain, difficulty swallowing. • Treated with antacids, H2 blockers (Tagamet, Pepsid, Zantac), proton pump inhibitors such as Prilosec, Prevacid; for side effects, see "Peptic Ulcer Disease," this chapter. Prokinetics (Reglan) used to tighten lower esophageal sphincter, help stomach empty more rapidly; prokinetics can cause nausea, diarrhea, sleeplessness, restlessness, drowsiness, fatigue. • Surgery uncommon, but usually aimed at narrowing stomach near weakened sphincter.

Interview Questions	• How does it affect you? • Will you feel comfortable lying down, especially if you have eaten recently? Should we raise your head or upper body, or have you lying on your side to be comfortable? • Treatment? Effects of treatment?
Massage Therapy Guidelines	• Position comfortably, consider side-lying, semi-reclining, seated position, especially after meals. • Adapt to effects of medications (see Figure 15-3), mostly well tolerated except for prokinetics (see Table 21-1 for other side effects of medications); if surgery recent, see Chapter 21.

IRRITABLE BOWEL SYNDROME (IBS)

Background	• Common, noninflammatory chronic bowel condition; abdominal pain, cramping, gas, bloating, diarrhea, constipation; symptoms can be mild, moderate or severe, intermittent. • Hemorrhoids can be aggravated by diarrhea and constipation. • Treated with dietary changes, fiber supplements, OTC antidiarrheal medication (Imodium), antispasmodic medication (Bentylol, Levsin), low dose tricyclic antidepressants or SSRIs (see Table 10-1). • Women with severe IBS may take alosetron (Lotronex) or lubiprostone (Amitiza) under strict supervision; potentially serious side effects of alosetron include constipation, bloating, abdominal pain, side effects of lubiprostone include nausea, diarrhea, incontinence.
Interview Questions	• Are you currently in a flare-up? What are your symptoms? • What is your preference for positioning on the massage table? Are there any positions to avoid, or any that are more comfortable than others, such as on your side? • What is your preference regarding massage or contact on your abdomen? • Treatment? Effects of treatment?
Massage Therapy Guidelines	• Gentle massage pressure, if tolerated, on abdomen; adjust massage positioning to avoid pressure at abdomen. • See Constipation, Diarrhea, Conditions in Brief. • Sensitivity about bathroom access and passing gas. • Adjust to side effects of medications (see Table 21-1), but do not use pressure >1 on abdomen without physician consultation if client is taking alosetron; immediate medical referral if side effects of alosetron have not been reported to client's doctor.

NAUSEA AND VOMITING

Background	• Unpleasant, queasy feeling in the stomach and forceful movement of stomach contents through esophagus and oral cavity; may include retching, the repeated rhythmic muscular contraction of the muscles of vomiting, without necessarily producing emesis, the contents brought up by vomiting. • Causes include gastroenteritis, ulcers, inner ear disturbance, brain injury, migraine headache, advanced cancer, hormonal changes during pregnancy, motion sickness, liver or kidney disease, medical treatments and medications such as chemotherapy, anesthesia. • Can lead to dehydration (see Diarrhea, Conditions in Brief), especially if individual is unable to keep fluids down for 12 hours or more. • OTC antinausea drugs (antiemetics) are antihistamines (Dramamine, Benadryl), used for motion sickness, may cause drowsiness, dry eyes, dry mouth. • Prescription antiemetics such as chlorpromazine HCl (Chlorpromanyl, Largactil), perphenazine (Trilafon), prochlorperazine maleate (Compazine, Compro, Nu-Prochlor), endansetron (Zofran), scopolamine (Scopace, Transderm Scop), metoclopramide (Apo-Metoclop, Clopra) are used; side effects include headache, insomnia, dryness, hypotension, dizziness, anxiety, depression. • Dehydration treated with replacement of electrolytes, IV fluid therapy.

Interview Questions	• Have you been vomiting as well as nauseated? For how long? • Have you been able to keep fluids down? If so, for how long? • Any chance you're dehydrated (list symptoms of mild, moderate, severe dehydration; see "Diarrhea," this Chapter)? • Do you know the cause? Have you reported it to your doctor? • Treatment? Effects of treatment? • Have you received any antinausea medication in the past few hours? Any through an IV or patch?
Massage Therapy Guidelines	• Investigate cause of nausea and vomiting and adapt massage to cause. • Avoid contact, or follow excellent infection control precautions, if cause is unknown, or could be contagious. • Medical referral for client who has been vomiting, especially if dehydration is a risk. • Advise urgent medical referral and postpone session if client has been vomiting 24+ hours, or unable to keep fluids down 12+ hours, has severe headache or pain, is vomiting blood or bile, or has fever or chills. See Diarrhea, Conditions in Brief, to identify mild, moderate, or severe dehydration. • For chronic, low-level nausea, use slow speeds, even rhythms, avoid joint movement; consider side-lying or semi-reclining positions for comfort. • Avoid massage if individual has been vomiting; if vomiting occurs, glove before handling emesis basin or when cleaning up afterward. • Adapt massage to side effects of antiemetics (see Table 21-1). • At sites of transdermal patch or recent injection, avoid circulatory intent.

PANCREATIC CANCER

Background	• Aggressive cancer that is most often (90%) diagnosed after metastasis, as tumors tend to be large before producing symptoms. • Symptoms include abdominal pain, back pain, which can be severe; other symptoms are weight loss, nausea, diarrhea, loss of appetite and weight, fatigue. • Tumors can block bile duct, producing jaundice, intense itching; pressure can also obstruct flow of stomach contents to small intestine, producing vomiting; obstruction of nearby veins can produce splenomegaly, esophageal varices, gastric varices, bleeding from rupture. • Usual spread is to liver, lung; can also metastasize to stomach, spleen, intestine, bones, other sites. • Treatments include surgery, radiation therapy, chemotherapy and targeted drug therapy (erlotinib), as well as experimental treatments (cancer vaccines, angiogenesis inhibitors). • Surgical bypass when intestines or ducts blocked by large tumor, stent insertion to keep ducts open. • Pain management usually requires strong painkillers (codeine, morphine) or nerve blocks. • Replacement of pancreatic enzymes with oral enzyme tablets; insulin therapy needed if diabetes develops.
Interview Questions	• Where is or was it in your body? How does it affect you? • Any complications? Any pressure of tumor on surrounding structures? Any swelling or congestion anywhere? • Is there any bone involvement? Effects on liver or lungs, other vital organs? • Do you have pain? What is your pain level, and where? How is your pain being treated? • What are comfortable positions for you? • Treatment? Effects of treatment?
Massage Therapy Guidelines	• Review "Cancer," Chapter 20, for massage therapy guidelines for cancer and cancer treatment. • Adapt to symptoms such as diarrhea, nausea, or vomiting (this chapter). • Adjust massage to sites of cancer spread, such as liver, lungs (follow Vital Organ Principle); limit pressure (2 max) at abdomen if spread to intestine, spleen. • If bone involvement, see "Bone Metastasis," Chapter 20; if pain, especially new, unfamiliar, or increasing pain, do not use pressure or joint movement at site until physician verifies that no bone metastasis is present. • Adapt position to pain, liver or spleen enlargement.

- If liver function impaired, avoid general circulatory intent, adjust position for liver enlargement; (see "Liver Cancer," Chapter 16).
- Follow DVT Risk Principle I indefinitely throughout active pancreatic cancer, advanced pancreatic cancer, treatment; if successful treatment completed, consider adding DVT Risk Principle II (see Chapter 11).
- Gentle overall session if profound weight loss, or if strong pain medications are used.

PANCREATITIS

Background	• Serious, chronic or acute inflammation or infection of the pancreas. • Typical causes are heavy alcohol use, gallstones (acute pancreatitis), other medical conditions and medications. • Symptoms usually develop quickly, ease after a few days, but can last several months (acute pancreatitis); can persist for years and destroy function of organ (chronic pancreatitis) • Symptoms include upper abdominal pain, often severe, possibly radiating to back, aggravated by eating, eased by leaning forward or moving to fetal position; also causes nausea, vomiting, fever, weight loss. • Fever may be present, or postural hypotension. • Complications include formation of fluid and tissue debris in pockets (pseudocysts) in pancreas, which can cause infection or rupture with bleeding; malnutrition, diabetes, respiratory failure, kidney failure, and shock can occur. • Movement of intestinal and stomach contents may stop, causing swelling in upper abdomen. • Chronic pancreatitis increases risk of pancreatic cancer. • Most cases require hospitalization with monitoring, fasting, IV fluids, aggressive pain relief. Alcohol and drug use are stopped, and alcohol dependence treated; dietary changes, supplementation with oral pancreatic enzymes, and nutrition to address malabsorption. • Surgery to remove bile duct obstruction, gallbladder removal, drainage or removal of diseased tissue from pancreas.
Interview Questions	• Is your pancreatitis current, or recent? Chronic or acute? • Is the cause known? • How does it affect you? Does it cause pain or any swelling? Where? Describe your pain level? • Have any complications occurred? Any infection, diabetes, or effects on breathing, kidney function? Any effects on blood pressure? Any fever? • Has the condition affected your digestion? • Treatment? Effects of treatment?
Massage Therapy Guidelines	• Pancreatitis pain can be severe and may make massage unwanted or poorly tolerated; physician consultation advised; gentle session overall (follow Compromised Client Principle) with intent to provide comfort. • High likelihood that condition is being treated, i.e., massage will be in hospital setting or home after discharge. • Adjust positioning for comfort, which may require the side-lying "fetal position." Slow rise from table if hypotension present. • No general circulatory intent if fever, infection, abdominal swelling, strong pain; limit pressure and joint movement overall if pain medications interfere with perception; limit pressure and joint movement at sites of current pain. • Adapt to failure of other organs: breathing difficulties in respiratory failure (position for optimum breathing) or chronic kidney failure (see Chapter 18), diabetes (see Chapter 17). • Adapt massage to treatment, effects of treatment (see "Analgesics," "Surgery,"Chapter 21).

PERITONITIS

Background	• Serious infection of peritoneum, caused by peritoneal dialysis, injury, infection, inflammation, abscess; rupture of appendix, colon, peptic ulcer (see "Peptic Ulcer Disease," this chapter), diverticula (see "Diverticular Disease," online); may also be caused by liver damage, such as in cirrhosis, in which ascites develop (see "Liver Failure," Chapter 16). • Causes pain throughout abdomen, abdominal distension with gas and fluid, hard and tender to touch; leads to fever, thirst, low urine output; inability to pass gas or have bowel movement, diarrhea, nausea, vomiting, fatigue.

- Complications include life-threatening sepsis, widespread inflammatory response, septic shock, multiple organ failure.
- Treatment with IV antibiotics to clean abdominal cavity, surgery to remove infected tissue.

Interview Questions	• When did it occur? How did it affect you? Still recovering or full recovery? • Treatment? Effects of treatment?
Massage Therapy Guidelines	• Signs or symptoms of peritonitis signal emergency medical referral. • For recent peritonitis, treated but still resolving, extremely gentle session overall; physician consultation advised (Follow Stabilization of an Acute Condition Principle) • Avoid general circulatory intent until infection resolved, client resumes normal activities. • Adapt to effects of treatment (see Table 21-1; "Surgery," Chapter 21)

STOMACH CANCER (GASTRIC CANCER)

Background	• Cancer of the stomach, most often of the epithelial cells of the stomach lining (adenocarcinoma), uncommon in United States. and declining; believed to be linked with *H. pylori* infection (see "Peptic Ulcer Disease," this chapter). • Tends to develop slowly over years; early stages cause vague symptoms that are easily dismissed, such as heartburn and abdominal pain; also causes bloating, nausea, vomiting, blood in vomit, stomach pain, weight loss, fatigue. • Complications include blood loss in vomit or stool. Anemia may occur. • Spreads to nearby organs: pancreas, spleen, colon, small intestine, esophagus. Distant spread to liver (most common), lungs, bone, other tissues/organs; often metastasis has occurred by the time cancer is detected; poor prognosis in most cases. • Treated with surgery (entire stomach—gastrectomy—or portion), chemotherapy, radiation.
Interview Questions	• Where is or was the cancer in your body? How does it affect you? • Have there been any complications of the cancer? Any effects on function of your liver or lungs? • Is there any bone involvement? • Treatment? Effects of treatment? • Any areas of swelling or discomfort? • What are comfortable positions for you? • Treatment? Effects of treatment?
Massage Therapy Guidelines	• Review Cancer, Chapter 20, for massage therapy guidelines for cancer and cancer treatment; follow Vital Organ Principle (see Chapter 3) if cancer has spread to liver, lungs. • Limit pressure at upper abdomen (level 2 max), position for comfort if client has pain, or if liver or spleen is enlarged (consider side-lying). • Adapt to symptoms such as diarrhea, nausea, or vomiting (this chapter). • If bone involvement, see "Bone Metastasis," Chapter 20; if pain, especially new, unfamiliar, or increasing pain, do not use pressure or joint movement at site until physician verifies that no bone metastasis is present. • If liver function impaired, avoid general circulatory intent, adjust position for liver enlargement; (see "Liver Cancer," Chapter 16). Follow DVT Risk Principle I indefinitely throughout active cancer, advanced cancer, treatment. For completed treatment, consider adding DVT Risk Principle II (see Chapter 11).

SELF TEST

1. List five factors that contribute to constipation, and four types of drugs that have constipation as a side effect.
2. What is the medical definition of constipation?
3. Describe four complications of constipation.
4. Which symptoms or signs of constipation suggest a medical referral and limited abdominal pressure?
5. Is the effectiveness of abdominal massage for constipation established by research? Describe research on this topic.
6. What is an ulcer, and what are the three common kinds of ulcers in peptic ulcer disease?
7. Define these conditions and explain the relationship between them: sepsis, peritonitis, peptic ulcer.
8. How is peptic ulcer disease treated? What are the side effects of treatment?
9. If a client with peptic ulcer disease complains of symptoms, how can you adapt the massage position and scheduling for the client's comfort?
10. What are the differences between mild, moderate, and severe ulcerative colitis?
11. Define and give four examples of extraintestinal ulcerative colitis.
12. What is a colostomy? Explain how the client's position might need to be modified for various colostomy placements.
13. Describe the side effects of mesalamine and Imuran, used for ulcerative colitis, and how you might adjust the massage for the side effects.
14. Regarding toxic megacolon, what are the symptoms, and how should you respond in the rare event that a client mentions them in a session?
15. How should you adapt massage pressure during a flare-up of ulcerative colitis? During remission? If the client is dehydrated from ulcerative colitis?

 For answers to these questions and to see a bibliography for this chapter, visit http://thePoint.lww.com/Walton.

16 Liver Conditions

It was at one time considered the seat of life; hence its name—liver, the thing we live with.

—AMBROSE BIERCE

The liver performs over 500 physiological functions. It neutralizes toxic materials, such as drugs and alcohol; produces bile for digesting fats and cholesterol; helps regulate blood sugar levels; and produces proteins that help blood clot. The liver is also an adaptive organ, shouldering the functions of the spleen and gallbladder if either of those organs is removed.

Because the functions of the liver are so diverse, liver disease can affect seemingly unrelated body functions, and it has a broad reach. The composition of the blood, stability of the tissues, and health of every other organ are affected by liver disease. There is a close relationship between the most common liver conditions: Diseases of inflammation (hepatitis) can lead to cancer (hepatocellular carcinoma), to liver failure, or to both. Likewise, liver failure can lead to cancer, or progression can happen in reverse.

This chapter addresses the following conditions at length, with full Decision Trees:

- Viral hepatitis
- Liver failure
- Liver cancer

Conditions in Brief in this chapter are: **cirrhosis, fatty liver disease** (nonalcoholic steatosis, nonalcoholic steatohepatitis), **alcoholic hepatitis**, and **autoimmune hepatitis**.

General Principles

For the massage therapist, an essential question when working with people with liver conditions is how well a client's liver is functioning. Liver function is not always impaired in liver disease, but because of the numerous functions of the liver, a variety of things can go wrong if it is unhealthy. Several layered interview questions about liver function can easily be fit into a short intake or a longer interview. In some cases, you may need direct communication with the client's doctor to determine whether liver function impairment requires modifications in the massage plan.

When asking about liver conditions, a general rule of thumb is to determine whether liver function is compromised enough to merit adjustments to massage. Questions are organized to assess whether the current level of liver function:

1. Produces symptoms, such as jaundice or GI discomfort;
2. Concerns the client's physician; or
3. Affects the client's activity level, energy level, or functions of daily living.

If any one of these is true for your client, apply three principles from Chapter 3: the Vital Organ Principle, the Filter and Pump Principle, and the Detoxification Principle.

There is some overlap between these principles, but each has important elements for a client with liver impairment. The Vital Organ Principle suggests a gentle session overall: Slow the speed, lighten up on pressure, even up the rhythms, and consider limiting the length of the session if necessary. When such an essential organ is not working properly, a gentle session makes the most sense. The Filter and Pump Principle is also used, because a compromised liver may not be able to filter blood as well as usual. In this case, refrain from general circulatory intent.

The Detoxification Principle is also in force when the liver is compromised. The liver is an organ of detoxification, and detoxification is commonly claimed as a benefit of massage and spa treatments. As of this writing, the question of whether massage and spa services *actually* speed the elimination of toxins is still open, and it is not established by research. Moreover, the term detoxification is loosely used. Claims of detoxification are not universally clear about which substances are thought to be toxins, or how massage and spa treatments work to hasten their exit from the body.

Until more is known about any detoxifying effects of massage and spa treatments, we rely on clinical observations: Clients with liver conditions frequently feel worse after vigorous massage, heat treatments, and some spa wraps. We also rely on common sense: It is not advisable to place additional demand on a weakened organ. Using this reasoning, we omit detoxifying treatments and techniques whenever liver function is compromised.

Besides these general principles from Chapter 3, there are additional massage adjustments to apply for the broad effects of liver impairment. Guidelines for liver and spleen congestion, the effects on the skin, and other factors are addressed in this chapter.

Viral Hepatitis

Hepatitis is inflammation of the liver. Causes of hepatitis include viral infection; the ingestion of excessive alcohol; drugs or other toxins; and autoimmune diseases. Viral hepatitis is discussed here, although signs, symptoms, and massage guidelines also hold true for other causes of hepatitis.

● BACKGROUND

As of this writing, six hepatitis viruses have been identified worldwide: hepatitis A, B, C, D, E, and G. The first three are more common in developed countries and are the focus of this chapter.

When hepatitis inflammation lasts more than 6 months, the infection is considered chronic. The chief differences between hepatitis A, B, and C are their mode of transmission, the onset of any symptoms, and tendency to produce long-term effects—a chronic state of infection that contributes to liver problems later. Table 16-1 summarizes characteristics of the three most common types of viral hepatitis.

In each case, the name of the virus is the same as the disease it produces. The three conditions are:

- *Hepatitis A*. The mildest form of viral hepatitis is **hepatitis A**. Infection with this virus can be asymptomatic, especially in young children who might have mild cases. In older children and adults, it tends to be more severe. The incubation period is often up to a month, and then the symptoms appear suddenly and may be mistaken for an intestinal flu. Symptoms of hepatitis A often clear quickly. Complete liver healing occurs within 1–2 months, although a person may have relapses over the next 6–9 months. Hepatitis A infection, while it can be uncomfortable and sometimes life threatening, is the most short-lived of the three. Most importantly, it does not produce a lingering chronic state, and it does not usually lead to later liver disease. The virus is transmitted through the fecal-oral contact. Unsanitary food preparation and diaper changing in child care settings are common modes of hepatitis A transmission.
- *Hepatitis B*. Infection with **hepatitis B** is more serious than hepatitis A, although the symptoms are similar. In hepatitis B, the symptoms appear more gradually, and last longer.

Many people are asymptomatic for months with hepatitis B, and some never develop symptoms. Adults usually recover fully from hepatitis B, but most infants and children, and about 5–10% of infected adults, develop chronic hepatitis. Chronic disease elevates the risk of long-term liver complications. The course of hepatitis B infection is shown in Figure 16-1. Hepatitis B virus is transmitted through blood and other body fluids (similar to the spread of HIV, although it is more highly infectious than HIV). It is a hardy virus and can survive outside the body for a week or more. IV drug use and unprotected sex with someone with hepatitis B increase the risk of transmission. Infants born to women with hepatitis B are also at increased risk.

- *Hepatitis C*. In **hepatitis C** infection, the individual may experience no symptoms, mild flu-like symptoms, or acute symptoms at first. Most people with hepatitis C infection do not develop symptoms for years after exposure. A person can be completely asymptomatic for decades, as Therapist's Journal 16-1 describes. Although symptoms may initially escape notice, hepatitis C infection is serious: A majority of individuals experience a chronic form of infection, and about two thirds of those go on to have long-term liver problems. The hepatitis C virus is blood-borne, and only rarely transmitted sexually. Instead, contaminated needles put people at risk, through accidental needle sticks in medical settings, or shared needles during IV drug use. Blood transfusions performed before 1992, before blood screening for hepatitis C was available, also put people at risk.

Signs and Symptoms

The cardinal signs and symptoms of hepatitis are abdominal pain, nausea, diarrhea, loss of appetite, dark urine, fatigue, and low-grade fever. Muscle pain and itching may occur. **Jaundice**, a feature of many liver conditions, is a yellow tint in the eyes and skin. It occurs when a yellow substance called *bilirubin* accumulates in the tissues. Because the liver is inflamed or injured, it is unable to metabolize this substance. In acute hepatitis, the liver is enlarged, called **hepatomegaly**. Spleen enlargement (**splenomegaly**) also occurs in some cases.

TABLE 16-1.	CHARACTERISTICS OF VIRAL HEPATITIS		
Virus	Hepatitis A	Hepatitis B	Hepatitis C
Transmission	From stool of one person to mouth of another; contamination through unsanitary food preparation, or diaper changing in child care settings	Blood and other body fluids, including saliva, tears, breast milk, urine, semen, vaginal fluid; sexual transmission, IV needle sharing, accidental needle sticks in medical settings, contact with other body fluids	Blood, most often through IV needle sharing
Chronic state	No	Yes, in 5–10% of cases	Yes, in 75% of cases
Contributor to later liver disease	No	Yes	Yes

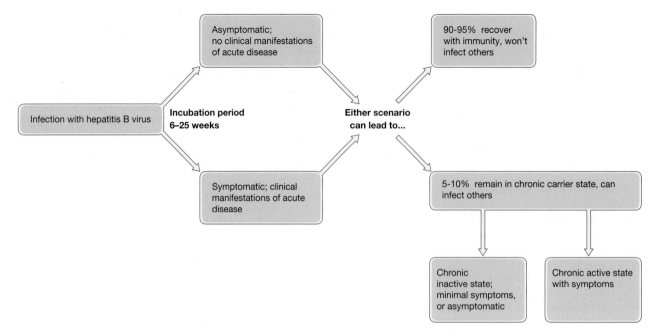

FIGURE 16-1. Course of hepatitis B infection in adults. Note the possibility of both symptomatic and asymptomatic presentations, and either a chronic active or chronic carrier state. Hepatitis C follows a similar course, but with a shorter incubation period (3–15 weeks), and a more likely chronic carrier state.

Complications

Complications of hepatitis can occur during the acute stage or later, in a chronic state that may follow acute infection. Advanced disease features **cirrhosis**, the replacement of normal liver cells with scar tissue (see Conditions in Brief), and liver failure can follow (see Figures 16-3 and 16-4), as well as liver cancer (see Figure 16-6).

Several scenarios are possible in the course of viral hepatitis infection:

- *Acute, life-threatening disease.* **Fulminant hepatitis** is a severe, rapid progression toward life-threatening liver failure. This progression is not common in hepatitis A; it is more likely in B and C.
- *Full recovery.* One can also recover fully with protective immunity, a successful "clearing" of the virus, which means it can't be transmitted to others. This is possible in all three infections, but it is nearly certain in hepatitis A, highly likely in hepatitis B, and much less likely in hepatitis C.
- *Lifelong carrier state.* Both hepatitis B and C can lead to a lifelong **carrier** state, with the possibility of infecting others unknowingly. This is especially likely when the disease is clinically silent, or symptoms are mild. In this scenario, hepatitis B or hepatitis C infection is discovered years or even decades later in the doctor's office when testing for other diseases.

Once an individual becomes a **chronic carrier**, capable of transmitting the virus, there are two possible clinical pictures: active and inactive. In a **chronic active** state, the liver inflammation has become constant; the most prominent symptom is profound fatigue, along with abdominal pain, muscle pain, and other milder symptoms of the acute form. In a **chronic inactive** state, the individual has no symptoms, but can transmit the disease. See Figure 16-1 for the course of infection in hepatitis B. Hepatitis C infection follows a similar course, although, as stated above, the proportions are different: a majority of those infected with hepatitis C virus develop chronic disease.

Treatment

There is no specific treatment for hepatitis A. Supportive measures are rest, good nutrition, and avoiding alcohol in order to minimize stress on the liver, thereby preventing permanent liver damage.

Treatment for hepatitis B, immediately after a known exposure, consists of an injection of hepatitis B immunoglobulin within the first 24 hours of contact with the virus, followed by a series of three shots with the hepatitis B vaccine. This can prevent an individual from developing hepatitis B.

For an individual with hepatitis B or C who has no signs, symptoms, or diagnosed liver damage, the condition may be monitored, not treated. With only slight liver abnormalities, chances of future liver problems are low.

If hepatitis is treated, five drug approaches are interferon, lamivudine, telbivudine, adefovir, and entecavir. Interferon is a strong treatment with strong side effects, some of which are also the signs and symptoms of hepatitis B. Depression, fatigue, body and muscle aches, fever, and nausea may occur with interferon, as well as low RBC production. Side effects of the other four antiviral medications tend to be minimal, although patients are monitored closely for their responses to these drugs.

Liver transplantation may be performed to treat hepatitis when extensive liver damage has occurred. This involves surgery, placement of the transplanted tissue, and long-term immunosuppressive drugs to prevent rejection (see Chapter 21). In hepatitis B infection with advanced liver disease, liver transplantation is usually unsuccessful because the infection quickly develops in the transplanted tissue with severe manifestations, but drugs can help. In hepatitis C, the infection can affect the transplanted tissue, but it tends to be milder, and asymptomatic, with high long-term survival rates.

● INTERVIEW QUESTIONS

1. What kind of hepatitis do you have, or did you have?
2. Has it resolved, or is it considered acute, chronic active, or chronic inactive/asymptomatic?
3. How does it affect you? Do you have symptoms?
4. Is the function of your liver currently affected? Does it affect your activity or energy level?
5. Are you tested regularly for liver function? Are doctors concerned about it?
6. Have any complications occurred? Has the condition caused cirrhosis or liver failure?
7. Do you have any areas of swelling or congestion? Any fluid retention?
8. How is it treated?
9. How does the treatment affect you?

● MASSAGE THERAPY GUIDELINES

Notice that the interview questions do not include a question about how the client became infected with hepatitis, although the type of hepatitis suggests how it might have been transmitted. The mode of transmission is not important to the massage session, and it can be a sensitive subject, broaching on sexual activity or drug use. Instead of asking for details of transmission, practice standard precautions. Standard infection control measures for healthcare settings are designed to protect against viral transmission during the session, regardless of whether you or the client has the virus. Of the three viruses, hepatitis A is the most easily transmitted by casual contact because it does not rely on blood transfer for transmission. Excellent hand washing is especially important to the prevention of transmission of hepatitis A and other diseases spread by contact.

The interview questions focus on the health of the client's liver and his or her overall health. Questions 1–3 help establish the status of the infection. It is important to know if the infection has completely resolved with full immunity, or if it is in a chronic state. If the client has no symptoms, and the liver is fully functioning, there may be no massage adjustments. As explained earlier, full resolution is usually the case after hepatitis A and many cases of hepatitis B; a chronic state is possible for some cases of hepatitis B and most cases of hepatitis C.

A client with acute hepatitis symptoms may not tolerate massage well, and is unlikely to be out and about, but massage may be welcome as a comfort measure. If the client has any symptoms of hepatitis, then the liver is still inflamed or injured. If this is the case, follow the Vital Organ Principle, the Filter and Pump Principle, and the Detoxification Principle.

> *The Filter and Pump Principle.* **If a filtering organ (liver, kidney, spleen, or lymph node), or a pumping organ (the heart) is functioning poorly or overworking, do not work it harder with massage that is circulatory in intent.**

Question 3 may cue answers such as fatigue, achiness, nausea, and loss of appetite. In these cases, keep all elements of massage gentle. Specific guidelines for these symptoms are in the Decision Tree (see Figure 16-2). If itching is present, use firm, stationary pressure.

Questions 3–7 are different ways of cueing the client to talk about the health of his or her liver. There is some repetition in these questions, and while it might not be necessary in some cases, it is good practice to use all of them to clarify whether the liver is still affected by the disease. If the client's symptoms are mild or nonspecific (such as fatigue), and you don't have a clear sense of how to proceed, Questions 4–7 are especially important. Review "General Principles," this chapter. If you get a sense that liver function is compromised, then follow the three principles from Chapter 3, mentioned above.

Question 6 about complications is most likely to signal cirrhosis or liver failure. These are addressed elsewhere in this chapter. Question 7 may reveal an enlarged liver or spleen, or even **ascites**, mild to severe abdominal swelling, then the prone and supine positions can be uncomfortable or impossible. If this is the case, see "Liver Failure," this chapter, for position guidelines.

Questions 8 and 9 about medical treatment could raise the issue of interferon or other antiviral approaches. Side effects such as fatigue, flu-like symptoms, fever, and nausea point to a gentler massage session (see Figure 16-2). The client may prefer nonmoving contact, rather than continuous stroking. If the client's RBCs are low, adapt the massage accordingly (see "Anemia," Chapter 12).

If the client has had a recent liver transplant, follow the massage precautions for someone with recent surgery, and a major transplant (see Chapter 21). No matter when the transplant

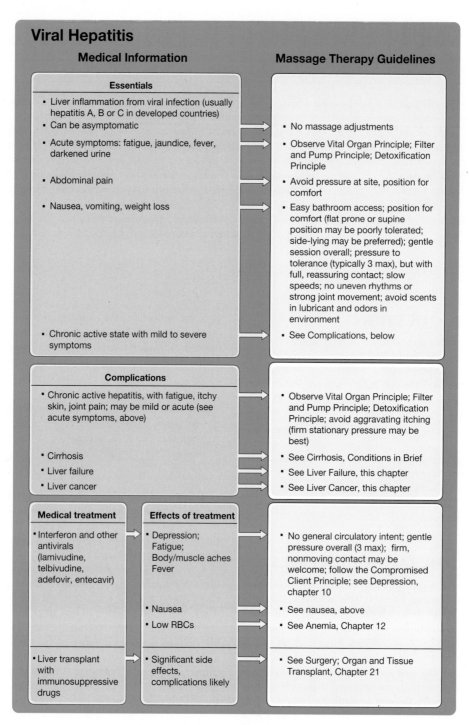

FIGURE 16-2. A Decision Tree for viral hepatitis.

was, the individual is likely to be taking immunosuppressive medications. Extra infection control measures, above and beyond standard precautions, may be in order, so inquire about them and adjust your own practices.

● MASSAGE RESEARCH

As of this writing, there are no randomized, controlled trials, published in the English language, on viral hepatitis and massage indexed in PubMed or the Massage Therapy Foundation Research Database. The NIH RePORTER tool lists no active, federally funded research projects on this topic in the United States. No active projects are listed on the clinicaltrials. gov database (see Chapter 6).

● POSSIBLE MASSAGE BENEFITS

Gentle massage may provide supportive care for people who are ill with symptoms of hepatitis. Chronic symptoms may make the person feel tired and overwhelmed, while continuing to keep a full or nearly full schedule. As well, there may be the stress of ongoing concern about worsening liver disease. Massage therapy may help with this stress and contribute to overall well-being in individuals with hepatitis. (See Therapist's Journal 16-2.)

THERAPIST'S JOURNAL 16-2 *Adapting Massage to Hepatitis C*

A couple of years ago, a new client came in to redeem a gift certificate. During the interview, she told me that she had hepatitis C. She didn't have any outward signs of it, and I wouldn't have known without her telling me. This is a good case for taking a good health history. In some other massage therapy settings, it might not have come up.

This client came in for a regular Swedish relaxation massage. I did not feel comfortable burdening her liver with any increase in circulation, so I lightened up my pressure on the Swedish strokes and did a fair amount of energy work. I worked all areas: head, face, neck, back, and extremities. She left the session feeling very satisfied and has returned to me every few months or so. She'll often return when she feels unwell, and says the energy work seems to make her feel more relaxed, but also more emotionally balanced. I continue using a conservative approach with her.

The client was about 55 years old when she was diagnosed. She had contracted the virus years before during a blood transfusion. She was asymptomatic for a very long time so she didn't even know she was infected, which is typical of hepatitis C. When she developed symptoms she felt pretty sick, and tests confirmed a hepatitis C diagnosis. She did try interferon treatment in the beginning, but it was hard to tolerate. She primarily uses complementary and alternative therapies. She sees a naturopath and receives regular massage, eats well, and doesn't tax her liver in any way—doesn't eat toxic foods or drink alcohol. She has a good support system, which seems to make a difference.

Her disease goes up and down—it's pretty cyclical. Periodically she can go a few months at a time feeling pretty good, then she is unwell again. But even during the good phases, she never feels completely normal, as she fatigues easily. Considering her condition, she's pretty functional. She describes herself as "healthy in mind, body, and spirit most of the time." She's an amazing woman. She works when she can and stays pretty upbeat. I've been glad to be part of her support system in some way.

Judi Railey Funaro
Sequim, WA

Moreover, because hepatitis B and C may have been transmitted through sexual activity or IV drug use, there can be a stigma associated with the disease. You are in a good position to provide supportive care with acceptance and without judgment.

Liver Failure

Liver failure is the severe loss of liver function, or the diminishment of liver function over time. It is the progression of liver disease to the point that other body systems are affected. Chronic liver failure develops gradually over months or years. Acute liver failure develops suddenly over days or weeks and is much less common than the chronic form. Although it sounds final, liver failure can be a temporary condition, and reversible. However, once a large portion of the liver has sustained permanent injury, liver failure is a common end point in many diseases.

● BACKGROUND

Liver failure has many causes, including cirrhosis (see Conditions in Brief); severe alcoholic hepatitis; chronic viral hepatitis; exposure to toxic chemicals and some medications such as acetaminophen; liver cancer; and other conditions.

Signs and Symptoms

Liver failure may be asymptomatic at first, then progress to mild, moderate, and severe signs and symptoms. The distinction between the signs/symptoms and complications is not always clear, and in some cases it is arbitrary. Liver failure may be more clearly described in terms of early and late symptoms. The early or first symptoms of liver failure are nausea, diarrhea, loss of appetite, and fatigue. Because these symptoms are not specific to liver failure, the individual may not seek medical attention, and the condition may go undiagnosed until it is more advanced.

Complications

Later in the disease, symptoms worsen. The liver becomes congested, tender on palpation, and enlarged. The spleen may also enlarge. Abdominal pain may occur in the upper right abdomen, along with fever, muscle/body aches, and dark urine. As the disease advances, the liver is less able to filter and clean the blood. It can no longer metabolize medications as well, and the result may be increased sensitivity to drugs.

Skin changes become evident, as jaundice appears. Bile salts are deposited in the skin and can cause intense itching, first in the hands and feet, then over the entire body. The liver has a role in blood clotting, so if it fails, easy bruising and bleeding may be noticeable on the skin, along with the formation of red spider veins.

Portal hypertension, the backup of blood in the portal vein, occurs during liver failure. Under normal conditions, blood from the intestines, pancreas, and spleen enters the liver through the portal vein. As cirrhosis scars and damages the liver tissue, blood cannot circulate as easily through the liver. Blood backs up, increasing pressure in the portal vein. Portal hypertension can lead to further backup in the blood vessels of the esophagus, stomach, and rectum, leading to **esophageal varices** or **gastric varices**. These are essentially internal varicose veins that have expanded. In their swollen, stretched state, they can spontaneously bleed. One sign of this is vomiting large amounts of blood. Because they are internal, blood loss can be massive, hard to prevent or treat, and fatal. Liver failure treatment may be focused on managing the varices.

As liver damage progresses, the liver becomes less able to regulate fluid levels. With portal hypertension, fluid leaks from the surface of the liver and the intestines. Ascites, the abnormal accumulation of fluid in the peritoneal space, occurs. Ascites can escape notice until about a quart of fluid accumulates, at which point swelling in the abdomen is visible in most cases. The swelling can be pronounced, and pressure on the diaphragm can make breathing difficult. Edema may form in the lower extremities, as well.

Failure of the liver to cleanse the blood leads to a particularly serious complication: hepatic encephalopathy. Toxins such as ammonia, building up in the blood, spill into the brain and cause injury to the tissues. This causes personality, mood, and behavior changes, as well as cognitive impairments such as confusion and forgetfulness. Delirium, coma, and death may result as the disease progresses.

Because the liver plays a role in blood sugar control, liver failure can lead to insulin resistance and type 2 diabetes (see Chapter 17). Liver failure also leads to kidney failure in some people, a poorly understood condition called *hepatorenal syndrome*. Osteoporosis (see Chapter 9) can result from liver failure because the liver cannot process the vitamin D and calcium needed for bone health. As bones thin, they may be susceptible to pathologic fracture.

Years of chronic liver failure increase the risk of liver cancer (this chapter). Chronic liver can progress to end-stage liver failure or *end-stage liver disease*, in which cirrhosis, portal hypertension, and functional impairment have become irreversible. Once hepatic encephalopathy or GI bleeding occurs, the disease tends to progress more quickly.

Treatment

Treatment of liver failure is aimed at preventing more liver damage and reducing or managing complications. Fluid retention is treated by avoiding or limiting alcohol, protein, and salt intake, and diuretics may be prescribed to draw off excess fluid. Bed rest is encouraged for ascites. Paracentesis, the insertion of a tube in the abdomen to draw off excess fluid, may be needed if ascites is severe. The sudden shifts in fluid and electrolyte balance from paracentesis can be destabilizing, causing dizziness, nausea, and weakness in the first 4–48 hours after the procedure.

Management of portal hypertension is a high priority, to prevent internal bleeding from gastric and esophageal varices. Blood pressure medications such as β-blockers may be prescribed to reduce strain on the vessels. Vasoconstrictors are also used. To prevent bleeding, bands may be inserted to "pinch off" the blood supply to the affected vessels. This is called endoscopic variceal band ligation. If stomach veins are bleeding, an adhesive substance may be injected into the vein, or a catheter may be inserted with a balloon that compresses the veins to stop bleeding. For recurrent bleeding, a transjugular intrahepatic portosystemic shunt can be inserted. In this procedure, the blood is shunted away from the swollen vessels and to another systemic vein to relieve the pressure. Bleeding vessels may be cauterized or injected with epinephrine.

Itching is treated with antihistamines and other medications. Hepatic encephalopathy is treated with a medication called lactulose, which reduces the absorption of ammonia from the intestines to the blood. By sending ammonia out in the stool, blood levels of ammonia are lowered. Lactulose is a laxative with few strong side effects, typically limited to GI discomfort such as bloating or gas.

A liver transplant may be performed, requiring the use of immunosuppressive medications (see "Organ and Tissue Transplant," Chapter 21). However, the waiting time for a liver transplant can be prohibitively long.

● INTERVIEW QUESTIONS

1. What is the cause of your liver failure? How does it affect you?
2. How well does your liver function? Is your doctor concerned about your liver function?
3. Does your doctor say you have portal hypertension? Are there any effects on your esophagus (esophageal varices) or stomach (gastric varices)?
4. Do you have any swelling in your abdomen? Swelling in your legs, caused by your liver condition?
5. Any swollen or congested organs, such as your liver or spleen? Is your breathing affected?
6. Is your skin affected? Any discoloration, easy bruising or bleeding, or itching?
7. Do you have any osteoporosis as a result? Has the condition affected your kidney function?
8. Has the liver failure affected any nervous system functions?
9. What would be the most comfortable position for you during the massage? In what position do you sleep? Does your doctor or nurse advise any particular sleeping or resting position?
10. How is your condition being treated? Are you taking any medications, or have you had any procedures?
11. How does treatment affect you?

● MASSAGE THERAPY GUIDELINES

Questions 1 and 2 can illuminate the extent of the disease. If the liver is compromised enough to produce symptoms, concern the physician, or affect activity or energy levels, then review "General Principles," this chapter. Apply the Vital Organ Principle, the Filter and Pump Principle, and the Detoxification Principle (see Chapter 3). Work gently during the session, toning down many of the elements of massage, and avoid general circulatory intent. Avoid spa services that are intended to release toxins from the tissues. Also avoid any non-massage services that raise core temperature or are intended to increase general circulation.

> *The Detoxification Principle. If an intent of a spa treatment is to detoxify, avoid using it when the client is significantly challenged by illness or injury, or is taking strong medication.*

Along with these general modifications, adapt the massage to any fatigue, loss of appetite, or GI symptoms that the client reports. Specific massage therapy guidelines are in the Decision Tree (see Figure 16-3).

Affirmative answers to Questions 3–8 suggest moderate to severe liver failure. Follow the relevant principles described above. If you are unsure about the level of liver function, consult the client's physician for help. Often a client's activity level and activity tolerance are the most useful in estimating massage tolerance.

Liver Failure

Medical Information	Massage Therapy Guidelines

Essentials

- Total loss of liver function or deterioration of liver function over time; can be asymptomatic, chronic (occurring over months, years), acute (developing over days, weeks); may be temporary; in many cases, is irreversible.

  → If symptomatic, avoid general circulatory intent (Filter and Pump Principle); provide gentle session overall (Vital Organ Principle); avoid spa therapies or massage techniques intended to accelerate detoxification (Detoxification Principle)

- Early symptoms:
  - Fatigue, loss of appetite
  - Nausea, vomiting

  → Gentle session overall
  → Easy bathroom access; position for comfort (flat prone or supine position may be poorly tolerated; side-lying may be preferred); gentle session overall; pressure to tolerance (typically 3 max), but with full, reassuring contact; slow speeds; no uneven rhythms or strong joint movement; avoid scents in lubricant and odors in environment

- Diarrhea

  → Easy bathroom access; gentle session overall; avoid contact or pressure at abdomen that could aggravate

Complications

- Jaundice

  → No specific massage adjustments for jaundice, beyond general massage adjustments for liver failure

- Itching

  → Avoid aggravating itching (firm stationary pressure may be best)

- Easy bruising and bleeding

  → Gentle pressure overall (usually level 2-3 max, depending on tissue stability)

- Portal hypertension, esophageal varices, gastric varices

  → Adapt position for comfort; consider sidelying, semireclining, or seated; avoid flat prone or supine position

- Ascites

  → Adapt position for comfort; consider sidelying, semireclining, or seated; avoid flat prone or supine position

- Edema, often in legs

  → Avoid circulatory intent at site

- Breathing problems

  → Position for comfort; sidelying, seated, or semireclining may ease breathing; avoid flat prone or supine position

- Hepatic encephalopathy

  → Gentle session overall; adapt massage and movements to changes in feedback due to confusion, perception

- Insulin resistance, type 2 diabetes

  → See Diabetes, Chapter 17

- Osteoporosis

  → See Osteoporosis, chapter 9

- Kidney failure (hepatorenal syndrome)

  → Avoid general circulatory intent; see Chapter 18

- Liver cancer

  → See Liver Cancer, this chapter

FIGURE 16-3. A Decision Tree for liver failure.

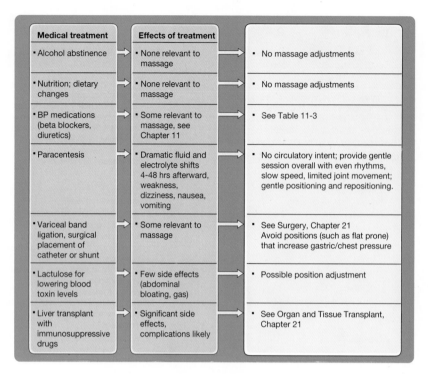

Medical treatment	Effects of treatment	
• Alcohol abstinence	• None relevant to massage	• No massage adjustments
• Nutrition; dietary changes	• None relevant to massage	• No massage adjustments
• BP medications (beta blockers, diuretics)	• Some relevant to massage, see Chapter 11	• See Table 11-3
• Paracentesis	• Dramatic fluid and electrolyte shifts 4-48 hrs afterward, weakness, dizziness, nausea, vomiting	• No circulatory intent; provide gentle session overall with even rhythms, slow speed, limited joint movement; gentle positioning and repositioning.
• Variceal band ligation, surgical placement of catheter or shunt	• Some relevant to massage	• See Surgery, Chapter 21 Avoid positions (such as flat prone) that increase gastric/chest pressure
• Lactulose for lowering blood toxin levels	• Few side effects (abdominal bloating, gas)	• Possible position adjustment
• Liver transplant with immunosuppressive drugs	• Significant side effects, complications likely	• See Organ and Tissue Transplant, Chapter 21

FIGURE 16-3. (*Continued*).

Massage adjustments tend to be similar across different causes of liver failure. General massage considerations for liver failure are highlighted in Figure 16-4.

Skin changes from liver failure almost certainly affect your massage plan. With moderate to severe disease, limit overall pressure to level 1–3, depending how easily the tissues bruise, and avoid too much friction or poorly tolerated lubricant if there is itching. Itching can be generalized, and extremely uncomfortable; firm, stationary pressure touch may be much better tolerated than stroking. It may be that any touch is unwelcome during this time.

If edema is present in the legs, or fluid is present in the abdomen, avoid circulatory intent in these areas. Fluid balance is already a problem in liver failure, and you don't want to aggravate it. Positioning, which may need to be adjusted for these conditions, is addressed below in Question 9.

If the liver failure has led to diabetes, see Chapter 17. See "Osteoporosis," Chapter 9, if the client has this complication of liver failure. If renal function is impaired, follow the Filter and Pump Principle, which you are already following because of liver failure. See "Chronic Kidney Failure," Chapter 18, for additional information. See "Liver Cancer," this chapter, if the client has developed this complication of chronic liver failure.

Question 8 about neurologic function is important, although if a client's CNS function is truly compromised, he or she is unlikely to be able to answer the question clearly. Direct your questions to a caregiver if the client's mental status is in question. In this case, adapt the massage to changes in perception and communication. Work gently, as comfort is your primary focus. Respond to nonverbal cues of discomfort.

Hepatic encephalopathy is serious, signaling severe liver impairment. If you notice behavior or personality changes, confusion or forgetfulness, and these symptoms haven't already been reported to the client's doctor, an immediate medical referral is essential.

Question 9 could bring up a variety of positioning needs. Adjust positioning to the presence of ascites or congested organs. Often a well-supported side-lying position, as shown in Figure 16-5, is much more comfortable than the flat prone or supine position. The semi-reclining position may also work; in nursing care, patients with ascites are often positioned in bed with the upper body inclined anywhere from 30–90 degrees, in order to ease the fluid pressure on the diaphragm and make breathing easier. These position changes may work for someone with portal hypertension, esophageal or gastric varices, variceal band ligation, and the mild abdominal discomfort from lactulose, as well.

Question 10 about treatments and their effects are important to take into account, but the effects of the disease and the effects of treatment become blurred in advanced liver disease. Follow massage modifications for clients taking BP medications (see Table 11-3), but note that liver disease, by itself, tends to produce stronger effects than the medications used to treat it. By already following the Vital Organ Principle, you will have taken care of the contraindications necessary for most BP medications.

The Vital Organ Principle. If a vital organ—heart, lung, kidney, liver, or brain—is compromised in function, use gentle massage elements and adjust them to pose minimal challenge to the client's body.

If paracentesis was performed recently, continue your gentle approach, since strong side effects occur in the hours and even days following the procedure. Adapt as you normally would to weakness, dizziness, nausea, and vomiting. If the client has had recent surgery for gastric or esophageal varices, see "Surgery," Chapter 21. If any of these procedures have been performed, or the client is medically frail, then a gentle, even approach is in order.

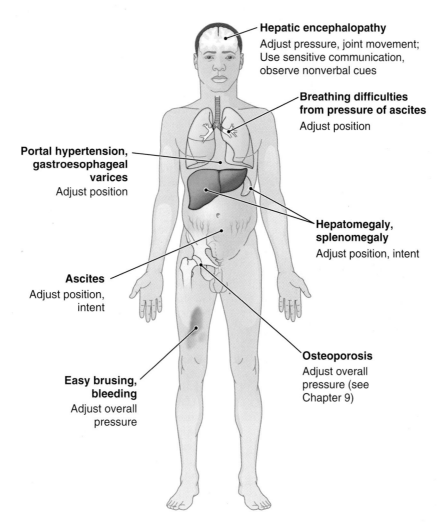

Hepatic encephalopathy
Adjust pressure, joint movement;
Use sensitive communication,
observe nonverbal cues

**Breathing difficulties
from pressure of ascites**
Adjust position

**Portal hypertension,
gastroesophageal
varices**
Adjust position

**Hepatomegaly,
splenomegaly**
Adjust position, intent

Ascites
Adjust position,
intent

Osteoporosis
Adjust overall
pressure (see
Chapter 9)

**Easy brusing,
bleeding**
Adjust overall
pressure

FIGURE 16-4. Liver failure: Selected clinical features and massage adjustments to consider. Specific instructions and additional massage therapy guidelines are in Decision Tree and text.

If a liver transplant has been performed, find out how well the new liver is functioning, and see "Organ and Tissue Transplant," Chapter 21, for specific massage adjustments.

● MASSAGE RESEARCH

As of this writing, there are no randomized, controlled trials, published in the English language, on liver failure and massage indexed in PubMed or the Massage Therapy Foundation Research Database. The NIH RePORTER tool lists no active, federally funded research projects on this topic in the United States. No active projects are listed on the clinicaltrials.gov database (see Chapter 6).

● POSSIBLE MASSAGE BENEFITS

Liver failure can become an extremely uncomfortable and disabling condition over the long term, as the disease advances. Massage therapy can be part of supportive care, perhaps facilitating sleep and easing pain. Liver failure may be due to cirrhosis, commonly caused by the overuse of alcohol, or it may follow chronic hepatitis infection. It is then classified as a "lifestyle disease," and an individual may experience social judgment, from the belief that he or she brought the disease on himself or herself. By approaching your client with compassion and without judgment, you may be able to provide healing companionship.

Liver Cancer

The liver is a common site of primary cancer, and an even more common site of cancer spread from other sites such as the breast, lung, GI tract, ovary, or pancreas. About 80–90% of primary liver cancers are called **hepatocellular carcinoma**, or *hepatoma*. If the liver is a secondary site, the condition is called metastatic liver disease or *liver mets* (see Chapter 20). Cancer exerts the same influence on liver function, whether

the liver is a primary or secondary site, so the massage therapy adjustments are also similar.

● BACKGROUND

Primary liver cancer is often a complication of cirrhosis and liver failure, which often results from chronic

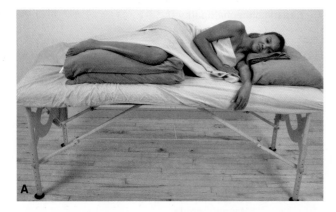

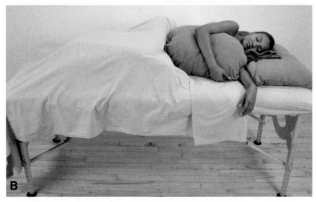

FIGURE 16-5. A well-supported side-lying position. To ease pressure on the abdomen, ample support can prevent the client from rolling into the prone or semi-prone position. (A) The client's top thigh, leg, and foot are given the support of two firm pillows. (B) An additional pillow is placed in front of the chest and abdomen.

hepatitis B or C, excessive alcohol use, or other inflammatory diseases of the liver.

Signs and Symptoms

Signs and symptoms of liver cancer include loss of appetite, weight loss, abdominal pain, right shoulder pain, fever, fatigue, and enlargement of the liver, with palpable masses. Spleen enlargement may also occur.

These signs and symptoms are not specific to cancer. Most of them could point to other, much less harmful conditions. Because many other conditions cause these signs and symptoms, and because early disease is often asymptomatic, diagnosis can be delayed. A delay in diagnosis means a poor prognosis in most cases of liver cancer. The 5-year survival rate for people with hepatocellular carcinoma is less than 20%.

Complications

If the liver is the primary site of cancer, as in hepatocellular carcinoma, metastases to other sites most often include the lungs, abdominal lymph nodes, and bone. For this reason, patients often present with shortness of breath or bone pain, signs that the cancer has advanced.

Liver cancer commonly leads to end-stage liver failure (see "Liver Failure," this chapter). Liver cancer can cause portal hypertension with esophageal varices, ascites, and profound weight loss.

Treatment

Although the prognosis for liver cancer is poor, if the tumors are small, localized, and slow growing, they may be surgically removable. Standard cancer treatments, such as chemotherapy and radiation, do not usually provide a cure by themselves, but they may shrink tumors to make them operable. Usually the treatment is focused on delaying end-stage liver failure rather than curing the cancer. Throughout, supportive care is aimed at managing symptoms.

Treatment may include cryosurgery, using metal probes to freeze the tumors under general anesthesia. The recovery from cryosurgery is usually rapid since serious complications are rare. Ethanol may be injected into tumor sites, dehydrating and destroying them under local anesthesia. Side effects of this procedure are fever and brief pain around the injection sites.

Sometimes chemotherapy is delivered directly to the liver via **chemoembolization**. In this procedure, the blood supply to the liver tumor is blocked and medication is delivered directly into the artery supplying the tumor area. The combination of depriving the tumor of oxygen and nutrition and focusing higher concentrations of medication directly at the tumor can shrink the tumor. Pain from the procedure is common, as is nausea, vomiting, fever, and fatigue. Individuals who have had the procedure can generally resume normal activities a week afterward but are told to watch for side effects, as fever and fatigue can linger.

A liver transplant might be performed, depending on size, location, and the degree of liver disease. The wait for a liver transplant can be long, often too long for the timeline of liver cancer and end-stage disease.

● INTERVIEW QUESTIONS

1. Where is the cancer in your body? Did your liver cancer begin in the liver or spread from somewhere else? Are there other sites of cancer in your body?
2. How does the condition affect you? What are your signs and symptoms?
3. How well does your liver function? Is your doctor concerned about your level of liver function?
4. Do any of your doctors say you have portal hypertension?
5. Do you have any swelling in your abdomen? Swelling in your legs, caused by your liver condition?
6. Any swollen or congested organs?
7. Is your skin affected by your liver function? Any discoloration, easy bruising or bleeding, or itching?
8. What would be the most comfortable position for you during the massage? In what position do you sleep? Does your doctor advise any particular sleeping or resting position?
9. Are there any complications of your cancer? Any effects on bone, lung, or brain?
10. How is your condition being treated?
11. How has the treatment affected you?

● MASSAGE THERAPY GUIDELINES

Working with liver cancer combines massage adjustments for liver failure and massage adjustments for cancer (see Chapter 20). Liver failure is addressed separately in this chapter. For a story of working with a client with metastatic liver disease, see Therapist's Journal online at http://thePoint.lww.com/Walton.

Question 1, always the first one in a case of cancer, establishes the location of any cancer in the body. Question 9 can reinforce this inquiry. A client reporting liver cancer could be referring to true, primary liver cancer, or to liver metastasis from another primary site. Whether the liver is a primary or secondary site is less important than knowing all of the sites of active cancer in the body. See Chapter 20 for ways to access this essential information, and for massage therapy guidelines for common sites of metastasis. As always, avoid pressure at any and all accessible sites of cancer, whether primary or secondary. For liver cancer, this means avoiding direct pressure on the area of liver that is accessible just under the ribs. But consider other sites, too. For example, take care at the abdomen if the tissues there are also involved.

Question 2 about the client's signs and symptoms can bring up many scenarios. In particular, with liver cancer, fatigue or fever may be present. If so, then provide a gentle session overall. If weight loss has been profound (*cachexia*), then pressure, positioning, and bolstering are adapted to accommodate protruding bony landmarks, and vulnerable nerve and vascular endangerment sites. Make any joint movement gentle because lost muscle mass causes joint instability. If abdominal pain or right shoulder pain is present, adapt the position accordingly, and consider the side-lying position for the massage.

Question 3 about liver function is important because a person can have primary liver cancer or liver metastasis without liver impairment. The lesions can be present in the tissue without affecting function. If this is the case, massage adjustments may be limited to pressure at active cancer sites, or organized around other features of the cancer. On the other hand, if liver function is impaired, the Vital Organ Principle, Filter and Pump Principle, and Detoxification Principle are in force along with any other relevant modifications. Questions 3–7 also point you to common massage adjustments for liver failure (this chapter). In particular, the tendency to bruise and bleed also requires lighter pressures overall.

> *The Unstable Tissue Principle.* **If a tissue is unstable, do not challenge it with too much pressure or joint movement in the area.**

Difficulty breathing or congested organs suggest positioning modifications. Splenomegaly or hepatomegaly may require positioning for comfort (see Figure 16-5 for suggestions). Strong abdominal pain may limit client positions, and pressure should obviously be avoided at the abdomen. Both abdominal pain and right shoulder pain might be eased in the side-lying position.

Question 8 helps you to determine the best position for the client. If cancer is also in the lungs, consider elevating the upper body. An inclined supine position or a seated position might be best.

Question 9 reflects the importance of asking about bone and lung involvement in at least two different ways, in order to be certain of a good answer. These common secondary sites call for serious consideration. If there is any possible bone involvement, bones may be unstable. Use gentle movement and pressure to avoid pathologic fracture (see "Bone Metastasis," Chapter 20). Treat any new or unfamiliar pain as possible bone involvement, and avoid pressure in the area. Determine from the client's physician how stable the bones are before pressing on them or moving joints.

Questions 10 and 11 could bring up a number of possible treatments. If cryosurgery or ethanol injections are being used, the side effects and complications tend to be minimal except at the incision/injection sites. On the other hand, chemoembolization is intense therapy; post-embolization side effects can be strong. Use extremely gentle massage, to respect fever and fatigue, with slow speeds and even rhythms for nausea. Additional adjustments for nausea are listed in the Decision Tree (see Figure 16-6). As the effects of chemoembolization fade, use the client's activity level to gauge the strength of your session. If your client has had a liver transplant, see Chapter 21 for the complex medical and massage issues that may be present.

Because liver cancer tends to be aggressive, often diagnosed in the later stages, clients with liver involvement may be quite ill. Apply these common massage adjustments for liver cancer and metastatic liver disease, but be alert for other health issues, as well. A good understanding of the issues raised in Chapter 20 is necessary to carry out massage safely in this population. As with any advanced cancer, the DVT Risk Principles (see Chapter 11) are advised, even if the client has easy bruising or bleeding.

● MASSAGE RESEARCH

Little research has been done on massage for people with liver cancer, and the data are not conclusive. One small study of 40 patients with primary liver disease, all undergoing arterial embolization, suggested that stress management could help patients manage the anxiety of this procedure. The procedure causes painful side effects (Lin et al., 1998). Stress management measures studied were back massage, muscle relaxation, and health education.

While liver cancer is not a focus of massage research, other studies on massage and cancer draw from a broad patient population, and the findings may be applicable to liver cancer. See Chapter 20 and the bibliography for mention of these studies.

● POSSIBLE MASSAGE BENEFITS

The median length of survival after a diagnosis of liver cancer is 8 months, reflecting how advanced the condition often is before symptoms prompt an individual to see a doctor. Primary hepatoma may follow years of carefully monitored chronic liver disease, and the sudden appearance and advancement of cancer can be a shock. At the same time, when the cancer is treatable, survival for years is possible.

Well-crafted massage therapy can be a blessing in either of these scenarios. Emotional support and gentle, positive touch against a backdrop of painful procedures can be beneficial. The body can change rapidly under the influence of such an aggressive cancer, and massage may "even things out," providing support for a positive body image, in the middle of disfiguring changes.

Liver Cancer

Medical Information	Massage Therapy Guidelines

Essentials

- Tumor formation in liver, either as primary tumor or metastasis from another primary tumor; may be asymptomatic, with no effect on function, or causing many symptoms. ·

  → - No direct massage pressure at/over site; if liver function is affected, follow Vital Organ Principle, Filter and Pump Principle, Detoxification Principle.
  - Review Chapter 20 for massage guidelines for cancer and cancer treatment

- Fever, fatigue → - Gentle session overall
- Weight loss → - Adapt pressure, position and bolstering to accommodate nerve and vascular endangerments, bony landmarks
  - Limit joint movement if joints unstable

- Splenomegaly, hepatomegaly → - Adapt position; consider sidelying, semi-reclining, seated

- Pain: abdominal, right shoulder → - Adjust position and bolsters for comfort

Complications

- Metastasis to bone → - Physician consultation to determine bone stability; avoid pressure and joint movement at fragile sites (see Chapter 20)

- Metastasis to lung → - Adapt positioning to breathing difficulties; consider semi-reclining, sidelying, seated

- Liver failure → - See Liver Failure, this chapter

Medical treatment	Effects of treatment	
· Surgery	· See Surgery, Chapter 21, for side effects, complications	· Follow the Procedure Principle; see Surgery, Chapter 21
· Cryosurgery, ethanol injections	· Mild, brief pain at site; fever	· Few massage adjustments except at site; gentle session overall for fever
· Chemoembolization	· Acute pain, nausea, vomiting, chronic fever, fatigue	· Easy bathroom access; position for pain relief (flat prone or supine position may be poorly tolerated; side-lying may be preferred); gentle session overall; pressure to tolerance (typically 2 max), but with full, reassuring contact; slow speeds; no uneven rhythms or strong joint movement; avoid scents in lubricant and odors in environment
· Liver transplant	· Significant side effects, complications likely	· See Surgery; Organ and Tissue Transplant, Chapter 21

FIGURE 16-6. A Decision Tree for liver cancer.

Other Liver Conditions in Brief

CIRRHOSIS

Background	• Replacement of healthy liver cells with scar tissue, causing impairment in function. • Commonly caused by chronic hepatitis B and C, alcoholic hepatitis, autoimmune hepatitis; less frequently caused by hemochromatosis (see Chapter 12). • May be asymptomatic in early stages; as more scar tissue forms, fatigue, loss of appetite, weight loss, nausea occur. • As function declines, chronic or acute liver failure occurs (see "Liver Failure," this chapter). • Treated with alcohol abstinence, addiction treatment, improved nutrition; treatments for liver failure (this chapter).
Interview Questions	• How long have you had the diagnosis of cirrhosis? How does it affect you? • How well does your liver function? Is your doctor concerned about it? Does it affect your activity or energy level? Does it cause symptoms? • Do you have portal hypertension? Swelling (ascites) in abdomen? Swelling in your legs from the condition? • Any swollen or congested organs? • Any effects on skin? Any discoloration (jaundice), easy bruising or bleeding, itching? • What would be the best position for you during the massage? • Treatment? Effects of treatment?
Massage Therapy Guidelines	• If cirrhosis produces symptoms, proceed as though chronic liver failure has occurred. Follow Filter and Pump Principle—avoid general circulatory intent; observe Vital Organ Principle. • Follow Detoxification Principle, avoiding general circulatory intent, avoid spa services intended to accelerate detoxification. • Limit overall pressure to 1–3, depending on bruising/bleeding tendency. • See "Liver Failure," this chapter, for massage guidelines for specific symptoms and complications. • Practice sensitivity, compassion for addiction and recovery.

FATTY LIVER DISEASE (NONALCOHOLIC STEATOSIS, NONALCOHOLIC STEATOHEPATITIS)

Background	• Mild liver damage due to accumulation of triglycerides in liver cells; can be from alcohol use, or from other factors. • Nonalcoholic steatosis (simple fatty liver) and steatohepatitis (fatty liver with inflammation) occur at any age; associated with obesity, hypertension, high cholesterol and triglycerides (metabolic syndrome), diabetes, some medications. • May cause no symptoms or complications, or may cause fatigue, malaise, upper right abdominal pain. • Without treatment and management, may progress to cirrhosis and liver failure. • Treated with weight loss, alcohol abstinence, diabetes management, stopping toxic medication.
Interview Questions	• Symptoms? Is the function of your liver affected? Are you tested regularly for liver function, or is your doctor concerned about it? • Have any complications occurred? Has the condition caused cirrhosis or liver failure? Any bruising or bleeding, or fluid accumulation? • Activity and energy level? • Treatment? Effects of Treatment?
Massage Therapy Guidelines	• If liver function is intact, or only mildly affected, adapt massage to activity and energy level. If liver inflammation or liver failure is present, follow Vital Organ Principle, Filter and Pump Principle, Detoxification Principle (see Chapter 3). • Medical consultation may be needed for assessment of liver function and appropriate massage adjustments. • See Cirrhosis, Conditions in Brief; see "Liver Failure," this chapter. • See "Hypertension," Chapter 11; "Metabolic Syndrome," "Diabetes," Chapter 17.

HEPATITIS, ALCOHOLIC

Background	• Liver inflammation from alcohol use. Usually caused by chronic overuse, but also from binge drinking or moderate, regular use. • Mild forms may present no symptoms; severe symptoms indicate progression to cirrhosis (see Conditions in Brief) and liver failure, including fever, hepatomegaly, jaundice, bleeding, portal hypertension (see "Liver Failure," this chapter). • Chronic condition progresses to cirrhosis, which persists unless alcohol use is stopped; if alcohol use ceases, inflammation resolves over weeks or months. • Treated with alcohol abstinence, good nutrition, especially B vitamins; vitamin K for bleeding; corticosteroids used in severe cases of liver inflammation.
Interview Questions	• Symptoms? Is the function of your liver affected? Are you tested regularly for liver function, or is your doctor concerned about it? • Have any complications occurred? Has the condition caused cirrhosis or liver failure? Any bruising or bleeding, or fluid accumulation? • Activity and energy level? • Treatment? Effects of treatment?
Massage Therapy Guidelines	• If liver function impaired, complications present, or alcohol use continues, follow Vital Organ Principle, Filter and Pump Principle, Detoxification Principle. • Medical consultation may be needed for assessment of liver function and appropriate massage adjustments. • Adapt massage to activity and energy level. • See Cirrhosis, "Liver Failure," this chapter, for additional massage therapy guidelines. • See "Corticosteroids," Chapter 21, for massage adaptations.

HEPATITIS, AUTOIMMUNE

Background	• Liver inflammation from autoimmune condition; often occurring in adolescence or young adulthood. • Disease can be mild with few symptoms; advanced disease includes liver failure and associated symptoms (jaundice, poor blood clotting, etc.) • Many patients also have other autoimmune conditions, such as type 1 diabetes, ulcerative colitis, thyroiditis; may be triggered by other diseases, drugs, or toxic exposure. • Treated with corticosteroid medication (prednisone) and immunosuppressant medication such as azathioprine (Imuran). See "Corticosteroids," Chapter 21, for prednisone side effects; Imuran can suppress WBC counts, cause nausea, reduce appetite.
Interview Questions	• Symptoms? Is the function of your liver affected? Are you tested regularly for liver function, or is your doctor concerned about it? • Have any complications occurred? Has the condition caused cirrhosis or liver failure? Any bruising or bleeding, or fluid accumulation? • Other autoimmune conditions, such as colitis, rheumatoid arthritis, diabetes? • Activity and energy level? • Treatment? Effects of treatment?
Massage Therapy Guidelines	• If liver inflammation present, liver failure has occurred, or any symptoms are present, follow Vital Organ Principle, Filter and Pump Principle, Detoxification Principle (see Chapter 3). • Medical consultation may be needed for assessment of liver function and appropriate massage adjustments. • Adapt massage to activity and energy level. • See Cirrhosis, Conditions in Brief, Liver Failure (Figure 16-3 and text); adjust massage to any other autoimmune conditions. • See "Corticosteroids," Chapter 21, for massage adaptations to prednisone side effects; for nausea, position for comfort, provide gentle session overall, pressure to tolerance, slow speeds; avoid uneven rhythms or strong joint movement; for WBC suppression, adapt to reduced immunity: use good infection control precautions (see Neutropenia, Chapter 12).

SELF TEST

1. Explain why the Vital Organ Principle, Filter and Pump Principle, and Detoxification Principle are used in work with clients who have liver conditions. How is each principle important?

2. Compare and contrast hepatitis A, B, and C in terms of mode of transmission and severity of symptoms, and the course of the disease. Which type of hepatitis is most likely to progress to a chronic active state, and long-term liver problems?

3. Compare the acute, chronic active, and chronic inactive states of hepatitis infection.

4. Describe the massage modifications necessary for a client taking interferon or other antiviral drugs to treat hepatitis.

5. How do you prevent transmission of hepatitis A during a massage session?

6. What does it mean to be a carrier of hepatitis? How long can a person with hepatitis remain in a carrier state?

7. How are hepatitis C, cirrhosis, and liver failure related?

8. What is the difference between chronic and acute liver failure? Which is more common?

9. List three common, later complications in liver failure, the symptoms caused, and the appropriate massage adjustments for each.

10. Which spa services should be avoided in a client with liver failure? Explain the reasoning behind this precaution.

11. What is portal hypertension, and how is it caused? Explain the gastric and esophageal complications of portal hypertension, and why they are serious.

12. How should massage be adapted for a client who has recently undergone an embolization procedure for liver cancer? Does research prove any benefit of massage for people undergoing embolization for liver cancer? Explain.

13. In the event that liver cancer causes profound weight loss, which massage elements should be adapted, and why?

14. Explain three ways that poor liver function can affect the skin in advanced liver cancer and other liver disease. How should massage be adjusted if this is the case?

15. Explain two causes of bone instability in clients with primary liver cancer, and how to adjust the massage if this is the case.

 For answers to these questions and to see a bibliography for this chapter, visit http://thePoint.lww.com/Walton.

17 Endocrine System Conditions

The process of living is the process of reacting to stress.

—STANLEY SARNOFF

The endocrine system, a system of glands, hormones, and target tissues, controls the internal environment of the body and adapts to changes that occur during everyday living. Together with the nervous system, the endocrine system regulates the basic physiological functions of metabolism, growth, fluid balance, and reproduction, among many others. The endocrine system responds each day to many *stressors*—whether internal or external. Internal stressors range from blood sugar elevation after eating to the need for more calcium in the bones. External stressors range from a chronically bothersome situation at work to the appearance of an oncoming car in the wrong lane.

Because the endocrine system is involved in maintaining **homeostasis**, the body's tendency, to return to balance in response to a stressor, can be problematic when the system itself is out of balance. Hormones can be overproduced

or underproduced—suggested by the prefix, "hyper-" or "hypo-"—thereby disrupting the body's equilibrium. In adjusting to a "new normal" state, the body compensates with a cascade of responses that are felt across other body systems.

In this chapter, three conditions are discussed at length, each reflecting an internal imbalance in the endocrine system. The conditions are:

- Diabetes mellitus
- Cushing syndrome (hypercortisolism)
- Hypothyroidism

In addition, a full discussion of **thyroid cancer**, including a Decision Tree, may be found online at http://thePoint.lww.com/Walton. Conditions in Brief addressed in this chapter are **Acromegaly**, **Addison disease** (hypocortisolism), **Hyperthyroidism**, **Hypoglycemia**, **Metabolic syndrome**, and **Stress**. Hypoglycemia is also discussed in the Diabetes Mellitus section of this chapter.

General Principles

There are no massage principles that are specific to endocrine conditions, but it is good to be mindful of the various ways that the body can be out of balance. By using common sense, and observing basic principles from Chapter 3, you can work safely and well, without adding further challenge to the body systems.

When endocrine conditions weaken the tissues, the Unstable Tissue Principle is used. And because several endocrine conditions affect blood pressure and other cardiovascular factors, the DVT Risk Principles and Plaque Problem Principle are often applied (see Chapter 11).

Diabetes Mellitus

Diabetes mellitus is a prevalent metabolic disorder that affects the level of glucose in the blood and tissues. High or low blood glucose levels cause a range of signs, symptoms, and complications.

● BACKGROUND

Blood glucose, or *blood sugar*, reflects the supply of fuel for the body's cells. To be used, glucose must be moved from the blood into the cells. Blood sugar is carefully controlled by two hormones produced by the pancreas: insulin and glucagon. **Insulin** lowers blood sugar, by moving glucose from the blood to the cells it supplies. **Glucagon** raises blood sugar, by prompting the liver to release its reserves of glucose to the blood.

There are several types of diabetes. Diabetes mellitus type 1 and 2 are the focus of this chapter. In **Type 1 diabetes mellitus**, an autoimmune process destroys the insulin-producing cells of the pancreas. The insulin deficiency causes glucose to

become trapped in the blood. The absence of glucose in the body's cells causes immediate problems, and blood chemistry changes occur over time. This form of diabetes used to be called *insulin-dependent diabetes* or *juvenile-onset diabetes*. Most people with type 1 diabetes develop the disease before age 30. It accounts for just 10% of diabetes in the United States.

In **Type 2 diabetes mellitus**, the most common form, insulin is produced, but the cells of the body do not respond to it. Again, glucose builds up in the blood. Type 2 disease is also called *insulin resistance*, because the cells of the body are resistant to the action of insulin. It used to be called *non–insulin-dependent diabetes mellitus*. The onset is gradual, and type 2 diabetes is often asymptomatic for years. It tends to develop in adulthood.

There are other notable differences between type 1 and 2 diabetes: the onset is different in each case. In type 1 diabetes, the first symptoms develop over a period of several days. It is thought that a viral or nutritional factor causes the immune system to destroy the insulin-producing cells in the pancreas, in an autoimmune process. The symptoms do not appear until the majority—about 90%—of the insulin-producing cells (called β *islet cells*) have been destroyed, but at that point, the symptoms appear rapidly. Almost overnight, the blood is crowded with glucose that it cannot release to the waiting cells. In contrast, symptoms of type 2 diabetes develop gradually, often over a period of years. Because insulin is still produced, but the body builds a slow resistance to it, early disease is not as dramatic as it is in type 1 diabetes.

The profile of type 2 diabetes is changing because of a strong link to obesity and sedentary lifestyle. With the increase in childhood obesity, type 2 diabetes in children is increasing at an alarming rate in developed countries. Table 17-1 compares diabetes type 1 and 2.

Prediabetes is a condition related to type 2. In this case, blood sugar levels are near but not at the defining level of a type 2 diagnosis. This is called *impaired glucose tolerance (IGT)* or *impaired fasting glucose (IFG)*. Although it is possible to correct the glucose levels, individuals with this condition are likely to progress to diabetes unless underlying health issues are addressed. Blood glucose levels in prediabetes may be part of the constellation of problems in metabolic syndrome (see Conditions in Brief), a condition characterized by high cholesterol, hypertension, and abdominal obesity. When prediabetes and metabolic syndrome are identified, individuals are encouraged to make diet and exercise changes to avert type 2 diabetes.

A related condition, *gestational diabetes*, occurs during pregnancy. Hormones produced by the placenta, especially in the second and third trimester, can make the pregnant woman's cells resistant to insulin. Testing for this form of diabetes is part of routine prenatal care, as it is often asymptomatic. It is typically treated successfully with diet, exercise, and medication to prevent complications. Gestational diabetes tends to resolve after childbirth.

Signs and Symptoms

One feature of diabetes is hyperglycemia (abnormally high blood glucose). When the blood has too much glucose in it, the effects on the rest of the body develop gradually.

The cardinal symptoms of hyperglycemia are polydypsia (excessive thirst); polyphagia (excessive hunger), and polyuria (excessive urination). Headache is another symptom. Because blood sugar concentration is so high, the body attempts to dilute the sugar by increasing water intake (excessive thirst). It also begins dumping excess glucose into the urine. When glucose is moved to the urine, the kidneys attempt to dilute it with water and increased urination results. Excessive thirst is aggravated by the water loss in the urine. Then, because calories are lost from the body through glucose in the urine, the individual becomes calorie deprived and hungry. Weight loss often occurs as the individual is unable to compensate for the calorie loss.

Another feature of diabetes is hypoglycemia (abnormally low blood glucose). When the blood glucose level becomes excessively low, and cells are deprived of glucose, the effects are immediate and dramatic. This is called an insulin reaction, and the term is used interchangeably with hypoglycemia. Some signs and symptoms of hypoglycemia are irritability, sudden mood changes, sudden changes in personality or behavior, slow or incoherent speech, confusion, and difficulties with attention. These and other hypoglycemia symptoms (see Table 17-2) reflect the poor function of cells when they are deprived of fuel. Those who live with people with hypoglycemia know the signs well and often are the first to notice them and link them with the need for blood sugar.

TABLE 17-1. TYPE 1 AND TYPE 2 DIABETES MELLITUS COMPARED	
Type 1 Diabetes Mellitus	**Type 2 Diabetes Mellitus**
Sudden onset	Gradual onset
10% of diabetes cases in the United States	About 90% of diabetes cases in the United States
Formerly called *insulin-dependent diabetes, juvenile-onset diabetes*	Formerly called *non–insulin-dependent diabetes, adult-onset diabetes*
Usually develops in people under 30	Usually develops in people over 30
Results from absence of insulin when insulin-producing cells of the pancreas are destroyed	Results from body cells becoming insulin resistant
Believed to be an autoimmune disease; common viral infections may also contribute	Tends to run in families; strongly linked to obesity, sedentary lifestyle, high blood pressure
Hypoglycemia is usually a side effect of insulin therapy, or a result of imbalance in insulin, food intake, exercise	Hypoglycemia can occur in early stages of the disease, may be a feature of diabetes itself
Hyperglycemia tends to lead to diabetic ketoacidosis (DKA), a blood chemistry change that gives a fruity odor to the breath; breathing quickens and deepens, and headache, nausea, dry mouth, vomiting, and fatigue occur. Can progress to coma and death	Hyperglycemia tends to lead to hyperglycemic-hyperosmolar state (HHS), a blood chemistry change in which fluid shifts from the tissues to the blood and then to the urine; causes dehydration, confusion, drowsiness, seizures and coma; can progress to coma and death
Treated with insulin therapy to move glucose out of blood and into cells	Treated with drugs that increase cell sensitivity to insulin, drug combinations, and insulin
Long-term complications: cardiovascular, neurological, kidney, immune (similar to type 2)	Long-term complications: cardiovascular, neurological, kidney, immune (similar to type 1)

Hyperglycemia and hypoglycemia are compared in Table 17-2.

Complications

People with diabetes struggle with blood glucose control, with varying levels of success. Blood sugar can often be too high or too low. These imbalances trigger other changes in blood chemistry that affect the cells and tissues supplied by the blood.

Hypoglycemia is a problem in both types of diabetes. In type 1 diabetes, hypoglycemia typically reflects an imbalance in insulin level, food intake, and exercise. Three major factors lower blood glucose levels: an increase in insulin, exercise, and skipping or delaying meals.

- Insulin lowers blood glucose by moving it out of the blood and into the body's cells. This can occur after an insulin injection or after another drug is taken to stimulate insulin production (see "Treatment," below).
- Exercise lowers blood glucose by creating a metabolic demand for it in the tissues, also shifting it out of the blood.
- When an individual delays or skips a meal, there is no dietary glucose to replenish the blood's supply of glucose on the schedule that the body needs.

Sometimes more than one of these factors is at play, reducing blood glucose levels significantly.

In type 2 diabetes, hypoglycemia may be an early symptom in the disease. It can also result from poor blood sugar control, as in type 1 diabetes. Some treatments for type 2 diabetes stimulate insulin production, leading to a drop in blood sugar (see Table 17-3).

Whatever the cause, hypoglycemia tends to come on suddenly, and it can quickly become a medical emergency and be fatal if untreated. Without new glucose in the blood, from tablets, sweets, or juice, the body's cells and tissues face a crisis in fuel supply, and eventually the tissues are unable to function. Common features of hypoglycemia—confusion, faintness, slow speech, mood and behavior changes—are signs that the brain is not getting the glucose it needs (see Table 17-2).

In contrast, hyperglycemia tends to cause change gradually, altering blood concentrations of fatty acids and triglycerides over time. Hyperglycemia causes one of two scenarios, depending on the type of diabetes. In type 1 diabetes, the body's cells are forced to use fat cells for fuel since they cannot access glucose. The by-products of fat cell breakdown are ketones, which accumulate in the blood and make it acidic.

TABLE 17-2.	**HYPOGLYCEMIA AND HYPERGLYCEMIA COMPARED**
Hypoglycemia (Insulin Reaction)	**Hyperglycemia**
LOW blood glucose	HIGH blood glucose
Symptoms worsen suddenly	Symptoms worsen gradually
Signs and Symptoms	Signs and Symptoms
<ul><li>Irritability</li><li>Sudden mood or behavior changes</li><li>Changes in personality</li><li>Slow or incoherent speech</li><li>Confusion</li><li>Difficulty paying attention</li><li>Faintness</li><li>Dizziness</li><li>Shakiness, trembling</li><li>Clumsy or jerky movement</li><li>Visual disturbances</li><li>Anxiety</li><li>Sweating</li><li>Pallor</li><li>Headache</li><li>Intense hunger</li><li>Rapid heartbeat</li><li>Nightmares</li><li>Night waking</li><li>Difficulty waking</li></ul>	<ul><li>Excessive thirst</li><li>Excessive hunger</li><li>Excessive urination</li><li>Headache</li></ul>
Complications:	Complications:
If untreated, fainting can occur. Can lead to coma and death.	In type 1 diabetes, can progress to diabetic ketoacidosis (DKA, see text for symptoms/signs). If untreated, can cause coma and death. In type 2 diabetes, can progress to hyperosmolar-hypoglycemic state (HHS, see text for symptoms/signs). If untreated, can lead to death.
Usual response to acute episode: administer sweets, glucose tablets; wait 10 minutes; administer again. If ineffective, emergency medical care.	Response to acute episode: emergency medical care.

A crisis point occurs when **diabetic ketoacidosis (DKA)** develops. DKA is a common problem in type 1 diabetes.

In DKA, the ketones give a fruity odor to the breath, and breathing quickens and deepens as the body tries to restore homeostasis in the blood. Other symptoms of DKA are headache, nausea, dry mouth, vomiting, and fatigue. The condition can progress to coma and death, and emergency medical attention is needed.

In type 2 diabetes, high blood sugar does not typically follow the same progression to ketoacidosis because some insulin is still produced. But blood sugar can be very high in type 2 disease, especially when there is an additional stress on the body, such as infection or drug use. In type 2 diabetes, a crisis point is reached when a **hyperglycemic-hyperosmolar state (HHS)** develops. In this fluid imbalance, fluid from the tissues shifts to the blood and to the urine, leading to dehydration, confusion, drowsiness, seizures, and a gradual loss of consciousness. HHS is less common than DKA, but it, too, can be life threatening, and immediate medical care is warranted.

DKA and HHS are acute, life-threatening conditions. But over time, advanced diabetes also causes chronic health problems. Common effects on other systems of the body are:

- *Cardiovascular complications.* Diabetes changes blood composition, causing **hyperlipidemia**, an excess of fatty substances in the blood. These substances, usually cholesterol and triglycerides, set up an environment for cardiovascular complications. Atherosclerotic plaque forms on arteries, causing circulation problems (see "Atherosclerosis," Peripheral vascular disease, Chapter 11). Heart disease, stroke, and erectile dysfunction follow.
- *Skin problems.* Narrowed vessels lead to poor wound healing, infection, and even gangrene, especially in the feet and hands. Skin may injure due to loss of feeling, and infections may form deep in skin, called **diabetic ulcers**.
- *Peripheral neuropathy.* Impaired function in peripheral nerves (see Chapter 10), also called **diabetic neuropathy**, often occurs in hands and feet. Symptoms are impaired sensation, motor weakness, and pain. Autonomic nerves that control the heart, blood pressure, digestion, and other functions may also be affected; this condition is called **autonomic neuropathy**. Poor autonomic function can lead to unstable blood pressure and heart rate, poor digestion, diarrhea, difficulty swallowing, and other problems.
- *Kidney complications.* Injury to renal vessels leads to loss of protein in the urine and impairment of kidney function. This can ultimately lead to kidney failure (see Chapter 18).
- *Impaired vision.* Small blood vessels that supply the retina, when damaged, lead to vision impairment and blindness. This is called **diabetic retinopathy**.
- *Changes in connective tissue.* Failure to metabolize glucose leads to thickening and contracture in connective tissue. This can contribute to conditions such as carpal tunnel syndrome (see Chapter 10).
- *Poor immunity.* White blood cell (WBC) function can be affected, increasing an individual's vulnerability to infection. This leads to increased skin infections (see above), urinary tract infections (see Chapter 18), as well as respiratory infections (see Chapter 14).

Treatment

Diabetes treatment includes long-term management of the disease as well as immediate responses to acute episodes.

An acute episode of hypoglycemia is typically addressed by ingesting sweets, such as glucose tablets, juice, hard candy, or any other form of easily digested sugar (see Table 17-2). If a person's symptoms do not respond to these measures, it is a medical emergency. In this case, the hormone glucagon can be injected, opposing the action of insulin: it acts on the liver, where excess glucose is stored. By accessing these reserves, it moves glucose from the liver to the bloodstream, raising blood sugar. People with diabetes may carry emergency syringes with glucagon, for this purpose.

Hyperglycemia can be a medical emergency as well, although it tends to appear gradually and will not resolve with sugar administration. DKA and HHS are dangerous and can worsen quickly, leading to unconsciousness and even death. Insulin is administered intravenously to decrease blood sugar as much as possible. Fluids and electrolytes are administered to replace losses from excessive urination.

Diabetes management includes proper diet and exercise to keep blood sugar levels in the normal range. In both type 1 and type 2, maintaining a healthy weight is important to disease management. In type 2, it can reverse or arrest the course of disease.

Insulin replacement is the essential foundation of type 1 treatment. It is also used as part of type 2 treatment, even though the body's cells are insulin resistant, to assist in the uptake of glucose from the blood to the cells. The balance of insulin and glucose can be delicate: Delivering too much insulin for the body's needs causes hypoglycemia, and too little insulin leaves the body hyperglycemic. People who take insulin monitor their blood sugar levels and their insulin needs throughout the day with quick needle sticks.

Insulin is usually injected into the layer of fat in the abdomen, thighs, buttocks, or upper arms (Figure 17-1). In general, insulin is absorbed most rapidly if administered into the abdomen, and more slowly if injected into the thighs, buttocks, or upper arms.

Injected insulin comes in four forms, designed for different needs. They are:

1. *Rapid-acting insulin,* which begins lowering blood glucose in about 5 minutes, peaks at about 30–90 minutes and fades in less than 5 hours. It may be used for emergencies, to

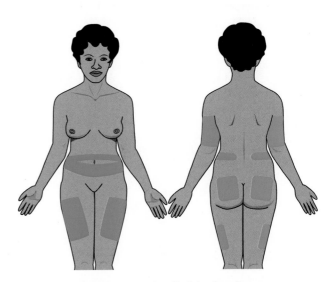

FIGURE 17-1. Insulin injection sites.

combat hyperglycemia. If an individual injects rapid-acting insulin before a meal, he or she typically needs to begin eating within 15 minutes. Brand names include NovoLog, Apidra, and Humalog.

2. *Short-acting insulin* or regular insulin takes 30–60 minutes to begin working in the bloodstream, peaks at 2–3 hours, and lasts about 3–6 hours. It is often used in anticipation of a meal in the next hour or to adjust the blood sugar in response to a high reading. Brand names include Humulin R and Novolin R.

3. *Intermediate-acting insulin* begins lowering blood sugar in 1–4 hours, peaks at 4–12 hours, and lasts 12–18 hours. This type of insulin is designed to be absorbed more slowly so that it provides insulin coverage for a good part of the day, or at night. Brand names include Humulin N and Novolin N.

4. *Long-acting insulin* begins working in the bloodstream at about 6–10 hours, has little or no clear peak of activity, and lasts up to 24 hours. It is used to provide a baseline of insulin coverage, and it is often taken at bedtime. Brand names include Lantus and Levemir.

Many people with diabetes use premixed, combined preparations, with more than one type of insulin. Insulin may be drawn up in a syringe, used in a cartridge or a pre-filled insulin pen. Insulin injection sites can become lumpy with frequent use, and sometimes injections must be discontinued at a site. People taking insulin usually rotate injection sites to avoid this problem.

Insulin can also be infused through a pump, attached through a needle to the abdomen (Figure 17-2). Continuous pumping more closely mimics the action of the pancreas, thus ensuring better blood sugar control.

Oral antihyperglycemic drugs are taken for type 2 diabetes to lower blood glucose levels if exercise, diet, and weight control are ineffective. There are several drug classes, and they are often given in combination. Oral *biguanides* such as Glucophage are usually first-line therapy. They overcome insulin resistance, to some degree, by forcing insulin to carry glucose into cells more effectively. They also help stop the liver from releasing glucose to the blood. The biguanides can cause stomach upset, nausea, and diarrhea. Sulfonylureas help lower blood sugar by stimulating the pancreas to produce

more insulin. A side effect is hypoglycemia. These and other medications for type 2 diabetes are listed in Table 17-3, along with common side effects.

● INTERVIEW QUESTIONS

1. What kind of diabetes do you have? How long have you had it? When were you diagnosed?
2. Do you ever experience the effects of acute high or low blood sugar levels? If so, what are they, how often, and when do they occur? What are your typical signs and symptoms? Have you ever been unaware of a rise in blood sugar or a drop, and someone else had to bring your attention to it?
3. If you have had an acute high or low blood sugar episode, how do you treat it? If you have an emergency response kit, where do you keep it and how do you use it?
4. Is your diabetes considered advanced? Do you have any diabetes complications?
5. Are there any effects of diabetes on your cardiovascular system? Do you have any high blood pressure, atherosclerosis, heart disease, angina, or areas of poor circulation, such as your legs?
6. Has your doctor expressed any concern about the health of your heart? Has your doctor put any medical restrictions on your activities, or exercise, or on the use of extreme heat such as saunas or hot tubs?
7. Do you have a history of stroke or mini-stroke (TIA)? Do you have any leg pain when walking or at rest?
8. Do your feet or legs ever turn blue or cold? Any swelling, heat, redness, or slow wound healing on your legs?
9. Do you have any areas of broken skin, bruising, poor healing, or infection?
10. Are there any effects of diabetes on your nervous system? Do you have any neuropathy? Any sensation changes or weakness anywhere such as hands or feet?
11. Any effects of diabetes on your kidney function? How serious is it, if so?
12. How is your immune system functioning? Are there any effects of diabetes on your immunity?
13. Is your diabetes well controlled? How is it treated? Any oral injected medication?
14. How does your diabetes treatment affect you?
15. If you inject insulin, how long does the medication take to be absorbed from the site? Is it short acting, long acting, or somewhere in between? Where and when was your last injection?
16. If you have an insulin pump, where is it? How can we best position around it for the massage session?
17. Does the timing of your most recent meal and medication support a pretty stable blood sugar level for the next hour or so?

Massage Therapy Guidelines

As with many conditions, be prepared for a range of clinical scenarios for clients with diabetes. One client could have excellent blood sugar control and no complications. Another client could have a number of complications, and great difficulty with blood sugar control, no matter how hard he or she tries. General health questions, along with questions about diabetes, should help establish the client's overall health, massage tolerance, and any massage contraindications.

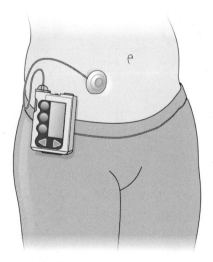

FIGURE 17-2. An insulin pump.

TABLE 17-3.	MEDICATIONS FOR TYPE 2 DIABETES MELLITUS*		
Medications	**Administration**	**How It Works**	**Possible Side Effects**
α-Glucosidase inhibitors, for example, acarbose (Precose), meglitol (Glyset)	Oral, with first bite of a meal	Blocks the breakdown of dietary starches into glucose in the intestine, slows the breakdown of some sugars; moderates increases in blood glucose after meals	Diarrhea, gas
Amylin mimetics, for example, pramlintide (Symlin)	Injection	Slows food absorption	Nausea
Biguanides, for example, metformin (Glucophage)	Oral	Decreases the liver's release of glucose reserves, makes muscle tissue more insulin sensitive	Stomach upset, nausea, diarrhea
DPP-4 Inhibitors, for example, sitagliptin (Januvia)	Oral	Prevents the breakdown of GLP-1, a natural substance in the body that stimulates the pancreas to release insulin	Upper respiratory tract infection, sore throat, diarrhea
Incretin mimetics, for example, exenatide (Byetta)	Injection	Stimulates the pancreas to release more insulin	Nausea
Meglitinides, for example, repaglinide (Pandin), nateglinide (Starlix)	Oral, before meals	Stimulates the pancreas to release more insulin	Hypoglycemia, stomach upset
Sulfonylureas, for example, chlorpropomide, glipizide (Glucotrol); glyburide (Micronase, Glynase, Diabeta); glimepiride (Amaryl)	Oral, before meals	Stimulates the pancreas to release more insulin	Hypoglycemia, weight gain
Thiazolidinediones, for example, rosiglitazone (Avandia), pioglitazone (Actos)	Oral	Assists insulin activity in muscle and fat tissue, decreases the liver's release of glucose	Swelling, weight gain; may increase risk of liver problems, heart failure; patients closely monitored

*Trade names are in parentheses. Not all medications and side effects are listed here. Not all medications cause all side effects.

Question 1 provides you with important background information, including the type of diabetes. The length of time since diagnosis is useful, as the likelihood of complications increases with the length of time the person has had the condition. If the client tells you that he or she has prediabetes, see Metabolic Syndrome, Conditions in Brief.

Questions 2 and 3 establish typical patterns of symptoms and what you need to do if you see signs of hypoglycemia in your client. Recall that some people with diabetes experience hypoglycemia without recognizing it, especially if they have had diabetes for a long time. By having this conversation up front, you will know how to respond if an acute episode happens during a session and the client is unable to tell you what to do. Be alert for any signs of blood sugar problems, listed under hypoglycemia (see Table 17-2). Typically, an episode of hypoglycemia calls for administering some sort of sugar source. Sweets will clear up hypoglycemia pretty quickly. If symptoms persist, call emergency services.

It is also important to be alert for signs and symptoms of hyperglycemia, although chronic, identified hyperglycemia is less likely to require an emergency response than acute hypoglycemia. However, if chronic hyperglycemia becomes complicated, the condition is serious. Review the signs of DKA or HHS. The symptoms and signs are in the Decision Tree, and an urgent or immediate response is necessary. You are more likely to encounter DKA than HHS, although with recent increases in obesity and type 2 diabetes, the incidence of HHS is expected to increase.

Questions 4–14 all concern the effects on body systems when diabetes is advanced. Questions 5–7 focus on cardiovascular conditions, and Question 6 is designed to catch heart conditions that could be taxed by high heat or exercise. If present, such a heart condition contraindicates spa therapies that raise core temperature, and general circulatory intent may be contraindicated, as well. These are layered questions, with built-in redundancy to be sure to catch any information for the massage session. If your client answers yes to any of Questions 5–7, review the relevant condition (see "Stroke [Cerebrovascular Accident]", Chapter 10; see "Atherosclerosis," "Hypertension," "Heart Disease [Coronary Artery Disease]," Angina, or Peripheral Vascular Disease, Chapter 11). Review the CV Conditions Often "Run in Packs" Principle for massage therapy guidelines.

Diabetes

Medical Information	Massage Therapy Guidelines

Essentials

- Metabolic disease affecting blood glucose levels
  - Type 1 – insulin production by pancreas impaired
  - Type 2 – insulin produced but cells resistant
- Hyperglycemia
  - Excessive thirst
  - Excessive hunger
  - Excessive unrination
  - Headache
- Hypoglycemia
  - Confussion
  - Clumsiness, slow, incoherent speech
  - Difficulty waking
  - Difficulty paying attention
  - Irritability
  - Sweating, pallor
  - Changes in personality, mood, behavior
  - Headache
  - Faintness
  - Dizziness or shakiness
  - Hunger
  - Rapid heartbeat

→ • Ask about blood sugar stability; be alert for signs of hypoglycemia and hyperglycemia, especially if unstable, poorly controlled

→ • Immediate medical referral

→ • Check with client before session about symptoms, proper emergency response; ask location of glucose tablets or other emergency glucose source
  - Typical emergency response is to give glucose substance, wait 10 minutes, administer again, contact emergency services if no improvement

Complications

- Diabetic ketoacidosis (in type 1): Excessive thirst, hunger, urination; weight loss, fruity odor to breath, nausea, vomiting, fatigue, may progress to coma and death

- Hyperosmolar-hyperglycemic state (in type 2): Dehydration, confusion, drowsiness, may progress to seizures, coma, and death

- Cardiovascular complications
  - Atherosclerosis
  - Peripheral vascular disease
  - Heart disease (e.g. angina, heart failure)
  - Stroke

- Skin problems
  - Poor wound healing
  - Diabetic ulcer; gangrene

- Neurologic complications
  - Diabetic neuropathy

  - Autonomic neuropathy
  - Unstable heart rate, BP

  - Poor digestion (diarrhea, difficulty swallowing)
- Kidney failure
- Vision impairment
- Poor immunity

→ • Immediate medical referral–emergency

→ • Immediate medical referral–emergency

→ • See Chapter 11

→ • See Chapter 10
  - Inspect tissue before massage, discuss any lesions with client; avoid contact, lubricant at open or infected skin

→ • Follow Sensation Principle; Sensation Loss, Injury Prone Principle; see Peripheral Neuropathy, Chapter 10

→ • Avoid general circulatory intent; no strong pressure (level 2-3 max); avoid strong joint movement, use slow speeds, predictable rhythms, gradual transitions; slow rise from table at end of session

→ • See Chapter 15

→ • See Chronic Kidney Failure, Chapter 18

→ • Sensitivity; clear, easy access

→ • Standard precautions; additional infection control precautions as necessary

FIGURE 17-3. A Decision Tree for diabetes mellitus.

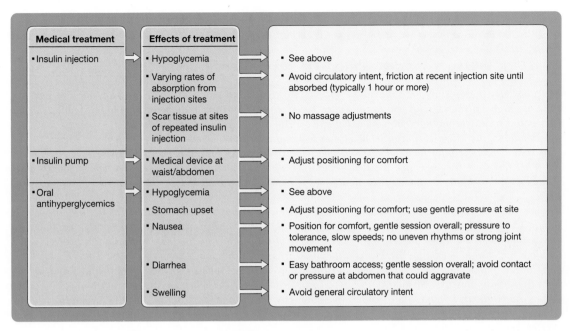

FIGURE 17-3. (*Continued*).

If any of your client's answers suggest that the condition is advanced, the best approach is to use caution on the lower extremities (DVT Risk Principles) and the neck (Plaque Problem Principle). This conservative approach is especially useful with one-time or first-time clients, where there is no clear follow-up or monitoring the client over a course of treatment.

> *The CV Conditions Often "Run in Packs" Principle. If one cardiovascular condition is present, the therapist should be on the alert for others.*

Question 8 specifically targets peripheral vascular disease, but together with Questions 9 and 10, it also highlights skin integrity issues for the massage therapist. In peripheral vascular disease, the skin of the extremities may heal slowly and ulcerate, and this can be compounded by losses in sensation due to diabetic neuropathy. This is especially true in the feet and lower legs. People with this constellation of problems can be:

- Unaware of ulcer formation
- Oblivious to injury from a pebble or foreign body in the shoe
- Unlikely to heal quickly, because of impaired blood flow

In these cases, always inspect the tissues before massaging, and alert the client to any compromised skin. As always, be cautious and avoid contact and lubricant at open lesions. Be gentle with your pressure in areas of bruising, pain, and impaired sensation. As suggested in Therapist's Journal 17-1, the health and integrity of the feet can be part of an ongoing dialogue between you and your client.

Question 10 is a catch-all question for neuropathy, stroke, or even retinopathy. If retinopathy impairs vision, be sensitive if extra assistance for the client is necessary. Maintain a clear path through your office and to the massage table, where possible. See Chapter 10 for more on peripheral neuropathy and stroke, and be prepared to follow the Principles of Sensation (see Chapter 3), if necessary. With autonomic neuropathy, because the blood pressure and heart rate can be unstable, you want to be gentle overall, avoiding circulatory intent and any unpredictable or strong pressures. If autonomic neuropathy affects digestion, see Chapter 15.

The client's answer to Question 11 about kidney function may change the intent of your massage. Diabetes can impair kidney function a little or a lot, and kidney failure is a possible result (see "Chronic Kidney Failure," Chapter 18). Be prepared to avoid general circulatory intent if the kidneys are not filtering well, respecting the Filter and Pump Principle. Follow the Vital Organ Principle, as well.

> *The Vital Organ Principle. If a vital organ—heart, lung, kidney, liver, or brain—is compromised in function, use gentle massage elements and adjust them to pose minimal challenge to the client's body.*

Question 12 could identify compromised WBC count or a client's complaint of frequent colds and flu. In diabetes, drops in WBC count are more likely to be slight than substantial. Always use good infection control measures, and follow any additional precautions if the client or client's doctor requests it. A client whose immunity is affected may not want to receive massage from you if you have symptoms of a cold. People with advanced diabetes have a higher risk of dying from the flu or other common infections.

Advanced diabetes presents numerous massage contraindications, and the interview questions provided here should identify most of them. Common clinical features and massage guidelines are summarized in Figure 17-4.

Questions 13–16 address the primary diabetes treatments. Medications for type 1 and 2 diabetes may differ considerably, so follow the client's account of treatment closely.

A principal concern with insulin injection is an insulin reaction, discussed above. Another concern is the injection site.

Typically, pharmaceutical companies that make insulin recommend avoiding exercising the muscles in the area of insulin

THERAPIST'S JOURNAL 17-1 *Foot Massage and Type 2 Diabetes*

I've been a massage therapist in a hospital and in private practice. I have a client I care for a lot, one I've seen for 6 years. She has type 2 diabetes, with poorly controlled blood sugar. This type of diabetes runs in her family: her mother and sister both had it. Her mother had a lower leg and several toes amputated before she died.

Understandably, this client is concerned about her feet and wants to take care of them. She doesn't want to lose them. She comes exclusively for foot massage and reflexology. She comes faithfully every 4 weeks.

At first, her feet were very sensitive to touch—even spreading lotion on the balls of her feet was uncomfortable and caused one foot to involuntarily quiver. Also, the tissues of her feet were discolored—the feet, ankles, and nail beds were pale.

There have been a few massage adaptations. I use a stepstool and help her onto my table, as her weight—around 350 pounds—makes it hard for her to lift herself onto the table, raise her legs, turn over, and so on. I give her a couple of pillows for her head and extra bolsters under her arms to effectively widen the table so that her arms can rest. I can tell that life is not easy in her body. Exercise is difficult. Movement is difficult.

I work for an hour session, using petrissage and effleurage as well as reflexology. She loves the full hand strokes. I use light to medium pressure. No knuckles or fists. Light pressure for the reflex points. In order to work on such a small area for a full hour, I do find that I change positions frequently, and stand for part of the session in order to use my body well. Also, this is a complete foot treatment. I work each toe thoroughly: lateral, medial, dorsal, and plantar aspects. Her feet get a good "workout."

I don't have to follow many other contraindications because my work is confined to her feet, which she uses to walk so that they already get significant pressure. She walks and travels a great deal. Even though there are complications of diabetes and her weight, the massage contraindications mostly apply to other parts of the body.

Although she could not take any pressure at first, after a few months she was able to tolerate good, solid, medium pressure, heavier than lotioning. After months of regular foot massage treatment, her feet weren't as sensitive. The discoloration faded, and the texture now feels good. The tissues look and feel healthy. I did notice that even though her feet improved, her ankles and lower legs remained discolored. In the last few months, she received acupuncture, and those tissues have started to look much healthier. I told her I'd never seen anything that dramatic. I do think because of her weight, it's hard for her to see all aspects of her feet, so it helps to have my feedback.

Most importantly, there's been a difference in her pain. In her first few years of sessions, she would tell me, at the beginning of every session, how much her feet hurt. Afterward, she always tells me how good they feel. And recently, she's made it clear that her chronic pain has eased.

My client and I have a wonderful relationship. She inspires me, and I tell her so. She travels a lot, much more than I do, and is very involved in her community. She's always telling me stories of her travels, her family, and her other adventures. It's been great to see her so regularly for so many years, and to feel like I am helping her, helping her feet carry her through a life that is not always easy, but is interesting and full.

Michelle Boutin
Tewksbury, MA

injection during the 1st hour following an injection. Often massage is discouraged at the site, as well. This recommendation is made to avoid speeding the absorption of the drug from the site. By this logic, any friction or circulatory intent around the injection site should be avoided during that timeframe. This is unlikely to be an issue with rapid-acting and short-acting injection, because a meal typically follows an injection, not a massage. You are more likely to encounter a recent injection of intermediate-acting insulin, which is absorbed more slowly. In the safest approach, avoid circulatory intent around the injection site until the medication is known to have peaked.

The above precaution is *local*, only around the site of the injection. There is no clear contraindication to *general* circulatory intent after an insulin injection, even though physical exercise is discouraged during the hour or so after an injection. Physical exercise is ill-advised during that period because muscle activity creates metabolic demand for glucose. Together with the injected insulin, physical activity can deplete the blood of glucose, causing an insulin reaction. In contrast, massage with general circulatory intent is unlikely to place the same demand on the tissues that exercise does. At most, massage might increase venous return of blood, speeding the *movement* of blood sugar through the vessels, but not the *utilization* of it.

Most clients with diabetes are skilled at maintaining blood sugar levels. As stated before, you will not usually have to be involved, beyond being alert for signs of hypoglycemia. You can ask Question 17 if you need additional reassurance about massage timing, but be diplomatic, so that the question is not perceived as meddlesome or patronizing.

Repeated insulin injections at the same site can cause scar tissue to form in the area—hard lumps or fat pads may build up. Although these should be approached with gentleness at first, in case of soreness, there are no notable massage adjustments in these areas.

If the client uses an insulin pump, it delivers a timed, low-level insulin infusion. Often the pump clips to the waistband but might lie loosely on the massage table during the session. Be

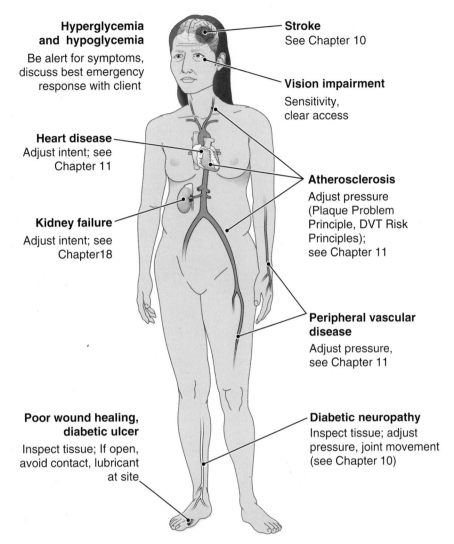

Poor immunity
Follow standard precautions, plus
any additional precautions as
necessary

**Hyperglycemia
and hypoglycemia**

Be alert for symptoms,
discuss best emergency
response with client

Stroke
See Chapter 10

Vision impairment
Sensitivity,
clear access

Heart disease
Adjust intent; see
Chapter 11

Atherosclerosis

Adjust pressure
(Plaque Problem
Principle, DVT Risk
Principles);
see Chapter 11

Kidney failure

Adjust intent; see
Chapter18

**Peripheral vascular
disease**

Adjust pressure,
see Chapter 11

**Poor wound healing,
diabetic ulcer**

Inspect tissue; If open,
avoid contact, lubricant
at site

Diabetic neuropathy

Inspect tissue; adjust
pressure, joint movement
(see Chapter 10)

FIGURE 17-4. Diabetes mellitus: selected clinical features and massage therapy guidelines to consider. Specific instructions and additional massage therapy guidelines are in Decision Tree and text.

aware of the whereabouts of the pump, tubing, and insertion site when you ask the client to turn, when you bolster, and when you draw the drape across the client's body (see Figure 17-2).

Some side effects of type 2 diabetes medications are listed in Table 17-3, and common side effects are addressed in the Decision Tree (see Figure 17-3). Adapt the massage to each side effect: If there is swelling, avoid massage with general circulatory intent; if there is GI distress, adjust the position for comfort and avoid pressure at tender areas. Plan for easy bathroom access, where possible. Look up any other side effects in Table 21-1, which also lists corresponding massage guidelines.

Medication Principle. Adapt the massage to the condition for which the medication is taken or prescribed and to any side effects.

● MASSAGE RESEARCH

As of this writing, there are few randomized, controlled trials (RCTs), published in the English language, on diabetes and massage indexed in PubMed or the Massage Therapy Foundation Research Database. The NIH RePORTER tool lists no active, federally funded research projects on the topic in the United States. No active projects are listed on the clinicaltrials.gov database (see Chapter 6), although the Karolinska Institute in Stockholm has just completed an RCT testing a course of massage in subjects with type 2 diabetes.

In one RCT, with 20 children with diabetes (Field et al., 1997), investigators looked at the effects of a 20-minute massage by each child's parents each night. The control intervention was relaxation therapy, again provided by the parents. The interventions continued for 30 days. The researchers reported reduced depression, along with reduced parent and child anxiety, in the massage group. The massaged children's insulin and diet compliance increased, and their blood glucose decreased. This study is too small to draw firm conclusions from, but if collaborating evidence appears from other groups, it might make a case for parental massage in this population.

Another recent RCT looked at a specific massage protocol for people with type 2 diabetes and peripheral artery disease (Castro-Sanchez et al., 2009). Using a sample size of 98 patients, investigators compared a very specific, standardized massage protocol (1-hour massage, twice per week, for 15 weeks) to a sham control procedure (magnetotherapy treatments from equipment that was not turned on). They found an increase in blood circulation in the lower extremities of the massaged patients, compared to the sham control patients. If this work is corroborated by further research, especially with different massage techniques and protocols, a growing evidence base may support an effect of massage on circulation at the site of application.

● POSSIBLE MASSAGE BENEFITS

As with many diseases, stress makes diabetes more difficult. Stress makes blood sugar control harder, and it can precipitate hypoglycemic episodes. Massage can play a vital role in stress management. Exercise, which is an important component of diabetes management, can be compromised by excess weight and muscle injury, and massage can support regular movement by maintaining flexibility and preventing muscle injury.

Diabetes can negatively affect a person's body image. An accepting, nonjudgmental massage therapist can welcome a client regardless of body type and illness, easing the emotional pain of a poor body image. Massage therapy supports the whole person in body, mind, and spirit.

As a massage therapist, you may also provide a timely referral. It is important to remember that many people with diabetes are undiagnosed. During the initial health interview, and in casual conversation about the client's health, symptoms of diabetes may come up. Recognizing the classic signs of hypoglycemia and hyperglycemia, you are in a good position to make a medical referral to someone who might need it.

Cushing Syndrome (Hypercortisolism)

Cushing syndrome or hypercortisolism is a collection of signs and symptoms caused by an excess production of cortisol. Cortisol is the major glucocorticoid produced by the adrenal cortex. Glucocorticoids are steroid hormones that regulate metabolism and inflammation. Cortisol is a strong anti-inflammatory, produced during times of chronic stress.

● BACKGROUND

Cushing syndrome is usually caused by a benign (noncancerous) pituitary tumor. This is called Cushing disease, or *pituitary Cushing*. The tumor causes the pituitary gland to produce too much adrenocorticotropic hormone (ACTH). ACTH stimulates the adrenal cortex to overproduce cortisol.

In a similar condition, *ectopic Cushing syndrome*, an excess of cortisol arises from overproduction of ACTH by tumors *outside* of the pituitary, as in small cell lung cancer (see Chapter 14), pancreatic cancer (see Chapter 15) or medullary thyroid cancer (online). In rare cases, cancer in the adrenal gland can cause Cushing syndrome. High doses of corticosteroids, used to treat asthma, lupus, or rheumatoid arthritis, can also lead to Cushing syndrome. The condition is more common in women.

Signs and Symptoms

The most striking symptom of Cushing syndrome is progressive, unintentional weight gain in the face, neck, trunk, and abdomen, with the extremities remaining thin. A person with Cushing syndrome has a noticeably moon-shaped face—round, full, and often red. Adipose tissue concentrates between the shoulders, forming what is called a buffalo hump. Striations, or stretch marks, appear at the sites of weight gain. Backache and headache are common.

Complications

In Cushing syndrome, the presence of excess cortisol breaks down tissues in several areas. The person may experience loss of muscle mass and weakness in the arms and legs, making it difficult, in combination with the core weight gain, to rise from a chair. The skin bruises easily and heals poorly, and osteoporosis can develop.

Levels of other hormones are also disturbed in Cushing syndrome, and women may grow facial hair or experience infrequent or absent menstrual periods. Infertility is common. If Cushing syndrome persists untreated or treatment is unsuccessful, fluid retention persists, contributing to hypertension, and putting strain on the heart. Osteoporosis can lead to pathologic fracture (see Chapter 9). Cushing syndrome predisposes an individual to kidney stones and increases a person's vulnerability to infection.

Cushing syndrome may cause glucose intolerance, thus leading to elevated blood sugar levels. This prediabetic condition can progress to type 2 diabetes mellitus (this chapter). Psychological complications include depression, panic attacks, crying spells, irritability, and sleep problems.

Treatment

Cushing syndrome can usually be treated successfully, but because there are several different causes, some involving tiny tumors that are hard to detect, it can take time to diagnose the cause.

If the cause is a corticosteroid medication for another condition, the dose is tapered and stopped where possible, or a substitute medication is used. Corticosteroid withdrawal is no small task and must be gradual. While taking corticosteroid medication, the body reduces its cortisol production and needs time to adjust to the absence of corticosteroid and ramp up its cortisol production. If the withdrawal of the drug is too abrupt, hypocortisolism (insufficient cortisol) may develop. See Addison disease, Conditions in Brief, for the signs and symptoms of this condition.

If a pituitary gland tumor is the cause, treatment includes surgery and radiation. Surgery is called transphenoidal adenectomy. The pituitary gland is accessed through the

Cushing Syndrome (Hypercortisolism)

Medical Information

Essentials

- Excess cortisol production by adrenal cortex

- Causes:
  - Benign pituitary tumor (Cushing disease)
  - Pancreatic cancer, non-small cell lung cancer, medullary thyroid cancer
  - Cancer in adrenal gland

  - High doses of corticosteroids

- Weight gain in face, neck, trunk, abdomen, formation of stretch marks
- Buffalo hump between shoulders
- Rounded, full face, often red

- Back pain

- Headache

Complications

- Loss of muscle mass, weakness in extremities

- Hypertension
- Fluid balance shifts, edema
- Osteoporosis
- Kidney stones
- Increased risk of infection

- Glucose intolerance, diabetes
- Mood changes (depression, panic attacks, irritability, crying spells, sleep difficulties)
- Menstrual changes, infertility

- Thin skin, poor wound healing

Medical treatment

- Gradual tapering of corticosteroids

- Surgery to remove pituitary gland

- Radiation therapy of pituitary gland

Effects of treatment

- Symptoms, signs of hypocortisolism

- Symptoms, signs of hypocortisolism

- See Surgery, Chapter 21, for side effects, complications

- See Chapter 20

Massage Therapy Guidelines

- Ask about cause and adapt massage; if cancer is cause, see Chapter 20

- If due to corticosteroid medication, ask four medication questions (see Chapter 4) and adapt massage accordingly

- No significant massage adjustments; avoid friction if stretch marks itch

- Careful positioning for back pain

- Position for comfort, especially prone; consider inclined table or propping; gentle session overall; pressure to tolerance; slow speed and even rhythm; avoid headache trigger; general circulatory intent may be poorly tolerated

- Limit joint movement if joints unstable

- See Chapter 11
- Avoid general circulatory intent
- See Chapter 9
- See Chapter 18
- Follow standard precautions; additional infection control if physician advises

- See Diabetes, this chapter
- Sensitivity and compassion; medical referral; see Chapter 10
- No massage adjustments unless severe bleeding (see Anemia, Chapter 12); see Infertility, Female, Chapter 19

- Gentle pressure overall (level 2-3 max); no contact, lubricant at open lesions

- See Addison Disease (Hypocortisolism), Conditions in Brief

- See Addison Disease (Hypocortisolism), Conditions in Brief
- Follow the Procedure Principle; see Surgery, Chapter 21

- See Chapter 20

FIGURE 17-5. A Decision Tree for Cushing syndrome (hypercortisolism)

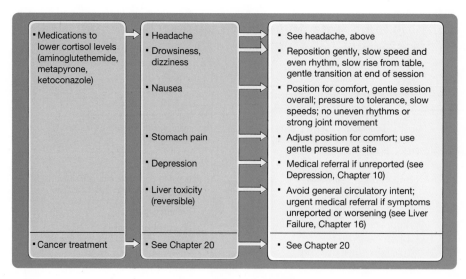

FIGURE 17-5. (*Continued*).

nose or by an incision above the front teeth and removed. If surgery is successful, cortisol levels can be very low for months afterward (hypocortisolism). If surgery is ineffective, surgical removal of the adrenal glands may be performed, thereby requiring lifelong adrenal hormone replacement.

Radiation therapy may follow surgery, in small doses over several weeks, or in a single *stereotactic radiosurgery* procedure. It can take months or even years for radiation of the pituitary gland to take effect, reducing cortisol production for good.

Until these other procedures are successful, medications aimed at the adrenal gland may be used to control cortisol and relieve acute symptoms. Medications may also be used ahead of other procedures in order to control symptoms and prepare the patient for surgery. Drugs include aminoglutethemide, metapyrone, and ketoconazole. The strongest side effects of these medications are well monitored, such as reversible liver toxicity, stomach pain, and depression. Many of the milder side effects, such as drowsiness, dizziness, weakness, headache, and nausea, tend to subside after a few weeks.

If a tumor in an adrenal gland is the cause, the affected gland is usually removed, leaving the other in place for cortisol production. If the tumor is benign, the condition is resolved. If it is malignant, typical cancer treatment—radiation and chemotherapy—follow. Adrenal carcinoma is a serious cancer, and the prognosis is often poor.

If the excess ACTH production was from a nonpituitary tumor, the tumor is removed. If this is not possible, medications can reduce the cortisol production, or both adrenal glands can be removed to eliminate it.

● INTERVIEW QUESTIONS

1. What is the cause of your Cushing syndrome?
2. How does it affect you?
3. Are there any effects on bone and skin strength/stability?
4. Are there any effects on your blood pressure?
5. Are you particularly vulnerability to infection?
6. Are there any effects on your blood sugar?
7. How is your energy level?
8. How is it being treated?
9. Is the treatment effective?
10. How does the treatment affect you?

● MASSAGE THERAPY GUIDELINES

Any time there is a significant disruption in fluid balance in the body, avoid general circulatory intent. Cushing syndrome features swelling, with sodium and fluid retention contributing to hypertension. Avoiding general circulatory intent is a good approach for a first or one-time session with a client; over time, you may modify this in response to improvements in the client's health and activity.

Question 1 about the cause helps determine whether there are other factors to consider in the massage session. With pituitary Cushing, there are no adjustments specific to the cause, but other causes, such as corticosteroid treatment or cancer, may require modifications in the massage plan.

If high doses of corticosteroids have caused Cushing syndrome, ask the Four Medication Questions (see Chapter 4). Another significant condition is likely to be present, such as rheumatoid arthritis or other autoimmune disease. Although the corticosteroid treatment is likely to be stopped, reversing the Cushing symptoms, you might need to adapt the massage to the other condition.

If cancer is causing Cushing syndrome, adapt the massage to the specific type of cancer (see "Lung Cancer," Chapter 14, "Pancreatic Cancer," Chapter 15, or "Thyroid Cancer," online at http://thePoint.lww.com/Walton). In general, review massage adjustments for the presence of cancer, other possible complications, and effects of treatment (see Chapter 20). These adjustments are also in order if adrenal carcinoma is the cause.

Questions 2–7 highlight other factors in the client presentation. If cortisol production is not yet under control, chances are that all of these factors are affected at least in some way. Pressure is a concern whenever tissues are unstable, a pattern in Cushing syndrome. Use gentle pressure overall, probably in the level 2–3 range, for easy bruising and poorly healing skin. With lost muscle mass, joint movement should be cautious, since muscles stabilize many joints. Pressure and joint movement should both be gentle for osteoporosis, gauged to the physician's assessment of bone stability and risk of pathologic fracture (see Chapter 9). Avoid friction over stretch marks, as they may itch. For back pain and headache, see the Decision Tree (Figure 17-5).

> *The Unstable Tissue Principle. If a tissue is unstable, do not challenge it with too much pressure or joint movement in the area.*

Always follow good infection control procedures. Depending on the client's vulnerability to infection, you might need to pay extra attention to infection control, by offering to reschedule, for example, if you have cold symptoms.

If blood pressure is affected, limit pressure to level 2 in the abdomen, and follow the Plaque Problem Principle. (See Chapter 11 for a full discussion of the massage issues associated with hypertension.) If the client has high blood sugar levels, leading to a prediabetic state, see "Diabetes Mellitus" or "Metabolic Syndrome," this chapter. See Chapter 18 if the client has developed kidney stones, a possible complication of Cushing syndrome. If there are effects on the client's menstrual cycle or fertility, see Chapter 19.

Adapt the massage to the client's energy level and mood, and be sensitive to any mood changes the client describes. Encourage the client to report mood problems to his or her doctor. See Chapter 10 if anxiety or depression seems to be present; both can occur with this condition.

Cushing usually has complex signs, symptoms, and complications. Common clinical features and factors, to consider in the massage plan, are summarized in Figure 17-6.

The last three questions can bring up a range of treatments. In some cases, Cushing syndrome is resolved easily, as when it is caused by corticosteroid medication. Ask about any effects from withdrawal, and side effects of a substitute drug. Review "Addison Disease (Hypocortisolism)," Conditions in Brief, for problems that occur when treatment is tapered or discontinued too quickly. If surgery to remove all or part of the pituitary gland was done recently, the loss of adrenal stimulation can also lead to hypocortisolism, which can last for months. Review the massage precautions to use after surgery in Chapter 21.

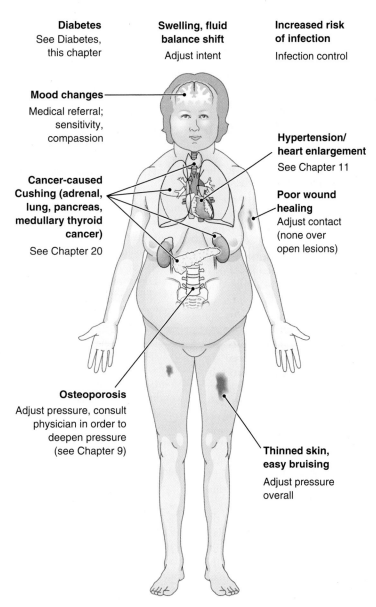

Diabetes
See Diabetes, this chapter

Swelling, fluid balance shift
Adjust intent

Increased risk of infection
Infection control

Mood changes
Medical referral; sensitivity, compassion

Cancer-caused Cushing (adrenal, lung, pancreas, medullary thyroid cancer)
See Chapter 20

Hypertension/ heart enlargement
See Chapter 11

Poor wound healing
Adjust contact (none over open lesions)

Osteoporosis
Adjust pressure, consult physician in order to deepen pressure (see Chapter 9)

Thinned skin, easy bruising
Adjust pressure overall

FIGURE 17-6. Cushing syndrome: selected clinical features and massage adjustments to consider. Specific instructions and additional massage therapy guidelines are in Decision Tree and text.

Cushing diagnosis and treatment can take a long time depending on the cause, and a client's extended story may take a bit more interview time. Treatment may be partially effective but on its way to be fully effective over a period of months. The online Therapist's Journal, "Cushing Disease, a Long Road," tells a story of the many layers of Cushing disease treatment. Adjust the massage to the effects of the treatment as well as the effects of the remaining influence of disease.

If cancer elsewhere in the body—such as the lung or pancreas—is the cause of the hypercortisolism, the person may be in cancer treatment for the primary cause. Review Chapter 20 for guidelines to incorporate into the massage plan.

Medications to reduce cortisol are often part of treatment. Question 10 may reveal side effects such as drowsiness or dizziness, calling for gentle repositioning and other small adjustments described in the Decision Tree (Figure 17-5). Specific guidelines for other side effects, including headache, nausea, stomach pain, and depression, are also listed in the Decision Tree. Liver toxicity, a complication of treatment, is typically monitored closely and is reversible. However, if it is a concern, avoid general circulatory intent, and be alert for unreported or worsening symptoms of liver failure (see Chapter 16).

If treatment was or is conventional cancer treatment, meaning radiation and chemotherapy, see Chapter 20 for specific questions and precautions before working with the client.

● MASSAGE RESEARCH

As of this writing, there are no RCTs, published in the English language, on Cushing syndrome and massage indexed in PubMed or the Massage Therapy Foundation Research Database. The NIH RePORTER tool lists no active, federally funded research projects on the topic in the United States. No active projects are listed on the clinicaltrials.gov database (see Chapter 6).

● POSSIBLE MASSAGE BENEFITS

The process of diagnosing Cushing syndrome, identifying the cause, and treating it effectively can be prolonged and frustrating. Treatment itself can take many months to work. The support of massage therapy may be welcome during this time. Body image can be affected. Sudden mood changes—crying spells, irritability, and so on—may be eased by the stress-relieving effects of massage, and someone suffering in this way can certainly benefit from the sensitive touch of a caring massage professional. In addition, there is the potential for massage therapy to facilitate good, restorative sleep—which can be hard to come by in Cushing syndrome.

The backache and headache of Cushing syndrome may respond to massage, although because the condition is due to an underlying cortisol imbalance, tissue manipulation may not have lasting impact. Still, massage therapy definitely counts as good supportive care.

Hypothyroidism

The thyroid gland, located at the base of the larynx in the anterior neck, releases hormones that regulate the metabolism of every cell in the body, controlling growth, temperature, blood pressure, heart rate, and reproductive function. In **hypothyroidism**, the thyroid gland does not produce adequate amounts of two hormones: **thyroxine (T4)** and **triiodothyronine (T3)**, which is converted from thyroxine. The deficiency in these two thyroid hormones has broad effects on the body. The condition is commonly called "low thyroid."

● BACKGROUND

The release of the thyroid hormones is triggered by **thyroid-stimulating hormone (TSH)**, which is produced by the pituitary gland. In most cases of *primary hypothyroidism*, the condition is due to a problem in the thyroid gland itself. In North America, the most common cause of primary hypothyroidism is **Hashimoto thyroiditis**, in which the thyroid gland is inflamed in a chronic autoimmune process. Primary hypothyroidism can also result from dietary iodine deficiency, although this is rare in developed countries, where table salt is iodized. Iodized salt provides the thyroid gland with the iodine necessary to produce its hormones.

In *secondary hypothyroidism*, an uncommon form, the pituitary gland fails to produce sufficient TSH to stimulate the thyroid gland, or the pituitary gland itself is not being stimulated properly by the hypothalamus. In these cases, the thyroid gland is intact. The focus of this chapter is primary hypothyroidism.

Signs and Symptoms

Some people with hypothyroidism have no symptoms, and in many cases, symptoms develop almost imperceptibly. They can be associated with the "slowing down" of aging or even mistaken for depression. Typical signs and symptoms are fatigue and lethargy, weight gain, and cold intolerance. Shortness of breath on exertion and decreased exercise tolerance are other characteristics. Digestion and elimination slow down, causing constipation. The skin and hair become coarse and dry, and hair loss commonly occurs from the scalp and lateral eyebrows. Women may experience heavy menstrual bleeding, called *menorrhagia*.

Muscle weakness, aches, and tenderness are symptoms of hypothyroidism, as are stiffness, swelling, and pain in the joints. Hypothyroidism is also thought to produce trigger points in the tissues, which tend not to resolve until the thyroid condition is treated.

Not all people with hypothyroidism have the same symptoms. But all of them need help with thyroid balance. Therapist's Journal 17-2 describes how a massage therapist can make an all-important medical referral and encourage a client to get needed care.

Complications

If hypothyroidism continues untreated, several complications can develop. **Goiter**, an enlargement of the thyroid gland, can form and impede swallowing and breathing. Hoarseness may occur. Coronary artery disease and other heart problems may develop, as cardiac contractions weaken and the heart

THERAPIST'S JOURNAL 17-2 *Encouraging a Client to Get Thyroid Help*

Hypothyroidism is very common in women (about 25% develop hypothyroidism by the age of 60), and people with low thyroid tend to seek out massage for fatigue and muscle pain, both of which are symptoms of hypothyroidism. I'm familiar with the problem because I've worked with my own thyroid imbalance for years.

Some people know their thyroid is low, and others don't. I had a client I'll call Eleanor, who was 65 when she first came to see me. With a history of many medical problems, she'd had lots of medical treatments. She knew she had low thyroid, but she didn't want to "take another pill," and she didn't have good rapport with her doctor.

Eleanor came to me with pain in her feet and certainty about what she wanted from massage therapy. She only wanted her legs and feet massaged. I did everything she told me to do massage-wise, and I avoided areas she didn't want me to work on. Slowly I gained her trust. Eleanor was slender, very high strung, and had a hard time sleeping. Lots of people have hypothyroidism without having the classic symptoms—sluggishness, weight gain, sleepiness, pain. In fact, my doctor tells me that some people with low thyroid convert T4 to T3 more quickly, creating anxiety, palpitations, insomnia, and weight loss. I talked with Eleanor about her hypothyroidism—not every session, but periodically. I kept encouraging her to see her doctor and to follow his advice. I let her know I understood the problems of hypothyroidism from my own experience, and how glad I was to get help with it for myself.

This went on for a few months and then Eleanor was assigned a new primary care physician, whom she seemed to like. She went ahead and got her thyroid tested again. Her TSH level was very high, which meant her pituitary gland was working extremely hard to stimulate her thyroid gland to produce thyroid hormones, and her thyroid gland was unable to do so.

Under the care of this new doctor, Eleanor agreed to start thyroid replacement therapy. Within a few weeks, the pain in her feet went away. She became a little more relaxed and less anxious. She began to sleep better, although she still has high energy and is a bit high strung. I worked with her for 7 years, until I moved away from the area 5 years ago. But she still calls me every 6 months or so to say hello, and she's still doing well at age 77. I'm always glad to hear from her.

I think massage is healing because it's a ritual. We do the same thing each time, with great deliberation. We set up the table, position the client, and apply oil. We often start with the same area—the head or the feet. Our strokes are slow and even. Massage is predictable and people can count on it. They can relax and feel safe in the routine of it. I imagine that safety occurred for Eleanor.

The gist of Eleanor's story is that she had lost her confidence in her doctor, and that was keeping her from getting medical help. She needed a lot of support to deal with her medical problem. She needed to feel safe. Often I think of massage therapists as being on the front line in health care because we have a whole hour with people, and they tell us things that they haven't yet told their doctor, or that they're afraid to mention or act on. As massage therapists, we have a chance to work with and support our clients in getting the care they need.

Patricia Rackowski
Dorchester, MA

becomes enlarged. Mental processes slow down, resulting in forgetfulness and confusion. Depression may develop. When thyroid disease goes untreated during pregnancy, the effects on the fetus can result in developmental and cognitive problems later on.

Longstanding hypothyroidism can lead to a skin and tissue disorder known as **myxedema**, characterized by swelling of the hands, feet, face, and eyes. The swelling can also occur in the heart or brain, affecting function. Cold intolerance increases. In rare cases, ordinary stimuli, such as an infection or the use of sedatives, can trigger a *myxedema coma*, which is life threatening. Common signs, symptoms, and complications of hypothyroidism are shown in Figure 17-7.

Treatment

Treatment for hypothyroidism involves **thyroid replacement therapy**, an oral medication that replaces the insufficient thyroid hormone with a synthetic form. This approach often makes people feel better in a couple of weeks, although it can take months. Typically, there are few side effects, although overreplacement of thyroid hormone can cause other problems (see *Hyper*thyroidism, Conditions in Brief).

● INTERVIEW QUESTIONS

1. When were you diagnosed with hypothyroidism?
2. How does it affect you?
3. Are there any complications, such as effects on your heart?
4. How is it being treated?
5. How does the treatment affect you?

● MASSAGE THERAPY GUIDELINES

Most people diagnosed with hypothyroidism are successfully treated or are on their way to restoring normal thyroid balance. Questions 1–5 are aimed at getting a good sense of the client's condition and whether any issues warrant your attention. Questions 2 and 3 could illuminate important massage adjustments. If the person is drowsy or fatigued, he or she will need a gentle massage session, with time to rise from the table slowly and change positions gradually. Cold intolerance obviously calls for extra draping and a comfortably warm room. Constipation doesn't require much adjustment unless it has been prolonged (see Chapter 15).

Hair loss obviously calls for extra sensitivity on your part, but it presents no massage precautions unless the client

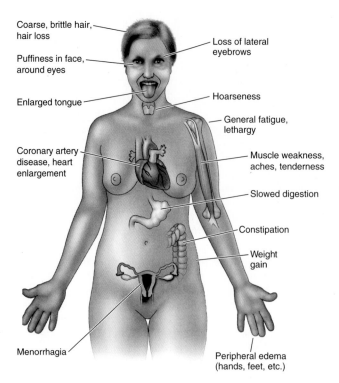

Coarse, brittle hair, hair loss

Loss of lateral eyebrows

Puffiness in face, around eyes

Hoarseness

Enlarged tongue

General fatigue, lethargy

Coronary artery disease, heart enlargement

Muscle weakness, aches, tenderness

Slowed digestion

Constipation

Weight gain

Menorrhagia

Peripheral edema (hands, feet, etc.)

FIGURE 17-7. Signs, symptoms, and complications of hypothyroidism. (Adapted from Werner R. *A Massage Therapist's Guide to Pathology*, 4th ed. Philadelphia: Lippincott Williams & Wilkins, 2009.)

prefers no pressure on the scalp. Dry skin may respond well to massage oil or lotion. If a client's menorrhagia has caused anemia, a gentle session overall and slow rise from the table are in order (see "Anemia," Chapter 12).

While muscle stiffness, pain, and trigger points all call for massage therapy, these symptoms may not resolve completely until the underlying thyroid condition is corrected. In the meantime, you may be able to provide some symptom relief.

If the client has a significant goiter, it might be uncomfortable in the prone position, so be sure the client's neck does not extend too much or collapse as the head rests in the face

cradle. Bolstering under the chest with a folded bath towel might make the client more comfortable.

If the client has atherosclerosis, coronary artery disease, and/or heart complications, it may be important to follow the Plaque Problem Principle and the DVT Risk Principles. Review the particular condition, interview questions, and massage adjustments in Chapter 11.

Low thyroid can cause depression, calling for added sensitivity and compassion. Review Chapter 10. Myxedema is unlikely to respond much to circulatory intent, but if the swelling is severe, then circulatory intent is contraindicated at the site. Use

---

THERAPIST'S JOURNAL 17-3 *Thyroid, Depression, Pain and Massage*

I worked with a client in her 40s who had hypothyroidism. She was employed in human services, working with at-risk kids and families. She loved this work, but it was very stressful. She had regular doctor visits for blood tests to monitor her thyroid medications, but still she struggled to bring her thyroid into balance. The most consistent symptom she would describe was the emotional and physical sense of heaviness that she felt. In addition, she was in chronic nonspecific pain.

I provided weekly half-hour massages. If we worked longer, the overload increased her fatigue. While she was on the table, we worked together—monitoring and adjusting for pressure and length of time in each area. As I worked her muscles, they would initially relax. If I stayed in that area for too long, they would become tense again and her skin would remain significantly reddened for a while thereafter.

I would love to say that regular massage directly helped decrease her pain. But I can't say that with confidence. Massage did, however, seem to ease her symptoms of depression, and perhaps her perception of pain, because with weekly sessions for over 2 years, she was able to be more active.

This client taught me a great deal about managing chronic issues. She drew from a constellation of stress-reduction methods, with massage as a primary tool, along with walks outside during her workday. With these tools, she was better able to cope. Sometimes it's more about managing health issues, rather than treating them. In this case, massage played a very important role.

Meg Robsahm
Monroe, WA

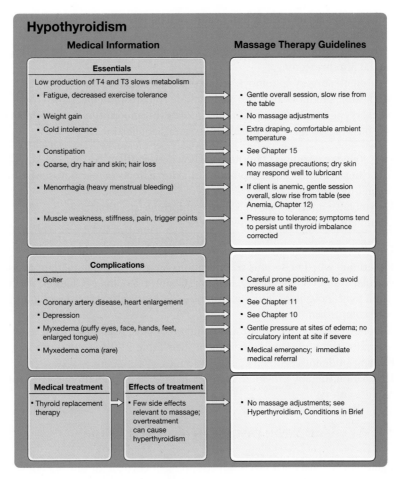

FIGURE 17-8. A Decision Tree for hypothyroidism.

gentle pressure. Myxedema coma is an extremely rare event, but signs of it obviously call for emergency medical attention.

If the client's slightly low thyroid is responding well to thyroid replacement medication and there are no side effects, there are unlikely to be massage adjustments for the medication. If the appropriate dose of replacement therapy is still being determined and there are signs of *hyper*thyroidism, adjust accordingly (see Conditions in Brief, this chapter).

● **MASSAGE RESEARCH**

As of this writing, there are no RCTs, published in the English language, on hypothyroidism and massage indexed

in PubMed or the Massage Therapy Foundation Research Database. The NIH RePORTER tool lists no active, federally funded research projects on the topic in the United States. No active projects are listed on the clinicaltrials.gov database (see Chapter 6).

● **POSSIBLE MASSAGE BENEFITS**

Massage is unlikely to specifically benefit the condition of hypothyroidism, but general support may be beneficial to the person with the condition. People with low thyroid can have pain and depression, and massage therapy may help with these symptoms, as Therapist's Journal 17-3 suggests.

Other Endocrine Conditions in Brief

ACROMEGALY

Background
- Overproduction of growth hormone (GH) by pituitary gland, or stimulation or direct production of GH by other glands. Usually caused by a tumor (adenoma) of pituitary gland.
- Increased bone size, often enlarged hands, feet, and face; enlarged nose, protruding jaw and brow, wide spaces between teeth.
- Symptoms of fatigue, muscle weakness, pain, limited joint mobility; deepening voice, snoring, sleep apnea from vocal cord and sinus changes, headaches, impaired vision; possible vital organ and spleen enlargement; "barrel chest."

- Skin changes include thickening, increased oil production, increased sweating, body odor.
- Untreated acromegaly can cause hypertension, osteoarthritis, diabetes, spinal cord compression; can be life threatening.
- Treatment: surgery to remove pituitary tumor, radiation therapy.
- Medications to block or lower GH include somatostatin analogues (octreotide), GH receptor blockers (pegvisomant), dopamine agonists (bromocriptine); side effects include headache, nausea, bloating, fatigue, lightheadedness, sinus congestion.

Interview Questions	• How long have you had symptoms? How does it affect you? • Any complications? Effects on bone or skin? Effects on cardiovascular function? Effects on vital organ function? • Do you have areas of pain? Certain comfortable positions? • Treatment? Effects of treatment?
Massage Therapy Guidelines	• Usually controlled by treatment; serious complications unlikely. • Determine whether serious complications have occurred and adapt massage to effects on cardiovascular system (Chapter 11), kidneys (Chapter 18), liver (Chapter 16), and spleen (Chapter 13). • Limit joint movement if joints unstable; use cautious pressure and joint movement if risk of spinal cord compression. • Adapt positioning to comfort and enlarged organs. Adapt lubricant to levels of skin oil. • Adapt to effects of strong medication. (See Table 21-1 for common drug side effects and massage therapy guidelines.) • If radiation therapy provided, review Chapter 20 for radiation; see Chapter 21 for guidelines for recent surgery.

ADDISON DISEASE (HYPOCORTISOLISM)

Background	• Failure of adrenal cortex to produce sufficient cortisol for normal body function, resulting in drop in blood cortisol levels; also called adrenal insufficiency. • May also involve insufficient production of aldosterone by adrenal glands. • Caused by atrophy of the adrenal cortex due to autoimmune disease (most common in developed countries), or infection such as TB, HIV (most common in developing countries). Also caused by tumor, trauma to the tissue, use of anticoagulant medication. Symptoms may appear after treatment for hypercortisolism (see "Cushing Syndrome [hypercortisolism]," this chapter) overcorrects, leading to low levels of cortisol. • Signs/symptoms develop gradually: loss of appetite, weight loss, nausea, vomiting, diarrhea, fatigue, sluggishness, muscle weakness, darkening of skin tone. • Serious complications: hypoglycemia, low BP, low blood sodium, fainting, irritability, depression. • Addisonian crisis (adrenal crisis) features acute failure of adrenals: dangerously low BP, low blood sugar, high blood potassium; sudden, severe vomiting, diarrhea, pain in low back, abdomen, lower extremities, mental confusion, loss of consciousness. • Treated by replacement of cortisol with low doses of corticosteroid, replacement of aldosterone with fludrocortisone; replacement at higher doses during stressful events such as surgery, minor illness. • Replacement dose of corticosteroid is lower than the anti-inflammatory dose (see "Corticosteroids," Chapter 21), avoiding the serious complications of the higher dose. Side effects can include insomnia and hypertension, closely monitored. • Treatment of adrenal crisis with emergency IV of strong corticosteroids, saline, glucose.
Interview Questions	• What is the cause of your Addison disease? • How does it affect you? Effects on blood sugar or blood pressure? • What is your energy level? Activity level? • Is condition well controlled? Any history of adrenal crisis? If so, what are your symptoms/signs? • Treatment? Effects of treatment?

| Massage Therapy Guidelines | • Adapt to causes such as tumor, anticoagulants, HIV.
• If blood sugar, blood pressure are not yet stable, provide gentler session overall (see "Diabetes Mellitus," this chapter).
• If blood pressure low, reposition gently, slow rise from table, gentle transition at end of session.
• Observe the Activity and Energy Principle; gentle session overall if weight loss is profound or muscle weakness is present.
• If nausea, vomiting, diarrhea present, see Chapter 15; if severe, immediate medical referral for possible adrenal crisis.
• If hypertension is a side effect of medication, adapt massage accordingly (see Chapter 11).
• With insomnia, use sedative intent at end of day, activating/stimulating intent at beginning. |

HYPERTHYROIDISM

Background	• Overproduction of thyroxine by thyroid gland due to Graves disease (autoimmune stimulation of thyroid), thyroiditis (inflammation), or benign thyroid tumor. • Causes sudden weight loss, rapid heartbeat, trembling, nervousness, irritability, anxiety, sweating, heat sensitivity, menstrual changes, fatigue, sleeping difficulty, increased bowel movement frequency; goiter (enlarged thyroid gland) may form. Complications include bulging eyes, light sensitivity, vision changes, osteoporosis, heart problems, and red, swollen skin on feet and shins. • Acute symptoms (thyrotoxic crisis) include fever, delirium, rapid heartbeat. • Treated by surgical removal of thyroid gland, RAI therapy (see "Thyroid Cancer," online), antithyroid medications (with possible liver toxicity, carefully monitored), β-blockers for rapid heart rate and other cardiovascular symptoms.
Interview Questions	• Cause? How does it affect you? Symptoms? • Any complications? Effects on heart, bone stability, skin? • Any effects on eyes/vision? Are there comfortable positions for you when you lie down? • Treatment? Effects of Treatment?
Massage Therapy Guidelines	• Adapt massage elements to cause, symptoms, and complications. • Medical referral if symptoms unreported, but diagnosed hyperthyroidism is usually being treated successfully; serious complications, from untreated disease, are uncommon. • Avoid contact, pressure, circulatory intent at site of swelling and skin changes. If eyes affected, position to incline head and avoid face cradle, possibly avoid prone position entirely; if goiter present, position to avoid pressure on it. • Avoid rapid speeds and uneven rhythms, sudden deep pressures. • Adapt to effects of medication, surgery. See "Thyroid Cancer," online, for RAI therapy; see Table 11-3 for β-blockers. If signs of liver toxicity appear (see Table 21-1), make immediate medical referral.

HYPOGLYCEMIA

| Background | • Low blood glucose, affects the brain (e.g., confusion, visual disturbances); causes other symptoms such as tremor, anxiety. See "Diabetes Mellitus," this chapter, for full list of signs/symptoms.
• Causes include diabetes mellitus (this chapter), some medications (e.g., quinine), excessive alcohol consumption, drug-induced hepatitis, kidney disease, tumors, enlargement of insulin-producing pancreatic cells, adrenal or pituitary gland disorders.
• May occur after meals (reactive or postprandial hypoglycemia), when body produces too much insulin in response to increased blood glucose.
• May progress to seizures, loss of consciousness, death.
• Treatment for early symptoms: consuming sugar such as candy, fruit juice, glucose tablets; treatment for severe symptoms may require IV glucose or glucagon injection to bring up blood sugar level.
• Recurrent hypoglycemia treated by changing or adjusting medication causing it; tumor of pancreas removed surgically. |

Interview Questions	• How long have you had it? Has your doctor diagnosed it? • How often do you have episodes? What do they look like? How can I recognize an episode? How do you treat it? What is the most effective thing for me to say and do if you seem to be having an episode? • Treatment? Effects of treatment?
Massage Therapy Guidelines	• Be alert for signs of hypoglycemia; bring them to client's attention. • Make medical referral if the client has not brought symptoms to his or her doctor's attention; urgent medical referral if symptoms recur, immediate referral if client complains of severe episodes or complications (see "Diabetes Mellitus," this chapter). • Follow the Emergency Protocol Principle; discuss the best course of action for the client if an episode occurs during the session. • Identify where client keeps sweets, glucose tablets, etc., in case they are needed. • Review "Diabetes Mellitus," this chapter, for signs and complications of severe hypoglycemia; make emergency medical referral if you observe them in the session.

METABOLIC SYNDROME

Background	• Cluster of risk factors for cardiovascular disease: obesity concentrated at waist, hypertension, high triglyceride levels, low HDL cholesterol, insulin resistance with high blood glucose levels; can increase tendency for blood to clot. • Often presents with prediabetes. • Strong predictor for the development of type 2 diabetes.
Interview Questions	• How long since it was diagnosed? How does it affect you? • Is your blood sugar under control and stable? • What is your blood pressure? Is it under control and stable? • Any history of heart disease or stroke? Any complications? • Treatment? Effects of treatment?
Massage Therapy Guidelines	• Adjust massage to hypertension and heart disease (see Chapter 11), and to risk of stroke (see Chapter 10); review Type 2 Diabetes (this chapter). • Follow the Plaque Problem Principle and DVT Risk Principles (see Chapter 11).

STRESS

Background	• A response to stressor, or effect of a stressor on the body. • Common use: an actual or perceived threat to survival or well-being that causes stress reaction involving autonomic, endocrine, immune factors; contributors to stress include medical illness. • Signs/symptoms include increased heart rate, rise in blood pressure, increased perspiration, dry mouth, pupil dilation, increase in tendency of blood to clot; blood diverted to essential body functions (brain, heart, skeletal muscle). • Cortisol, epinephrine produced in increased amounts in "fight-or-flight" response to acute stress; may become chronic over time. • Increased cortisol changes metabolism, suppresses inflammation and immune response, degrades tissues, leads to delayed wound healing, increased vulnerability to infection. • Conditions/signs/symptoms of chronic stress: headache, clenched muscles, muscle pain, shortness of breath, GI upset (pain, constipation, diarrhea), low energy, sleep problems, skin eruptions (acne, eczema, herpes), hypertension, cognitive difficulties (forgetfulness, errors in judgment, decreased attention to detail), emotional reactions (irritability, anxiety, depression), behavioral problems (compulsive or addictive behavior, increased aggression, accidents). • Treatment includes relaxation therapy, massage, bodywork, movement therapy, psychotherapy, pharmalogic treatment with anti-anxiety and antidepressant medications.

Interview Questions	• On a scale of 0–10, 0 being no stress, and 10 being the worst stress imaginable, how much stress do you feel in the moment?
	• How does stress affect you?
	• Any effects of stress on your digestion?
	• Any cardiovascular effects such as high blood pressure or heart palpitations?
	• Does stress affect your muscles? If so, where? Any headache, low energy, or sleep problems?
	• Any effects of stress on your skin?
	• Treatment? Effects of treatment?
Massage Therapy Guidelines	• Use sensitivity, compassion; avoid strong statements about stress causing physical conditions that might be interpreted as judgments.
	• Instead, define clear role of massage therapy: "If stress has any role in aggravating your symptoms, or if your symptoms themselves are stressful, it's possible regular massage can help. At the very least, massage can support you while you manage your condition and treatment."
	• Avoid sudden increases in pressure; consider gradual warm-up of muscles at pressure levels 1–3; focus gently on muscles in spasm if client requests, check in about pressure.
	• Use slow speeds, even rhythms, use gradual transitions; adjust ambient music, level of conversation to client comfort.
	• Follow massage therapy guidelines for specific stress-related conditions: headache (see Chapter 10), GI upset (see Chapter 15), skin problems (see Chapter 7), hypertension (see Chapter 11), anxiety or depression (see Chapter 10).
	• Adjust massage to effects of anti-anxiety, antidepressant medications (see Chapter 10).

SELF TEST

1. What is the function of insulin, and how do type 1 and type 2 diabetes affect that function?
2. Describe two complications of diabetes and massage adjustments needed for each.
3. How is insulin therapy administered? Describe specific adjustments in massage therapy for the two different methods of delivery.
4. Although diabetes is not a cardiovascular condition, how and why is the CV Conditions Often "Run in Packs" Principle applicable? The Filter and Pump Principle?
5. How could massage help a person with diabetes? Does research support the use of massage in people with diabetes?
6. Compare Type 1 and Type 2 diabetes mellitus in terms of the usual age of onset, the causes or risk factors, and the treatment approaches.
7. Of the many signs and symptoms of hypoglycemia, list six that are true *signs* of the condition (things that you could recognize by observing the client, without having to be told about them).

8. How do individuals with hypoglycemia typically relieve an acute episode?
9. What are the signs, symptoms, and body changes that occur during Cushing syndrome? What are the possible benefits of massage for a person with Cushing syndrome?
10. List and describe three causes of Cushing syndrome.
11. Explain why you might avoid general circulatory intent in Cushing syndrome.
12. What are three reasons for following the Unstable Tissue Principle while working with a client who has Cushing syndrome? Which tissues might require lighter pressure, and which might limit joint movement?
13. What is primary hypothyroidism, and what causes it?
14. List the symptoms and signs of hypothyroidism, and the body functions that are slowed or impaired in the condition.
15. Describe myxedema and the corresponding massage therapy guidelines.

 For answers to these questions and to see a bibliography for this chapter, visit http://thePoint. lww.com/Walton.

18 Urinary System Conditions

The coordinated physiological processes which maintain most of the steady states in the organism are so complex and so peculiar to living beings—involving, as they may, the brain and nerves, the heart, lungs, kidneys and spleen, all working cooperatively—that I have suggested a special designation for these states, homeostasis.

—WALTER BRADFORD CANNON

In the day-to-day function of the body, balance is made possible, in part, because of the actions of the kidneys. The kidneys carry out many complex functions, all in the service of homeostasis. Among them are the filtration of blood, maintenance of fluid balance, and regulation of blood pressure (BP). The kidneys produce *erythropoietin*, which stimulates red blood cell (RBC) production in the bone marrow. They also produce other substances, responsible for bone growth and mineralization.

Structurally, the urinary system consists of the kidneys, ureters, urinary bladder, and urethra. The kidneys and ureters make up the upper urinary tract, and the bladder and urethra make up the lower urinary tract. When the kidneys are not functioning properly, it can throw off fluid balance and BP. It can also result in anemia, because of the failure to produce normal levels of erythropoietin. Bone loss can occur when the kidneys are unable to help mineralize bone. Imbalances resulting from kidney and urinary disease can be felt across body systems.

This chapter addresses the following conditions at length, with full Decision Trees:

- Urinary tract infection
- Kidney stone
- Chronic kidney failure

Conditions in Brief in this chapter are **acute kidney failure** (acute renal failure), **bladder cancer**, **glomerulonephritis,** (nephritic syndrome), **nephrotic syndrome, polycystic kidney disease (PKD)** (renal cystic disease), and **kidney cancer** (renal cell carcinoma).

General Principles

Under normal conditions, the kidneys filter and cleanse the blood, so the Filter and Pump Principle is applied when they are compromised by disease. Because disease can also weaken the kidneys' ability to regulate BP, principles from Chapter 11 (cardiovascular conditions) are often used, as well. In this chapter, we add another principle:

The Fluid Balance Principle. *If fluid balance is off, causing either systemic swelling or dehydration, massage with general circulatory intent is contraindicated.*

Healthy body function depends on fluids being in the right place at the right time, with tissues properly hydrated, and the correct distribution of fluids among organ systems. Fluid imbalances can be due to kidney problems or other conditions, and they are often very serious.

Enhanced fluid movement is a commonly claimed benefit of massage, but it is not a wise goal when the body is struggling to maintain homeostasis on its own. Instead, respect the fluid imbalance, the disease at the root of it, the body's ongoing efforts to correct or adapt to it, and any medical treatments organized to correct the imbalance. If systemic swelling or dehydration is present, steer clear of general circulatory intent, to avoid introducing any further strain on the body.

Urinary Tract Infection

A **Urinary tract infection (UTI)** is an infection of any of the urinary system structures. A lower UTI affects the urethra, bladder, or both; an upper UTI affects the ureters, kidneys, or both. **Pyelonephritis** is a kidney infection; a bladder infection is called **cystitis**.

● BACKGROUND

Most infections of the urinary tract are caused by bacteria. UTIs commonly begin in the lower urinary tract, when normal bacteria from the anus or vagina are transferred to the urethra. This can happen during improper bathroom hygiene, or during sexual intercourse, especially when a diaphragm or spermicide is used. If untreated, the infection often ascends to the upper urinary tract. This becomes a serious situation if the kidneys become involved, as complications can occur. In the absence of complications, the typical course of infection is 6 days.

Most UTIs occur in women, because of the proximity of the urethra to the anus and vagina (Figure 18-1). In men, UTI frequency increases with age, and one cause is an enlarged

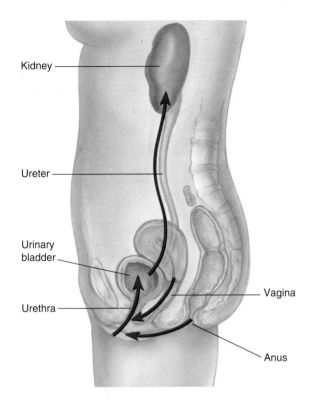

FIGURE 18-1. Routes of urinary tract infection. Movement of bacteria from the vaginal and anal areas can lead to infection in the urethra. From there, bacteria may travel up through the bladder and ureters to the kidney. (Adapted from Anatomical Chart Co.)

(Image labels: Kidney, Ureter, Urinary bladder, Urethra, Vagina, Anus)

prostate gland, pressing on the urethra and interfering with voiding the bladder. For both sexes, another potential source of infection occurs with the therapeutic use of a **urinary catheter**, a tube inserted in the urethra to help drain the bladder.

Incomplete emptying can contribute to UTI because the urine left behind in the bladder becomes a site for infection. Waiting too long to urinate can weaken bladder muscles over time, leading to incomplete emptying of the bladder. Structural problems that interfere with emptying the bladder and urethra can contribute to UTI, especially in young children. People with diabetes, or a weakened immune system, are at higher risk of getting a UTI. Less commonly, fungi can cause UTIs; in these cases, the organisms are usually sexually transmitted.

Signs and Symptoms

The symptoms of a UTI are fatigue, fever, and shakiness. A lower UTI causes pain and burning with urination, as well as urinary urgency and frequency. Even with the urgency, only a small amount of urine may be passed. The urine may have blood in it—a condition called **hematuria**, or it may be cloudy. Although older adults with UTI may also experience urinary incontinence, a diagnosis of UTI in older adults can be difficult, because the UTI is often asymptomatic. In older adults, sometimes mental changes or confusion is the only sign.

The pain of a UTI can vary. A sharp pain may be felt above the pubic bone as the bladder empties, or after it is emptied. **Flank pain**, in the region between the lowest ribs and the pelvis, including the upper abdomen, side, and back, may be felt on one side. Pain may also extend to the pelvis, and men may feel pain in the penis or scrotum. If pain is strong, or there

is a fever, it may be a sign of kidney infection, and immediate medical attention is needed.

Complications

A complication of a lower UTI is an upper UTI, in which the bacteria have migrated upward, from urethra, to bladder, to ureters, to kidney. If this happens, fever, chills, nausea, and vomiting often occur. Acute kidney failure can result (see Conditions in Brief).

Kidney infection is serious, because it can result in the release of bacteria to the blood, causing **sepsis**, a life-threatening blood infection. Symptoms of sepsis are increased heart and respiration rates, fever or abnormally low temperature, and altered mental status.

UTIs can become chronic. In this case, chronic kidney failure can result.

Treatment

Treatment of a UTI is typically a short course of antibiotics. The side effects are usually minimal, limited to nausea and headache. Sometimes antibiotics don't clear the infection, and a relapse occurs, or reinfection is caused by a different organism. Individuals who are chronically plagued by reinfections may be on a longer dose of antibiotics over 6 or more weeks.

Some people self-treat by drinking lots of fluids, especially acidic liquids such as cranberry juice or blueberry juice. Sitz baths may be recommended, as well, although some patients are discouraged from regular tub baths because of the risk of infection. Surgery may be necessary to address any structural problem that contributes to repeated UTIs.

● INTERVIEW QUESTIONS

1. How long have you had it? Which part of the urinary tract is affected?
2. Is the infection getting worse, staying the same, getting better, or has it resolved?
3. How does it affect you? Do you have any fever, or blood in your urine? Do you have any low-back or flank pain, or severe pain when urinating? Any chills, nausea, or vomiting?
4. Has your kidney function been affected by this or any previous infections?
5. Have you seen a doctor for this condition?
6. How was or is it being treated, and where are you in the course of treatment?
7. How does the treatment affect you?

● MASSAGE THERAPY GUIDELINES

During an acute UTI, bladder urgency and frequency may make lying on a table for a massage impractical, and discomfort may make massage, or any kind of touch, poorly tolerated and unwelcome. If you *are* providing massage to someone with UTI, make sure there is easy access to a bathroom. Obviously, pressure on the lower abdomen should not exceed level 1, although even minor, gentle contact might not be welcome in the area. Heavy or focused pressure over the kidneys is also contraindicated, so limit your pressure to level 2 over the lower ribs.

Questions 1–3 give you an idea of the seriousness of the infection and how compromised the client might be feeling. The higher up the infection is in the urinary tract, the more serious it is, although even in a lower UTI, the risk of kidney infection is very real.

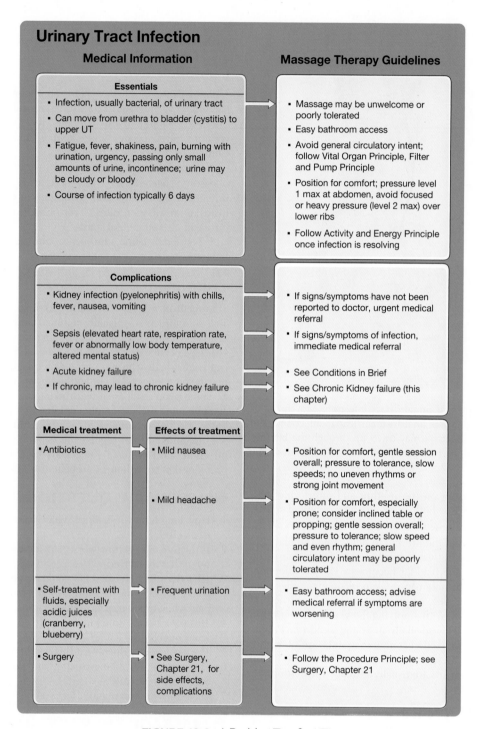

FIGURE 18-2. A Decision Tree for UTI.

No matter which structures are infected, work gently. Although it is highly unlikely that general circulatory intent would drive bacterial migration up through the urinary tract, avoid general circulatory intent because it's too vigorous for someone fighting an infection, and because the system is responsible for filtering blood. Respect the infection, the proximity and potential involvement of a vital organ (the kidney), the immune system, and the body's need for support rather than further challenge. Follow the Vital Organ Principle.

On the other hand, if the condition has improved over several days, or has resolved completely, general circulatory intent may be well tolerated.

The Filter and Pump Principle. If a filtering organ (liver, kidney, spleen, or lymph node), or a pumping organ (the heart) is functioning poorly or overworking, do not work it harder with massage that is circulatory in intent.

The client's responses to Questions 2 and 3 about symptoms also give you a sense of how gentle your overall massage plan should be. If symptoms have subsided, with no fever or fatigue, a stronger session with level 3 pressure may be well tolerated. Follow the Activity and Energy Principle. If the client mentions fever or fatigue, or even shakiness, a gentler session is advised, with no general circulatory intent. If the client is experiencing low-back or flank pain, or the pain is severe when urinating, an urgent medical referral is strongly advised, especially if the client has not yet brought it to the attention of the doctor (Question 5). Kidney involvement can be very serious, with the risk of sepsis and kidney failure. In addition, pyelonephritis is extremely painful, so touch may be poorly tolerated.

> *The Activity and Energy Principle. A client who enjoys regular, moderate physical activity or a good overall energy level is better able to tolerate strong massage elements—including circulatory intent—than one whose activity or energy level is low.*

Be alert for complications. If Question 3 or 4 yields any signs or symptoms of sepsis, immediate medical attention is needed to prevent *septic shock*, which can be fatal. Ask about fever, chills, abnormally low body temperature, rapid heartbeat, or rapid breathing, and if any one is present, make an emergency medical referral. Obvious changes in mental status indicate a referral, as well. If kidney function has been impaired by chronic UTIs over time, then see "Chronic Kidney Failure," this chapter.

Question 5 should always be asked as a matter of course, but is especially important with UTI symptoms, because many people self-diagnose. Question 6 about treatment is important because some people self-treat UTIs, preferring to avoid anti-biotic treatment where possible. In this case, acute symptoms may still be present because self-treatment can take longer to work than antibiotic treatment. Provide conservative massage, as described above. Bathroom access will be important for the client who is drinking lots of fluids and urinating frequently.

If antibiotics are administered, they will relieve symptoms in just a day or two. Although the side effects of antibiotics are minimal, ask Question 7 as a matter of course. Massage adjustments for side effects are listed in the Decision Tree (see Figure 18-2). See Table 21-1 for massage therapy guidelines for any other side effects that occur. In the unusual event of surgical treatment for a structural problem, adapt the session to surgery (see Chapter 21).

● MASSAGE RESEARCH

As of this writing, there are no randomized, controlled trials (RCTs), published in the English language, on UTI and massage indexed in PubMed or the Massage Therapy Foundation Research Database. The NIH RePORTER tool lists no active, federally funded research projects on this topic in the United States. No active projects are listed on the clinicaltrials.gov database (see Chapter 6).

● POSSIBLE MASSAGE BENEFITS

Specific benefits of massage for UTI are unlikely and the stimulation of massage may be too overwhelming for someone coping with one. However, in some cases, the soothing comfort of massage therapy may be welcome.

Kidney Stone

A **kidney stone**, also called a *renal calculus*, is a hardened mineral deposit that forms in the tubes of the kidneys, and *nephrolithiasis* refers to the presence of stones in the kidney. The crystals consolidate to form small, hard masses, called stones, in the bowl-shaped *renal pelvis*.

● BACKGROUND

Different types of stones form from different minerals. Calcium stones are the most common, forming from calcium and oxalate, a compound that comes from high oxalic acid foods, such as dark green vegetables. Calcium stones are shown in Figure 18-3. Uric acid stones, formed from by-products of protein metabolism, can develop from an excessively high-protein diet. Certain types of chemotherapy, and genetic predisposing factors, can also lead to uric acid stones. Other types of stones are most likely to develop in women with chronic UTIs. These *staghorn calculi* are large and pointed, and can significantly damage kidney tissue along with tissue in the tubes as they descend.

Kidney stones are more likely to form when the urine is concentrated, as in hot climates where perspiration leads to fluid loss. Low dietary fluids can also contribute to stones. Some people have a hereditary condition that predisposes them to kidney stone formation. In others, the cause is unknown.

Signs and Symptoms

Some small kidney stones pass through silently: they pass out of the renal pelvis, through the ureters, bladder, and urethra without damaging tissue or causing pain. However, kidney stones are known for causing severe pain, and the pain from a larger stone is excruciating. Waves of severe pain are referred to as **renal colic**. It often begins as flank pain. As the stone moves down the left or right ureter, the pain may be felt in the lower abdomen, groin, and genitals on that side. The pain may stop when the stone stops moving.

Other signs and symptoms include nausea and vomiting, urinary urgency, and bloody, cloudy urine. The urine might have a foul smell.

Complications

A large stone can cause a urinary obstruction, blocking urine flow through the kidney, ureter, or urethra. The abnormal accumulation of urine in the kidney leads to *hydronephrosis*, or swelling of the kidney with impaired function. Infection is a complication, along with injury to the involved structures. If an infection is also present, fever and chills will often develop. Scarring can leave the person susceptible to stones in the future. In the worst case, permanent damage to the kidney tissues can occur. Chronic kidney failure may follow.

Treatment

To help the stone pass, people with kidney stones are encouraged to drink several quarts of liquids a day and be as physically active as possible. If a patient is nauseated and vomiting, unable to keep fluids down, IV fluids are administered instead. Stones smaller than 5 mm in diameter, and even some up

Calcium stones

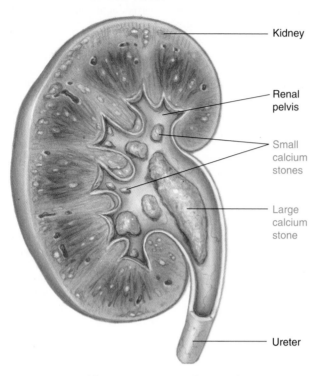

FIGURE 18-3. Kidney stones. Stones form in the renal pelvis, shown. Depending on their size, they may cause injury to the tissues and excruciating pain as they pass through the ureters, bladder, and urethra. (Adapted from Anatomical Chart Co.)

to 9 or 10 mm, often pass on their own, without treatment. Pain relievers include oral or IV nonsteroid anti-inflammatory drugs (NSAIDs). Stronger pain medication is often prescribed in the form of opioid analgesics.

Lithotripsy is commonly used to treat kidney stones. In this procedure, shock waves are delivered while the patient, lightly sedated, lies on a cushion or is partially submerged in a tub of water. It can take weeks for smaller fragments to clear, and they can cause pain as they pass, depending on their size. *Laser lithotripsy*, in which the energy of a laser is used instead of shock waves, is another technique.

Percutaneous nephrolithotomy, the surgical removal of a stubborn or large stone, may be done in some cases. A small incision is made in the back and a fiber optic instrument is inserted to view the inside the kidney; the stone can be removed through a tube. A similar technique enables the removal of a stone lodged in a ureter. Sometimes a **ureteral stent**, a flexible tube, is inserted to keep the ureter open or bypass a stone, restoring urine flow. The stent may be in place for a few weeks to a few months and can cause some discomfort, urgency, or pain in the flank, groin, or genitals. Therapist's Journal 18-1 describes working with a client after surgery for kidney stones and the placement of a ureteral stent.

Prevention is critical to anyone with a history of kidney stones, in order to avoid a repeat performance. Dietary changes, avoiding risky foods such as salt or animal protein, and maintaining a high fluid intake seem to help prevent stones. Medications to regulate the chemistry of the kidneys and the urine may also help avoid stones.

THERAPIST'S JOURNAL 18-1 *Massage Relief Following Kidney Stone Surgery*

I have a female client in her mid-40s with recurring kidney stones. She has other chronic health issues as well, and uses acupuncture and chiropractic for symptom relief and support. She manages her complex health problems as positively as she can.

She's had three kidney stone episodes over the last few years, and they've recurred even after lithotripsy. Twice over that time she had surgery, and had a ureteral stent implanted for several weeks to keep the passageways open.

Although a stent is a flexible tube, people feel it deep inside them and it can be uncomfortable. It's definitely "there." I adapt positioning for her while the stent is in place. Side-lying has been more comfortable for her. I teach and provide prenatal massage, so I tend to use that position often. We start with the stent side down and her ribcage supported with a contoured body cushion.

I've worked with her postsurgery for general relaxation as well as relief of neck and shoulder tension from her stays in the hospital bed. I do intercostal work on the "up side," doing ribcage releases and trigger point work on that side and whatever I can reach on the "down side." Along with some gentle friction and tensile stretching, this approach seems to help her. I also work briefly and superficially over the "down side" just for integration of that area. This helps her a lot after her surgeries, and we think we also help her body recover from the anesthesia.

After the stent is removed and she is kidney stone free, we resume our regular massage and attend to the proper scar work. Although she usually sees other MTs, calling my side-lying position "weird," she'll often see me after surgery and when her condition is vulnerable. I'm glad to be here for her at those times. She uses massage to feel well and whole. As MTs, we have an important role: to support people while they deal either with their symptoms or with the effects of their medical treatments.

Linda Hickey
Calgary, AB, Canada

● INTERVIEW QUESTIONS

1. What is the status of your kidney stone? Is it current, recent, or has it passed?
2. How does it affect you, or how did it affect you?
3. Have there been any complications? Has your kidney function been affected by this stone, or by any past occurrences? Has there been any associated infection?
4. How was (or is) it treated?
5. How does (or did) the treatment affect you?

● MASSAGE THERAPY GUIDELINES

Questions 1–5 are written in both the past and present tense because it is unlikely that a client in an acute situation will seek massage. In general, the pain of kidney stones is too excruciating to welcome or tolerate additional stimulation. Therapist's Journal 18-2 recounts a story of an exception to this, a client who chose to receive massage while waiting for stones to pass.

If the client is in pain, the massage session should be extremely gentle overall, with limited joint movement. Favor stationary pressure, rather than strokes involving movement. Avoid general circulatory intent if the client is in pain, if kidney function is affected, or if there is urinary obstruction or infection. In the unusual event that there are signs of infection, but the client has not seen his or her doctor regarding them, advise an urgent or immediate medical referral.

You may have a client who recently passed a stone, or one who is in the limbo of having had lithotripsy, but is waiting for the fragments to pass. Use the answers to Questions 1–3 to determine how well the client has recovered or is recovering from the experience, and to gauge the strength of the massage session. Ask more about any complications of kidney stones; see "Chronic Kidney Failure," this chapter. The Activity Questions (see Chapter 4) will help you assess the client in this case. Obviously, if the client is drinking a lot of fluids, easy bathroom access will be appreciated.

Opioid analgesics, necessary in some cases for pain control, come with strong side effects (see "Analgesics," Chapter 21). In addition, overall pressure will need to be gentle because of diminished pain perception, and joint movement should be similarly cautious. But these elements should be gentle anyway if the client is ill enough to require that type of medication.

There are no specific massage adjustments for recent lithotripsy, aside from those described above when stones are passing. If the client has had recent surgery, see Chapter 21. If the client has a ureteral stent, take time to find the right massage position, one that minimizes discomfort.

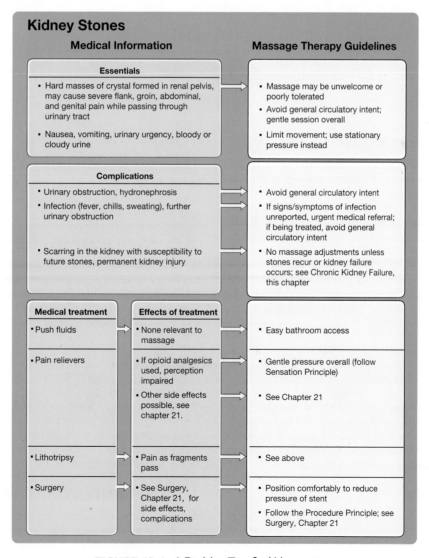

FIGURE 18-4. A Decision Tree for kidney stones.

THERAPIST'S JOURNAL 18-2 *Passing the Stone in My Office!*

My client was a businessman, with an office across town. I had been giving him general relaxation massage and deep tissue work for years. One day he came in complaining of severe low-back pain on the right side. It had bothered him for 3 days. He asked, "what can you do for me?" I said, "let's see what's going on." I put him through some routine assessments—bending, side flexing, and so on. He was very guarded bending to the right, but no injury was suggested.

I worked with him on the table for 30 minutes, just some general relaxation work and some stretching. Nothing was working. So we put him in the hot tub for about 20 minutes, isolating the jets to his low back. Then I had him back on the table, lying on his left, side flexed to the left about 30 degrees (my hydraulic table folds in the middle) with some slight flexion in the low back.

Sometimes the best thing you can do for a client is provide a medical referral. I told him, "You need to see your doctor—nothing here is helping." He did, and indeed, tests showed several kidney stones. He had lithotripsy, which was unsuccessful in releasing the stones. A few days later he was back, looking for pain relief. Although he was taking Vicodin, then Oxycontin, he was still in pain.

I had to adapt positioning with this client. He could not lie supine or prone, just side-lying, and he had to move slowly between positions. I angled the table as before. I had no illusions that massage would help release the stones, just that I might help him with his pain level. He needed to rest, to sleep. I hoped massage would help with that. My attention went to his quadratus lumborum. Massage was barely tolerable, so I used hydrotherapy at first. Then I worked the QL, a series of holds and releases. Mind you, the anatomy had to be pretty precise for pressure in this area. And reduced pain perception, from the effects of pain meds, meant I had to be extra careful. I drew on both my nursing and massage therapy background, and I wouldn't recommend these techniques to less experienced therapists. But the hydrotherapy can be done with less skill and may help a lot.

At one point, he yelped on the table, and left for the bathroom. It was a good thing he carried his basket with him because he captured half a dozen stones! He was triumphant, relieved, and, in the next session, dramatic: He threw his wallet on my massage table and offered me everything in it. He was so happy to be out of that kind of pain. And he could rest.

Sharon Thompson
Raleigh, NC

● MASSAGE RESEARCH

As of this writing, there are no RCTs, published in the English language, on kidney stones and western massage techniques indexed in PubMed or the Massage Therapy Foundation Research Database. The NIH RePORTER tool lists no active, federally funded research projects on this topic in the United States. No active projects are listed on the clinicaltrials.gov database (see Chapter 6).

There is one small RCT of 50 subjects, testing acupressure to relaxation points in the ear (Mora et al., 2007), prior to lithotripsy treatment for kidney stones. The study looked at anxiety levels in elderly patients after a relaxation and sham intervention were carried out in the ambulance on the way to

the hospital. In the active treatment group, the investigators reported less anxiety, the anticipation of less pain, and more optimism about the outcome than in the sham group. If additional, larger studies support these outcomes, perhaps this simple intervention will be broadly applied to other urgent and emergency medical situations.

● POSSIBLE MASSAGE BENEFITS

As suggested in Therapist's Journal 18-2, some massage intervention may be welcome to relax muscles and provide pain relief in clients with kidney stone pain. In particular, massage may be welcome after a stone has passed, to ease fatigue and promote overall relaxation.

Chronic Kidney Failure

Chronic kidney failure, also referred to as *renal insufficiency*, is an irreversible and often progressive condition resulting in the permanent loss of kidney tissue. Destruction of the nephrons, the kidney's basic functional components, impairs filtration and other essential processes.

● BACKGROUND

Unlike acute kidney failure (see Conditions in Brief), chronic kidney failure is gradual and irreversible. It is most often caused by diabetes mellitus. It can also be brought on by hypertension, urinary obstruction, other kidney diseases (e.g., PKD, pyelonephritis, and glomerulonephritis), lupus erythematosus, sickle cell disease,

and toxic exposure. Some antibiotics, chemotherapy, and pain relievers may lead to kidney failure, and the contrast dyes used in some diagnostic tests are implicated. Blockage of a renal artery supplying a kidney can also injure the tissue and cause chronic kidney failure (see "Atherosclerosis," Chapter 11).

● SIGNS AND SYMPTOMS

Although the word "failure" suggests that the organ has completely failed, symptoms may be mild or absent until kidney function has dropped below 20–25% of normal. In fact, survival for years is possible with chronic kidney failure. Careful monitoring over time is designed to track the level of function.

Early signs and symptoms of kidney failure are decreased urination, fatigue, unintentional weight loss, nausea, vomiting, headache, itching, and decreased mental function. Later, the effects of advancing disease become evident on the skin: Itching worsens, and *uremic frost*, the formation of white crystals of urea on the skin, occurs as the kidneys are unable to clear the blood of excess urea. Bruising and bleeding occur easily, and may be evident on the skin. Blood can appear in the vomit or stool.

Fatigue and mental function worsen, with drowsiness, confusion, and delirium. In most cases, advanced disease leads to hypertension. Systemic swelling appears, notably in the extremities.

Neuromuscular effects also occur: there is muscle twitching and cramping, and neuropathy causes decreased sensation in the hands and feet. Seizures may occur. Insomnia interferes with restful sleep, making it difficult to cope with other disease factors.

● COMPLICATIONS

Like many progressive diseases, there is no firm distinction between the signs and symptoms of chronic kidney failure, and the complications. Osteoporosis develops over time. Anemia also develops, as the kidney's erythropoietin production falls off, thereby diminishing RBC production. Fluid backup creates problems in other systems: cardiovascular complications include worsening hypertension, congestive heart failure (CHF), and pericarditis. Breathing difficulty is common, from fluid accumulation in the lungs (pulmonary edema).

At some point, chronic kidney failure can lead to **end-stage renal disease (ESRD)**, when the kidney is functioning at less than 10–15% of normal function, complications are evident, and aggressive treatment is required. ESRD, also called *end-stage renal failure*, leads to death if treatment does not occur.

● TREATMENT

Early and late in the disease, treatment of chronic kidney failure often involves treating the underlying condition: improved blood sugar control in diabetes, or better BP control in hypertension.

Treating chronic kidney failure may include renal **dialysis**, also called *hemodialysis*, a method of cleaning the blood externally through filters (Figure 18-5A). This typically requires three visits to a dialysis center each week, each visit requiring 3–5 hours. Because repeated needle insertions are necessary, some sort of venous access device is needed, such as an **arteriovenous fistula** in the wrist, elbow, forearm, or upper arm (Figure 18-5B). This *AV fistula*, as it is often called, is formed by surgically attaching an artery directly to a vein. This increases the blood flow through the vein, which makes the vein grow stronger and larger, and better able to withstand repeated needle insertions during dialysis. The AV fistula is less likely than other venous access devices to become infected or form blood clots.

If an AV fistula cannot be performed at the site, a small synthetic tube called an *arteriovenous graft* may be implanted, instead (Figure 18-5C). This tube connects the artery and vein, thus providing a site for repeated needle placement. If neither of these procedures is feasible, a central venous catheter may be placed in the neck or groin for access to a vein.

In another form of treatment, *peritoneal dialysis*, the blood is cleaned inside the body, several times each day. The peritoneal cavity is filled with fluid through a catheter in the abdomen, then drained a few hours later, after drawing waste products from the blood flowing through nearby vessels.

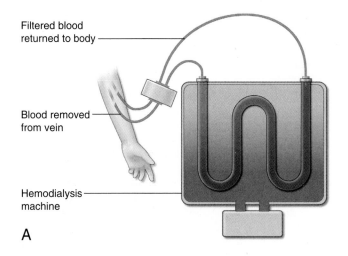

Filtered blood
returned to body

Blood removed
from vein

Hemodialysis
machine

A

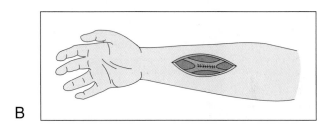

B

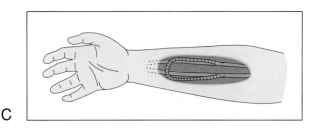

C

FIGURE 18-5. Hemodialysis. In (A), a dialysis machine filters impurities from the blood and returns it to the body. In (B), an arteriovenous fistula and in (C), an arteriovenous graft are shown, providing venous access for repeated needle insertions. (A: Adapted from Premkumar K. *The Massage Connection Anatomy and Physiology.* Baltimore: Lippincott Williams & Wilkins 2004. B and C: Adapted from LifeART.)

Between the filling and draining periods, the individual can carry out normal activities around the home, or at work.

Dialysis has some side effects, but most of them are also signs and symptoms of the kidney failure itself, and many side effects fade as treatment goes on. Problems can arise with the access sites, such as infection or blood clot formation, and the sites are monitored carefully. Hypotension can occur with dialysis. Over the long term, after years of dialysis, carpal tunnel syndrome, arthritis, and bone cysts may develop.

A kidney transplant may be performed. This involves surgery, placement of an organ from a living donor or cadaver, and strong medication to limit organ rejection.

● INTERVIEW QUESTIONS

1. What is the cause of your kidney failure?
2. How well are your kidneys functioning? Are any of your doctors concerned about your level of kidney function?
3. What is your activity level?

4. How does the condition affect you? Do you have any nausea, vomiting, or headaches?

5. Are there any effects on your muscles, such as pain, cramping, or twitching?

6. How is your skin? Do you have any itching, bruising, or deposits on your skin? Do you bruise or bleed easily? Is there any swelling?

7. Are there any neurological effects of your condition, such as seizures? Has your condition affected your ability to think clearly? Do you have any sensation changes—numbness, or "pins and needles?"

8. Do you have any associated conditions, such as diabetes or hypertension? Are there any heart or lung problems? Do you have any form of anemia?

Chronic Kidney Failure

Medical Information	**Massage Therapy Guidelines**
Essentials	
• Gradual, irreversible loss of kidney function	• Avoid general circulatory intent; work gently overall • Follow the Activity and Energy Principle, use physician input if a stronger session is desired.
• Caused by diabetes, hypertension, other kidney diseases, autoimmune conditions, sickle cell disease, toxic exposure, some medications, renal artery blockage	• Adapt massage to cause (see Diabetes, Chapter 17; Hypertension, Chapter 11; Autoimmunity, Chapter 13; Sickle cell disease, Chapter 12)
• Weight loss	• No massage adjustments unless weight loss profound
• Fatigue	• Gentle session overall
• Nausea and vomiting	• Easy bathroom access; position for comfort (flat prone or supine position may be poorly tolerated; side-lying may be preferred); gentle session overall; pressure to tolerance (typically 3 max), but with full, reassuring contact; slow speeds; no uneven rhythms or strong joint movement; avoid scents in lubricant and odors in environment
• Headaches	• Position for comfort, especially prone; consider inclined table or propping; gentle session overall; pressure to tolerance; slow speed and even rhythm; general circulatory intent may be poorly tolerated
• Muscle pain, twitching, cramping	• Full, firm contact; position to avoid cramping; avoid strong joint movement or stretches
• Itching	• Avoid aggravating itching (firm stationary pressure, with no friction, may be best) ; watch for open skin from scratching; avoid contact at open lesions
• Urea crystals on skin (uremic frost)	• Glove for session
• Bruising, bleeding	• Gentler pressure overall, level 1-3 max
• Swelling (generalized)	• Avoid general circulatory intent
• Decreased mental function	• Communicate simply and clearly, adapt massage and movements to changes in feedback due to confusion, impaired perception
• Hypertension	• See Chapter 11
• Neuropathy	• Observe Sensation Principle (see Chapter 3)
• Seizures	• See Chapter 10
• Insomnia	• When appropriate, use sedative intent at end of day, activating/stimulating intent at beginning

FIGURE 18-6. A Decision Tree for chronic kidney failure.

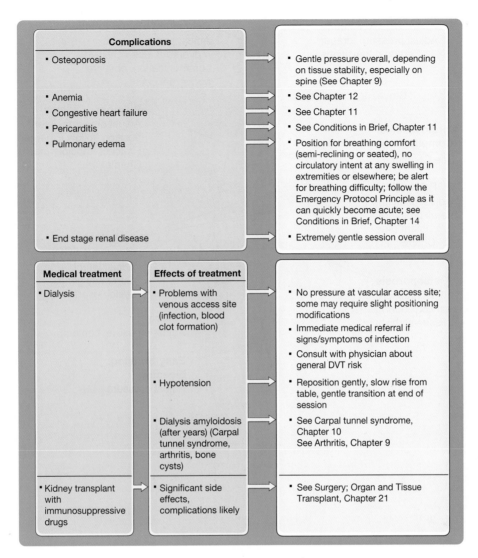

FIGURE 18-6. (*Continued*).

9. Do you have any other urinary or kidney conditions? Any lupus or sickle-cell disease, or anything else thought to contribute to the condition?
10. Have there been any other complications of your condition? Any osteoporosis, or anemia?
11. Is your sleep affected?
12. How is your condition treated? Are you on any medications for management of your symptoms?
13. How do the treatments affect you?
14. If you undergo dialysis, where is the access?

● MASSAGE THERAPY GUIDELINES

The effects of chronic kidney failure occur across many organ systems, with many considerations for the massage plan. Question 1 about the cause of kidney failure could point you to any number of other serious conditions, such as diabetes or hypertension. Refer to the appropriate chapter in each case, listed in the Decision Tree (Figure 18-6).

Question 2 suggests that the most significant determinant of the massage plan is the function of the kidney. For diagnosed disease, avoid general circulatory intent and provide a gentle session overall. This adjustment is more or less universal for chronic kidney failure, even for clients on dialysis.

However, if the client's activity level suggests a more robust picture, and his or her doctor supports a more vigorous session, you might gradually increase the pressure or intent over a course of massage treatment, when you can monitor the client's response to massage. Question 3, and additional Activity and Energy Questions (see Chapter 4) should help you assess this.

Questions 4–11 could reveal several signs or symptoms that do not require significant massage changes: weight loss, or changes in skin color, for example. But other mild effects of kidney failure require massage adjustments, broadly summarized in Figure 18-7. Adjust the strength of the session to the level of fatigue. For nausea, vomiting, or headache, see the Decision Tree (Figure 18-6).

In kidney failure, muscle twitching, cramps, and pain are due to metabolic waste buildup, rather than normal tension in muscles. In this event, your hand contact should be gentle but firm. Use bolsters and positions that ease cramps, and do not overstretch muscles or perform strong joint movement.

Of special interest is the condition of the client's skin, in Question 6. Obviously, if itching is present, you will want to avoid aggravating it with your lubricant or strokes. Massage should be firm, stationary and without friction, if it is welcome at all. But be mindful that where there is itching, there is

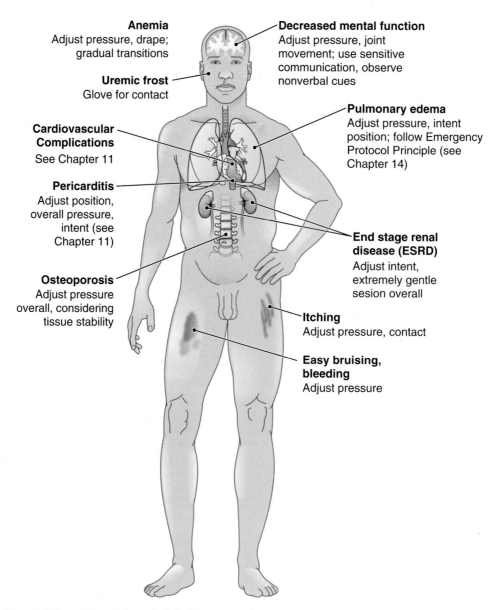

Anemia
Adjust pressure, drape;
gradual transitions

Uremic frost
Glove for contact

**Cardiovascular
Complications**
See Chapter 11

Pericarditis
Adjust position,
overall pressure,
intent (see
Chapter 11)

Osteoporosis
Adjust pressure
overall, considering
tissue stability

Decreased mental function
Adjust pressure, joint
movement; use sensitive
communication, observe
nonverbal cues

Pulmonary edema
Adjust pressure, intent
position; follow Emergency
Protocol Principle (see
Chapter 14)

**End stage renal
disease (ESRD)**
Adjust intent,
extremely gentle
sesion overall

Itching
Adjust pressure, contact

**Easy bruising,
bleeding**
Adjust pressure

FIGURE 18-7. Chronic kidney failure: Selected clinical features and massage adjustments to consider. Specific instructions and additional massage therapy guidelines are in Decision Tree and text.

usually scratching, and be alert for areas of open skin. Always avoid contact with open lesions.

If white urea crystals are deposited on the skin (uremic frost), massage therapists are advised to glove (Wible, 2009, personal communication). If there is bruising, then overall pressure should be in the 1–3 range, depending on tissue stability.

The presence of swelling in the feet, legs, hands, or face suggests that excess water has collected in the body. This, along with the kidney impairment itself, presents another argument for avoiding general circulatory intent.

The Fluid Balance Principle. **If fluid balance is off, causing either systemic swelling or dehydration, massage with general circulatory intent is contraindicated.**

You might need to direct Question 7 (as well as other interview questions) to a caregiver as well as the client, if the client's

mental status has been affected. If the client has mild problems with mental acuity, reminders about appointments might be appropriate. If his or her mental function has deteriorated further, then clear communication is in order, with simple yes-no questions, or communication through a caregiver. Continue to work gently, in the absence of the usual feedback about your pressure or movements. Be alert for nonverbal cues of comfort and discomfort. Avoid strong stretches and adapt your pressure to any areas of sensation loss, as you do in neuropathy.

The Sensation Principle. **In an area of impaired or absent sensation, use caution with pressure and joint movement.**

Questions 8–10 concern other serious conditions, causes, and complications of chronic renal failure. Your massage plan for the kidney failure itself is already conservative enough to encompass most of the massage adjustments for these other conditions. But to be sure you have covered everything, ask your client about each condition that comes up. Consult the Decision Tree (Figure 18-6) and other relevant chapters for further direction for hypertension, seizures, osteoporosis, anemia, and several other conditions that arise.

Question 11, about sleep, points up the fact that kidney failure often causes insomnia. Massage therapy may help support good quality sleep, especially if relaxation massage is done near the end of the day. At the beginning of the day, you might use more stimulating strokes, and use a more sedating approach at the end of the day.

Your client's answers to Questions 12–14 may be extensive. Many medications are used for the conditions that cause kidney disease or result from it. For this reason, follow the Medication Principle (see Chapter 3), and always ask the Four Medication Questions for each drug (Chapter 4). Common side effects of medications are listed in Table 21-1, along with massage therapy guidelines.

> *The Medication Principle. Adapt massage to the condition for which the medication is taken or prescribed, and to any side effects.*

Treatment for chronic kidney disease itself usually amounts to dialysis or kidney transplant. If the client undergoes dialysis, ask him or her to point to the AV fistula, graft, or catheter, and avoid pressure in the region of vascular access. As shown in Figure 18-5, this could be the forearm. You do not want to displace equipment or weaken the structure. For some clients, a slight position adjustment might be needed to reduce pressure at the site.

Although problems such as infection and blood clot formation sometimes occur with access sites, these are usually well monitored and treated. Follow the usual guidelines for infection (urgent or immediate medical referral if there are symptoms or signs of it). Consult the client's doctor about whether the DVT Principles should be in force, in the event that a blood clot forms at the access site. If hypotension is a side effect of dialysis, then reposition the client gently, and urge a slow rise from the table or chair after massage. Some long-term complications of dialysis, such as carpal tunnel syndrome or arthritis, may require slight massage adjustments: gentle pressure or limited joint movement at the affected sites should suffice.

If the client has had a kidney transplant, adapt the session to the effects of ongoing immunosuppressant medications (see "Organ and Tissue Transplant," Chapter 21). If the transplant was recent, see "Surgery," Chapter 21.

● MASSAGE RESEARCH

As of this writing, there are no RCTs, published in the English language, on chronic kidney failure and western styles of massage indexed in PubMed or the Massage Therapy Foundation Research Database. The NIH RePORTER tool lists no active, federally funded research projects on this topic in the United States. No active projects are listed on the clinicaltrials.gov database (see Chapter 6).

However, two studies, published by the same research group, suggest that acupressure points may help patients with ESRD. One RCT, a study of 98 patients, suggested that a course of twelve sessions over 4 weeks, using 9 minutes of acupressure preceded by 5 minutes of unspecified "warm-up" massage, helped relieve insomnia (Tsay et al., 2003). This is promising information since insomnia is a persistent problem in people with kidney failure.

Another RCT, with 62 dialysis patients, reported improvements in depression and fatigue in the subjects who received acupressure (Cho and Tsay, 2004). In this RCT, the active treatment was acupressure/massage three times a week, for 4 weeks. The sessions were 15 minutes each, with 12 minutes devoted to acupressure points, followed by 3 minutes of leg massage. If the results of these studies are corroborated in future investigations, then there could be a strong case for providing these sessions, and for teaching patients how to stimulate the acupressure points themselves.

● POSSIBLE MASSAGE BENEFITS

There is no cure for chronic kidney failure. It can go on for years, often progressing to ESRD, which can also go on for years. The wait for a kidney transplant can be prolonged, as well, if there is no eligible donor in the client's family. Chronic kidney failure comes with a long list of signs, symptoms, and life-threatening complications, and it can feel like a chronic crisis. Dialysis is time consuming and energy draining.

These factors add up to a stressful condition. In the face of this, MTs can be part of compassionate, supportive care. Massage may ease pain and help sleep. Over time, we may learn of many other ways for thoughtful massage therapy to help clients manage stress, and cope more easily with chronic kidney disease.

Other Urinary and Renal Conditions in Brief

ACUTE KIDNEY FAILURE (ACUTE RENAL FAILURE)

Background	• Sudden, reversible loss of kidney function, often following severe injury or complicated surgery. Progresses rapidly if not treated; death can occur in 3–4 days. Signs/symptoms are low urine volume, swelling in lower extremities, drowsiness and confusion, breathing difficulty, fatigue, seizures.
	• Complications include chronic kidney failure if tissues fail to heal when treated, or ESRD if damage is severe.
	• Changes in potassium levels can cause arrhythmia; pericarditis possible. Easy bruising and bleeding occur.
	• Treatments are dialysis and medications to balance blood potassium levels; side effects are hypotension, headache, nausea, vomiting. Temporary dietary restriction of fluid and protein while kidneys heal.

Interview Questions	• Cause? When did occur? Has it resolved or is it resolving? How did or does it affect you? • Complications? Blood counts? Effects on immunity or blood clotting? Easy bruising or bleeding? Breathing difficulty? Swelling? • How is kidney function now? Any long-term effect on kidneys? • Treatment? Effects of treatment? Do you have a dialysis access site?
Massage Therapy Guidelines	• Acute kidney failure is unlikely to be seen in most massage settings; past episode is more likely. • If still acute, avoid general circulatory intent, provide extremely gentle session overall in consultation with physician; adjust massage to other health issues causing condition. • Adapt pressure to bruising; adapt position to breathing difficulty, side-lying or semi-reclining. • Avoid pressure near dialysis site, sometimes a catheter in neck, and adapt positioning if needed. • Gentle massage overall if symptoms of hypotension. • If recent and resolving, adjust to kidney function by following Vital Organ Principle, Filter and Pump Principle. • If chronic or end stage, see "Chronic Kidney Failure," this chapter. • Adjust massage plan to side effects of medications (see Table 21-1).

BLADDER CANCER

Background	• One of several types of carcinoma beginning in the lining of the bladder, most common (discussed here) is transitional cell carcinoma (TCC); typically diagnosed in older adults. • Progresses to surrounding organs, usually causes symptoms before metastasizing to distant organs; often caught early enough for successful treatment. • Symptoms include blood in urine (hematuria), urinary frequency, urinary urgency and incontinence, pain and difficulty during urination, slowing of urinary stream. • Can lead to anemia, blockage of ureters and urine flow; considered complicated when locally advanced, invading nearby organs/tissues such as sigmoid colon, rectum, uterus, prostate gland, bones of pelvis. • Commonly metastasizes to lung, liver, bone; high rate of recurrence. • Treated with surgery (transurethral resection or cystectomy) to remove involved tissue, destruction of cells with laser or electrical current; may be followed with urostomy (collection of urine in external pouch) or bladder reconstruction (internal). • Radiation and chemotherapy may follow (radiation therapy less common in the United States than other countries); radiation therapy may lead to bladder and bowel incontinence, diarrhea. • Biologic therapy (immunotherapy) may be used (see Chapter 20) to prevent recurrence; side effects include flu-like symptoms, fever, bladder irritation.
Interview Questions	• Where is cancer in your body? Does it affect any organs or tissues next to the bladder? • What are your signs and symptoms? Any urinary difficulties (incontinence, urgency)? • Do you have anemia? How are your blood counts? Is energy level affected? What is your activity level? Activity tolerance? • Is there any bone involvement? Any effects on colon, liver, lungs, brain or spinal cord? • Treatment? Effects of treatment? Any surgery and/or catheterization, medical devices?
Massage Therapy Guidelines	• Review "Cancer," Chapter 20, for massage therapy guidelines for cancer and cancer treatment. • Adjust massage to sites of cancer spread, such as liver, lungs; limit pressure (2 max) at abdomen if spread to colon, rectum, reproductive organs; adjust positioning to minimize uncomfortable pressure at lower abdomen if needed. • If bone involvement, see "Bone Metastasis," Chapter 20; if pain, especially new, unfamiliar, or increasing pain, do not use pressure or joint movement at site until physician verifies that no bone metastasis is present. • If liver function impaired, avoid general circulatory intent, adjust position for liver enlargement; (see "Liver Cancer," Chapter 16); if metastasis to lungs, position for breathing difficulty (see "Lung Cancer," Chapter 14). • If anemia present, provide gentle session overall and slow rise from the table (see "Anemia," Chapter 12).

- Position around urine collection bag, often attached to the thigh; collection bag may need to be lower than bladder to prevent backflow of contents from gravity; easy bathroom access may be necessary for bladder urgency, incontinence.
- Adapt to effects of biological therapy with gentle overall session, avoid general circulatory intent.

GLOMERULONEPHRITIS (NEPHRITIC SYNDROME)

Background	• Inflammation of glomeruli in kidney, may follow infection, or be caused by autoimmune or allergic stimulus, toxic exposure; in adults, often associated with systemic lupus erythematosus, vasculitis, bacterial infection, viral infections such as measles, mumps, mononucleosis, hepatitis, endocarditis. • Early symptoms include protein in urine, low urine volume, bloody or foamy urine, swelling of face and extremities, generalized swelling, hypertension, malaise, headache, muscle and joint pain, blurred vision. • Short-term acute infection subsides in weeks to months after treatment; long-term progressive condition can lead to nephrotic syndrome (see Conditions in Brief) and to acute, chronic, and end-stage kidney failure (this chapter). • Treatment with bed rest, dietary changes, antibiotics for infection, corticosteroids and other anti-inflammatories, BP medication (ACE inhibitors, angiotensin II receptor blockers, diuretics), other treatments for kidney failure.
Interview Questions	• Cause? Chronic or acute? Is kidney function intact? • How does it affect you? What is your activity level? How is your kidney function? Any chronic or acute kidney failure? • Any complications? How is your BP? • How is it treated? How does treatment affect you?
Massage Therapy Guidelines	• Avoid general circulatory intent; gentle session overall; follow Fluid Balance Principle (this chapter) if swelling present. Avoid circulatory intent at site of swelling. • Investigate cause and adjust massage accordingly (see "Autoimmunity," Chapter 13). Medical referral for worsening signs/symptoms of infection. • Depending on kidney function, see "Chronic Kidney Failure" (this chapter) or Acute kidney failure (see Conditions in Brief). • Adjust massage plan to hypertension and BP medication (Table 11-3). • Adjust overall pressure to corticosteroid medication (see Chapter 21), side effects of antibiotics (see Table 21-1).

NEPHROTIC SYNDROME

Background	• Disturbance in fluid balance resulting from excessive protein loss from blood to urine (proteinuria). • Can be primary (affecting only kidneys) or associated with other kidney diseases; can be autoimmune in origin, or result from diabetes, sickle-cell diseases, systemic lupus erythematosus, some types of cancer, drug and allergic reactions, IV drug use, or infection (malaria, HIV, herpes zoster). • Symptoms are foamy urine; swelling in eyelids, hands, feet, knees, abdomen; general systemic swelling; muscle weakness, wasting, and fatigue; ascites, abdominal pain; difficulty breathing; low or high BP. • Complications are infection (including pneumonia), chronic and acute kidney failure, atherosclerosis, CHF, pulmonary edema, renal vein thrombosis, DVT. • Treatment of underlying condition may resolve condition; can include corticosteroids, diuretics, BP medications, blood thinners.
Interview Questions	• Cause? Any associated conditions (causes or complications)? • How does it affect you? Any swelling? Where? • Effects on BP? Is it well controlled? • Any effects on breathing? Comfortable positions for breathing or abdominal discomfort? • Complications, such as acute kidney failure or infection? • Treatment? Effects of treatment?

| Massage Therapy Guidelines | • Avoid general circulatory intent (follow Fluid Balance Principle, this chapter); avoid circulatory intent at individual sites of swelling.
• Adapt to cause (see Sickle-cell disease, Chapter 12; Autoimmunity, HIV, Chapter 13; "Diabetes Mellitus," Chapter 17).
• Adapt position for breathing or abdominal discomfort, consider side-lying, seated, or semi-reclining.
• Adapt massage to hypertension (see Chapter 11); for hypotension, encourage slow rise from table at end of session, gradual position changes.
• Gentle joint movement if muscle weakness or wasting.
• Adapt massage to kidney failure (see Acute kidney failure, Conditions in Brief).
• Gentle overall session if infection; consider DVT Risk Principles, especially if other DVT risk factors present (see Chapter 11)
• Adjust massage to BP medication, blood thinners (see Chapter 11), corticosteroids (see Chapter 21). |

POLYCYSTIC KIDNEY DISEASE (PKD, RENAL CYSTIC DISEASE)

Background	• Hereditary disorder, infant or adult onset, causing cysts in kidney: fluid-filled cavities with degeneration of normal renal tissue. • Asymptomatic if single cyst; multiple cysts cause chronic abdominal or flank pain, bloody urine, fever. • Complications include chronic kidney failure, kidney stone, UTI, hypertension, increased risk of brain aneurysm and stroke, diverticulosis, liver cysts; risk of complications increases in older adults. • If polycystic, hypertension treated with BP medication; low-protein diet to forestall kidney failure; acetaminophen for pain; antibiotics for UTI treatment. • Surgical removal or drainage of cysts in rare cases.
Interview Questions	• Single or multiple cysts? Large or small? One side or both? • Any symptoms, such as pain? Where? Fever? • How is your kidney function? Any effects on BP? • Any associated conditions such as diverticulosis, liver problems, or aneurysm? • Treatment? Effects of treatment?
Massage Therapy Guidelines	• If cysts are asymptomatic, no complications, then minimal massage adjustment. Avoid general circulatory intent if disease affects kidney function or BP, causes fever, produces blood in urine, causes pain (see "Chronic Kidney Failure," this chapter), or impairs liver function (see Chapter 16). • If fever, gentle session overall; be alert for complications affecting other organs, especially in older adults, and adjust massage (see "Diverticular Disease," Chapter 15; "Stroke [Cerebrovascular Accident]," Chapter 10; "Urinary Tract Infection," "Kidney Stone," this chapter). • Adapt massage to hypertension and BP medications (see Chapter 11); see NSAIDs, "Surgery," Chapter 21. For antibiotics and other medications, see common side effects in Table 21-1.

KIDNEY CANCER (RENAL CELL CARCINOMA)

| Background | • Most common type of kidney cancer; begins in cells lining the tubules of nephrons; often spotted during procedures for other conditions.
• Symptoms are blood in urine; pain in flank, abdomen, or back; fever, fatigue, weight loss, enlargement of abdomen.
• Metastasis is common to lung, bone, liver, other kidney; other complications include hypertension, anemia, polycythemia, DVT.
• Treatment includes surgery, hormone therapy, biologic therapy, targeted therapies.
• Chemotherapy and radiation therapy are not often used for renal cell carcinoma. |

Interview Questions	• Where is or was it in your body? How does it affect you? • Have there been any complications? Any effects on function of your liver or lungs? Is there any bone involvement? • Are there any effects on your BP or blood, such as hypertension, anemia, polycythemia, or blood clots? • Any areas of swelling or discomfort? What are comfortable positions for you? • Treatment? Effects of treatment?
Massage Therapy Guidelines	• Review "Cancer," Chapter 20, for massage therapy guidelines for cancer and cancer treatment; follow Vital Organ Principle, Filter and Pump Principle. • Adjust massage to sites of cancer spread; adapt position for comfort if abdominal swelling present, or if breathing difficulty (consider side-lying, seated, semi-reclining); gentle focus on muscles of breathing may assist respiration. • If bone involvement, see "Bone Metastasis," Chapter 20; if pain, especially new, unfamiliar, or increasing pain, do not use pressure or joint movement at site until physician verifies that no bone metastasis is present. • If liver function impaired, avoid general circulatory intent, adjust position for liver enlargement (see "Liver Cancer," Chapter 16). • Adapt to polycythemia, anemia (see Chapter 12); follow DVT Risk Principles (see Chapter 11). • Adjust to hypertension and BP medication (see Chapter 11)

SELF TEST

1. Describe four functions of the kidneys, and how the body is affected in each case, when the kidneys are not functioning properly.
2. Explain the Fluid Balance Principle, the reasons behind it, and an example of a urinary condition in which to apply it.
3. How and where does a UTI usually begin? At what point is it considered the most serious?
4. What is the difference between pyelonephritis and cystitis?
5. Where is pain felt during a UTI?
6. Describe the common treatments for kidney stones.
7. Describe three complications of kidney stones.
8. Describe the research in support of massage therapy or bodywork for people with kidney stones. Have Swedish massage strokes been tested in this research?
9. Compare chronic and acute kidney failure in terms of the causes, symptoms and signs, the course of disease, and whether or not the conditions are reversible.
10. List three ways that chronic kidney failure may be evident in the skin. What are the massage adjustments for each?
11. How does chronic kidney failure affect the blood and cardiovascular system?
12. How are muscles affected by chronic kidney failure, and how do you adapt your massage to the effects on muscle?
13. Name the three venous access devices used in dialysis, their typical sites of placement on the body, and the massage adjustment needed for each.
14. How could massage therapy be helpful to a client with kidney failure? Describe any available research that supports massage in this population.
15. If advanced kidney failure affects mental status, how might you need to change the way you work with the client?

 For answers to these questions and to see a bibliography for this chapter, visit http://thePoint.lww.com/Walton.

The reproduction of mankind is a great marvel and mystery.

—MARTIN LUTHER

This chapter concerns the female and male reproductive systems, with a focus on the internal reproductive structures. The reproductive system, especially in the female, is dynamic, with active tissues and a swirl of hormones affecting the internal environment. Many factors must line up well in order to carry out normal reproductive function. Conversely, many things can go wrong to produce dysfunction.

This chapter addresses the following conditions at length, with full Decision Trees:

- Female infertility
- Breast cancer
- Prostate cancer

Conditions in Brief in this chapter are **benign prostatic hyperplasia** (prostate gland enlargement), **cervical cancer**, **dysmenorrhea**, **endometrial cancer** (uterine adenocarcinoma), **endometriosis**, **fibroids** (uterine fibroids), **male infertility** (male factor infertility), **miscarriage** (spontaneous abortion), **ovarian cancer** (ovarian epithelial carcinoma), **pelvic inflammatory disease (PID)**, **polycystic ovary syndrome/disease (PCOS)** (ovarian cysts), **pregnancy**, **premenstrual syndrome (PMS)**, and **testicular cancer**.

Normal, uncomplicated pregnancy is discussed in Conditions in Brief, where only the basic safety essentials are described. Other textbooks, focused solely on prenatal massage, address safety guidelines in much more detail, including normal, high-risk, and complicated pregnancy (Osborne, 2011; Stager, 2009; Stillerman, 2007). If your client's pregnancy becomes complicated and you are not trained to work specifically with the condition, additional training is advised; at minimum, a close reading of a prenatal massage textbook is in order, along with communication with the client's physician (see Chapter 4).

Space limits discussion of other normal or common reproductive conditions, such as amenorrhea, PMS, and menopause. In these cases, patient education resources are widely available, and building a Decision Tree is a straightforward process.

General Principles

Many of the principles presented in previous chapters apply here, and a new one is introduced: the Privacy Principle. This principle is particularly important for working with people with reproductive conditions.

The Privacy Principle. *When asking about sensitive or emotionally charged health matters, avoid stray interview questions.*

Focus on questions that figure into the massage plan, explain why they're necessary, and use a warm, matter-of-fact tone.

Stick to questions you need to ask for massage purposes. Some strong medical treatments are used for reproductive conditions, and they must be explored in order to arrive at the most appropriate massage.

Female Infertility

Infertility, or *subfertility* as it is often called, is the biological inability to conceive within a year of attempting to get pregnant. It is different from **sterility**, which is the complete inability to conceive due to a physical problem. Infertility occurs in both women and men, and a proper diagnosis and workup in a heterosexual relationship involve both partners. The diagnostic process can be time-consuming.

● BACKGROUND

There are many factors that can interfere with female fertility, and they may be structural or physiological. Causes include endometriosis, uterine fibroids, and polycystic ovary syndrome. Inflammation can play a role in infertility, as well. Contributing inflammatory conditions are *endometritis*, inflammation of the uterine lining; pelvic inflammatory disease, *cervicitis*, chronic inflammation of the cervix; and *salpingitis*, inflammation of the fallopian tubes. Sometimes, an autoimmune response can destroy ovarian tissues, resulting in loss of eggs and premature ovarian failure.

Common causes of infertility are hormonal. The hypothalamus or pituitary gland can be deficient in stimulating *ovulation*, or the timing can be off over the course of the menstrual cycle. In these cases, development, maturation, and release of an egg are affected. Hormonal problems include imbalances in **gonadotropins**, hormones produced that stimulate the function of the ovaries and testes. In female infertility, gonadotropin imbalances include the abnormal pituitary secretion of **follicle stimulating hormone (FSH)** and **luteinizing hormone (LH)**. FSH is a pituitary hormone that stimulates the growth of *ovarian follicle* cells to grow in the female and the production of sperm cells in the male testes. LH is another pituitary hormone that stimulates the growth and maturation of eggs in the female and sperm cells in the male. Another cause of infertility is elevated prolactin, a pituitary hormone that stimulates the production of breast milk and inhibits hormones necessary for ovulation.

Infertility may occur when a woman's immune system produces antibodies to sperm, thus preventing conception. Certain medications, cancer treatments, thyroid problems, or other diseases can also affect fertility. Early menopause, with or without a clear cause, may explain infertility.

Signs and Symptoms

Besides the obvious lack of signs of being pregnant, there may be no other signs or symptoms of infertility. Irregular menstrual periods, pain during menstruation, and/or pain during intercourse may signal conditions that are associated with infertility.

Complications

Although infertility can be addressed successfully by a number of different treatments, a constellation of emotions may surface in a woman trying to become pregnant, or between partners. Among them is depression. Other problems include guilt, disappointment, anger, blame or resentment, diminished self-esteem, and fear of losing a partner or relationship. Infertile individuals and couples often experience deep grief.

Treatment

A number of fertility treatments exist for women. Fertility drugs are often tried first. Most of them address hormonal imbalances, boosting ovulation.

Clomiphene (Clomid, Serophene) is often the first-line fertility drug. It stimulates ovulation by causing the pituitary gland to release more FSH and LH. Clomiphene can cause hot flashes, headaches, and mood swings. It may also cause lightheadedness or dizziness.

Several fertility medications are designed to replace the function of natural gonadotropins. These drugs, also called gonadotropins, increase LH and FSH production from other sources. Commonly used gonadotropins include:

- *Follicle-stimulating hormone (FSH)*. Available as Fertinex, Follistim, Gonal-F, and Bravelle, this medication stimulates the ovaries to produce mature eggs.
- *Human chorionic gonadotropin (hCG)*. Available as Novarel, Ovidrel, and Pregnyl; this substance is structurally similar to LH and triggers ovulation.
- *Human menopausal gonadotropin (hMG)*. Available as Repronex, Pergonal, and Menopur, this drug contains both FSH and LH.

A principal side effect of gonadotropin medications is ovarian hyperstimulation syndrome (OHSS). In 10–20% of cases, the mild form of this occurs, and the ovaries are enlarged, causing abdominal bloating and pain. The woman is monitored closely so that the condition doesn't worsen; severe OHSS can lead to life-threatening complications: blood clots, kidney failure, fluid accumulation in the abdomen and chest, and severe electrolyte imbalance. Signs and symptoms of severe complications are swelling in the extremities and abdomen, rapid weight gain, shortness of breath, nausea, and vomiting. Mild cases of OHSS resolve quickly on their own if menstruation starts; if pregnancy occurs, they take weeks to go away. Severe cases are monitored and treated in the hospital.

A significant number of pregnancies resulting from hormone therapies are multiple: twins, triplets, and higher order pregnancies, which can lead to additional complications. *Ectopic pregnancy*, a life-threatening condition if untreated, is more likely with fertility treatments. In this case, the embryo grows outside of the uterus, usually in the fallopian tube, ovary, cervix, or in the pelvic cavity.

Other drugs for fertility include GnRH analogues, or substances that behave like gonadotropin-releasing hormone (GnRH), in the body. GnRH is usually produced by the hypothalamus, signaling the pituitary gland to secrete LH and FSH. GnRH is available by prescription as Factrel, targeted at triggering ovulation. As of this writing, Factrel is not available in the United States. GnRH analogues may cause short-lived hot flashes, headache, mood changes, and vaginal dryness.

Other drug therapies are bromocriptine and metformin. The drug bromocriptine (Parlodel) suppresses prolactin production and can help infertility caused by excess prolactin. It has several side effects, including headache, nausea, abdominal discomfort and bloating, diarrhea, fatigue, dizziness, lightheadedness, and sinus congestion. Another drug, metformin (Glucophage), also used in insulin-resistant diabetes, may help when insulin resistance interferes with conception. It is often used in women with polycystic ovary syndrome (see Conditions in Brief). It may cause GI disturbance, including abdominal discomfort, nausea, and vomiting. With both drugs, bothersome side effects tend to lessen over time.

Some fertility drugs are oral, and some are injectable. The timing of injectable drugs during specific points in the menstrual cycle is critical. Many injectable drugs increase the chance of multiple births and pregnancy complications. Fertility treatment often involves being beholden to a schedule—of ovulation, injections, diagnostic procedures, and either sexual intercourse or inseminations.

Surgery may be tried, depending on the cause of the infertility. The fallopian tubes can be unblocked, and endometrial growths and adhesions can be removed to restore healthy structure and function to the reproductive organs.

Assisted reproductive technology (ART) is a group of techniques in which both sperm and eggs are manipulated outside the body to facilitate pregnancy. Typically, hormone treatments are required, then eggs are removed for treatment with sperm, then one or more embryos are implanted in the uterus.

The most common and effective type of ART is in vitro fertilization (IVF). Mature eggs are retrieved from a woman, fertilized in a dish with a man's sperm, and implanted in the uterus several days later. To increase the chances of fertilization, IVF requires the woman to inject hormones to optimize the number of follicles carrying eggs that can then be exposed to sperm.

Intracytoplasmic sperm injection (ICSI) involves adding a step to the standard IVF procedure, in which a single sperm cell is injected into an egg to achieve fertilization. Assisted hatching involves a small puncture to the outermost membrane of the embryo, allowing it to more readily implant in the uterine lining once it is inserted. As with any invasive procedure, bleeding or infection may result from ART.

In ART, several fertilized eggs are often implanted in order to enhance the chances of pregnancy. As with hormone treatments by themselves, multiple pregnancies occur in ART, and the parent or parents may choose to reduce the number of fetuses to improve the survival chances of the others. This process, called *multifetal pregnancy reduction*, obviously involves serious emotional and ethical decision making.

Pregnancies from ART may result in low birth weight and birth defects. Research is ongoing on birth defects and ART.

● INTERVIEW QUESTIONS

1. Are there any other conditions, such as endometriosis, fibroids, polycystic ovary syndrome, or previous medical treatments, associated with the infertility?
2. How is it being treated?
3. How does the treatment affect you?
4. Are there any signs of ovarian hyperstimulation with your treatments?
5. Are any of your medications injected? Have you injected any in the last 24 hours? If so, where?

● MASSAGE THERAPY GUIDELINES

When working with a client in fertility treatment, *always* adjust massage to the possibility of pregnancy, whether or not the client reports she is pregnant. This saves asking the client, "Is there any chance you might be pregnant?" at each session and helps preserve her privacy.

> *The Privacy Principle. When asking about sensitive or emotionally charged health matters, avoid stray interview questions. Focus on questions that figure into the massage plan, explain why they're necessary, and use a warm, matter-of-fact tone.*

The Privacy Principle is especially important for anyone going through fertility treatment, where intimate reproductive and sexual functions become medical matters: the focus of numerous diagnostic tests and procedures, and discussions with health care providers.

In assuring the client that you will always adjust the massage plan for the possibility of pregnancy, explain that you avoid any techniques that are thought to compromise early pregnancy. For example, you will obviously avoid pressure at the abdomen, as well as focused work on certain acupressure and reflexology points. See Pregnancy, Conditions in Brief, for a short list of pregnancy massage essentials.

Because pregnancy following fertility treatment may be considered high risk, communicate clearly with the client's prenatal care provider about the massage care plan during that time. The format for physician communication, described in Figures 5-2 and 5-3, can be easily adapted to a high-risk pregnancy. In addition, seek out textbooks and training focused on pregnancy massage (see Bibliography, online at http://thepoint.lww.com/walton) for more elaboration.

In Question 1, rather than focusing on cause and effect of fertility, a gentler approach is to ask whether there are any associated or related conditions. Fertility treatment is often focused on the cause, and this can be an emotionally raw subject. Most causes are found in this chapter, and others, such as the long-term effects of cancer treatment, are in other chapters.

Questions 2–4 will have several possible responses since side effects are common with fertility treatments. Adjust the massage to any side effects of clomiphene and the gonadotropins: hot flashes obviously require adjustments in room temperature and draping. Headaches require a gentler session overall, as described in the Decision Tree (Figure 19-1). If the client has mood swings, she will welcome your compassion, sensitivity, and patience. Dizziness calls for gradual repositioning and a slow rise from the massage table after the session.

OHSS, if mild, may require some adjustments to the prone position to accommodate abdominal bloating. Slight padding above and below the abdomen may be welcome, or the side-lying position may be most comfortable. Even though swelling is not extensive, follow the Fluid Balance Principle (see Chapter 18) until signs and symptoms pass. If more serious OHSS side effects develop, such as swelling in the extremities, shortness of breath, or rapid weight gain, an emergency medical referral is in order.

> *The Fluid Balance Principle. If fluid balance is off, causing either systemic swelling or dehydration, massage with general circulatory intent is contraindicated.*

Side effects and massage adjustments for bromocriptine and metformin are described in the Decision Tree. Recall that side effects of these medications tend to be worse when the drugs are started, easing over time. Check in regularly with your client about side effects.

If your client has had recent surgery to unblock fallopian tubes or remove adhesions, ask how extensive the surgery was, and review "Surgery," Chapter 21, for massage guidelines.

If the client is using ART to become pregnant, she will likely be taking fertility drugs. In addition, her schedule can be disrupted by her menstrual cycle, ovulation tests, and daily ultrasounds around the time of expected ovulation. A shared understanding of her scheduling challenges is a good idea, since last-minute cancellations of massage appointments may occur.

Some ART procedures are more invasive than others. Overall, work gently before and after procedures. The waiting time for a pregnancy test is a particularly tender and hopeful time. During fertility treatment, your massage intent is to ease stress and support her body's integration of the treatments, not to bring about ambitious changes in muscle tension or circulation.

If signs of infection arise, make a medical referral. Even though ART procedures are much less invasive than surgery, bleeding may occur, and it's a good idea to consider the DVT Risk Principles (see Chapter 11).

If a multiple pregnancy occurs, this qualifies as a high-risk pregnancy. Review texts on pregnancy massage and communicate closely with the client's prenatal health care provider about the massage care plan.

Question 5 alerts you to respect recent injection sites, which are often intramuscular. Avoid circulatory intent at the most recent site for about a day, to give the medication time to be absorbed at its own pace.

● MASSAGE RESEARCH

As of this writing, there are no randomized, controlled trials (RCTs), published in the English language, on fertility and classical massage indexed in PubMed or the Massage Therapy Foundation Research Database. The NIH RePORTER tool lists no active, federally funded research projects on this topic in the United States. No active projects are listed on the clinicaltrials.gov database (see Chapter 6).

Female Infertility

Medical Information	Massage Therapy Guidelines

Essentials

- Inability to conceive within 1 year of trying to get pregnant

- Contributing factors: endometriosis, uterine fibroids, polycystic ovary syndrome, blocked/inflamed reproductive structures, cancer treatment, hormonal problems, other medical conditions

→ • Follow the Privacy Principle; apply massage guidelines for first trimester pregnancy (see Conditions in Brief) if client is actively trying to become pregnant, or if status unknown

→ • Adapt to cause (see endometriosis, fibroids, polycystic ovary syndrome, Conditions in Brief)

Complications

- Emotional effects include depression, grief, guilt, diminished self-esteem, fear of judgment, feelings of isolation

→ • Sensitivity, warmth; follow Privacy Principle

Medical treatment	Effects of treatment	

- Fertility medications (Clomid, Serophene)

  → • Hot flashes
  → • Headache

  → • Dizziness, lightheadedness
  → • Mood changes

→ • Adjust ambient temperature, drape; avoid hot pads

→ • Position for comfort, especially prone; consider inclined table or propping; gentle session overall; pressure to tolerance; slow speed and even rhythm; general circulatory intent may be poorly tolerated

→ • Gentle repositioning, slow rise from table

→ • No specific massage adjustments; patience, compassion

- Gonadotropins (follicle-stimulating hormone, human chorionic gonadotropin, human menopausal gonadotropin)

  → • Injectable
  → • Ovarian hyperstimulation syndrome

    • Mild (abdominal bloating, discomfort)

    • Severe (blood clots, kidney failure, fluid accumulation in chest and abdomen, electrolyte imbalance)

→ • Avoid circulatory intent at recent injection site

→ • Adjust for discomfort in lower abdomen (padding above and below for prone position, or use sidelying)
→ • No general circulatory intent (see Fluid Balance Principle, Chapter 18)

→ • Immediate or emergency medical referral (see text for signs and symptoms)

- Bromocriptine

  → • Headache
  → • Nausea

  → • Abdominal discomfort, bloating
  → • Diarrhea

  → • Fatigue
  → • Dizziness, lightheadedness

  → • Sinus congestion

→ • See above
→ • Position for comfort, gentle session overall; pressure to tolerance, slow speeds; no uneven rhythms or strong joint movement

→ • Adjust for discomfort in lower abdomen (padding above and below for prone position, or use sidelying)
→ • Easy bathroom access; gentle session overall; avoid contact or pressure at abdomen that could aggravate

→ • Gentle session overall
→ • Reposition gently, slow speed and even rhythm, slow rise from table, gentle transition at end of session

→ • Limit flat prone position; consider inclined table or change in position

- Metformin

  → • Abdominal discomfort
  → • Nausea
  → • Diarrhea

→ • See above

- Surgery (removal of adhesions, endometrial growths; unblocking tubes)

  → • See Surgery, Chapter 21, for side effects, complications

→ • Follow the Procedure Principle; see Surgery, Chapter 21

FIGURE 19-1. A Decision Tree for female infertility.

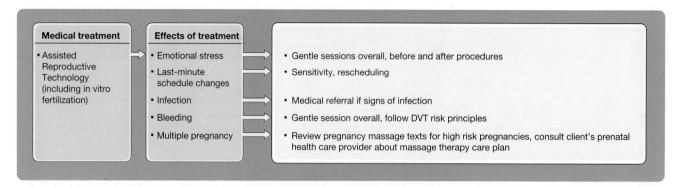

Medical treatment	Effects of treatment	
• Assisted Reproductive Technology (including in vitro fertilization)	• Emotional stress	• Gentle sessions overall, before and after procedures
	• Last-minute schedule changes	• Sensitivity, rescheduling
	• Infection	• Medical referral if signs of infection
	• Bleeding	• Gentle session overall, follow DVT risk principles
	• Multiple pregnancy	• Review pregnancy massage texts for high risk pregnancies, consult client's prenatal health care provider about massage therapy care plan

FIGURE 19-1. (*Continued*).

A small RCT examined the effects of acupressure on 104 women undergoing laparoscopy during a course of fertility treatment (Harmon et al., 1999). Investigators compared the stimulation of the P6 (Neiguan) point on the anterior forearm/wrist with a sham acupressure procedure, and noted that the incidence of nausea or vomiting was 42% in the sham group and 19% in the true acupressure group. In their report in the *British Journal of Anesthesia*, they concluded that the acupressure point deserved further study in this population. As of this writing, there does not appear to be a published follow-up study.

● POSSIBLE MASSAGE BENEFITS

The challenges of infertility can be difficult and prolonged, and massage therapy can be a wonderful support to women and men during this important time. Self-care is paramount, and stress may be relieved by massage. A massage session might be the only appointment all week or all month that is focused, *not* on fertility, but on the whole person, and such a respite from the experience may be welcome.

Be careful about linking stress to infertility, though, because people often feel judged by the ideas and opinions of others, who offer simplistic solutions, such as "Reduce your stress and you'll get pregnant!" or "Stop focusing on it and you'll get pregnant!" Instead, offer massage as a way of relieving stress during the journey. Good listening, without offering advice or observation, can be highly therapeutic, as the online Therapist's Journal describes (see http://thePoint.lww.com/Walton).

Breast Cancer

Breast cancer is any type of malignancy that begins in the breast tissue. It is the most common type of female cancer in the United States. In addition, although fewer than 1% of breast cancer diagnoses occur in males, the incidence of this disease in men has increased 25% over the past 25 years.

● BACKGROUND

Most breast cancers develop in the ducts that convey milk to the nipple (ductal carcinoma), in the milk-producing sacs (lobular carcinoma), and in other breast tissue that is not glandular. **Inflammatory carcinoma** is a form of breast cancer in which the cancer cells block lymph vessels in the breast tissue, causing redness and swelling. This form of breast cancer accounts for just a small percentage (1%) of total breast cancer cases; it is fast growing and spreads quickly, and therefore is difficult to treat.

There are several slow-growing types of breast cancer, representing about 8% of total cases. These include *medullary carcinoma, mucinous carcinoma,* and *tubular carcinoma*. About 1–4% of breast cancer cases are called *Paget disease of the breast*. Unrelated to Paget disease affecting bone, this disease affects the nipple and areola.

Like other types of cancer, breast cancer is staged, which generally describes the size and behavior of the tumor, and the movement of it beyond its home tissue. Breast cancer **in situ**, refers to a tumor "in its original place," or *noninvasive*. The cancer is early and has not spread to neighboring tissue.

Examples are **ductal carcinoma in situ (DCIS)** and **lobular carcinoma in situ (LCIS)**. DCIS generally requires treatment and has a high cure rate; without treatment, it usually leads to invasive breast cancer in 10 years. LCIS does not require treatment but does raise the individual's risk of later cancer in other areas. In situ cancers do not usually require whole-body treatments such as chemotherapy.

In contrast, *invasive* breast cancer has moved beyond its place of origin to other tissues in the breast. *Locally advanced* breast cancer has not progressed beyond nearby lymph nodes; in some classifications, the chest wall or skin of the breast is affected. In advanced breast cancer, the disease has spread to distant sites such as the bones, lungs, liver, and brain. It can even spread to the ovaries and adrenal glands.

Signs and Symptoms

The most common sign of breast cancer—a painless lump or thickening of tissue in the breast—may go unnoticed, or it might be picked up during a breast self-examination or by a mammogram or ultrasound scan. A **needle biopsy**, the removal of tissue or fluid with a needle, is often performed to test the tissue and determine whether further action is needed.

Other possible symptoms are a change in breast size or shape; a change in the skin of the breast, such as flattening, indentation, scaling, redness, warmth, or dimpling; an indentation or retraction of the nipple; or discharge from the nipple, either clear or bloody.

Complications

As already mentioned, breast cancer can metastasize to the bones, lungs, liver, brain, or the chest wall, affecting the structure and function of the tissues. Bone is the most common site of metastasis; 25% of breast cancers spread there first. Bone involvement is a grave concern because it can compromise the structure of the bones, making them vulnerable to pathologic fracture. This problem is compounded when an individual has osteoporosis, and some forms of treatment for breast cancer increase the risk of osteoporosis.

When bones are affected by bone metastasis, the spine (and nearby spinal cord) are chief concerns. Spinal cord compression occurs when bone lesions press into the spinal canal, impinging on the spinal cord or nerve roots. Cord compression can also occur when weakened vertebrae fracture and slip out of place, pressing against the same CNS structures (see "Bone Metastasis," Chapter 20).

After bone, lungs are the next most common area of metastasis, and the liver is the third. Other secondary sites are the ovaries, bone marrow, eyes, and adrenal glands. A recurrence of breast cancer is possible months or years after successful treatment. At that time, it might be a local recurrence, confined to the breast, or it may be in the chest wall or involve distant metastases.

Symptoms and signs of distant spread depend on the organ or organs involved. A site of metastasis may be clinically silent at first, then eventually affect organ or tissue function.

As is true of many cancers, when breast cancer advances, it raises the risk of deep vein thrombosis. Blood clots can form, often in the lower extremities.

Treatment

Surgery is both diagnostic and therapeutic. Surgery might be performed to remove only the tumor, the tumor and nearby lymph nodes, or additional breast tissue.

In a lumpectomy, the tumor itself is removed, along with a small amount of healthy tissue around it to ensure all the cancer is removed. In a mastectomy, much more tissue is removed. In a partial mastectomy, the surgeon removes the tumor, along with more surrounding soft tissue in the area. In a total mastectomy, the entire breast is removed, but the muscle tissue underneath the breast is preserved.

Axillary lymph node dissection (ALND) is the removal of some number of lymph nodes from the axilla (armpit), to prevent further cancer spread, and to stage the cancer. As in many cancer surgeries, a sentinel node biopsy (SNB) may be performed first, to test whether ALND is necessary. In this case, the surgeon removes the first lymph node or nodes that the tumor cells are likely to spread to from their starting point. If these sentinel nodes do not contain cancer, there is no need to remove additional nodes, further down the line. See "Surgery," Chapter 20, for discussion of this procedure.

Lymphedema (see Chapter 13) is an uncomfortable and disfiguring cycle of swelling that is a side effect of lymph node removal, usually from the axilla. In breast cancer, lymphedema can appear in the upper extremity and trunk on the side of lymph node removal. It may appear soon after surgery, but it can also appear years or even decades later, and the risk of lymphedema is lifelong.

It is impossible to predict whether a given individual will develop lymphedema after surgery, although other factors such as higher body weight, subsequent injury, or a later infection in the upper extremity all aggravate the risk. Removing fewer nodes, as in SNB, lowers the risk of lymphedema but does not eliminate it. In a study of 936 women at the 5-year mark after breast surgery, researchers found that 16% of patients had developed lymphedema following ALND, compared with 5% after SNB (McLaughlin et al., 2008). Even the small risk accompanying SNB is clinically significant. Effective treatment for lymphedema is limited; see Chapter 13 for specialized manual techniques that ease lymphedema.

Removal of the axillary lymph nodes can reduce mobility at the shoulder joint. Physical therapy (PT) is therefore often part of the treatment plan. In an ideal situation, a cancer rehabilitation program is available, including PT and supervised exercise to rebuild strength and flexibility after breast surgery. Research in lymphedema patients after breast surgery suggests that carefully supervised exercise may help control lymphedema (Schmitz et al., 2009). However, further study is needed to determine whether such programs *also* help to prevent lymphedema from occurring in the first place.

Some patients choose additional surgery after breast cancer treatment is complete: the reconstruction of breast tissue. Several procedures are used to create a breast out of muscle or adipose tissue from another part of the body, or implants may be used.

Surgery for breast cancer may also include a hysterectomy and removal of the ovaries to limit the body's natural production of estrogen. Estrogen creates a favorable environment for the growth of some types of breast cancer, and the surgery can reduce the risk of recurrence.

A lumpectomy or a partial mastectomy is usually followed with radiation therapy. External beam radiation may be delivered to the breast, chest, and axilla. Radiation of the axilla can injure lymph nodes, placing the person at lifelong risk of lymphedema.

Chemotherapy is also common for breast cancer. It is usually most effective as a combination of drugs. Strong side effects are possible, although they vary based on the type of chemotherapy, the dose, and the individual's tolerance of the drug. See Chapter 20 for more information about side effects of radiation therapy and chemotherapy.

Because female sex hormones such as *estrogen* and *progesterone* may encourage the growth of most forms of breast cancer, hormone therapy is used to limit the influence of these hormones. Hormone therapy is often used for several years after successful treatment, to prevent recurrence of breast cancer. These drugs include anastrozole (Arimidex), exemestane (Aromasin), and letrozole (Femara). These are *aromatase inhibitors*. They can cause heart problems, joint pain, and osteoporosis. Other drugs are tamoxifen (Nolvadex), raloxifene (Evista), and toremifene (Fareston). These *selective estrogen receptor modulators* (SERMs) cause a number of side effects, including fatigue, hot flashes, night sweats, and mood swings. Serious complications include blood clots, stroke, and increased risk of endometrial cancer. Finally, there is one *estrogen receptor downregulator*, working similarly to SERMs, called fulvestrant (Faslodex). Side effects include hot flashes, nausea, vomiting, diarrhea, and constipation.

Targeted therapies are treatments for active cancer that focus on unique features of cancer cells: for example, the synthesis of specific proteins that allow the cells to grow rapidly. Certain targeted therapies used in breast cancer include trastuzumab (Herceptin), lapatinib (Tykerb), and bevacizumab (Avastin). These drugs target those proteins and slow the growth of the cancer cells. Mild, common side effects of herceptin are flu-like symptoms, such as fever, chills, nausea, and muscle aches, which tend to pass after the first treatment.

Patients are monitored for serious side effects such as heart problems. Avastin chokes off the blood supply to tumors. It is usually well tolerated, but it can cause blood clotting problems that lead to poor wound healing and nosebleeds, as well as high blood pressure (BP). Tykerb may cause side effects including diarrhea, vomiting, and fatigue. Tykerb is given in combination with a chemotherapy drug called capecitabine (Xeloda), so side effects may be caused by chemotherapy as well as Tykerb, itself.

● INTERVIEW QUESTIONS

1. Where is (or was) the cancer in your body? Is it active or has it resolved?
2. How does the condition affect you? What are your signs and symptoms?
3. Have you had any complications? Has there been any bone involvement?
4. Has there been any lung, liver, or brain involvement? Has the function of any of these organs been affected?
5. How is or was your condition treated?
6. How has treatment affected you?
7. Did you have any lymph nodes removed? Was radiation part of your treatment? If so, where?
8. Have you had any swelling (lymphedema) as a result of cancer treatment? Have you been told you were at risk of lymphedema? Are there any precautions you were instructed to follow, such as avoiding BP readings on your arm on one side?

● MASSAGE THERAPY GUIDELINES

Consult Chapter 20 for massage adjustments related to cancer diagnosis, history, and treatment. Question 1, always an important one for any client with cancer, establishes the exact location of the cancer and whether it is active. Position for comfort, and avoid pressure and joint movement at accessible sites. Since many people find their way to massage after surgery or other successful treatment, you might not be concerned with the primary tumor. Instead, positioning, pressure, and joint movement are adapted to incisions or other areas of discomfort resulting from surgery.

A primary tumor of the breast usually causes minimal signs and symptoms, such as a painless lump in the breast, or a change in breast size, shape, or the skin of the breast. If the client reports symptoms outside of these (Question 2), chances are that the cancer is advanced, meaning distant metastasis is present. As in any advanced cancer, follow the DVT Risk Principles (see Chapter 11). In general, avoid pressure or movement that disturbs any primary or secondary lesions, and adjust the massage plan to the effects of cancer spread.

The DVT Risk Principle I. If there is an elevated risk of thrombosis, such as in the lower or upper extremities, use extremely cautious pressure (level 1 or 2 maximum) on areas of risk and avoid joint movement in those areas.

The DVT Risk Principle II. Continue to follow DVT Risk Principle I until the client's physician has assessed the client's risk of DVT, understands the potential for pressure or joint movement to disturb a blood clot at the site, speaks directly to these massage concerns, and approves the use of added pressure and joint movement in the area.

Questions 3 and 4 are arranged in descending order of the likelihood of metastasis.

If the cancer has spread to bone, you will need information about the locations and stability of bone lesions from the client's doctor in order to design a safe massage plan. Limit your overall pressure to level 1 until you have had this communication. One of the most serious complications of advanced breast cancer is bone fracture. This consequence can be due to effects on bone stability from metastasis, and the problem can be compounded by osteoporosis, which may be a complication of hormone therapy for breast cancer. See "Bone Metastasis," Chapter 20, for essential detail about adjusting massage, recognizing possible symptoms of bone involvement and communicating specific questions to the client and client's doctor.

If your client complains of neurological symptoms (numbness, weakness, burning pain), especially in the lower trunk or lower extremities, or bladder or bowel incontinence, ask the client whether she has reported these symptoms to her doctor. Your specific concern is spinal cord compression, which can indicate an extremely fragile spine. In this situation, pressure, joint movement, and even position changes could worsen the situation. If the client hasn't already spoken to her doctor, suggest an immediate phone call to the doctor's office or a visit to the emergency room.

If your client has already brought the symptoms to her doctor's attention, and the doctor has not found pathologic fracture, you can move forward with the massage. However, limit your pressure and joint movement in the affected area, and continue to communicate with the client and physician about the overall bone stability.

If lung, liver, or brain function is affected, follow the Vital Organ Principle (see Chapter 3). If breast cancer has spread to the lungs, breathing problems and coughing may be problematic. If this is the case, inclined or side-lying positioning may be best for the client. If liver function is affected, follow the Filter and Pump Principle, avoiding general circulatory intent. See "Liver Metastasis," Chapter 20, for further massage therapy guidelines when cancer involves the liver.

There is no single massage adjustment for brain function impairment because of the range of signs and symptoms that occur. Instead, different adaptations are necessary for dizziness, headaches, seizures, or other problems (see "Brain Metastasis," Chapter 20).

Common clinical features and massage therapy guidelines for breast cancer are summarized in Figure 19-3.

The client's response to Questions 5 and 6 about treatment will usually include a surgery history. You are likely to hear about chemotherapy and radiation, as well. If surgery was in the last few days, there may be one or more surgical drains. Be aware of the drain when repositioning and draping the client. See Chapter 21 for massage therapy guidelines for general surgery, and Chapter 20 for massage guidelines for cancer surgery and chemotherapy.

Adjust the massage to the effects of any drugs, and recognize that some medications, such as hormone therapy, are prescribed for several years after successful cancer treatment. With hormone therapy, you are likely to encounter symptoms such as hot flashes and joint pain. If joint pain is a side effect, limit pressure at the site, but do not be discouraged from simple "laying on of hands" at those areas. If hot flashes are an issue, make obvious adjustments to draping and room temperature. For other side effects, consult Table 21-1.

The safest approach to a slight increase in blood clot risk is to follow the DVT Risk Principles, especially if a client has other risk factors for DVT. Of the hormone therapies listed, tamoxifen has received the most attention with regard to DVT risk, and the risk is slightly elevated.

If the client is receiving targeted therapies, flu-like symptoms require a gentle session overall at first—the symptoms often resolve with successive doses of medication. Pressure should probably be limited to level 2, with limited joint movement, even rhythms, and slow speeds. If hypertension

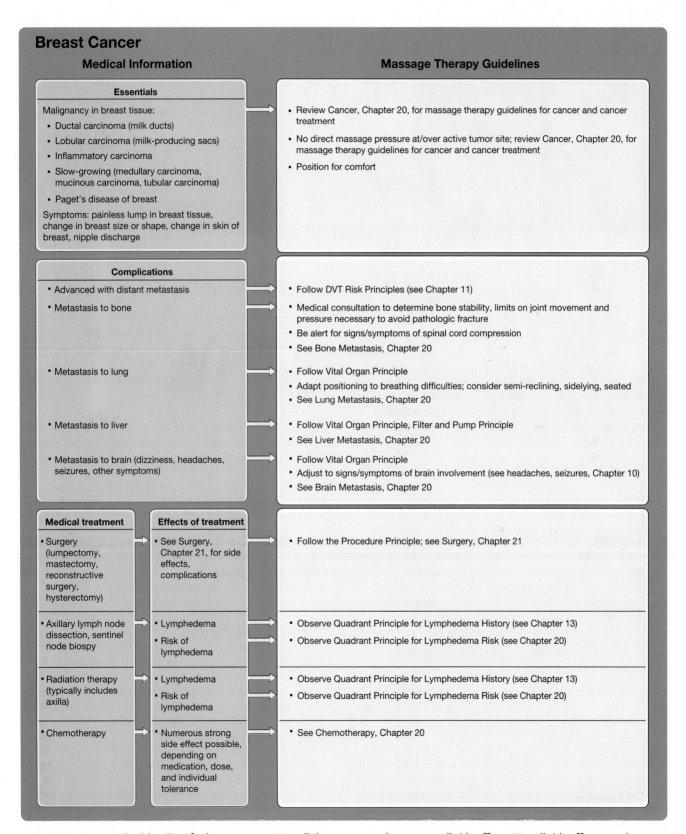

FIGURE 19-2. A Decision Tree for breast cancer. Not all drugs or procedures cause all side effects. Not all side effects are shown.

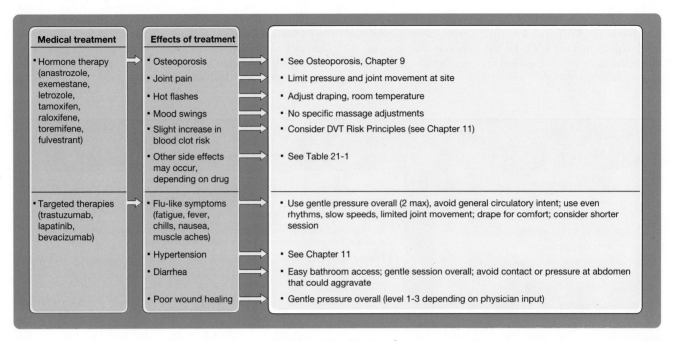

FIGURE 19-2. (*Continued*).

is a problem, see Chapter 11 for massage therapy guidelines. Simple massage adjustments for a client with diarrhea are described in the Decision Tree (see Figure 19-2). Poor wound healing calls for gentle pressure overall, in the level 1–3 range.

Questions 7 and 8 are designed to identify lymphedema or lymphedema risk. This issue may also arise in the client's answer to Question 6. If the client has experienced lymphedema, there are strict massage therapy guidelines regarding pressure, heat, friction, and positioning. This is a client with a lymphedema *history*, and you will follow the Quadrant Principle for Lymphedema History (see Chapter 13).

The Quadrant Principle for Lymphedema History. In an area of lymphedema history, as well as the associated trunk quadrant, use extreme caution to avoid aggravating lymphedema. In these areas, follow any precautions specified by the client's lymphedema therapist and health care team, limit pressure to level 1, and avoid reddening the tissues. Also avoid circulatory intent, friction, joint movement, and excessive focus on the area, and any client positions known to compromise lymph flow

Even if the client has not experienced lymphedema, Questions 7 and 8 about lymph node removal, radiation, and lymphedema are essential, because she may be at risk of it. Ask the client to point to any areas of lymph node treatment. If one or more lymph nodes in the axilla were removed or irradiated, but the client has no history of lymphedema, she is still at risk, and the risk is lifelong. Follow the Quadrant Principle for Lymphedema *Risk*, in Chapter 20. Even if only a single sentinel node was affected by treatment, and there is no history of swelling, the Quadrant Principle for Lymphedema Risk is the safest approach.

The Quadrant Principle for Lymphedema Risk. Avoid pressure above 2, reddening of the skin and strong joint movement in the at-risk region of an area of cervical, axillary, or inguinal lymph node removal or radiation therapy. This includes the extremity as well as the trunk area, anterior and posterior, drained by the affected lymph nodes.

If the client objects to your conservative approach, ask if she was ever discouraged by her nurse or doctor from having BP readings or needle sticks on the at-risk arm, and gently point out the parallel concerns about massage pressure and friction. If the client was told by a health care provider not to worry about lymphedema because her risk is minimal, let the client know that you will still tailor the session to the risk by being gentle on that side.

The principle is limiting, and in some cases, it is not well received, but it is vital. See Therapist's Journal 20-1 for a story of effective therapeutic massage, within the bounds of the Quadrant Principle for Lymphedema Risk.

● MASSAGE RESEARCH

A small flurry of research studies have focused on massage for women with breast cancer. Among them are studies in Sweden, Germany, and the United States. A few recent studies are mentioned here, and additional citations are in the Bibliography, but at the time of this writing, more data are needed to draw firm conclusions about massage in this population.

One small RCT, carried out in Sweden, tested 20-minute massage sessions in a sample of 39 breast cancer patients (Billhult et al., 2007). They reported that five sessions led to improvements in the patients' experience of nausea but not in anxiety or depression. The same researchers tested ten 20-minute effleurage sessions in an RCT of 22 women in a radiation therapy setting and found no differences between groups in immunity, cortisol, anxiety, depression, or other

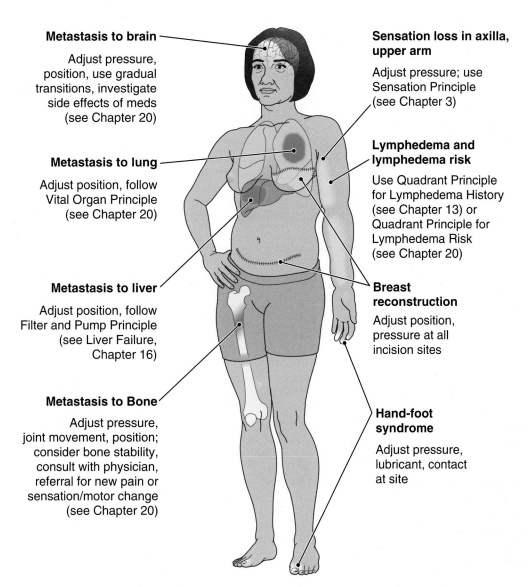

Metastasis to brain

Adjust pressure, position, use gradual transitions, investigate side effects of meds (see Chapter 20)

Metastasis to lung

Adjust position, follow Vital Organ Principle (see Chapter 20)

Metastasis to liver

Adjust position, follow Filter and Pump Principle (see Liver Failure, Chapter 16)

Metastasis to Bone

Adjust pressure, joint movement, position; consider bone stability, consult with physician, referral for new pain or sensation/motor change (see Chapter 20)

Sensation loss in axilla, upper arm

Adjust pressure; use Sensation Principle (see Chapter 3)

Lymphedema and lymphedema risk

Use Quadrant Principle for Lymphedema History (see Chapter 13) or Quadrant Principle for Lymphedema Risk (see Chapter 20)

Breast reconstruction

Adjust position, pressure at all incision sites

Hand-foot syndrome

Adjust pressure, lubricant, contact at site

FIGURE 19-3. Breast cancer: selected clinical features and massage adjustments to consider. Specific instructions and additional massage therapy guidelines are in Decision Tree and text.

factors (Billhult et al., 2008). In another study of 86 breast cancer patients, biweekly 30-minute massage sessions over 5 weeks were associated with reductions in discomfort, fatigue, and mood disturbance (Listing et al., 2009).

In surveys completed by 36 patients at the Mayo Clinic, all felt massage helped with relaxation (Pruthi et al., 2009) In addition, most felt positive changes in muscle tension, fatigue, wellness, sleep quality, and thinking clearly.

Increasing focus on massage for women with breast cancer will undoubtedly yield more research. The data will be of interest to therapists, consumers, and health care professionals in oncology and women's health.

● POSSIBLE MASSAGE BENEFITS

Depending on the stage of breast cancer and the success of treatment, the client may have a very good prognosis. But surgery is nearly always involved in a breast cancer diagnosis, and even a lumpectomy can bring on challenging body image issues. In the face of this, massage therapy may support a positive body image.

As prevalent as breast cancer is, it can be a lonely disease, and the companionship of massage therapy may be deeply welcome.

Prostate Cancer

The **prostate gland** is a small gland near the base of the penis that produces seminal fluid (semen). In **prostate cancer**, cells in the prostate become malignant, and they can remain localized, confined to the prostate gland itself, for years. Most types of prostate cancer are slow growing.

● BACKGROUND

Localized prostate cancer affects about one third of men around age 60, and the percentage increases as men get into their seventies and eighties. Years or even decades can elapse before the cancer grows outside of the prostate gland capsule. Because of screening, most cases of prostate cancer are detected before symptoms develop. Screening for prostate cancer is done with a blood test called a **prostate-specific antigen (PSA) test** and by a digital rectal exam.

Signs and Symptoms

Like many types of cancer, there are few noticeable signs and symptoms in the early stages of prostate cancer. When symptoms are felt, they are often noticed in the urine stream. It can be difficult to start the stream, or the stream might be less forceful, or a man may have difficulty passing urine at all. Urinary frequency and urgency may occur. A man might experience repeated urinary tract infections (UTIs) (see Chapter 18), or notice blood in the urine or semen. Advanced prostate cancer produces additional symptoms, described below as complications.

Complications

Prostate cancer most often spreads to the lymph nodes, bones, lungs, liver, or brain. Figure 19-4 shows the path traveled by the cancer cells in the prostate toward surrounding tissues. In advanced cases, it usually spreads to the bones, and most often to the lower spine and pelvis. At that time, it may produce pain in the spine, ribs, hips, or elsewhere. Neurological symptoms, resulting from compression of the spinal cord, include weakness and numbness in the legs or feet; bladder or bowel incontinence; and erectile dysfunction.

Prostate cancer and breast cancer present similar problems, the doubled threat of bone metastasis (from the disease itself) and osteoporosis (a complication of hormone treatment). Bone metastasis can cause severe, debilitating bone pain, but it can also be clinically silent. A sudden fracture, with no warning,

indicates damage that has already been done and is difficult to repair (see "Bone Metastasis," Chapter 20).

Treatment

Because prostate cancer often progresses slowly, the physician may adopt a **watch and wait** treatment approach, in which the cancer is monitored with regular tests, but not treated. A blood test for *prostate-specific antigen (PSA)* is used in prostate cancer screening and monitoring.

Two forms of radiation therapy are used to treat prostate cancer: standard external beam radiation and internal radiation. In internal radiation, or **brachytherapy**, small radioactive seeds called **radiation implants** are inserted into the prostate using a needle. Placing radioactive material directly inside a tumor, or a short distance away, allows close targeting of the tumor.

Either form of radiation can cause impotence, diarrhea, rectal bleeding, urinary urgency and frequency, and urinary incontinence, but the external form tends to cause more side effects. Radiation implants deliver a higher dose of radiation to the urethra, and this may cause slowed, painful, or more frequent urination. Medications or self-catheterization can help.

Most of the time, side effects of radiation fade when treatment is complete, but sometimes they persist. With brachytherapy, the patient is often told to stay at least 6 ft away from pregnant women or children for the first couple of months, until the radioactivity eases. In general, the radiation doesn't escape the body in significant doses that are a danger to others, but children, pregnant women, and a developing fetus are more vulnerable to it.

Surgical treatment, called a **radical prostatectomy**, is removal of the entire prostate gland. Depending on the surgery, nearby pelvic lymph nodes may be removed and tested for cancer. Complications of surgery include impotence and

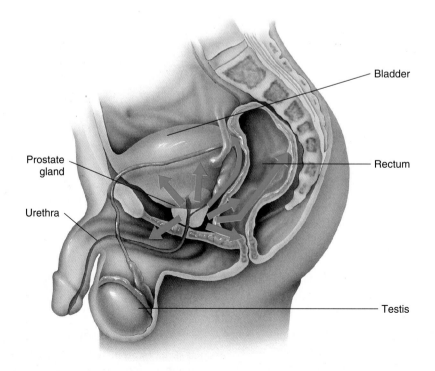

FIGURE 19-4. Prostate cancer spread.

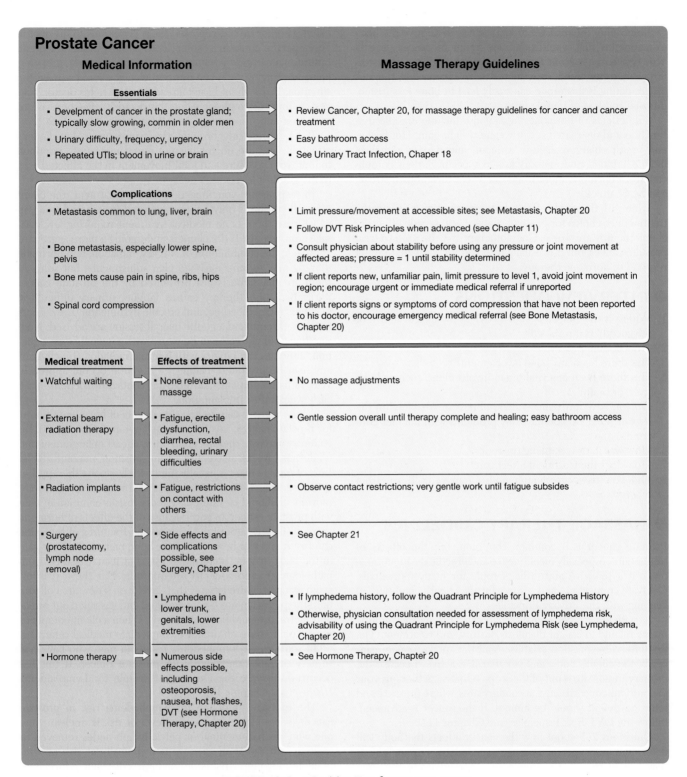

FIGURE 19-5. A Decision Tree for prostate cancer.

urinary incontinence. Infection may occur, as well; the signs are malaise, chills, fever, and sweating. Surgery and sometimes radiation can also elevate the risk of lymphedema in the genitals, lower trunk, or lower extremities.

If the tumor is large or the cancer has spread to other organs, a type of hormone therapy called **androgen-deprivation therapy** may be used. In this approach, the levels of testosterone and other male sex hormones (androgens) are reduced, or their actions are blocked by specific drugs. This therapy deprives the tumor of hormones that would otherwise stimulate it to grow. By shrinking the tumor in this way, it may be more amenable to surgery or radiation. This approach is sometimes called *chemical castration*. Hormones may be injected (Eligard, Lupron, Viadur, Zoladex, Trelstar), or oral (Casodex, Eulexin, Nilandron). Hormone therapy might follow surgery or radiation to kill any remaining cancer cells.

Removal of the testicles is another way to deprive the body of hormones that would otherwise promote cancer growth. This procedure, *orchiectomy*, prevents the release of testosterone into the blood. In either of these approaches, the lack of circulating testosterone can easily lead to bone loss (osteoporosis) and loss of muscle mass.

Side effects of hormone therapy also include erectile dysfunction and decreased sex drive and weight gain. Hot flashes and breast enlargement are frequent, and nausea, diarrhea, fatigue, anemia, and memory loss may occur. Serious complications of hormone therapy are deep vein thrombosis, stroke, and heart attack.

Even with these side effects, hormone therapy is usually the treatment of choice for prostate cancer because side effects of chemotherapy are worse. Chemotherapy may be used to treat prostate cancer, but it is usually reserved for cases that do not respond to hormone therapy.

● INTERVIEW QUESTIONS

1. Where is the cancer in your body? Is the cancer active or advanced? Is it resolved?
2. How does it affect you?
3. Has there been any bone involvement?
4. Has there been any vital organ involvement, such as lung, liver, or brain?
5. Do you have any pain? Any numbness or weakness in the legs or feet? Do you have any problems with bladder control?
6. How was it, or is it, being treated?
7. How does the treatment affect you?
8. Did you have any lymph nodes removed? If so, from where?

● MASSAGE THERAPY GUIDELINES

Prostate cancer is a common condition, but the effects of treatment—especially incontinence and erectile dysfunction—make it a sensitive and difficult topic for many individuals. Cultivate compassion and respect for the client's condition, in keeping with the Privacy Principle.

As with any cancer, consult Chapter 20 for massage adjustments related to cancer diagnosis, history, and treatment. The first interview question establishes all the known sites of cancer in the client's body, and whether it is active. Because the primary tumor site is out of the scope of massage therapy, your precautions concern active secondary sites, where pressure and joint movement should be limited. If the cancer is advanced, follow the DVT Risk Principles (see Chapter 11).

Questions 2–5 about how the cancer affects the body will determine more specific massage adjustments. Distant spread may call for many adjustments, and for following the Vital Organ Principle if the cancer has affected the function of the lungs, liver, or brain.

Questions 3 and 5 are aimed at one of the most serious consequences of advanced prostate cancer—bone fracture—either due to bone metastasis or due to osteoporosis that is caused or aggravated by hormone therapy. You need the client's doctor's input to determine the best pressures to use; stick with pressure level 1 until this dialogue has occurred, and see "Bone Metastasis," Chapter 20.

If your client complains of neurological symptoms (numbness, weakness, burning pain), especially in the lower trunk or lower extremities, or bladder or bowel incontinence, ask the client whether he has reported these symptoms to his doctor. Your specific concern is spinal cord compression, which can indicate an extremely fragile spine. In this situation, pressure, joint movement, and even position changes could worsen the situation. If the client hasn't already spoken to his doctor, suggest an immediate phone call to his doctor's office or a visit to the emergency room (see "Bone Metastasis," Chapter 20).

If he has already brought the symptoms to his doctor's attention, and the doctor has not found metastasis, continue to limit your pressure and joint movement in the affected area to the gentlest levels.

In response to your questions about treatment, the client may tell you he is only being monitored (watch and wait), in which case there is no medical treatment requiring any massage adjustments. If the client is undergoing a more aggressive approach, the combination of surgery, radiation, and hormone therapy may require massage plan adjustments, but some of them are the same issues presented by the prostate cancer itself. Radiation therapy causes fatigue, urinary difficulties, diarrhea, rectal bleeding, and erectile dysfunction. Easy access to the bathroom and a gentle overall session are advised. Note that these side effects can be worse with external beam radiation, although the fatigue with internal radiation (brachytherapy) can be profound, calling for a gentle overall approach. With radiation implants, observe any contact restrictions in the early weeks after implantation.

Adjust the massage to any side effects of hormone therapy for prostate cancer. See "Hormone Therapy," Chapter 20, for common massage therapy guidelines. Breast enlargement and tenderness might make the prone position uncomfortable. Loss of muscle mass is usually mild with hormone therapy, but if it is severe, the joints become unstable. In this case, joint movement should be limited. Osteoporosis is common in men with prostate cancer, in part because of the effects of hormone therapy (GnRH agonists). Compression fractures of the spine can result and can be mistaken for bone metastasis. New pain in the back may be bone metastasis, but it may also be from pathologic fracture due to osteoporosis. For these reasons, avoid using pressure greater than level 2 on a new area of pain until the physician has been consulted and has ruled out osteoporotic fracture and bone metastasis. When a client complains of new pain, make an urgent or immediate medical referral.

In some cases, lymphedema results in men who have had surgery or radiation therapy for prostate cancer. If this has occurred, observe the Quadrant Principle for Lymphedema *History* (see Chapter 13).

The massage guideline for lymphedema *risk* in prostate cancer is less clear because the level of risk is unclear. Anyone who has had inguinal or pelvic lymph nodes removed or treated with radiation therapy is technically at risk of lymphedema on the at-risk side, or both sides, but information and statistics about lymphedema following prostate cancer treatment are scarce. It is not as common as lymphedema after breast cancer treatment. Prostate cancer patients are often advised to take good care of the skin of the lower body, to prevent lymphedema, but these precautions are not as central to medical practice as they are after breast cancer treatment.

In the most conservative massage plan, you would follow the Quadrant Principle for Lymphedema Risk (see Chapter 20). However, it is difficult to find supporting information in the medical literature for this precaution, making it difficult to determine the best massage practice. For many patients after prostate cancer treatment, the Quadrant Principle for

THERAPIST'S JOURNAL 19-1 *My Alternative Experience of Prostate Cancer*

In July of 2002, I graduated from massage school. Three months later, when I was just 58 years old, I was diagnosed with prostate cancer. So at the same time I'd finally found something I wanted to do with my life, I felt that quite possibly my life was over.

I had had a couple of years of elevated PSA tests in my annual physical, although the manual examination continued to suggest there wasn't a problem—the prostate was of normal size. Because of the elevated PSA, my doctor sent me to a urologist, who did a PSA test. The results of that test indicated there was need for further investigation. He ordered a biopsy, an outpatient procedure. For the biopsy, they gave me a local anesthetic and Valium—it's important to be relaxed for the procedure. They used ultrasound to guide it and took multiple tissue samples. There are usually few side effects—just blood in urine and ejaculate. Out of the six sections of the prostate tested, two had active tumors, but the tests showed that the cancer was confined to the prostate and had not broken free of the capsule. So there was no need for lymph node sampling or other images for looking at spread.

After the biopsy, I had to come to grips with the idea of having active cancer. I talked a lot to my urologist. Being a surgeon, his recommendation was surgery. But he also had written about treating the prostate naturally. I bought his book and talked with him about supplements and dietary changes. I have a lot of respect for my urologist. He is such a peaceful spirit. His office reflects the life that he leads and his practice of other forms of healing.

I was no fan of surgery, so I opted for this other approach. I went for it.

My urologist wanted to do a second biopsy after a year. I didn't want to do anything that early or frequently. I waited until 4 years later. The second biopsy showed that there were no signs of cancer in the sampled tissue. My urologist reminded me that this didn't mean there was none in my body, just no cancer in the samples. I see him every 6 months to monitor my PSA. It's lower, still a bit high, but no one's very concerned about it.

I consider myself healthy and cancer free. I go on working at keeping myself stress free, too. There have been no massage contraindications because of the prostate cancer. In fact, massage, acupuncture, and Reiki have played a big part in my stress management. I have been getting far away from the idea of managing stress. I don't want to manage it—I just want to not have it in the first place. So I work hard to create my life with as little stress as possible. The experience of cancer taught me a lot that I bring to my clients. Cancer isn't just something that invades the body—it reflects a dysfunction in the body. I choose to treat the underlying dysfunction.

I like helping my clients pay close attention to their lives, and the things that are happening when they're experiencing pain or illness. Many times my older clients take on so much—care of spouses or parents, care of others—while not seeing to their own needs. They're tired, lacking sleep and good food and time for themselves. They look outside for things to adjust in their lives—a medical treatment, a new mattress that might help their sleep or pain. One client realized she didn't need the mattress; she needed to interrupt the cycle of stress and care for others, to address the dysfunction. Massage helped her sleep. She sent me a beautiful card, something to the effect that, "What a blessing my massage was today. I am so grateful. It's just what the Lord ordered today and my body is much relaxed tonight."

Lemuel Sherman
Raleigh, NC

Lymphedema Risk is probably too conservative, but for some, it is a better fit. When in doubt, the client's doctor should be consulted about the client's level of risk and the advisability of pressure in the areas of tissue drained by the missing or damaged lymph nodes. Because this could include both lower extremities, review discussion in Chapter 20 on lymphedema and consult the physician.

● MASSAGE RESEARCH

As of this writing, there are no RCTs, published in the English language, on prostate cancer and massage indexed in PubMed or the Massage Therapy Foundation Research Database. The NIH RePORTER tool lists no active, federally funded research projects on this topic in the United States. No active projects are listed on the clinicaltrials.gov database (see Chapter 6).

One study noted that little information was available on complementary and alternative medicine CAM therapies in patients with prostate cancer (Kao and Devine, 2000), and that they were surprised when their survey of 50 prostate cancer patients suggested that 37% were using CAM therapies. Of those, 18% were utilizing massage therapy or chiropractic care. If this small study reflects massage utilization in the larger population of men with prostate cancer, then studies on massage benefits should follow.

● POSSIBLE MASSAGE BENEFITS

Prostate cancer can be as challenging as any other cancer experience, even without treatment. Individuals finding themselves in a phase of "Watch and Wait" describe it as essentially waiting for things to get worse, but hoping they don't. Massage can provide wonderful support and reconnection to the body for clients with prostate cancer, no matter what the status or outlook may be. Therapist's Journal 19-1 is a story of prostate cancer, stress, and the role of massage.

Other Reproductive System Conditions in Brief

BENIGN PROSTATIC HYPERPLASIA (PROSTATE GLAND ENLARGEMENT)

Background	• Enlarged prostate gland presses on proximal end of urethra, causing difficulty starting urine stream, weak stream, urinary frequency and urgency, stopping and starting, incomplete bladder emptying, blood in urine; common with advancing age. • Complications include UTI, bleeding (uncommon), kidney damage (uncommon). • Treatment for moderate cases includes medications—α-blockers to relax muscles at neck of bladder, or testosterone blockers to shrink gland. • α-blockers cause dizziness, fatigue, hypotension; testosterone blockers work slowly, can cause erectile dysfunction. • Treatment to shrink prostate uses microwave therapy, radiofrequency therapy, electrovaporization, or laser therapy; prostatic stent can widen urethra. • Surgical removal for severe cases; includes transurethral removal of excess prostate or incisions in gland to make way for urethra; open prostatectomy for severe cases.
Interview Questions	• Is bathroom access necessary? Any bladder infection or kidney damage? • Any pain in low back, pelvis, or upper thighs? Do you ever have any symptoms of UTI? Fever, chills, etc.? • Treatment? Effects of treatment?
Massage Therapy Guidelines	• Provide easy bathroom access. • Adapt massage to bladder infection or rare kidney damage (see Chapter 18). Medical referral if unexplained low-back, pelvis or upper thigh pain; immediate medical referral if signs of infection. • Slow rise from table if dizziness, hypotension present; gentle session overall for fatigue.

CERVICAL CANCER

Background	• Slow-growing cancer of the cervix; uncommon in the United States due to early detection (Pap smear). • Asymptomatic in early stages, can cause changes in vaginal discharge, abnormal bleeding, spotting after intercourse. • Advanced cases can cause anemia, pain in pelvic area and low back, swelling of legs, loss of appetite, unintended weight loss. • Complications include spread to vagina, ureters, pelvic wall, bladder, rectum; common distant sites include liver, lung, bone. • Treatments of noninvasive cancer include cone biopsy, laser surgery, cryosurgery, and loop electrosurgical excision; often no other treatment is needed. • Invasive cancer treated with surgery (several levels of hysterectomy; may cause pelvic pain, bowel and bladder difficulty). • If radiation therapy is given to pelvic area, side effects include nausea, stomach upset, diarrhea, and bladder irritation. • Low-dose chemotherapy often used with radiation; higher-dose chemotherapy for more advanced cases. • Prevalence of diagnosed lymphedema in cervical cancer survivors may be around 12.2%; undiagnosed lower limb swelling about 14% (Beesley et al., 2007).
Interview Questions	• Where is it in your body? How does it affect you? • Symptoms? Complications? Any effects on liver, bone, or lung? • Treatment? Effects of treatment? Any lymph nodes removed?

| Massage Therapy Guidelines | • Review Chapter 20, for massage therapy guidelines for cancer and cancer treatment.
• If noninvasive, minor surgical procedure used to treat, no specific contraindications except postsurgery (see Chapter 21).
• If advanced, follow DVT Risk Principles (see Chapter 11).
• Adjust massage to sites of cancer spread; avoid circulatory intent at sites of swelling (often lower extremities).
• Follow Vital Organ Principle if lungs or liver involved (see Chapters 16 and 20); adjust position for breathing difficulty (consider side-lying, seated, semi-reclining); gentle focus on muscles of breathing may assist respiration.
• If bone involvement, see "Bone Metastasis," Chapter 20; if pain, especially new, unfamiliar, or increasing pain, do not use pressure or joint movement at site until physician verifies that no bone metastasis is present.
• If liver function impaired, avoid general circulatory intent, adjust position for liver enlargement; (see "Liver Cancer," Chapter 16).
• If lymphedema present, follow Quadrant Principle for Lymphedema History (see Chapter 13).
• If no lymphedema history, seek physician input to determine lymphedema risk after surgery and radiation, advisability of Quadrant Principle for Lymphedema Risk (see Chapter 20). |

DYSMENORRHEA

Background	• Painful menstruation; primary, with no known pelvic cause; secondary to endometriosis, uterine fibroids, pelvic inflammatory disease (PID). • Symptoms include cramps, nausea, diarrhea, headache, and fatigue/malaise; pain prior to menstruation, subsides 12–72 hours after. • Treatment usually NSAIDs, perhaps low-dose oral contraceptives, which can cause bloating, nausea, stomach upset, headache.
Interview Questions	• Painful cramps now? Cause? Is an underlying cause known and/or treated? • Any special positioning for massage? • Treatment? Effects of treatment?
Massage Therapy Guidelines	• Adapt positioning; side-lying might be best. • Avoid abdominal pressure; pressure on low back, hips, upper thighs OK if well tolerated. • Adapt massage to cause (see Endometriosis, Fibroids, and Pelvic Inflammatory Disease, this chapter). • See "NSAIDs," Chapter 21; see Table 21-1 for massage guidelines for oral contraceptive side effects.

ENDOMETRIAL CANCER (UTERINE ADENOCARCINOMA)

Background	• Cancer of uterine lining or uterine muscle; usually develops after menopause. Often found at early stage, symptoms include abnormal vaginal bleeding (bleeding between menstrual periods or after menopause), irregular or heavy periods, unusual vaginal discharge. • Symptoms of advanced disease include pelvic pain, swelling/fullness in abdomen, urinary difficulty or pain, bowel or bladder problems, swelling in groin. • May spread to vagina, bladder, bowel; distant metastases include lung, liver, bone, brain. • Treatments are surgery (hysterectomy and removal of ovaries and fallopian tubes), internal radiation therapy, and/or external radiation therapy. • Hormone therapy, chemotherapy used, typically if spread is beyond uterus. • Prevalence of diagnosed lymphedema in uterine cancer survivors may be around 8.2%; undiagnosed lower limb swelling about 14% (Beesley et al., 2007).
Interview Questions	• Where is it in your body? How does it affect you? • Symptoms? Complications? Any anemia? Effects on liver, bone, lung, or brain? • Treatment? Effects of treatment? Lymph nodes removed?

Massage Therapy Guidelines	• Review Chapter 20 for massage therapy guidelines for cancer and cancer treatment. • If cancer noninvasive, minor surgical procedure used to treat, no specific massage adjustments except postsurgery (see Chapter 21). • If advanced, follow DVT Risk Principles (see Chapter 11). • Adjust massage to sites of cancer spread; avoid circulatory intent at sites of swelling (often lower extremities). • Follow Vital Organ Principle if brain, lungs, or liver involved; adjust position for breathing difficulty (consider side-lying, seated, semi-reclining); gentle focus on muscles of breathing may assist respiration. • If bone involvement, see "Bone Metastasis," Chapter 20; if pain, especially new, unfamiliar, or increasing pain, do not use pressure or joint movement at site until physician verifies that no bone metastasis is present. • If liver function impaired, avoid general circulatory intent, adjust position for liver enlargement; (see "Liver Metastasis," Chapter 20; "Liver Cancer," Chapter 16). • If brain involvement, adjust massage to complications (see "Brain Metastasis," Chapter 20). • If lymphedema present, follow Quadrant Principle for Lymphedema History (see Chapter 13). • If no lymphedema history, seek physician input to determine lower extremity lymphedema risk after surgery and radiation, advisability of Quadrant Principle for Lymphedema Risk (see Chapter 20), and whether any precaution should be unilateral or bilateral.

ENDOMETRIOSIS

Background	• Formation of endometrial (uterine lining) tissue outside the uterus, usually in the pelvis; common sites are the surface of the ovaries, uterine ligaments, fallopian tubes, bowel, bladder. • Displaced tissues build up and bleed during menstruation; resolves during menopause. • Symptoms are heavy or frequent menstrual periods, premenstrual spotting, blood in urine. Pain occurs during menstruation, intercourse, urination, bowel movements. Pain may be constant or cyclical, with the menstrual period. • Infertility is the main complication (about one third of women who have difficulty becoming pregnant have endometriosis). • Treatment for pain is NSAIDs; oral contraceptives used to limit menstrual flow and ease symptoms for a period of time; symptoms resume when therapy is stopped. • Hormonal therapies include GnRH agonists and antagonists, progestins (injected Depo-Provera), danazol; generally used to stop menstrual period for 6 months or more, and/or shrink spots of endometriosis by limiting the effects of estrogen on the tissue. • Hormonal therapies may cause symptoms of menopause, weight gain, bloating, depressed mood, fatigue, bone loss, and other symptoms. • Surgical removal of endometrial growths by laparoscopy or major surgery; hysterectomy is done as last resort.
Interview Questions	• How does it affect you? How is it affecting you today? What are your symptoms? Any complications? • Are you comfortable lying face down? Are there other positions that would be more comfortable? How do you sleep? • Treatment? Effects of treatment?
Massage Therapy Guidelines	• Adjust position for comfort; consider side-lying position, which may be the most comfortable if dysmenorrhea is present. • Limit abdominal massage pressure to level 2 in most cases. • Be sensitive to fertility issues (see "Female Infertility," this chapter) • Adjust to effects of NSAIDs (see Chapter 21), oral contraceptives (see Table 21-1). Adjust to breast tenderness with padding above, below, and possibly between the breasts for prone position.

• Adjust massage to effects of GnRH agonists (see "Depression," Chapter 10; other side effects, Table 21-1). Adapt to hot flashes by adjusting draping, ambient temperature. See "Surgery," Chapter 21.

FIBROIDS (UTERINE FIBROIDS)

Background	• Common, often asymptomatic benign growths of uterine smooth muscle tissue, projecting into uterine cavity (submucosal fibroids) or outside uterus toward other organs (subserosal fibroids).
	• Symptoms include heavy, prolonged menstruation and bleeding between periods; pain in pelvis, low back, and legs; constipation; urinary frequency and incontinence.
	• Anemia, fatigue, and infertility possible.
	• GnRH may be used (leuprolide, goserelin), also hormonal contraceptives (progestins), or raloxifene (see Breast Cancer) to temporarily shrink fibroids; side effects are menopausal hot flashes, weight gain, headaches, mood changes, acne, or unwanted hair growth. Surgical options are myomectomy (removal from uterine wall), resection through vagina, arterial embolization, or hysterectomy.
Interview Questions	• How does it affect you? Symptoms? Any anemia?
	• Which positions are comfortable for you when lying down?
	• Treatment? Effects of treatment?
Massage Therapy Guidelines	• Position for comfort (flat prone position may be poorly tolerated); limit pressure at abdomen to level 1–2.
	• Adapt to side effects of treatments (see "Female Infertility," this chapter, for massage adjustments for GnRH; "Breast Cancer" for massage adjustments to raloxifene.
	• If anemic, Gentle session overall; reposition gently, slow speed and even rhythm, slow rise from table, gentle transition at end of session; adjust ambient temperature; drape for warmth.

MALE INFERTILITY (MALE FACTOR INFERTILITY)

Background	• Inability to conceive, usually caused by problems with sperm including poor movement or shape, low concentration, impairment by high temperature within the testicle, or inability of the testicle to produce sperm.
	• In 5–10% of cases, may be hormonal in cause: inadequate testosterone production; may be caused by treatment for hypertension.
	• Sexual problems such as erectile dysfunction, premature ejaculation can impair sperm delivery, or blockage of ejaculatory ducts.
	• Complications include low self-esteem, inadequacy, guilt, depression, anxiety, problems with sleep, sexual problems.
	• Treatment of general sexual problems, surgical treatment of structural problems, hormone treatments (oral, injected, or skin gels/patches).
	• Hormonal treatments are FSH, hCG, hMG (see "Female Infertility," this chapter), with side effects including acne, breast enlargement, enlargement of penis and testes, irritability, restlessness.
	• Clomiphene citrate, bromocriptine cause side effects similar to use in female infertility (this chapter).
Interview Questions	• Are there any other associated medical conditions or treatments, such as treatment for high BP?
	• Any recent surgery for the condition? Any injection site, or sites of skin applications such as gels or patches?
	• Treatment? Effects of treatment?
Massage Therapy Guidelines	• If caused by antihypertensive medication, adapt massage to medication and hypertension (see Chapter 11).
	• For injected medications, avoid circulatory intent at injection site for several hours, or until drug peaks.

- Avoid disturbing drug patches; if medication is a gel, avoid direct contact with the area of application, or glove to avoid absorbing it through the skin of your hands.
- Adapt to side effects of medications (see "Female Infertility" this chapter).

MISCARRIAGE (SPONTANEOUS ABORTION)

Background	- Termination in 15% of recognized pregnancies; usually occurs in first 12 weeks. - Symptoms include vaginal spotting, bleeding, or discharge of fluid, mucus, clots, or tissue; cramping in abdomen; low-back pain. - Can be due to abnormal fetal development, uncontrolled diabetes or thyroid disease, hormonal problems, structural problems in uterus or cervix, blood clotting disorders. - Threatened miscarriage is bleeding with no cervical dilation, and pregnancy often proceeds to term. - With cervical dilation, a contracting uterus, and bleeding, miscarriage is inevitable. - Complications include infection, fever, chills, severe pain, intense bleeding. Treatment may include D&C: dilation of cervix and curettage or scraping to remove remaining pregnancy tissue, including fetus.
Interview Questions	- When did it occur? Do you feel like your body has stabilized since then? - Have you had more than one miscarriage? - Did you have a lot of pain, or any complications such as infection? - Do you have any associated conditions such as diabetes or blood clotting problems? - Were you treated afterward with surgical procedure?
Massage Therapy Guidelines	- Use warmth and compassion and respect privacy during questioning; gentle session overall following miscarriage. - If bleeding is still occurring, or miscarriage was recent (last 12 weeks), recurrent, or associated with thrombophilia, follow DVT Risk Principles (see Chapter 11). - Adjust to identified cause (see "Diabetes Mellitus," "Hypothyroidism," and "Hyperthyroidism," Chapter 17; "Female Infertility," this chapter; "Thrombophilia," Chapter 11). - No pressure above level 2 on abdomen.

OVARIAN CANCER (OVARIAN EPITHELIAL CARCINOMA)

Background	- Cancer of the ovary; most common (85–90%) in the epithelial covering. - Asymptomatic in early stages, or vague, nonspecific symptoms: abdominal bloating, fullness, or pain; pelvic pain or discomfort; urinary urgency is most common; other symptoms are indigestion, nausea, change in bowel or bladder habits, unintended weight loss, fatigue, low back pain, pain during intercourse, swelling in lower extremities. - Can spread to uterus, fallopian tubes, peritoneum, other abdominal structures; distant spread most common to lungs, liver, bones; metastasis to brain less common. - Advanced ovarian cancer usually recurs. - Treated with surgery (hysterectomy plus removal of ovaries, fallopian tubes). - Diagnosed lymphedema prevalence in ovarian cancer survivors may be low (around 5%). - Prevalence of diagnosed lymphedema in ovarian cancer survivors may be low, around 5%; undiagnosed lower limb swelling about 16% (Beesley et al., 2007). - Strong chemotherapy may be systemic (IV) or regional (directly into peritoneal cavity), with strong side effects (see Chapter 20); radiation therapy not a primary treatment; if used, it can cause fatigue or bowel obstruction.
Interview Questions	- Where is it in your body? How does it affect you? - Symptoms? Complications? Effects on liver, bone, lung, or brain? - Treatment? Effects of treatment? Lymph nodes removed?
Massage Therapy Guidelines	- Review "Cancer," Chapter 20, for massage therapy guidelines for cancer and cancer treatment. - If advanced, follow DVT Risk Principles (see Chapter 11). - Adjust massage to sites of cancer spread; avoid circulatory intent at sites of swelling (often lower extremities).

- Follow Vital Organ Principle if brain, lungs, or liver involved; adjust position for breathing difficulty (consider side-lying, seated, semi-reclining); gentle focus on muscles of breathing may assist respiration.
- If bone involvement, see "Bone Metastasis," Chapter 20; if pain, especially new, unfamiliar, or increasing pain, do not use pressure or joint movement at site until physician verifies that no bone metastasis is present.
- If liver function impaired, avoid general circulatory intent, adjust position for liver enlargement; (see "Liver Cancer," Chapter 16).
- If brain involvement, adjust massage to complications (see "Brain Metastasis," Chapter 20).
- If in treatment, ask about vascular access device or intraperitoneal infusion site and avoid pressure around site.
- If lymphedema present, follow Quadrant Principle for Lymphedema History (see Chapter 13).
- If no lymphedema history, seek client's physician's input to determine lower extremity lymphedema risk after surgery and radiation, advisability of Quadrant Principle for Lymphedema Risk (see Chapter 20).

PELVIC INFLAMMATORY DISEASE (PID)

Background

- Inflammation from bacterial infection of any upper reproductive organs: cervix, uterus, fallopian tubes, ovaries; can be chronic or acute.
- Bacteria (usually those that cause gonorrhea or chlamydia) may enter during sexual activity, or during douching, vaginal birth, or medical procedure.
- Can be asymptomatic or cause cyclical symptoms at end of menstrual period or for few days following.
- Chronic symptoms include mild pain, in lower abdomen, low-back pain, irregular menstruation, lethargy, pain during intercourse, heavy vaginal discharge with unpleasant odor.
- Acute PID includes more severe pain in lower abdomen, fever, vaginal discharge, irregular bleeding; later, high fever, discharge with pus. Complications include blocked, swollen, abscessed fallopian tubes; irregular bleeding, and pain in lower abdomen; can progress to peritonitis: nausea, vomiting, dangerously low BP (shock), and then sepsis.
- May spread from fallopian tubes to tissues surrounding liver, with pain in upper right abdomen.
- Complications also include adhesions that cause infertility; later tubal pregnancy possible.
- Treated with antibiotics, unless its symptoms are severe or don't respond to treatment; pain relievers until symptoms improve, usually in 10–14 days on antibiotics.
- Abscesses may be drained surgically.

Interview Questions

- When diagnosed? Chronic or acute? How does it affect you?
- Which structures affected? Any complications?
- Treatment? Effects of treatment?

Massage Therapy Guidelines

- Have compassion and respect privacy, as complications include infertility and cause includes sexually transmitted disease.
- If infection is chronic, gentle overall session, avoiding pressure above 2 in lower abdomen.
- If infection acute, avoid general circulatory intent, avoid pressure >1 at lower abdomen if infection resolved, general circulatory intent okay, but no pressure above level 2 in lower abdomen or any other affected area (e.g. around liver).
- Adapt massage to recent surgery (see Chapter 21) and side effects of pain medication, antibiotics (see Table 21-1).

POLYCYSTIC OVARY SYNDROME/DISEASE (PCOS; OVARIAN CYSTS)

Background

- Fluid-filled sacs (cysts) on ovaries due to excess pituitary production of LH, causing increased androgen (male hormone) production by ovaries and adrenal glands.
- Caused by increased insulin production (as in metabolic syndrome, diabetes), hereditary factors.
- Abnormal hormone activity impairs follicle formation and release of eggs during ovulation.

- Symptoms are pelvic pain; skin changes (excess oil, acne, and darkened skin); abnormal vaginal bleeding.
- Possible male features include body hair growth, increased skeletal muscle mass, deepening voice.
- Complications: PCOS is most common cause of infertility in the United States and elevates risk of miscarriage; increased risk of metabolic syndrome, type 2 diabetes, hypertension, fatty liver disease, gestational diabetes, pregnancy-induced hypertension.
- Treatment with metformin (Glucophage) for insulin levels, dietary changes, weight loss.
- Low-dose oral contraceptives regulate menstruation and androgen levels; a male hormone blocker reduces excess body hair but may increase urine production and cause hypotension and fainting.
- Surgery to remove cysts is last course of treatment.

Interview Questions	- How does it affect you? Any particular large cysts that concern your doctor? Cause? - Complications involving diabetes or other endocrine problems? Any cardiovascular complications? - From your doctor or nurse, any mention of blood clot risk due to treatment or other factors? Any pain or positioning preferences? - Treatment? Effects of treatment?
Massage Therapy Guidelines	- No abdominal pressure above 2 with active cysts; position for comfort. - For related conditions, adapt massage to fatty liver disease (see Chapter 16); metabolic syndrome, diabetes (see Chapter 17); CV conditions (see Chapter 11). - Slow rise from table with hypotension, fainting; easy access to bathroom for increased urine production. - See "Diabetes," Chapter 17, for side effects of metformin.

PREGNANCY (NORMAL, UNCOMPLICATED)

Background	- Condition of carrying a fetus; trimester 1 = weeks 0–12; trimester 2 = weeks 13–24; trimester 3 = weeks 13–birth, after last menstrual period. - Dramatic cardiovascular changes include increased cardiac output beginning at 6 weeks, increased blood volume beginning in 1st trimester, decreased BP in trimesters 1 and 2 as peripheral vessels dilate to divert blood to uterus, increase in blood coagulability in trimester 3. - Supine hypotensive syndrome (nausea, dizziness, poor blood flow to fetus) may occur in flat supine position.
Interview Questions	- How far along is your pregnancy? What is your due date? - What kind of prenatal care are you receiving? - How are you feeling? How has your pregnancy been going? What kinds of symptoms have you noticed? - Have you had any problems or complications with your pregnancy, or with previous pregnancy? Are there any risk factors or problems that your doctor is monitoring closely? - Are you taking any medications or undergoing any procedures as part of your prenatal care?
Massage Therapy Guidelines	- For normal pregnancies, use conservative approach overall. - For complicated or high-risk pregnancies, see Osborne (2011); Stager (2009); Stillerman (2007). - No abdominal pressure above 1–2 in first trimester (some advise no contact at all with abdomen, as a liability precaution) - Observe point contraindications, below, and any others thought to affect gland function or stimulate preterm labor; to avoid inadvertent stimulation of points, avoid focused, deep pressure on the feet and hands. - Point contraindications include Hoku acupressure point (Stomach—36) at the web of the thumb and index finger; Spleen—6 acupressure point, on the medial low leg, about four finger-widths proximal to the malleolus; Kidney—3 acupressure point, at top of the medial malleolus; Liver—3 acupressure point, where the first and second metatarsal bones meet; reflexology points for the ovaries and uterus, located inferior and posterior to the lateral and medial malleolus, respectively. - Position for safety and comfort. - 1st trimester: supine, prone, side-lying, semi-reclining, seated are safe; prone may require padding to reduce pressure on tender breasts

- 2nd trimester: supine up to week 22, position supine with slight elevation under right hip (such as a folded bath towel or small pillow) to shift fetus off of inferior vena cava; discontinue prone and supine at week 22, or when client is uncomfortable, or when client's doctor advises, whichever comes first.
- 3rd trimester: side-lying, seated, or semi-reclining with client's back at minimum 45-degree angle with massage surface.
- Consider DVT Risk Principles (see Chapter 11), especially if additional risk factors exist; be alert for signs of DVT; always avoid pressure above 2 on medial thigh, medial low leg, or at any sites of varicose veins on lower extremities
- For heartburn, position for comfort, schedule massage well after meal where possible.
- For relaxed ligaments, limit joint movement: no strong stretches or ROM; no ROM at hips if pubic symphysis pain/separation has occurred.
- For swelling of wrists, ankles, feet: avoid circulatory intent at swollen ankles, lower legs without MD consultation about DVT risk; massage may ease pain at wrists.
- For high risk and complicated pregnancies, refer to texts on massage and pregnancy (Osborne, 2011; Stager, 2009)
- If client reports signs/symptoms of complicated pregnancy (vaginal bleeding/discharge, strong headache, vision disturbances, systemic edema, rapid weight gain, severe vomiting, back pain that does not resolve with position change, frequent urination, excessive hunger or thirst, early contractions, pelvic pain or cramping, low weight gain, decreased fetal movement, or anything else unusual), refrain from massage and urge immediate medical referral.

PREMENSTRUAL SYNDROME

Background	- Symptoms are fluid retention, breast tenderness, abdominal bloating, weight gain, mood swings, depression, anxiety, stress, irritability, crying spells, anger, insomnia, muscle and joints, food cravings, for up to one week prior to start of menstrual bleeding. - Treatments are dietary and lifestyle changes, pain relievers (NSAIDs), antidepressants, oral contraceptives.
Interview Questions	- Are you experiencing PMS now? How does it affect you? - Treatment? Effects of treatment?
Massage Therapy Guidelines	- Be sensitive and keep steady demeanor for mood problems. - Position comfortably for breast tenderness. - Adapt to effects of treatment (see NSAIDs, Chapter 21; antidepressants, Chapter 10; all other side effects, see Table 21-1).

TESTICULAR CANCER

Background	- Most common cancer in American males age 15–34; subtypes seminoma (40–45% of all testicular cancers; slow growing), nonseminoma (other types of tumors); more than 95% of men diagnosed with testicular cancer survive the disease. - Symptoms include lump or enlargement in testicle; feeling of heaviness, pain, or discomfort in testicle or scrotum; fluid accumulation in scrotum, dull ache in abdomen or groin also possible. - Other symptoms are fatigue, malaise, and development of excess breast tissue. - Complications include metastasis to retroperitoneal lymph nodes (located in abdomen); sites of distant spread include lungs, liver, brain, and bones, especially spine. - Treatment: surgery, radiation therapy, and chemotherapy. - Retroperitoneal lymph node dissection (removal of abdominal lymph nodes) may be done during surgery, or may follow other therapies if concern about cancer spread remains. - Information about lymphedema prevalence after testicular cancer is limited, but lymphedema has been documented following treatment. - Complications of treatment include infertility, erectile dysfunction.

Interview Questions	• Where is it in your body? How does it affect you? • Symptoms? Complications? Effects on liver, bone, lung, or brain? • Treatment? Effects of treatment? Lymph nodes removed?
Massage Therapy Guidelines	• Review "Cancer," Chapter 20, for massage therapy guidelines for cancer and cancer treatment. • If advanced, follow DVT Risk Principles (see Chapter 11). • Adjust massage to sites of cancer spread. • Follow Vital Organ Principle if brain, lungs, or liver involved; adjust position for breathing difficulty (consider side-lying, seated, semi-reclining); gentle focus on muscles of breathing may assist respiration. • If bone involvement, see "Bone Metastasis," Chapter 20; if pain, especially new, unfamiliar, or increasing pain, do not use pressure or joint movement at site until physician verifies that no bone metastasis is present. • If liver function impaired, avoid general circulatory intent, adjust position for liver enlargement; (see "Liver Cancer," Chapter 16). • If brain involvement, adjust massage to complications (see "Brain Metastasis," Chapter 20). • If lymphedema present, follow Quadrant Principle for Lymphedema History (see Chapter 13). • If no lymphedema history, seek physician input to determine lower extremity lymphedema risk after surgery and radiation, advisability of Quadrant Principle for Lymphedema Risk on one or both sides (see Chapter 20).

SELF TEST

1. Why should you follow massage precautions for pregnancy when working with a female client undergoing fertility treatment?
2. List three side effects of fertility medications and corresponding massage therapy guidelines.
3. How can you best support clients who are dealing with the stress of infertility and its treatment?
4. Define the term *in situ* and compare the two common types of breast cancer *in situ*.
5. Why do you pay close attention to whether a client with breast cancer has had any lymph nodes removed? Compare and explain the two principles you would follow if so, and when you would follow them.
6. Compare hormone therapies and targeted therapies in the treatment of breast cancer. Which group is primarily used to prevent recurrence? Which drugs tend to cause hot flashes?
7. How should you adjust a massage for flu-like symptoms caused by targeted therapies?

8. What is the most likely site of metastasis in breast cancer? How do you adapt the massage plan in this case?
9. Does research prove a benefit of massage therapy in women with breast cancer? Describe the suggested benefits of available research.
10. List four symptoms of prostate cancer.
11. Describe two common treatments for prostate cancer.
12. Describe the radiation implants used in prostate cancer and the contact precautions to follow for several weeks after they are inserted.
13. Explain two reasons why bone fracture may occur in prostate cancer.
14. Where does bone metastasis often cause pain in patients with prostate cancer? How should you adjust massage in this case?
15. How and why do prostate cancer treatments focus on testosterone?

 For answers to these questions and to see a bibliography for this chapter, visit http://thePoint.lww.com/Walton.

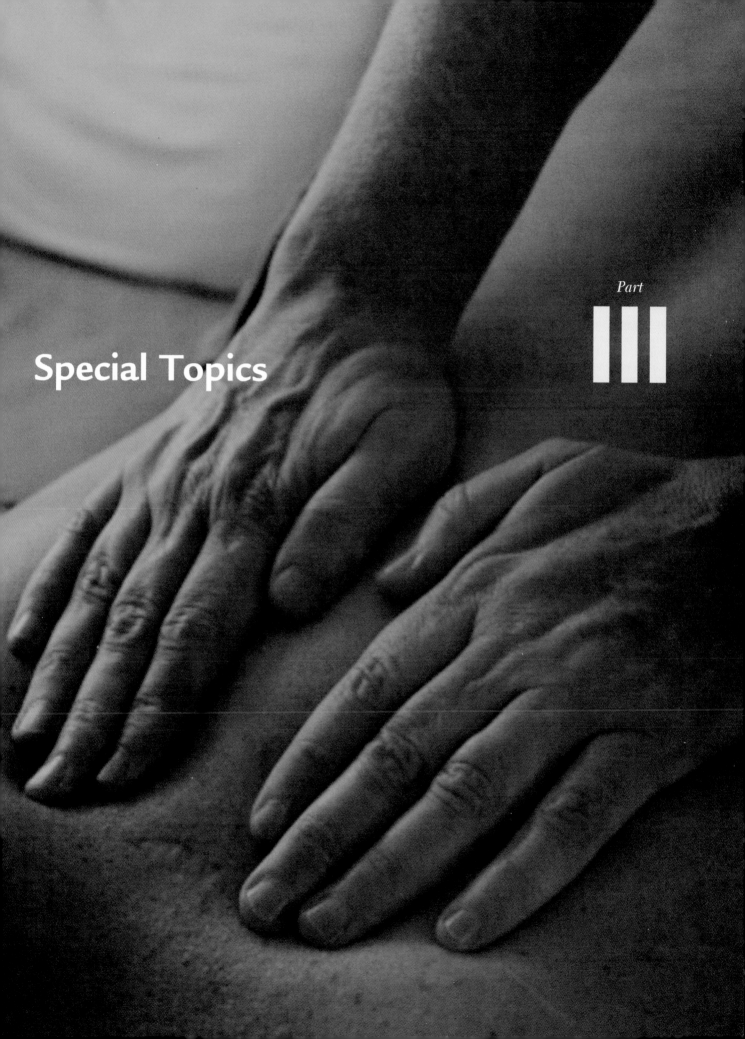

Special Topics

20 Cancer

Massage therapy is not contraindicated in cancer patients. Massaging a tumor is, but there is a great deal more to a person than the tumor.

—BERNIE SIEGEL

Many massage therapists work with people who have cancer, and many people with the disease seek out massage throughout treatment, at end of life, in survivorship, and during diagnosis. Bernie Siegel, the well-known patient advocate, speaks to the wholeness of the person with cancer, above and beyond his or her medical condition. Massage therapists are drawn to this wholeness, and the potential of massage to make a difference in the well-being of cancer patients.

At the time of this writing, a groundswell of interest in massage for people with cancer is evident: research and training are increasing, and growing numbers of hospitals and treatment centers offer massage to patients and families affected by cancer. The Society for Oncology Massage was recently formed to provide standards of practice, education, and advocacy. These and other developments reflect a broadening acceptance of massage, as well as the desire of massage therapists, clients, and patients alike to have comforting touch during a challenging time.

Several cancers have been discussed in this book so far, as Conditions in Brief, or with full Decision Trees. These specific cancer types have specific massage guidelines, but all refer the reader to this chapter for general principles, interview questions, and massage therapy guidelines. The concepts presented in this chapter can and should be applied to many client scenarios. Some complications of cancer treatment linger, affecting people months or even decades after treatment is complete. Therefore, selected massage therapy guidelines apply to those with cancer histories, as well.

General Principles

This chapter introduces several cancer-specific principles to use with people with cancer and cancer histories. In addition, familiar principles from previous chapters will apply. The commonly used cancer-specific principles are the Massage Contraindication and Cancer Principle; the Tumor Site Principle; the Bone Metastasis Principle; and the Quadrant Principle for Lymphedema Risk:

1. **The Massage Contraindication and Cancer Principle.** *Skilled massage therapy is safe for people with cancer and will not spread the disease. Specific massage adjustments are based on* clinical presentations *of cancer, not the presence of a cancer diagnosis.*

    This principle counters an old myth that persisted in massage and bodywork for years: that massage was flatly contraindicated for cancer because massage might spread it. The misconception was never clear about the type of massage strokes that were problematic. It was based on the notion that massage was sufficiently circulatory in effect to increase the rate of cancer spread. It was also based on an early theory that cancer cells spread mechanically from point A to point B, powered by the movement of blood and lymph.

    During the 1990s, two authors questioned this misconception in the literature (Curties, 1993; MacDonald, 1999). These authors looked closely at the mechanism of cancer spread, which is a complex series of physiological events, not simply a mechanical trip through the vessels that progresses more quickly or slowly with changes in blood and lymph flow.

Increases in blood and lymph flow are normal, occurring many times each day in response to movement and increased heart rate. Shifts in blood flow occur across body tissues in response to metabolic demand, notably after meals or during activity. Oncologists generally encourage cancer patients to engage in movement and exercise, which are expected to increase the circulation rate more than massage. With this important comparison to exercise, the concern about promoting cancer spread is being put to rest in massage therapy. Massage therapists avoid disturbing tumor sites with direct pressure or movement, as long as those sites are in tissues within reach. But the threat of metastasis, by itself, does not contraindicate massage with general circulatory intent.

Unfortunately the myth persisted for decades in the profession, and many potential clients were turned away. Today, in fact, some massage therapists still face fear among their clients, other health care professionals, other massage therapists, and even themselves about possible cancer spread. Massage educators might continue to propagate the myth if they themselves haven't been exposed to different information. Some training programs consign "cancer massage" to continuing education rather than to the standard curriculum because the issues are too complicated to include in a basic training. The reality of working with people with cancer is no different than working with other complex conditions: Massage decisions are based on the clinical presentation of the client, not the name of the disease. In the United States, Gayle MacDonald identified massage site, pressure, and positioning of the client as central issues in the care of people with cancer. With this change in thinking, massage has begun to return to its rightful place in cancer care.

2. **The Tumor Site Principle.** *Do not press directly on a tumor site if it is accessible to the hands, and do not move joints if movement would mechanically disturb a nearby tumor.*

   The reasoning behind this principle is that mechanical pressure might disturb any kind of lesion, particularly a space-occupying one like a solid tumor, which could already be exerting pressure on surrounding tissues, and thus causing symptoms. Additional pressure from massage could disturb the tumor or aggravate those symptoms. And, just as surgeons are careful to limit mechanical disturbance of a tumor to contain its spread, so should massage therapists.

   Whether or not mechanical pressure actually promotes cancer spread remains to be seen. However, therapists should approach the area with strict pressure and movement limits for accessible tumors, as they would for an inflammation site or other lesion. "Accessible" is the operative word. Massage would no more easily disturb tumors buried deep in the body (e.g., lung, pancreas, brain, and kidney) than would the normal activities of daily living, such as breathing and flexing the spine. It is *direct pressure* on tumors that is discouraged.

   Massage therapists may be concerned that moving joints and soft tissue in one area of the body can translate into disturbance of a tumor in another area. But it's important not to take this principle to an extreme. The idea is to avoid disturbing unstable tissue at the site. Here is another way to state this important point: The mere act of moving a joint within range, adding a gentle stretch to joints a few inches away, or massaging adjacent muscles is unlikely to promote the spread of a nearby primary tumor. After all, people with cancer are not instructed to remain completely still to avoid dislodging a few cells from the primary site. If you still have questions about your techniques and the likelihood of tumor spread, ask the client's doctor and nurse for their recommendations.

3. **The Bone Metastasis Principle.** *If cancer involves the bone, determine the bone stability in order to apply safe levels of pressure and joint movement.*

   A variation on the Unstable Tissue Principle (see Chapter 3), this principle is one of the most critical for working with clients with cancer. Careful interviewing and often a medical consultation are necessary. The reasoning is that one or more bone lesions place bones at risk of pathologic fracture. This is similar, though not identical, to the risk inherent in advanced osteoporosis. A massage therapist needs reliable information about areas of bone instability in order to adjust the pressure and joint movement correctly in the session. The client position may also need to be modified in some cases of bone metastasis.

4. **The Quadrant Principle for Lymphedema Risk.** *Avoid pressure above 2, reddening of the skin, and strong joint movement in the at-risk region of an area of cervical, axillary, or inguinal lymph node removal or radiation therapy. This includes the extremity as well as the trunk area, anterior and posterior, drained by the affected lymph nodes.*

   The reasoning behind this principle is that some massage elements are similar to other activities that are contraindicated in someone with lymphedema risk. Massage pressure, like a blood pressure cuff, may place an increased load on the lymphatic system. Like a sauna or hot tub, reddening the skin with massage friction or heat treatments can cause the same problem. Joint movement that is too strong, causing trauma to the tissues, may also overload regional lymphatic structures. These and other activities are typically contraindicated for people who are at risk for lymphedema.

   The principle applies to the area drained by the missing or injured lymph nodes on the at-risk side, posterior and anterior. This area includes, for cervical nodes, that side of the head, the neck to the midline, down to the clavicle. For axillary nodes, it includes the upper right or left quadrant (level of the clavicle to the level of the lowest rib), plus the shoulder and arm. For inguinal nodes, the area includes the lower right or left quadrant (lowest rib level downward) and the lower extremity (see Figure 20-7).

   A similar principle, the Quadrant Principle for Lymphedema History, was introduced in Chapter 13. Although the areas of concern are the same in each case, the Quadrant Principle for Lymphedema *Risk* is less conservative than the Quadrant Principle for Lymphedema *History*.

   The Quadrant Principle presented here is designed to *prevent* a first occurrence of chronic lymphedema. The Quadrant Principle from Chapter 13 is designed to avoid *aggravating* lymphedema that has already occurred.

Background

The term **cancer** collectively refers to a group of more than 100 diseases whose common factor is the uncontrolled, abnormal growth of cells. The cells usually appear in a lump, mass, or solid **tumor**. A tumor that is capable of invading other tissues is cancerous, or **malignant**; a tumor that is noncancerous is **benign**. Alternate names for cancer are *neoplasm* and *malignancy*. A cancer of the blood-forming tissues, bone marrow, or lymphoid tissue is referred to as a **hematologic malignancy**. In these conditions, the cancer cells are distributed in the bone marrow, blood, or lymphatic system. Leukemia, lymphoma, and multiple myeloma are all hematologic cancers. (see Chapter 12 and 13).

In cancer, the tissue of origin is called the *primary site*, and a mass at a primary site is called a **primary tumor**. Solid primary tumors are grouped into two main categories, according to the tissue type from which they arise. If they come from epithelial tissues, such as those in the skin, in organ linings and coverings, or glands, they are called **carcinomas**. Connective tissue, such as adipose, bone, or cartilage, gives rise to **sarcomas**.

The process of cancer spread is **metastasis**, and the sites to which it spreads and implants are sometimes referred to as **metastatic lesions (mets)**. A site of metastasis may be called a *secondary site* or *secondary tumor*. When hematologic cancers spread to organs and tissues, causing injury and loss of function, it is not considered a true metastatic process. Instead, the process is described as *infiltration*.

Invasive cancer refers to a primary tumor that has grown beyond its starting place and invaded nearby tissues. In metastatic cancer, cells have moved beyond a primary solid tumor to another area or areas of the body. This is also referred to as *distant spread*, and metastatic disease is considered *advanced cancer*. Tumor cells travel through nearby lymphatic vessels, then through the bloodstream. In some cases, tumor cells move directly to the bloodstream, bypassing the lymphatic system.

A tumor is named for its primary site, not its secondary site. For example, cancer of the prostate gland that has spread to the bones is still called prostate cancer, not bone cancer. And cancer of the breast that has spread to the lungs is called breast cancer, with mets to the lung.

Because primary and metastatic tumors often behave differently physiologically, and because metastatic lesions retain characteristics of the tissue of origin, it is usually possible for the oncologist to distinguish between a site of metastasis and a primary site. For example, a lesion on the lung will usually be clearly identifiable as either a primary tumor or a metastasis site.

However, sometimes the distinction between the primary and secondary site is not obvious. Occasionally a cancer lesion shows up in a tissue, clearly behaving as a metastatic tumor would, but without evidence of where it came from. In this case, it's called a cancer of unknown primary (CUP). Often CUPs are eventually identified as arising from the lung, intestinal tract, or pancreas. But other times, unknown primaries resist even the best diagnostic tests and remain unknown. The tumor may be too small and indistinct to be detected on a scan.

Cancer staging is a method of describing how far the disease has advanced, for the purpose of diagnosis and treatment. Cancer stages describe the size of tumor and whether it is present in nearby tissues, regional lymph nodes, or distant sites. There are several different staging systems, and different systems are preferred for different primary cancers. In the stage I-IV system, the lower the number is, the better the prognosis, and the simpler the treatment. Stage I typically describes cancer that is confined to its primary site. Stage IV describes cancer that has advanced from its primary site to nearby tissues, to nearby lymph nodes, and has also spread to distant sites (metastasized). Stage IV treatment often addresses metastatic cancer as a chronic disease, as in stage IV breast cancer. Stage IV can also involve supportive care at the end of life. The treatment approach depends on clinical features, the results of tests, and the type of cancer.

The *TNM system* of cancer staging describes the condition in terms of tumor (T), node involvement (N), and metastasis (M). Numerical ratings with the letters indicate the extent of the tumor, the extent of lymph node involvement, and the extent of distant metastasis.

● SIGNS AND SYMPTOMS

Cancer has very few indicators that serve as early signs or symptoms. Tumors often develop slowly and gradually, and cancer is frequently not diagnosed until after it has advanced. As cancer advances, loss of tissue or organ function occurs, and the pressure of a tumor on surrounding structures causes pain and can lead to serious problems.

The seven main warning signs/symptoms of cancer create the acronym CAUTION:

C: *Change* in bowel or bladder habits (possible sign of colorectal cancer, among others)
A: *Area* or sore that does not heal (possible sign of skin or mouth cancer)
U: *Unusual* bleeding or discharge (possible sign of colorectal, bladder, prostate, or cervical cancer)
T: *Thickening* or lump in tissue (possible sign of breast or testicular cancer, among others)
I: *Indigestion* or difficulty swallowing (possible sign of throat, esophagus, stomach, or oral cancer)
O: *Obvious* change in a wart or mole (possible skin cancer)
N: *Nagging* cough or hoarseness (possible sign of lung or throat cancer)

In addition to these easily remembered warning signs, cancer can cause diverse symptoms and complications (described below). Symptoms, signs, and complications depend on the tissue affected. For example, a lesion on the brain can cause a seizure, or stroke-like symptoms. A lesion on the skin can bleed. A tumor can cause constipation; another tumor can cause symptoms of menopause. A massage therapist may be the first to hear about these symptoms: a new pain, a persistent cough, a lump, or a change in bowel habits. A timely medical referral can be lifesaving.

● COMPLICATIONS

As cancer advances, it can affect many different tissues and body functions. The main complications of cancer are discussed here.

Vital Organ Involvement

Both primary and secondary tumors can affect the vital organs: the liver, kidneys, lungs, brain, or heart. Of these, the heart is a rare site of primary tumor and an occasional site of metastatic disease. The brain is more commonly a site of metastasis than of primary tumor.

The mere presence of a primary or secondary lesion in a vital organ does not mean it affects the function of that organ, but function usually becomes impaired as the disease progresses.

Metastasis

By definition, metastasis is a complication of cancer. It means that the disease can cause dysfunction at two different sites in the body: the primary and secondary sites. Cancer can spread to almost any tissue or organ, but cancer cells tend to spread to four places: the bones, liver, lungs, and brain.

Primary tumors display certain patterns of metastasis. Primary lung cancer commonly spreads to the brain or bones, and prostate cancer tends to spread to the bones. Breast cancer metastasizes to the bones, lungs, liver, or brain. These patterns are attributed to tissue affinities between certain cancer cells and tissues at their preferred secondary sites.

Bone Metastasis

Bone is the third most common site of distant metastasis, and the most relevant to massage therapists. Because bones and joints are manipulated along with adjacent soft tissues, it is important for bone involvement to be considered in the massage plan.

Bone metastasis occurs in many types of cancer, and in some more than others. In North America, primary tumors of the breast are the most common cause of bone metastasis, followed by cancer of the prostate, lung, colon, stomach, bladder, uterus, rectum, thyroid, and kidney.

Most bone mets occur in adults, and the vertebrae are the most common sites, followed by the pelvis, proximal femur, ribs, proximal humerus, and the cranium. About 70% of spine metastases occur in the thoracic vertebrae. The hands and feet are rare sites of bone metastasis.

The pain of bone metastasis is one of the most feared symptoms of cancer. Bone mets cause other complications, too: pathologic fracture, nerve impingement, stiffness and limited movement, and excess calcium in the blood.

Pain may be the first noticeable symptom of bone involvement, and when the disease is extensive, people often have several areas of pain, or migrating pain. If it affects the long bones of the arms or legs, the pain may increase with activity or be relieved with rest. Pain may be felt at the site of the metastasis, or the pain can refer, as when metastasis in the hip region is felt around the knee. If a bone lesion presses on the spinal cord, it is called spinal cord compression. In this case, back pain may be felt, which can worsen at night or with bed rest.

Bone lesions destroy tissue and make the bones vulnerable to pathologic fracture. As in osteoporosis, pathologic fracture can lead to severe pain and disability when bone fragments press on adjacent nervous system structures. Spinal cord compression is likely when vertebrae fracture, causing sensation loss, motor weakness (especially in the lower extremities), and impairment of autonomic functions, such as bowel and bladder activities. Numbness from cord compression often occurs in the lower extremities or abdominal/pelvic area.

In some cases, bone metastasis is clinically silent; there are no symptoms until a fracture occurs. In fact, about one third of individuals with metastasis in the spine may not complain of bone pain at all. It is this mysterious, asymptomatic aspect that makes bone metastasis a high priority for the massage interview.

Not all bone metastasis is equal. In some cases, lesions are widely distributed but tiny, with little or no impact on the integrity of the bone. In other cases, lesions are more significant but are located in areas that do not receive the stress of bearing weight, so fracture is unlikely. In still other situations, a single large lesion or multiple lesions make an area of bone highly unstable. When bone is eroded, it can lead to hypercalcemia, elevated blood calcium levels. This serious condition can tax the kidneys in their attempt to clear the blood of the excess calcium.

Liver Metastasis

The liver is the most common site of distant cancer spread. In liver metastasis, lesions tend to form in more than one area of the organ, yet even with extensive liver involvement, metastatic liver disease may be asymptomatic.

As the disease advances, liver function is affected (see "Liver Failure," Chapter 16). Liver enlargement, jaundice, weight loss, and ascites (swelling of the abdomen) occur, often with swelling of the lower extremities.

Lung Metastasis

The lungs are the second most common site of distant metastasis. Primary cancers of the bladder, colon, breast, and prostate commonly spread to the lungs.

Lung metastases are often asymptomatic, but when lesions affect lung function, signs and symptoms include shortness of breath, pain in the chest or ribs, cough, weakness, and unintended weight loss.

Brain Metastasis

The brain is the fourth most common site of distant cancer spread. Primary tumors of the lung, breast, and kidney often spread to the brain. Colorectal cancer and melanoma also tend to spread to the brain.

When brain function is affected, signs and symptoms include headache, seizures, cognitive dysfunction, and motor dysfunction. Of these, headache and seizure are the two most common symptoms. Sometimes a morning headache occurs, accompanied by nausea and vomiting. Changes in sensation and vision occur. Balance may be affected. Most signs and symptoms of brain metastasis develop gradually. Acute symptoms can appear when brain lesions cause bleeding in the brain, as in a stroke.

Thrombosis and Embolism

The risk of thrombosis and embolism is increased in patients with cancer, notably primary cancer of the pancreas, lung, ovary, prostate, breast, and gastrointestinal (GI) tract. Of those, the lung is the most closely associated with thrombosis and embolic events. The mechanism of this risk is not entirely understood, and the medical literature does not agree on which types of cancer elevate DVT risk. Moreover, it is not always clear whether the risk is elevated by the primary tumor, the presence of metastasis, a paraneoplastic syndrome (PS) (discussed below), or some other factor. With this ambiguity, massage therapists should be aware of elevated DVT risk for clients with primary cancers of the organs listed above, and for *any* case of advanced cancer, regardless of the tissue of origin.

Paraneoplastic Syndrome

Apart from the possibility of pressing on other tissues and spreading, a primary tumor can cause a variety of symptoms and problems, seemingly unrelated to the cancer itself. These are collectively called paraneoplastic syndrome (PS). For example, a tumor might elicit an immune response, resulting in an autoimmune condition, with inflammation and destruction of normal tissue. Tumors can release physiologically active substances, such as hormones, precursors to hormones, enzymes, and other protein substances that cells use to communicate with each other. The abnormal or excessive production of these substances can have wide ranging effects, impairing the function of tissues in many systems of the body.

Fever and fatigue are examples of nonspecific PS symptoms associated with leukemia and lymphoma, as well as other cancers. Pancreatic cancer or prostate cancer can lead to abnormal production of antidiuretic hormone (ADH), which in turn causes fluid retention, muscle cramps, seizures, and other problems. Multiple myeloma or colorectal cancer can lead to arthritis. Ovarian cancer may cause an ectopic Cushing syndrome (see Chapter 17). Even profound weight loss—cachexia—can be a PS symptom in certain types of cancer.

Statistics about the incidence of PS range widely, from just a few percent to one fifth of people with cancer. These complications may prompt the doctor's visit that leads to a cancer diagnosis.

● TREATMENT

The treatment of cancer focuses on the removal, destruction, or control of the primary tumor and metastatic lesions, the management of symptoms, and limiting the damage to tissues and organs in advanced cancer. Because cancer treatment is strong medicine, additional treatments are often necessary to control side effects. Supportive care is part of the picture, whether during treatment or at end of life.

Treatment for a solid tumor typically involves some combination of surgery, chemotherapy, and radiation therapy. Treatment of hematologic tumors is addressed in Chapters 12 and 13. For some cancers, stem cell transplant is performed; for others, biological therapy or hormone therapy is used.

Adjuvant therapy is any treatment that follows the primary treatment for cancer; it increases the chance of a cure or lowers the chance that the cancer will recur. Examples are chemotherapy, radiation therapy, and other approaches that follow surgery. A course of hormone therapy for a period of years after the successful treatment, designed to prevent cancer recurrence, is another form of adjuvant therapy. **Neoadjuvant therapy** is given before the primary therapy to "pave the way," increasing the chance that the primary therapy goes well. An example of neoadjuvant therapy is the use of radiation or chemotherapy to shrink a large tumor prior to surgery, to minimize the potential for damaging nearby nerves or blood vessels.

Surgery

Surgery for cancer is used for both diagnostic and therapeutic purposes. Surgery is also performed to remove metastatic lesions or to relieve pain caused by a bulky tumor pressing on adjacent structures. In this case, the surgery might be strictly part of supportive care: not expected to cure the disease but to make the patient more comfortable and add to quality of life. Surgery can address the complications of cancer. It might be performed after other cancer therapies to restore tissue function or appearance, as in reconstructive surgery. Surgery may also be performed to insert or remove medical devices, such as catheters.

A **biopsy** is the removal of a sample of tissue or fluid for the purpose of diagnosis. In cancer surgery, a small part of the tumor may be biopsied, or the entire tumor is removed if it is feasible. By removing a tumor for analysis, the physician can diagnose its type, verify its size, and determine its stage. Biopsies range in invasiveness, from a simple **needle biopsy**, in which a small amount of tissue is aspirated into a hollow needle and examined, to open surgery for sampling tissue from multiple sites. In an **incisional biopsy**, part of a tumor is removed, and in an **excisional biopsy**, the whole solid tumor is removed.

The surgical removal of a tumor for diagnosis can also be the first line of cancer treatment. The surgeon removes the tumor itself and enough adjacent tissue to obtain *clear margins*, cancer-free tissue surrounding the tumor site.

Cancer surgery may be preceded by **lymph node mapping**. In this procedure, a dye and/or radioactive substance is injected into the tumor before surgery. These materials are followed through the lymphatic vessels to identify which lymph nodes they reach first. These "front-line" **sentinel nodes** drain the tissue surrounding the cancer and are the first to receive any cancer cells from the primary tumor. In a **sentinel node biopsy (SNB)**, these nodes are surgically removed first, then examined for the presence of cancer. Figure 20-1 shows lymph node mapping before breast surgery, along with SNB and removal of the primary tumor.

If no cancer is found in the one or more sentinel nodes identified through lymph node mapping, then the surgeons can usually avoid a **lymph node dissection (LND)**, the removal of a greater number of lymph nodes from the area. The status of the sentinel lymph nodes typically reflects the status of the other nodes in the area. On the other hand, if the sentinel lymph nodes are positive, subsequent lymph nodes are removed. Figure 20-2 shows lymph node mapping for melanoma at three different primary sites; the tumor sites are mapped to three different clusters of lymph nodes in different quadrants of the body. By pinpointing the locations of sentinel nodes, other lymph nodes are more likely to be conserved.

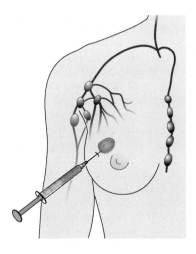
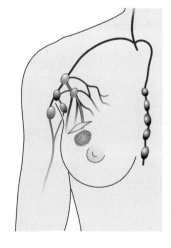
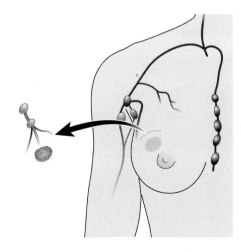

A   B   C

FIGURE 20-1. Sentinel node biopsy (SNB) in breast cancer surgery. The removal of one or more sentinel nodes begins with lymph node mapping (A) in which a dye, radioactive substance, or both are injected into the tumor. In (B), the dye or radioactive substance moves through the channels usually traveled by the tumor and is received by the first sentinel node or nodes in its path. In (C), the surgeon removes one or more of these sentinel nodes identified by the dye/radiolabel, and the tissue is checked for cancer cells. The tumor is also removed. If the sentinel node or nodes do *not* contain cancer cells, then no further nodes are removed. If the sentinel node or nodes *do* contain cancer cells, the surgeon removes additional nodes identified as cancerous.

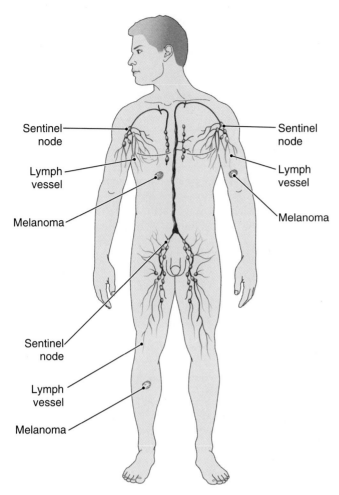

FIGURE 20-2. Comparison of lymph node mapping in different body regions. Three primary sites of melanoma are shown. After dye or radioactive substance is injected into a primary site, it is traced to the corresponding axillary or inguinal sentinel node. In a sentinel node biopsy (SNB), the first node or nodes to receive the dye/substance are removed and tested for the presence of cancer cells.

Labels in figure:
- Sentinel node
- Lymph vessel
- Melanoma
- Sentinel node
- Lymph vessel
- Melanoma
- Sentinel node
- Lymph vessel
- Melanoma

LYMPHEDEMA

One lingering complication, unique to some kinds of cancer surgery, is a type of swelling called **lymphedema**. This is an accumulation of fluid in the tissues, caused by faulty drainage through the lymphatic system. Over time, proteins concentrate in the tissues; this stagnation draws and holds swelling in the area. Lymphedema is discussed fully in Chapter 13.

Lymphedema after cancer surgery is associated with LND. The greater the number of lymph nodes removed in LND, the greater the risk of lymphedema. SNB lowers the risk significantly, but it does not eliminate it entirely. Lymphedema is a common occurrence after axillary lymph node dissection (ALND). It is less common after inguinal lymph node dissection (ILND). It is much less frequent after dissection of the cervical lymph nodes (for example, in thyroid cancer surgery). In the neck, gravity is thought to facilitate the downward movement of lymph, even when nodes and vessels are missing. Lymphedema can also occur after the removal of pelvic or abdominal lymph nodes, as in gynecological cancer surgery, but the level of risk is poorly understood.

The onset of lymphedema can be decades after cancer surgery, and the risk of it is lifelong. There is no cure for the condition, although there is treatment to manage it (see Chapter 13). Lymphatic anatomy can vary from person to person, so it is not easy to predict an individual's exact risk level of lymphedema at the time of surgery. Some people have adequate *collateral* pathways for lymph to travel through when principal routes are damaged. Risk statistics vary.

While lymph node removal sets up an environment favoring lymphedema, the onset of lymphedema usually follows another event, usually an increase in circulation somewhere in the tissues served by the missing lymph nodes. Inflammation, injury, or some other circulatory event increases the load on the lymphatic system, beyond the capacity of the collateral pathways and any remaining lymph nodes. Fluid then backs up in the tissues and lymphedema results. Because the balance of lymphatic capacity and flow can be so fragile, even a small event can precipitate lymphedema, such as an infected hangnail, a limb overheated in a hot tub, the pressure of a blood pressure cuff on the tissues, or an overused muscle.

Lymphedema is painful, disfiguring, and can lead to other problems such as infection, so great efforts are directed at preventing it, where possible. People at risk of lymphedema are often given strict activity precautions to follow, with instructions to follow them indefinitely. Care is taken with the entire area drained by the missing lymph nodes, not just the immediate site of lymph node removal. This is called the *at-risk area* or at-risk side.

Lymphedema prevention measures focus on the at-risk area. Common precautions are described in Table 20-1, and they can significantly affect an individual's quality of life. In particular, limits on physical activity may be difficult for active individuals to adjust to, and always shifting heavy bags off of the at-risk side brings logistical challenges. At the time of this writing, the longtime recommendation against lifting more than 5 pounds with the upper at-risk limb is being revisited; many professionals in cancer care believe a gradual, supervised return to exercise, including weightlifting with the at-risk limb, may *prevent* lymphedema.

These precautions for lymphedema prevention are still being debated, and they are unevenly applied. One patient with a SNB might be told to follow precautions to the letter, while another patient with the same clinical presentation is told that he or she doesn't need to be so careful. One patient with nine lymph nodes removed in an axillary dissection might be told to follow the lymphedema precautions, and another with the same presentation might be told not to worry about them.

There is not uniform education of patients about lymphedema, and not every patient hears the information correctly. Moreover, many people are aware of the risk but choose not to follow the precautions, citing them as too restrictive for daily living. Although facilities, clinicians, and researchers do not all agree on the exact precautions for all patients, most agree that some care must be taken to avoid lymphedema.

OTHER SIDE EFFECTS AND COMPLICATIONS OF SURGERY

Surgery obviously causes pain or soreness at the incision site, and infection is a possible complication. Respiratory infection is also a risk. Recent surgery, especially in the prior 12 weeks, elevates DVT risk. Cancer surgery, especially with any kind of amputation, can diminish body image, possibly leading to depression. General side effects and complications of surgery are covered in Chapter 21.

TABLE 20-1.	LYMPHEDEMA PREVENTION MEASURES AND EQUIVALENT MASSAGE PRECAUTIONS FOR PATIENTS AT ELEVATED RISK OF LYMPHEDEMA.

Activity Precautions for the At Risk Area	Equivalent Massage Therapy Precautions
Do not have blood pressure readings, blood draws, or IVs in the area.	Use cautious pressure (typically maximum level 2).
Take care to avoid overusing the limb; for upper extremity risk, do not carry heavy bags or luggage, and avoid shoulder straps that press into the skin. For lower extremity risk, avoid fatiguing muscles by overexercising.	Avoid resisted exercises if they are fatiguing.
Do not engage in activities that overwork the muscles, or could cause injury to the area. Instead, begin exercising gently, gradually increasing intensity and duration, including frequent rest periods and monitoring the at-risk area for swelling; a medically supervised exercise program is recommended.	Do not stretch or manipulate the area in any way that could cause injury. Avoid active or resisted stretching unless you are trained in exercise instruction for patients with lymphedema risk.
Avoid extreme hot or cold temperatures, such as ice applications, hot water, saunas that increase circulation to the skin in the area. Avoid freezing weather that causes chapped skin.	Avoid hot and cold applications, avoid steam or sauna treatments.
Do not hang the at-risk limb over the edge of a chair or table.	Do not hang the at-risk limb over the edge of massage table for long periods
For upper extremity risk, use gloves during dishwashing, gardening, and other activities where cuts, burns, and exposure to dirt occur.	Maintain short, filed fingernails for massage; remove jewelry.
Avoid inflammation: insect bites and burns, including sunburn, in the area.	Avoid friction or any pressure that raises redness on the skin in the area.
Practice meticulous skin and nail hygiene and lubrication, to avoid chapping and cuts that could introduce infection.	Inspect skin for open lesions before introducing contact and lubricant.
Avoid tight-fitting jewelry, tight undergarments, and other restrictive clothing, but use customized, well-fitting compression garments for activity and air travel.	No comparable massage adjustments.

Chemotherapy

Chemotherapy is the systemic use of drugs to treat cancer by impeding the growth of cancer cells. Many types of chemotherapy have been developed to shrink tumors or eliminate them entirely, hold off the spread, defeat cells that have already spread to secondary sites, and even to relieve cancer symptoms.

Chemotherapy agents work via slightly different methods and have different uses. *Alkylating agents* such as cyclophosphamide (Cytoxan) are used for the hematologic cancers as well as cancer of the breast, ovary, and lung. *Antimetabolites* such as capecitabine (Xeloda), 5-fluorouracil (5-FU), and gemcitabine (Gemzar) are typically used for leukemias and tumors of the breast, ovary, and intestine. *Topoisomerase inhibitors* include topotecan and mitoxantrone; these drugs are used for GI, ovarian, and lung cancers, among others. *Mitotic inhibitors*, such as paclitaxel (Taxol) and vincristine (Oncovin), are a class of drugs used for many types of cancer. These are known for causing peripheral nerve damage, as in neuropathy.

Chemotherapy is administered on an outpatient or inpatient basis. It is generally delivered in cycles of doses alternating with rest periods. Medication can be taken orally or administered intravenously by **infusion**. A device called an **implantable access port (IAP)** can be surgically implanted to distribute drugs into the bloodstream, eliminating the need for repeated needle sticks or IVs. A common port site is the chest, as shown in Figure 20-3. A port may also be implanted in the abdominal cavity for **intraperitoneal infusion** (Figure 20-4).

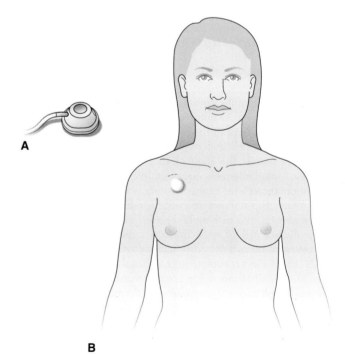

FIGURE 20-3. A port (implantable access port, or IAP) for chemotherapy. (A) A port. (B) Port surgically implanted in pectoral area, for delivery directly to the superior vena cava.

In some cases, a chemotherapy drug is introduced directly into an area of cancer in the body so that it contacts the tumor at full strength, before it is diluted in the bloodstream.

The kind of chemotherapy and the dose are typically determined by a *medical oncologist*.

Medications might be administered once every 2–3 weeks, weekly, or several times a week. Some are infused continuously over a few days. Oral pills might be taken daily or less often.

SIDE EFFECTS OF CHEMOTHERAPY

Chemotherapy is delivered systemically, and because the drugs are in the bloodstream, they can have strong effects on normal cells in the body. Some of the primary side effects are described below, and some are referenced and fully discussed in other chapters:

1. *General effects.* Fatigue can range from slight tiredness to profound, chronic exhaustion.
2. *Myelosuppression.* Chemotherapy diminishes blood cell production by the bone marrow, an effect called **myelosuppression**. As a result, blood levels of one or more blood cell types (red blood cells [RBCs], white blood cells [WBCs], or platelets) may be affected. When all three blood cell populations are abnormally low at once, it is called **pancytopenia**. Blood cell counts are monitored closely before each chemotherapy infusion to determine whether the treatment can proceed. Consequences of myelosuppression include thrombocytopenia (see Chapter 12) and easy bruising or bleeding; anemia (see Chapter 12), along with fatigue, light-headedness, and cold intolerance; and neutropenia (see Chapter 12), with a heightened vulnerability to infection. For each blood cell type, the severity of side effects depends on the degree of cytopenia. Platelets can be slightly low, with no detectable effect on bruising. Or they can be profoundly low, with easily bleeding gums or the danger of *bleeding out* (hemorrhage). Neutropenia can be mild or severe, requiring the use of masks and gloves to avoid infecting the person. Anemia can be mild, or can be severe enough to strain the heart.
3. *Gastrointestinal effects.* Side effects of chemotherapy that affect the GI tract include nausea, vomiting, diarrhea, and constipation. Mouth sores, known as **stomatitis** or *mucositis*, make chewing food difficult. Loss of appetite is common with chemotherapy and can be due to mouth sores, nausea, and changes in taste and smell.
4. *Effects on the skin and hair.* Hair loss **(alopecia)** is probably one of the most devastating side effects of chemotherapy, because it affects body image and because it is the most outward sign of cancer treatment. In **hand-foot syndrome**, a response to some chemotherapy treatments, the feet and hands become swollen, irritated, chapped, and peeling. Toenails or fingernails may become discolored, or fall off. This condition can compromise walking and the use of the hands.
5. *Neurological effects.* Peripheral neuropathy is common in the hands and feet and may extend further up the extremities (see Chapter 10). **Chemobrain** (or *brain fog*) is a chronic loss of memory, attention, and focus, specifically attributed to chemotherapy. Both neuropathy and chemobrain typically fade in the weeks and months after chemotherapy is completed, but in some people, they persist indefinitely.

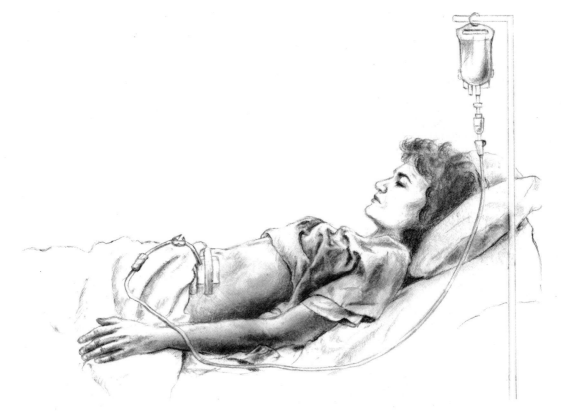

FIGURE 20-4. Intraperitoneal chemotherapy infusion. Medication is delivered from a drip into the peritoneal cavity. (From *Lippincott's Nursing Procedures*, 4th Edition. Ambler: Lippincott Williams & Wilkins, 2004).

Radiation Therapy

There are several types of radiation therapy, an approach that exploits the tendency of cancer cells to proliferate rapidly by damaging the genetic material that controls their growth. Cancer cells repair themselves poorly, so they tend to be destroyed when damaged by radiation. Radiation is aimed at cancer cells, but it might affect nearby tissues in the radiation field, or field of treatment.

Methods of radiation therapy include external radiation, internal radiation, and stereotactic radiation therapy, in which intensely focused beams are targeted from multiple directions, often on brain lesions. Stereotactic radiation therapy is usually a single session.

The most common type of radiation is external beam radiation therapy (EBRT), for which the source of radiation is a *linear accelerator*, a machine that delivers a beam of radiation aimed at the tumor. EBRT can be used to shrink a tumor before surgery (neoadjuvant therapy), to prevent recurrence after surgery (adjuvant therapy), or to relieve pain from a tumor (palliative). It can also help stabilize bone metastasis and reduce the risk of fracture. A typical course of EBRT is 5 days a week for 6 or 7 weeks. In palliative care, the daily radiation might be given over 2–3 weeks.

In internal radiation therapy, also called brachytherapy, small radiation implants are placed inside the body next to the tumor cells. A higher dose of radiation is possible, and it can be focused right at the tumor site, without damaging too much nearby tissue. Surgically implanted seeds may be left in rather than removed, as in the treatment of prostate cancer. To treat gynecologic cancer, a radioactive substance may be placed intravaginally in a tube and then removed. In thyroid cancer, radiation is often ingested, as in radioactive iodine therapy (see "Thyroid cancer," online).

SIDE EFFECTS OF RADIATION THERAPY

Radiation injures cells in the radiation field—nearby tissues, or the tissues through which a beam passes on its way to the tumor. This cell injury is responsible for the side effects of treatment. One of the most obvious effects of radiation is on the skin. The skin can redden, darken, swell, and turn dry, and it might itch. Hair loss generally occurs in the radiation field.

Fatigue during radiation therapy is common. It often begins after several treatments and subsides a few weeks or months after the treatments end.

Other side effects depend on the size and location of the radiation field. If radiation covers the head or neck, pain may be felt in the mouth and throat, causing difficulty eating. Mouth sores and dry mouth can also occur. If radiation is delivered to the neck or chest, it may cause shortness of breath and coughing. Radiation delivered to the abdomen can cause nausea, vomiting, diarrhea, bladder pain, and burning. Radiation over a large area, such as the thorax or pelvis, can also cause myelosuppression.

Radiation of lymph nodes puts one at risk for lymphedema. The risk is increased if lymph nodes were also surgically removed. As with surgical removal, radiation of cervical, axillary, or inguinal nodes can affect their function. Radiation to the pelvis can result in lymphedema, as well.

Radiation implants require a period of contact precautions. The quarantine period can be extremely isolating. An individual can be prone to loneliness and depression, especially when the other side effects of radiation, such as fatigue, are strong.

Over the long term, radiation may increase one's susceptibility to a second cancer, or it may cause infertility, lung scarring, cardiac issues, or GI problems, depending on where it is delivered. It can also cause neurological problems and osteoporosis.

Biologic Therapy

Biologic therapy, which is also called *immunotherapy*, is used to treat some types of cancer by stimulating the body's own immune mechanisms. Several therapies have been developed, with different immune mechanisms. Immunotherapy can also stop the transformation of normal cells into cancer cells or interfere with cancer cell spread. "Biologics," as these medications are called, may facilitate the body's normal repair mechanisms, helping to heal tissues injured by chemotherapy or radiation.

There are several types of biologic therapy. Some stimulate the immune system to fight cancer and others introduce components of the immune system, such as antibodies, into the body to fight cancer. Monoclonal antibodies are a class of drugs that include trastuzumab (Herceptin), used in breast cancer; rituximab (Rituxan), used in non-Hodgkin lymphoma; and bevacizumab (Avastin), used in colorectal, breast, and kidney cancer, among others. These are sometimes called targeted therapies because they bind directly to cancer cells, making it easier for other cancer therapies to selectively destroy them. At the time of this writing, they are the most widely used form of biologic therapy.

Interferon alpha is a class of biologics that slow the growth of cancer cells or alter their character to behave more normally. These drugs may also stimulate other cells of the immune system to fight cancer cells. Interferon alpha is used in some hematologic cancers, AIDS-related Kaposi sarcoma, melanoma, and kidney cancer. Brand names are Roferon-A and Intron-A. Interleukins (such as Proleukin) are a class of drugs that also occur naturally in the body, acting to stimulate immune cells to destroy cancer cells. They are used most often in kidney cancer and are also approved to treat melanoma.

Side effects of biologics include strong flu-like symptoms. Fever, chills, nausea, vomiting, fatigue, and loss of appetite may occur, as well as bone pain. Weight gain and low blood pressure are common. Interferon side effects can be severe. Low WBC counts may occur, as well as thinning hair.

Hormone Therapy

Any time hormones are used in medical treatment, it is called hormone therapy. In cancer treatment, hormones or hormone-blocking drugs are used to alter the internal environment so that it is less favorable to cancer growth. Cancers of the breast, endometrium, and prostate are treated with hormone therapy. Certain breast cancers grow more readily in the presence of hormones, such as estrogen or progesterone, and test positive for receptors for estrogen. Most prostate cancers grow more readily in the presence of testosterone. For breast cancer, hormone therapy might block the action of normally occurring estrogen on the cancer cells, or the ovaries might be surgically removed so that they do not produce estrogen. For prostate cancer, testosterone-blocking drugs may be used, or the testes might be surgically removed so that they do not produce testosterone.

Hormone therapy can slow the growth and spread of primary tumors and is often used after major cancer treatment has ended, to prevent recurrence of the cancer. A widely used drug is the *selective estrogen receptor modulator* tamoxifen (Nolvadex), typically prescribed for 5 years following breast cancer treatment in order to prevent recurrence. It does not interfere with estrogen production but with the effects of estrogen on the growth of cancer cells in the breast.

In prostate cancer, drugs that diminish the effects of testosterone are used. Drugs called LHRH analogs, including leuprolide (Lupron) and goserelin (Zoladex), are injected, and antiandrogens, such as bicalutamide (Casodex), are given orally. The testes might also be removed surgically (orchiectomy) to reduce the natural production of testosterone in the body.

Side effects of hormone therapy vary according to the specific drugs and individual responses to them. These side effects include hot flashes, fatigue, nausea, vomiting, loss of sex drive, and blood clots. Both sexes may experience symptoms of menopause, including hot flashes, and men may experience breast enlargement. See "Breast Cancer" and "Prostate Cancer," Chapter 19, for more discussion of hormone therapy and side effects.

Stem Cell Transplant

A **stem cell transplant** (also called a *bone marrow transplant*) is the infusion of stem cells into the blood of a patient to treat a number of conditions, especially hematologic cancers—lymphoma, leukemia, and multiple myeloma (See Chapter 12). **Stem cells**, which are unspecialized cells with the potential to develop into needed blood cells, may be drawn from the bone marrow or peripheral blood. They are treated, and then placed into the bloodstream of the patient. The stem cells are introduced in order to repopulate the patient's bone marrow and restart its production of healthy blood cells. A primary reason for a stem cell transplant is to restore or "rescue" the bone marrow after high doses of chemotherapy or radiation have destroyed the existing bone marrow.

In an **autologous transplant**, the stem cells are the patient's own cells; they are removed and treated, then delivered back (usually a 3-week hospital stay). In an **allogeneic transplant**, cells are harvested from a member of the patient's genetic family or an unknown, closely matched donor from the bone marrow registry. (In a *syngeneic transplant*, the stem cells are donated by an identical twin.) In an allogeneic transplant, the inherent differences between the tissue of the patient (the host) and the tissue of the donor (the graft) make the possibility of tissue rejection a major medical issue.

The transplantation of stem cells, combined with the associated chemotherapy, medications, and sometimes radiation, is one of the strongest medical treatments known. There are many possible complications, including **graft-vs.-host-disease (GVHD)**, in which the donated cells mount an immune response against the patient. The inflammation from GVHD can manifest in the skin, liver, and GI tract. Acute GVHD often follows transplantation, and it can be life threatening. Chronic GVHD can be a lifelong issue, producing tissue scarring, reduced mobility, and other compromised functions.

High-dose chemotherapy and radiation of the whole body, called **total body irradiation (TBI)**, often accompany a stem cell transplant, and there are many side effects and possible complications of these treatments. In particular, the consequences of high-dose chemotherapy are profound. Because infection control is of paramount concern, *isolation precautions* are typically in force initially. Gowns, masks, and gloves may be required to visit or care for the patient. After patients are discharged from the hospital, they may be restricted to the home for months, with limited contact with others. Limits on contact with pets, small children, and anyone with symptoms of infection are in force, and patients describe the feeling of being under "house arrest."

Many medications are prescribed during stem cell transplant and in the months following it. These medications are used to suppress immunity and manage symptoms, and they can have many different side effects (see "Organ and Tissue Transplant," Chapter 21).

Medications Used in Supportive Care

People with cancer may be on several medications to manage symptoms and prevent complications. There are many possibilities. Analgesics are taken for pain. Antiseizure drugs are taken for seizures, often in brain involvement. **Bisphosphonates** such as palmidronate (Aredia) and zoledronic acid (Zometa) are taken for bone metastasis or to mitigate the bone-thinning effects of cancer drugs (see "Osteoporosis," Chapter 9).

Side effects of cancer treatments are notorious, and additional drugs are administered to counter them. Patients might be taking **antiemetics** such as dexamethasone (Decadron) or ondansetron (Zofran). Such corticosteroids (Decadron) and *serotonin-receptor antagonists* (Zofran) are highly effective and well tolerated; headache, drowsiness, and orthostatic hypotension might result. Other antiemetics include prochlorperazine (Compazine), which also causes drowsiness and orthostatic hypotension, and metoclopramide (Reglan), which can cause drowsiness, restlessness, and diarrhea. Antianxiety drugs such as lorazepam (Ativan) are also helpful for nausea; drowsiness is a common side effect.

Individuals with cancer may take colony-stimulating factors (see Chapter 12) to stimulate the bone marrow to restore diminished blood cell populations. In the case of neutropenia, filgrastim (Neupogen) or long-acting pegfilgrastim (Neulasta) may be used. Side effects include headache and nausea. In anemia, epoietin alfa (Epogen, Procrit) may be prescribed. In both types of colony-stimulating factors, bone marrow expands, causing pain in the sternum and the ends of long bones.

Some drugs used in cancer treatment are multiuse. A drug called megestrol (Megace) is used to treat breast cancer and endometrial cancer but can also increase appetite. Decadron is a corticosteroid medication that can stimulate appetite, reduce nausea, reduce inflammation, and dampen an allergic response to chemotherapy. Pain medication is prescribed for neuropathic pain, muscle aches, bone metastasis, mouth sores, or headache. Nonsteroidal anti-inflammatory drugs (NSAIDs) might be used, but opioids are a mainstay of pain management. A transdermal fentanyl patch (Actiq, Duragesic) may be used.

These medications, in turn, can have side effects, but the drugs are chosen carefully by the doctor and patient because the symptom relief outweighs the additional effects they cause.

● INTERVIEW QUESTIONS

1. Have you had massage therapy before? If yes, was it since your cancer diagnosis?
2. What is the cancer status at this point in time?
3. What type of cancer is/was it? Where was or is it in your body?
4. Have you had any recent diagnostic tests, or do you have any scheduled? If so, what is being tested? What kinds of findings were there, or are they looking for?

5. Is there any bone involvement? If so, where? What is your activity level? Are there any medical restrictions on activities or movements? Have any of your health care team—doctors, nurses, physical therapists, or occupational therapists—expressed concern about the stability of your bones?

6. Are there any areas of pain or discomfort? If so, where? Is this new or unfamiliar, or familiar and well managed from the past? Is it sharp, or radiating?

7. Are there any areas of weakness, numbness, or sensation changes?

8. How does the cancer affect you?

9. Is there any vital organ involvement? [List the five vital organs for the client.] Is any vital organ *function* affected by cancer or by the cancer treatment?

10. Are there any effects of cancer or cancer treatment on your blood counts? Are you vulnerable to infection or anemic?

11. Are there any effects of cancer or cancer treatment on blood clotting? Do you have any bruising or bleeding?

12. Are there any complications or other problems caused by cancer?

13. What is your activity or movement level like, day to day and week to week? What is your activity tolerance? Describe your energy level.

14. Are there any medical restrictions on your activity or movement?

15. Are you currently in treatment? Recently? Or are you between treatments?

16. How was or is the cancer treated?
    - Surgery? When and where on your body? Complications afterward? Were any lymph nodes removed? Any sentinel node biopsy? If so, did your doctor talk with you about risk of lymphedema? Did your doctor or nurse discuss restrictions on blood pressure or anything else in that area?
    - Chemotherapy? When and how often? How does it affect you? How are your blood counts? (Ask at each session.) Do you have a port or other medical device? If so, where?
    - Radiation therapy? Where on your body? Any markings? How does it affect you? If there is an active or recent radiation field, do you want me to rest my hands on it through the sheet? Were any lymph nodes treated with radiation [list neck, underarm, groin, pelvis/abdomen], or included in the radiation field?
    - Other treatments, such as stem cell transplant, biologic therapy, hormone therapy, or others?
    - Any other medications? Any other medications to prevent cancer recurrence or to manage your symptoms or side effects? (Ask the Four Medication Questions if so.)

18. How does (or did) the treatment affect you? Are there any complications or side effects?

19. Are there any lingering effects of cancer treatment?

Massage Therapy Guidelines

Be prepared to explain the Massage Contraindication and Cancer Principle to allay any fears the client or family members might have. Even someone seeking massage might have heard the misconception about massage and cancer, and many people have been turned away from massage therapy by this old belief. Explain that massage is not contraindicated and will not spread the disease. Use the analogy to movement and exercise (see "General Principles," this chapter). Mention that many prominent cancer centers, smaller hospitals, and clinics offer massage to cancer patients; this supports the fact that the misconception is growing obsolete.

> *The Massage Contraindication and Cancer Principle. Skilled massage therapy is safe for people with cancer and will not spread the disease. Specific massage adjustments are based on clinical presentations of cancer, not the presence of a cancer diagnosis.*

Question 1 is an all-purpose question to ask clients in order to get agreement on expectations for the treatment. Clients might not know about the need to modify massage for cancer or cancer treatment, and they will need some sensitive, clear education on various contraindications. Clients might even expect to be refused treatment based on an old contraindication. Or they received massage following cancer treatment from someone who was unaware of the massage adjustments or was too careful. Often, clients undergoing cancer treatment will expect a normal massage session, and in fact might be indignant that they are being treated differently, massage-wise, because they have cancer. In such a case, it pays to take the lead and direct the session, explaining the reasons for each contraindication.

This is especially true for a first-time session with a client. Say something helpful, such as, "Maybe we could use firmer pressure over time, and I can keep track of how massage affects you. But for right now, you're in strong treatment, and this is the first time I'm working with you, so I think we should start gently. The last thing we'd want is for you to feel worse after this session rather than better! What do you think?"

Questions 2–4 are about the status and type of cancer, as well as the location. The "where?" answer will guide massage pressure at a certain site or sites. If the tumor is superficial enough to be reached with direct massage pressure (as in a breast lump or vertebral body) or disturbed by any joint movements (as in the acetabulum of the hip, with hip range of motion [ROM] or stretches), then avoid these actions. Cancer essentials and complications are summarized in a Decision Tree, Figure 20-5.

> *The Tumor Site Principle. Do not press directly on a tumor site if it is accessible to the hands, and do not move joints if movement would mechanically disturb a nearby tumor.*

This principle applies, as well, to sites of metastasis. In general, tumors in vital organs are too deep to be disturbed by most massage pressures but those in the lower GI tract or elsewhere in the abdomen or pelvis may be reachable depending on the massage focus. If a tumor is reachable, avoid reaching it. Hematological cancers do not typically feature a discrete site; instead, cancer cells are widely distributed and are unlikely to spread from place to place with massage. Review "Leukemia," "Non-Hodgkin Lymphoma," and "Multiple Myeloma" for particulars (Chapters 12 and 13).

Cancer Essentials and Complications

Medical Information	Massage Therapy Guidelines

Essentials

- Uncontrolled, malignant growth of abnormal cells, with potential to invade adjacent tissues or spread to distant sites
  - Carcinoma (solid tumor of epithelial tissue)
  - Sarcoma (solid tumor of connective tissue)
  - Hematologic malignancy (nonsolid cancer cells; affect bone marrow, blood, or lymphoid tissue)

May be asymptomatic; signs/symptoms include: change in bowel or bladder habits; area or sore that does not heal; unusual bleeding or discharge; thickening or lump in tissue; indigestion or difficulty swallowing; obvious change in wart or mole; nagging cough or hoarseness

→

- No pressure or joint movement that disturbs a solid tumor
- If client does not know primary site, limit overall pressure to level 1-2, limit joint movement to well within normal range
- If client has cancer of unknown primary site (CUP), there may be no overall pressure limitation, but consult with the physician to be certain
- Ask periodically about diagnostic tests for updates on cancer status, location

- If client reports symptoms, or you notice signs, bring to client's attention; medical referral

Complications

- Metastasis to Bone
  - May be asymptomatic
  - Pain
  - Possible pathologic fracture risk

  - Fracture
  - Spinal cord compression; sensation changes, impairment of bowel and bladder function; motor weakness

→

- Adjust pressure and joint movement to tissue stability per client's doctor; when in doubt, pressure level = 1 max
- Adjust massage to comparable medical restrictions on activity, if any
- Position may need to be adjusted for client comfort, to ease pressure at site
- For new, unfamiliar, or worsening pain, avoid pressure and joint movement near site; urgent medical referral
- For known fracture, position for comfort; no pressure at site
- For new symptoms, immediate medical referral; no massage
- For known cord compression, follow Sensation Principles (see Chapter 3) and any joint movement/position recommendations from the health care team

- Metastasis to Liver
  - Impaired liver function
  - Ascites

→

- Follow Filter and Pump Principle, Vital Organ Principle; see Liver Failure, Chapter 16
- No circulatory intent at site; adapt position for comfort; consider sidelying, semireclining, or seated; avoid flat prone or supine position

- Metastasis to Lung
  - Poor oxygenation of tissues; weakness
  - Breathing difficulties

→

- Follow Vital Organ Principle; possible shorter session, pressure to tolerance (level 3 maximum); see Lung Cancer, Conditions in Brief, Chapter 14
- Gentle pressure on thorax, slow speeds, even rhythms, gradual transitions; position to facilitate breathing: inclined upper body, seated, sidelying

- Metastasis to Brain
  - Seizures
  - Dizziness
  - Headaches
  - Blurred vision
  - Nausea
  - Mental status changes

→

- Follow Vital Organ Principle
- See Seizures; Seizure disorders, Conditions in Brief, Chapter 10; follow Emergency Protocol Principle (see Chapter 3)
- Reposition gently, slow speed and even rhythm, slow rise from table, gentle transition at end of session
- Position for comfort, especially prone; consider inclined table or propping; gentle session overall; pressure to tolerance; slow speed and even rhythm; avoid headache trigger; general circulatory intent may be poorly tolerated
- No massage adjustments
- Position for comfort, gentle session overall; pressure to tolerance, slow speeds; no uneven rhythms or strong joint movement
- Communicate with caregiver; verify client's consent; watch for nonverbal cues during the session

- Metastasis to other tissues, organs

→

- Investigate loss in function, tissue stability; adapt massage accordingly (consider Vital Organ Principle)
- If blockage or pain, adapt positioning for comfort
- Easy bathroom access if bowel, bladder control affected

- Thrombosis, embolism

→

- Follow DVT Risk Principles (see Chapter 11)
- Be alert for signs/symptoms of DVT, follow suspected DVT Principle

- Paraneoplastic syndrome (including fever, fatigue, fluid retention, seizures, arthritis, weight loss, and other complications)

→

- Adjust to signs/symptoms, dysfunction in organ or tissue; avoid general circulatory intent if fluid retention present

FIGURE 20-5. A Decision Tree for cancer essentials and complications.

If the client cannot tell you where the tumor site is, then adjust your overall pressure to the level 1–2 range. You may find this situation among individuals who choose not to treat their disease with conventional medicine. In most cases, people making these treatment choices still receive regular scans and other tests to know the cancer status, but some people go completely outside of conventional medicine. Still others are unaware of their status because the details do not interest them, or they do not have the capacity to understand the information or relay it correctly to you. In these cases, unless you have regular information from the physician or a family member, limit your overall pressure to level 1–2, as well.

If the client has a CUP site, this pressure limit may not apply. Usually the primary tumor is too tiny, diffuse, or indistinct to be detectable on a scan, and would not be affected by massage pressure any more than the usual pressure from sitting, standing, or lying down. If you are unsure, communicate with the client's doctor about the best overall pressure.

You might find out, in answer to Questions 2 and 3, that the condition was in the past and there is no tumor present to adjust to; it may be a non-issue. You might, instead, need to make a simple pressure adjustment near an incision site, or adapt to the lingering effects of cancer treatment, described below.

Question 4 about diagnostic tests is a useful question to ask periodically, perhaps at each visit. Diagnostic tests are used to determine cancer status. By updating this information, you can adjust your pressure and joint movement for new lesions. Questions about diagnostics also help you to gauge whether there are new areas of concern, as tests are also ordered when new symptoms appear, and when the doctor suspects the cancer has spread. Adapt massage to the medical concern—known or suspected. This is referred to as "borrowing the medical concern," and it might mean avoiding pressure on new areas that are being checked out, until test results come back. Treat suspected lesions like established ones, following the Waiting for a Diagnosis Principle.

> *The Waiting for a Diagnosis Principle.* **If a client is scheduled for diagnostic tests, or is awaiting results, adapt massage to the possible diagnosis. If more than one condition is being investigated, adapt massage to the worst-case scenario.**

Diagnostic tests can be stressful, and some are painful. Often the client must hold still for a time, which can increase muscle tension and anxiety. Massage may be a welcome, comforting diversion, as well as a source of tension relief.

Questions 5–12 concern the effects of cancer on the client's body. Question 5, about bone involvement, is vital information for the massage plan. Bone metastasis deserves special consideration, and it is important to ask each one of the follow-up questions even though there is some repetition. The client's responses should inform you about any bone stability concerns that the client's health care team might have, and your pressure and joint movement should mirror these concerns. Here are some scenarios:

- If the client is very active, the doctor is aware of the client's activity level, and there are no restrictions on activity, it might be possible to provide pressure at a level 3 or 4 overall, with much less pressure around known lesions.

- If the client has been told by his or her doctor or nurse to move carefully, use a cane, or step gently downstairs for fear of hip fracture in specific places, your overall pressure will most likely be in the level 2–3 range, with pressure at level 1–2 near known lesions.

- If bone lesions are widely disseminated, with significant impact on bone stability, your overall pressure limits will likely be at level 1–2, and severe instability may require only the softest holding at pressure level 1, with no stroking.

These scenarios reflect pressure ranges, not specific directives for specific clients you might encounter. The client's doctor and nurse provide the final, authoritative word on bone stability and the best pressures for the client. The pressure scale (see Chapter 2) can be very useful when you communicate with them about bone involvement and massage.

> *The Bone Metastasis Principle.* **If cancer involves the bone, determine the bone stability in order to apply safe levels of pressure and joint movement.**

Be sure to adjust your joint movement and positioning to reflect the pressure recommendations. Strong stretches may be ill-advised, and in some cases, even gentle joint movement could be too much for a nearby lesion. Position the client to ease discomfort.

If you work in a high-volume setting, with a likely one-time client and no opportunity for dialogue with the physician or monitoring over time, use extremely conservative pressure. Pressure level 1 is best to use whenever you feel you do not have complete information about a client's bone stability.

Questions 6 and 7 are important in their own right, but they also relate to Question 5. Any of these symptoms are red flags and could indicate new bone lesions. Specifically, if a client with active cancer, a recent cancer history, or continued follow-up reports any new, unfamiliar, or worsening pain, adjust your massage plan. Avoid pressure or joint movement in the area until the client's doctor has ruled out new lesions of any sort, especially bone metastasis. Encourage your client to bring his or her symptoms to the doctor. This is an urgent medical referral.

Heighten your concern even further if the client reports any of these symptoms:

- Pain that is sharp, shooting, or radiating
- Sensation changes such as numbness, pins and needles, or burning
- Motor weakness

Any of these could indicate nerve involvement: bone metastasis or pathologic fracture that has compressed on the spinal cord or nearby peripheral nerves. An *immediate* medical referral is in order because the client might require immobilization to limit the damage and prevent further injury. Paralysis is a grave concern in this scenario, and massage is inappropriate at this time. "This could be very serious, or it could be nothing at all; I'm not qualified to say either way. But this is not a good time for a massage. Instead, let's call your doctor's office and ask about the best course to follow."

Although these scenarios are not all that common in massage practice, they do occur, and clients often bring musculoskeletal pain to a massage therapist's attention before they approach their health care team. Your referral can be vital in getting the client needed medical care. For known cord compression, follow relevant Sensation Principles and positioning restrictions to protect the area.

Questions 8 and 9 address the possibility that cancer or cancer treatment might affect other functions in the body. Combining cancer with cancer treatment in one question saves time in the interview. Liver, lung, and brain are common sites of metastasis and can be sites of primary tumor, as well. Recall that cancer can be present in an organ without appreciably affecting organ function, but if it does, see Figure 20-5, and follow the Vital Organ Principle.

> *Vital Organ Principle. If a vital organ—heart, lung, kidney, liver, or brain—is compromised in function, use gentle massage elements and adjust them to pose minimal challenge to the client's body.*

For each organ involved, there are special concerns: Liver metastasis may cause ascites to form, requiring a change in position and intent (see "Liver Failure" and "Liver Cancer," Chapter 16). Follow the Filter and Pump Principle if function is impaired. Lung mets can cause breathing difficulties, which also indicate special positioning (see "Lung Cancer," Chapter 14). Brain metastasis, or even a primary tumor of the brain, can cause severe symptoms: seizures, dizziness, headaches, vision changes, and nausea are possible complications. Each of these is addressed in the Decision Tree (see Figure 20-5). If there are mental status changes, your health questions should be directed to the client's caregivers, and it will be important to establish that you have the client's consent for the session. Nonverbal cues will help you determine whether your work is welcome, the pressure is appropriate, and so on.

If other tissues or organs are affected by metastasis or by the primary tumor, inquire about any loss in organ/tissue function. Ask if it causes any blockage or pain and how massage and positioning might be helpful. Question 8, or any other general questions you ask, might bring up problems caused by paraneoplastic syndrome. People do not often recognize that term, and you don't need to use it, but symptoms such as headache and fever are encompassed in PS. Take careful notes, and consult appropriate Decision Trees in this book. Adjust the massage plan accordingly. If fluid retention is a result, avoid general circulatory massage.

Be alert for DVT risk. Recall that *any* advanced cancer could raise the risk of DVT, regardless of the primary site, but be especially careful in primary cancer of the lung, ovary, prostate, GI tract, or pancreas. Apply both DVT Risk principles to these situations, and potentially to anyone with active cancer. One way to apply these principles is to communicate with the physician through a written care plan (see Figure 5-3 for an example). You can address DVT risk explicitly on the form, and ask specifically about the advisability of pressure above 1 or 2 on the lower extremities. You might decide to use this form with every client in cancer treatment and within a standard timeframe after the end of treatment (1 year is typical). By communicating in this way, you can encourage dialogue about other massage adjustments for cancer and cancer treatment, as well. As always, be alert for DVT signs and symptoms.

Questions 10 and 11 about blood counts again combine the effects of cancer and cancer treatment into each question, thereby saving time. It is a good idea to ask some version of these questions at each session, since counts can change quickly.

Hematologic cancers (see Chapter 12) and even some solid tumors can affect bone marrow function, and chemotherapy is notorious for its injury to bone marrow. If the client's counts are affected, recall that low platelets (thrombocytopenia) indicate less pressure, as does any other clotting deficiency. Low WBCs (neutropenia) indicate careful infection control, and low RBCs (anemia) indicate adjustments for dizziness, fatigue, and cold intolerance. See Figure 20-8 for specific approaches.

Some precautions for neutropenia are good practice for anyone in cancer treatment, since it is not a good time for a patient to catch a cold or any other infection. Monitor your own health, and offer clients the chance to reschedule without penalty if you have symptoms that could indicate infection.

Question 12 about complications is open-ended and may already have been answered at this point in the interview, but it is good for reinforcement. Many answers to this question are possible, including various PS symptoms, end of life complications, emotions such as grief or anxiety, cancer pain, limits on activity, and so on. Whatever the client's answers, think carefully about whether a major organ or tissue function is impaired. Usually answers to this question suggest gentle pressure, a short session, gentle joint movement, and a compassionate manner.

Questions 13 and 14, the Activity and Energy Questions (see Chapter 4), help you assess how much the client is affected by cancer or cancer treatment, and gauge the proper massage strength for the first session. Answers here are invaluable. The activity questions may help you decide on a "normal" session of moderate strength, but always err on the gentler side if you're unsure. Also, if there are activity prohibitions, follow the Medically Restricted Activity Principle. This is an example of "borrowing the medical concern" of the client's health care team. For example, a physician might tell a client to take it easy after cancer surgery, possibly for 1–2 months, so you would work gently for that period of time. Another client, who sustained damage to her heart from radiation therapy 25 years ago, could have lifelong activity restrictions. This is also a time to begin gently, and without general circulatory intent.

> *Medically Restricted Activity Principle. If there are any medical restrictions on a client's activities, explore and apply any equivalent massage contraindications.*

Question 15, about treatment status, also points to gentle work overall if the client is in treatment, between treatments, or has recently completed a full course. Draw a distinction between major cancer treatments here (surgery, radiation, chemotherapy, stem cell transplant) and other, less strong follow-up treatments to prevent recurrence, such as hormone therapy. There is a common observation: "It can take a year to recover from cancer treatment." Respect this, and start gently; even if a client is 10 months out of major treatment, he or she might still be getting his or her strength back. On the other hand, treatment that ended 18 months ago might be barely noticeable, and the client is now playing basketball regularly. The Activity and Energy Questions can help you determine the right place to start, and with monitoring over time, it is possible to tailor the sessions to the client's responses.

Question 16 about various cancer treatments can open up a long series of follow-up questions. These can take time when done verbally, and a form with all of the possibilities generally

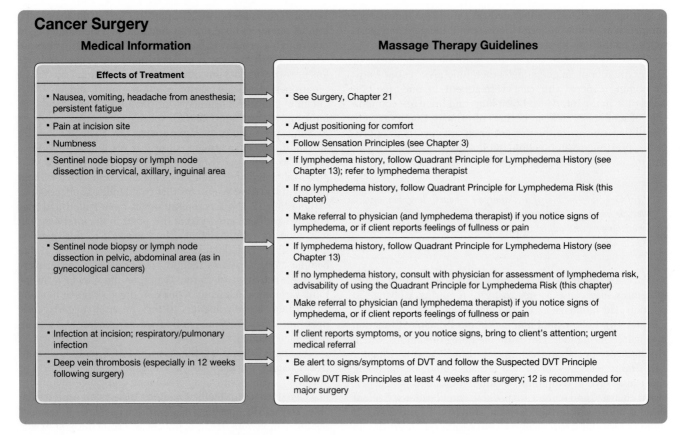

FIGURE 20-6. A Decision Tree for cancer surgery.

saves time. For a full list of massage guidelines, refer to the Decision Tree for each of the common cancer treatments. Highlights from each Decision Tree are discussed below.

There are three principal complications of cancer surgery to be alert to: infection, thrombosis, and lymphedema (Figure 20-6). The two most serious complications postsurgery are infection and thrombosis, and individuals are given careful aftercare guidelines to prevent and identify them. You are in a good position to make an immediate referral to the client's physician if you notice any signs or symptoms of infection at the incision site, or if the client shows any signs of respiratory infection. Keep an eye out for DVT signs and symptoms, and follow the Suspected DVT Principle if you observe any (see Chapter 11). Follow the DVT Risk Principles for at least 4 weeks after surgery, and 12 weeks after major surgery (see "Surgery," Chapter 21).

Minor swelling after surgery can resemble lymphedema if it occurs in key areas, but it usually resolves quickly and is not considered true lymphedema. Recall that chronic lymphedema can appear at any time after surgery when key lymph nodes are removed. For a client with lymphedema, either current, or in the past, follow the Quadrant Principle for Lymphedema History (see Chapter 13).

Where lymphedema is a risk, plan your session to avoid precipitating an episode. If one or more cervical, axillary, or inguinal lymph nodes were removed, even if it was just a SNB, follow the Quadrant Principle for Lymphedema Risk (this chapter). This precaution is lifelong. In the at-risk area, steer clear of heat treatments involving hot stones, hot packs or steam that could redden the skin. The at-risk regions, areas of caution for each site of lymph node removal, are shown in Figure 20-7.

The Quadrant Principle for Lymphedema Risk. Avoid pressure above 2, reddening of the skin, and strong joint movement in the at-risk region of an area of cervical, axillary, or inguinal lymph node removal or radiation therapy. This includes the extremity as well as the trunk area, anterior and posterior, drained by the affected lymph nodes.

If you notice signs of lymphedema, bring them to the client's attention for an urgent medical referral, and a referral to a lymphedema therapist. Make the same referral if the client complains of pain, fullness, or heaviness in the area. Do not try to treat the swelling with classical massage techniques such as effleurage and petrissage; they are unlikely to help lymphedema and can easily worsen the condition.

If SNB or LND was performed in the pelvic or abdominal area, the massage precaution is less clear, because little is known about the level of lymphedema risk in these areas. The safest course of action is to consult the client's physician about lymphedema risk before using pressure greater than 2 on the lower extremities. Again, if you notice signs of the condition, make appropriate referrals.

It can be difficult to explain this conservative massage plan to a client, and the massage adjustments can feel lopsided to both of you. The best approach to use is to compare the massage precautions to other activity precautions in wide use (see Table 20-1). If the client has been told that blood pressure should not be taken on that side, remind the client that your own pressure precautions mirror that medical concern. If the client has been

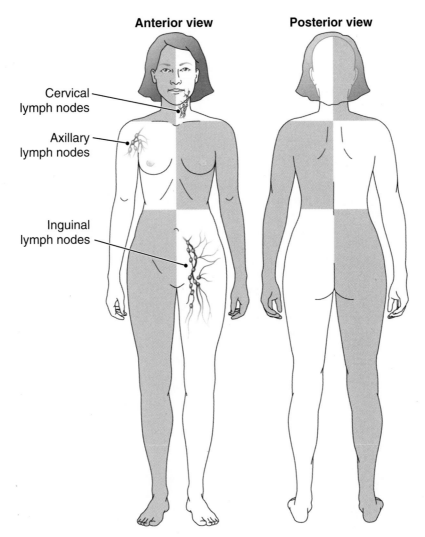

Anterior view   **Posterior view**

Cervical
lymph nodes

Axillary
lymph nodes

Inguinal
lymph nodes

FIGURE 20-7. Areas defined by the Quadrant Principle for Lymphedema Risk. Lymphedema risk is elevated when lymph nodes are removed or treated with radiation during cancer treatment. Each unshaded quadrant shows the area of massage caution that corresponds to the missing or injured lymph nodes.

told not to soak his legs in a hot tub, remind the client that you should avoid introducing heat, friction, or too much pressure in your work on those areas.

If you are working with a client who was *not* warned against these activities, or who chooses not to follow them, you can tell them that your massage adjustments parallel the activity precautions that are most widely used. Recall the disparities in medicine about the best approach to lymphedema prevention. Without consistent agreement on which medical precautions to follow, it makes sense to follow the most conservative massage approach.

Although the Quadrant Principle for Lymphedema Risk seems strict, there are still many possibilities for healing touch. See Therapist's Journal 20-1 for wonderful therapeutic results within the pressure limits of this principle.

If your client is in chemotherapy, or is still feeling the effects of it, your massage plan may include a number of adjustments. For a client with a port (see Figure 20-3), you might need to modify or avoid the prone position. Using a couple of hand towels as padding around a port, creating a depression or "nest," may be comfortable for some people.

Others barely notice their port and have no problem lying in any position.

Numerous, strong side effects of chemotherapy are discussed in the Treatment section, above. In general, avoid general circulatory intent with a client in chemotherapy, placing as little demand on the body as possible. Over a course of massage sessions, you might be able to work less carefully but only after monitoring the client's responses. Chemotherapy can cause profound fatigue. A client's energy level can change from week to week, even day to day, so do not be too ambitious. Moreover, avoid spa treatments or massage techniques that are thought to have a detoxifying effect (see "General Principles," Chapter 16). Avoid, as well, treatments that include strong exfoliation. These approaches are not recommended and may be too taxing for someone who is dealing with strong medication. Your intent should be to support the client's body, not add another demand on it.

*The Detoxification Principle. **If an intent of a spa treatment is to detoxify, avoid using it when the client is significantly challenged by illness or injury, or is taking strong medication.***

THERAPIST'S JOURNAL 20-1 *Healing within the Bounds of the Quadrant Principle*

A 45-year-old woman was diagnosed with an aggressive form of breast cancer. She had a mastectomy with axillary LND. The surgeon removed 33 lymph nodes from under her arm. This was followed by radiation to the area and chemotherapy.

Like many people after this kind of surgery, this client found it difficult to raise her arm to reach up, bring it back to put on a sweater, and so on. One day at a follow-up her surgeon said, "Raise your arm for me, please." She replied, "No! You took 33 lymph nodes out and I can't! It hurts!" This problem persisted even though, unlike many breast cancer survivors, she had received regular physical therapy (PT). She decided to try massage therapy in conjunction with her PT.

As a patient at the cancer treatment center where I worked, she decided to avail herself of the integrative services. Her goals at the time of our first meeting were to help with the discomfort and decreased ROM of her right arm. She also wanted to use massage to help with anxiety.

Although this client had no lymphedema, I am well aware of the risk of it in anyone with LND. I followed the Quadrant Principle carefully. I used Swedish strokes at very gentle pressure—levels 1 and 2 on her right upper trunk quadrant, and "energy holds" over the whole quadrant. I also know some acupressure and used an acupressure protocol for upper back and shoulder tension, making the proper adjustments for this modality as well.

One may wonder if this feels lopsided, but I concentrated on giving firm, reassuring, "I am here" touch throughout, no matter what the pressure, keeping the flow of healing intent in my hands. She never mentioned that the session felt uneven to her. She always felt relaxed after her sessions.

I followed this protocol for several weeks. My client began to raise her arm over her head. It was slow but steady progress. After a couple of months she said, proudly, "I can now do the 'itsy-bitsy spider' motions all the way up the waterspout!" an exercise that her doctor had initially suggested. As importantly, she began to reach up and back, change clothes more easily, and move through her work and life with less pain and full ROM.

It has been 4 years since we first worked together, and although I no longer see her at the integrative clinic, she continues to see a massage therapist who also has training in manual lymph drainage. Her massage therapist and I have communicated every now and then, and she follows the same principles on pressure limits as I started.

She is, and will always be, at risk of lymphedema, and these limits honor that fact. Massage within these limits still serves her.

Sometimes I think we get too attached to deep pressure in our profession and forget how helpful gentle work can be. We feel "pressured by our clients to apply pressure," so we don't explore all of the possibilities at the lighter end of the pressure spectrum. In any case, this client clearly benefited. And I feel very much blessed to have been part of helping her reach her goals.

Bambi Mathay
Melrose, MA

As seen in the Decision Tree (Figure 20-8), chief concerns during chemotherapy are low blood counts, GI side effects, and effects on the skin and nervous system. Brief massage therapy guidelines for low platelets, WBCs, and RBCs are outlined, and each condition is discussed more fully in Chapter 12. Other problems are straightforward: If hair loss has occurred, take care with your lubricant around a wig or headscarf, as wigs are expensive to wash. GI effects of chemotherapy are briefly described in the Decision Tree; they are common conditions discussed throughout this book, and in detail in Chapter 15. If mouth sores are a problem, avoid pressure on the face, from massage or the face cradle.

If hand-foot syndrome is a problem, take care with your pressure, and avoid contact with open lesions. When neuropathy is a side-effect of chemotherapy, review that section in Chapter 10. If the client reports having chemobrain, or seems to exhibit signs—forgetting appointments, repeating questions, lack of focus—consider making reminder calls before appointments. Take time with scheduling, and repeat important information if needed. Do not make the mistake of identifying with the client—"I forget things all the time!" or "That sounds just like menopause!"—as statements like these can seem dismissive.

The effects of chemobrain are profound and often terrifying, much greater than occasional forgetfulness. In general, be sensitive to the range of possible responses to chemotherapy, as Therapist's Journal 20-2 suggests.

If the client is in radiation therapy, review the Decision Tree in Figure 20-9. Most massage adjustments for radiation therapy are based on common sense: Avoid friction, pressure, anything but hospital-issue lubricant, and in most cases direct contact over the radiation field. Some clients might welcome gentle hands over the field through a drape during treatment, and some might find relief from pain or itching that way. But for the most part, the healing skin at a radiation site should be treated as such, and most massage techniques are contraindicated.

Adjust your massage plan to the effects of radiation in specific areas: You might have to incline the client's position if radiation to the chest has produced shortness of breath, or skip the face cradle if radiation has been delivered to the head or neck. If there has been radiation to the lower abdomen, the client's position might have to be adjusted for pain, and easy bathroom access might be necessary. If the radiation field is large, it may affect blood counts, as chemotherapy does; see Figure 20-8 for massage adjustments if so.

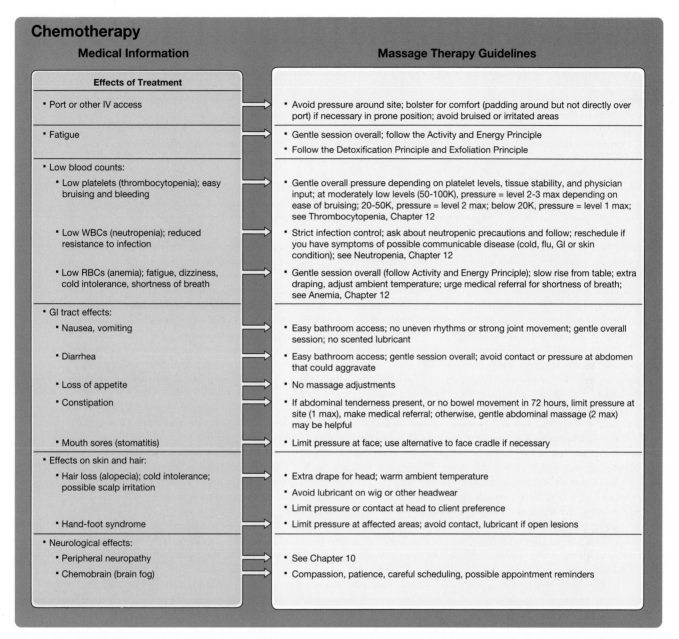

FIGURE 20-8. A Decision Tree for chemotherapy. Not all side effects are shown. Not all drugs cause all side effects.

Some radiation markings are permanent tattoos, but they may be darkened with a semipermanent marker. For these and other temporary radiation markings, avoid rubbing them with oil or lotion. The markings might be in the radiation field, outside of it, or even on the other side of the body because they are used to line up equipment. If radiation is internal or ingested, as in implants or radioactive iodine, follow the contact precautions given by the client's nurse and doctor.

Although less is known about it, radiation treatment of lymph nodes can cause lymphedema, just as surgical removal can. One of the two Quadrant Principles (Chapter 13; this chapter) may be in order. Review the lymphedema sections in this chapter carefully, and refer to the Decision Tree (Figure 20-9) for guidelines.

Remember that radiation can be terribly fatiguing as it goes on, and consider a gentle session overall, especially as the course of therapy progresses and the client begins to feel the cumulative effects of repeated radiation treatments.

If the client is having biologic therapy—strong immunotherapy—massage may need to be adapted to flu-like symptoms. Figure 20-10 shows massage guidelines for these and other side effects of biologic therapy. Gentle pressure, probably in the 1–2 range, is advised, and stationary contact may be the only welcome stimulation. The side effects of some biologics can be very strong, and touch is likely to be poorly tolerated when symptoms are acute.

Hormone therapy can be a primary cancer treatment or an adjuvant therapy to prevent recurrence. Massage guidelines for some effects of hormone therapy are shown in the Decision Tree in Figure 20-11. Note that hot flashes may be a side effect, calling for sensitive, layered draping. Breast enlargement calls for padding above and below the breasts when prone, or other helpful positioning. A skin reaction contraindicates friction at the site and possibly contact. And for any hormone therapy, investigate the risk of thrombosis, any other thrombosis risk factors the client might have, and

THERAPIST'S JOURNAL 20-2 *A Range of Responses to Chemotherapy*

When working with clients who have cancer, I try to remember that each person will respond differently to cancer and cancer treatment. The variety of responses to chemotherapy is the most striking example. Some people are profoundly weakened by chemotherapy and are very sick, and others sail through it, maintaining nearly normal activity levels.

From this variation, I've learned two things. The first is to question clients closely about their treatment and responses to it. When a client says, "I've been really tired and sick, and I haven't been able to do much at all during chemotherapy," what does that mean, exactly? Sometimes I've asked clients to elaborate, and I've been surprised by their activity levels. For one client, the definition of "I've been a slug because I'm so tired" meant doing just three work-outs at the gym that week, lifting weights, and climbing stairs. Before cancer treatment, she went to the gym daily, so this was a marked change. For another client, fatigue from chemotherapy meant he only attended two yoga sessions in a week instead of his usual five. For another, it meant "I am on the couch, literally all the time." And for another, working part-time and parenting took every ounce of energy and strength she had left after chemotherapy. She was completely spent. For most people, chemotherapy is completely consuming. All people in chemotherapy need to be treated with hands of kindness.

While I always begin with the gentlest of sessions for clients undergoing chemotherapy or any kind of strong treat-ment, there are moments that it might be possible to add a tiny bit more intensity if they wish. This might mean spending a couple of minutes longer in an area, or increasing overall pressure from level 2 to 2½. Later in the course of treatment, it's important to use less demanding pressures as the effects of chemotherapy are cumulative.

At the first session, it's very important to err on the gentler side, with all clients. I tell them, "I haven't worked with you during chemotherapy before. We don't know how you'll respond to the combination of chemo and massage. We need to be gentle, especially at first, and see how you do." Along the way, I make very fine adjustments, using intuition as well as information about the client's activity level.

The second thing I've learned is that neither of these responses—robust or frail—to cancer treatment is better or worse. They're just different. This is important because we tend to admire and marvel at the folks who are strong through chemo-therapy, who don't miss a beat, who keep working and fighting and keep on keeping on. We tend to idealize their strength, sometimes at the expense of others who are home on the couch, who are very, very sick and can barely move. We become tempted by simplistic theories: this person is doing well because she has a positive attitude, for example, or that person is sick because he is hopeless or weak. Too easily, we assign blame, praise, or meaning to our clients and their experiences. By doing so, we do them a disservice. Cancer, treatment, and healing are more complex than any one theory or belief system. We all have different bodies and different lives. We all respond differently.

Seeing this range in responses to chemotherapy has strengthened me as well—in compassion, understanding, and clinical judgment. My hands have learned how to let up when they need to, how to lean in very gently when they can, and how to know the difference. With everyone, I sit quietly for a time, with soft, still hands holding a head, or a shoul-der. I place one hand at the sacrum, the other between the scapulae. I bear witness to the courage and spirit of the per-son on the table. With my hands, I wish them strength and support for the next treatment, and the next step on the path.

Tracy Walton
Cambridge, MA

consider the DVT Risk Principles (see Chapter 11). Fatigue, nausea, and headache, common side effects of many drugs, call for simple adjustments to the massage plan. These are described in the Decision Tree.

If your client has had a stem cell transplant (Figure 20-12), you may have to make several massage adjustments. First, review the side effects and complications of chemotherapy and multiply those effects to extraordinary proportions for the high-dose chemotherapy scenario in a stem cell transplant. Adjust your massage accordingly. Second, if radiation is involved, the client may be recovering from total body irradiation (TBI) or another form. The effects of TBI are similar to those of chemo-therapy, and some are the same as with smaller radiation fields. Consider massage guidelines for radiation therapy, and amplify them for TBI. Third, the client is likely to be profoundly immunosuppressed for some time after the treatment. Follow the lead of the client's health care team and caregivers in terms of infection control precautions. These may be very strict and

not intuitively obvious. Read up on them, check with the cli-ent's caregivers about these guidelines, and work well within them. Clients may be taking immunosuppressive medications long after the treatment. Fourth, if chronic GVHD is a real-ity, avoid contact at the site of skin GVHD. If GVHD is also affecting the liver, or organs of the GI tract, adjust the massage accordingly, depending on symptoms.

A client who has had a stem cell transplant may be taking many medications (see Therapist's Journal 21-1 for one patient's story). It is necessary to ask the Four Medication Questions about each one and adapt accordingly (see Chapter 4). See Figure 21-7 for numerous side effects of medications, and corresponding massage guidelines.

No matter what kind of cancer treatment your client tells you about, ask if the client is taking any additional medications to manage cancer symptoms or side effects. This last, "catch-all" question may capture any further massage concerns. Ask the Four Medication Questions about each one (see

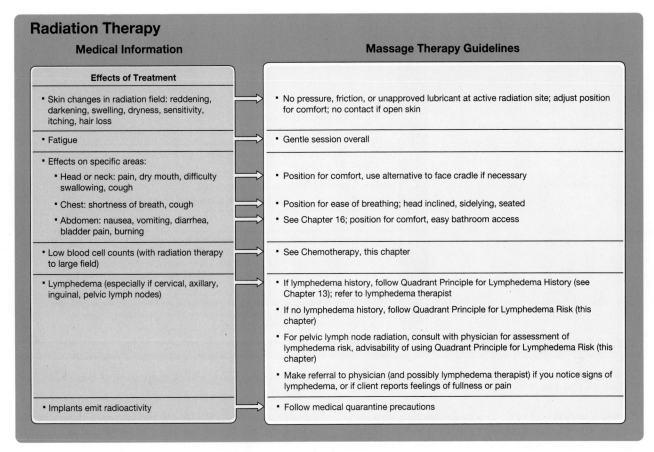

FIGURE 20-9. A Decision Tree for radiation therapy.

Chapter 4), and use the Medication Principle. As suggested in the Decision Tree for supportive care measures (Figure 20-13), adapt your massage to the side effects of drugs such as antiemetics, colony-stimulating factors, pain relievers, anti-seizure drugs, and bisphosphonates.

The Medication Principle. Adapt massage to the condition for which the medication is taken or prescribed, and to any side effects.

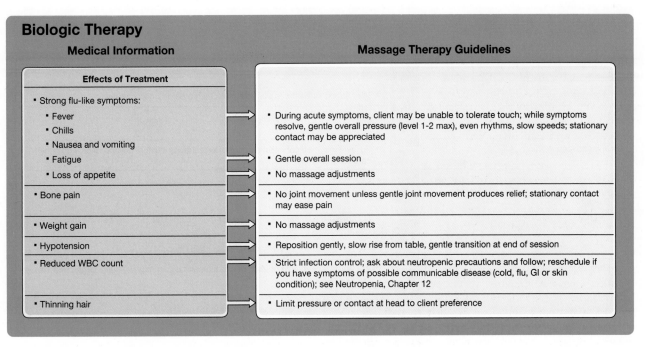

FIGURE 20-10. A Decision Tree for biologic therapy. Not all side effects are shown. Not all drugs cause all side effects.

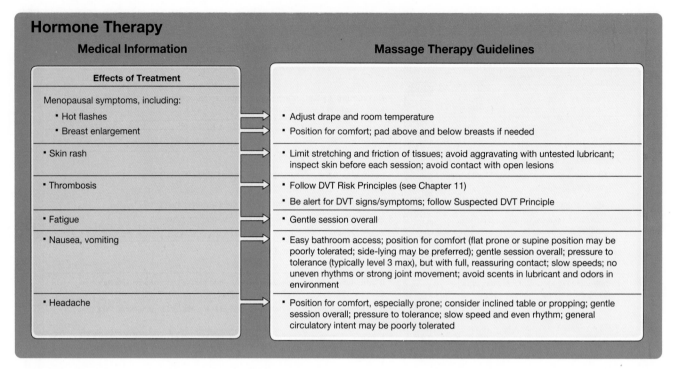

FIGURE 20-11. A Decision Tree for hormone therapy. Not all side effects are shown. Not all drugs cause all side effects.

Finally, Questions 18 and 19 provide another chance to capture any side effects not already mentioned, and an invitation to talk about long-term effects of cancer or treatment. Lymphedema history or risk is an obvious one. Scar tissue, reduced mobility, pain, lingering neuropathy, lingering chemobrain, and others may play a prominent role in a person's life when recovering from cancer treatment, and in the years beyond it. Emotional scars may also remain, and the year following the end of treatment can be an especially vulnerable time in terms of anxiety and depression. Once treatment ends, there is "less to do," and

the pace slows down. People can feel aimless without something to focus on, and in the absence of this drive and purpose, other feelings can creep in. Massage therapy can be an especially good resource during this time. Be sensitive to a client's challenges during that 1st year.

Cancer can be one of the most medically complex conditions to manage in massage therapy practice. There are many factors to consider in planning massage for someone with active cancer, in cancer treatment, and even in the weeks, months, and years following treatment. Some of common chief massage concerns

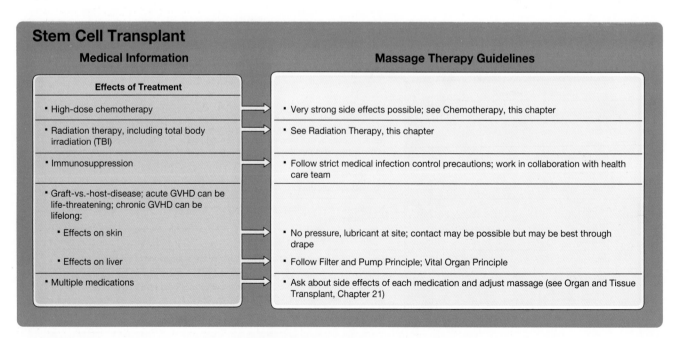

FIGURE 20-12. A Decision Tree for stem cell transplant.

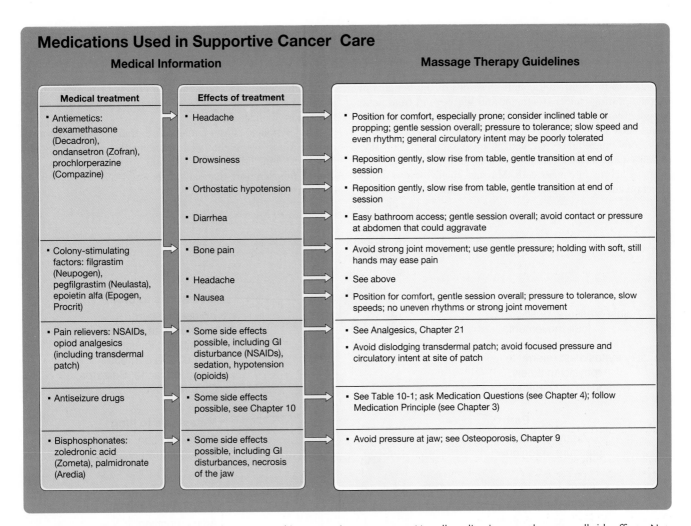

Medications Used in Supportive Cancer Care

Medical Information   **Massage Therapy Guidelines**

Medical treatment	Effects of treatment	Massage Therapy Guidelines
• Antiemetics: dexamethasone (Decadron), ondansetron (Zofran), prochlorperazine (Compazine)	• Headache	• Position for comfort, especially prone; consider inclined table or propping; gentle session overall; pressure to tolerance; slow speed and even rhythm; general circulatory intent may be poorly tolerated
	• Drowsiness	• Reposition gently, slow rise from table, gentle transition at end of session
	• Orthostatic hypotension	• Reposition gently, slow rise from table, gentle transition at end of session
	• Diarrhea	• Easy bathroom access; gentle session overall; avoid contact or pressure at abdomen that could aggravate
• Colony-stimulating factors: filgrastim (Neupogen), pegfilgrastim (Neulasta), epoietin alfa (Epogen, Procrit)	• Bone pain	• Avoid strong joint movement; use gentle pressure; holding with soft, still hands may ease pain
	• Headache	• See above
	• Nausea	• Position for comfort, gentle session overall; pressure to tolerance, slow speeds; no uneven rhythms or strong joint movement
• Pain relievers: NSAIDs, opiod analgesics (including transdermal patch)	• Some side effects possible, including GI disturbance (NSAIDs), sedation, hypotension (opioids)	• See Analgesics, Chapter 21 • Avoid dislodging transdermal patch; avoid focused pressure and circulatory intent at site of patch
• Antiseizure drugs	• Some side effects possible, see Chapter 10	• See Table 10-1; ask Medication Questions (see Chapter 4); follow Medication Principle (see Chapter 3)
• Bisphosphonates: zoledronic acid (Zometa), palmidronate (Aredia)	• Some side effects possible, including GI disturbances, necrosis of the jaw	• Avoid pressure at jaw; see Osteoporosis, Chapter 9

FIGURE 20-13. A Decision Tree for medications used in supportive cancer care. Not all medications are shown, or all side effects. Not all drugs cause all side effects.

are summarized in Figure 20-14. The list of symptoms, complications, treatments, and side effects may seem overwhelming, but remember that these reflect the spectrum of possibilities, not the clinical presentation of every client. Communication with the client's physician, using the care plan format (see Figure 5-3), is strongly recommended. By using the Decision Tree, you can sort the client's presentation into smaller, easy to manage parts, and adjust your massage plan to each one. Once you assemble them into a massage plan, direct your focus to what you *can* do, and what massage can offer, rather than what is contraindicated.

Massage Therapy Research

At the time of this writing, the effects of massage on people with cancer have received a fair amount of attention in massage therapy research, but it is not yet possible to draw firm conclusions about benefit.

Two of the largest studies in massage therapy have focused on people with cancer. One group of investigators compared professional massage therapy to simple touch provided by laypeople. The two forms of touch were provided in weekly sessions to 380 people with advanced cancer (Kutner et al, 2008). Both interventions were found to have immediate benefit on pain and mood, with professional massage having a greater effect. However, the results were not sustained over time.

In another observational study of 1290 patients at the Memorial Sloan-Kettering Cancer Institute in New York City, significant reductions in pain, fatigue, nausea, anxiety, and depression were found in patients with cancer, when post-massage and pre-massage self-assessments of symptoms were compared. However, this was not a controlled trial, so there was no comparison group.

In review papers on the topic, no firm conclusions could be drawn (Ernst, 2009; Jane et al., 2009). Numerous smaller studies suggest benefit from massage (Grealish et al., 2000; Post-White et al., 2004), and the list of studies is growing. Numerous controlled trials in progress are in evidence at clinicaltrials.gov and the NIH RePORTer database. It is a good idea to check the research literature periodically, as the body of research on massage and cancer is growing quickly.

Possible Massage Benefits

Clients and therapists tell countless stories of the benefits of massage during cancer treatment and life beyond treatment. Massage can provide comfort before procedures and treatments such as surgery and chemotherapy and may help heal a poor body image after treatment. Cancer symptoms and side effects—pain, nausea, fatigue, anxiety, and depression—are major concerns in cancer care. Massage might have a direct effect on any of these, providing welcome relief to a client and his family. Moreover, the relaxation effects of massage might promote sleep, which can make other side effects and symptoms more manageable.

The companionship of massage therapy has the potential to ease a host of psychosocial problems that arise during any life-threatening health crisis: isolation, stigmatization, fear, and grief. Clients report that skilled massage can do wonders to ease the cancer journey.

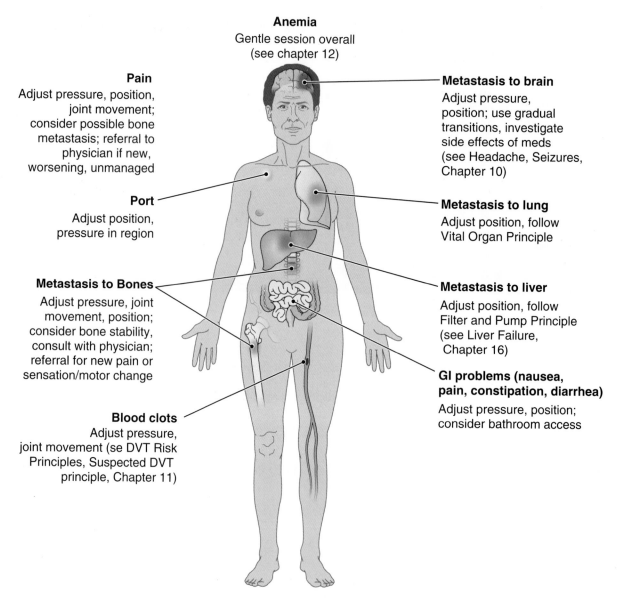

Anemia
Gentle session overall
(see chapter 12)

Pain
Adjust pressure, position, joint movement; consider possible bone metastasis; referral to physician if new, worsening, unmanaged

Port
Adjust position, pressure in region

Metastasis to Bones
Adjust pressure, joint movement, position; consider bone stability, consult with physician; referral for new pain or sensation/motor change

Blood clots
Adjust pressure, joint movement (se DVT Risk Principles, Suspected DVT principle, Chapter 11)

Metastasis to brain
Adjust pressure, position; use gradual transitions, investigate side effects of meds (see Headache, Seizures, Chapter 10)

Metastasis to lung
Adjust position, follow Vital Organ Principle

Metastasis to liver
Adjust position, follow Filter and Pump Principle (see Liver Failure, Chapter 16)

GI problems (nausea, pain, constipation, diarrhea)
Adjust pressure, position; consider bathroom access

FIGURE 20-14. Cancer: selected clinical features and massage therapy guidelines. Specific instructions and additional massage therapy guidelines are in Decision Trees and text.

SELF TEST

1. Describe the prevailing misconception that existed for many years about massage therapy and cancer, and the origins of it. Explain how current thinking about cancer spread overturns this myth.

2. How is the word "accessible" significant to the Tumor Site Principle?

3. Explain the Bone Metastasis Principle. Which massage elements may be modified when this principle is applied?

4. What are the four most common sites of cancer metastasis? Of these, which are vital organs?

5. Explain the difference between a primary and a secondary site of cancer.

6. What is the most common site of bone metastasis in adults? Why is knowledge of bone metastasis important to the massage plan?

7. Regarding a client with bone metastasis, what information do you use to determine the best pressure? What questions do you ask the client and/or physician? Describe which pressure level to use if you do not have that information.

8. What is a sentinel node biopsy (SNB), and in what ways is it helpful? What is the relationship between lymph node mapping and a SNB?

9. Why are increased circulation to the skin and inflammation risky for someone who is at risk for lymphedema?

10. Compare the Quadrant Principle for Lymphedema History and the Quadrant Principle for Lymphedema Risk. For each principle, describe one client presentation to which you would apply it. Describe the differences in massage adjustments in each case.

11. Explain how the Detoxification Principle relates to chemotherapy.

12. What is the purpose of radiation therapy?

13. Describe graft-vs.-host-disease (GVHD). How do you adjust massage for this condition?

14. Explain the purpose of hormone therapy in cancer treatment.

15. What is the purpose of biologic therapy? List three side effects and appropriate massage therapy adjustments for biologic therapy.

 For answers to these questions and to see a bibliography for this chapter, visit http://thePoint. lww.com/Walton.

Where a man feels pain, he lays his hand.

—DUTCH PROVERB

In Western medicine, medications and procedures work deeply and sometimes strongly to eliminate disease and manage symptoms. Medical treatments can also affect normal physiological function, resulting in unintended side effects, complications, and adverse reactions. Unintended, negative effects of drugs and other treatments create additional concerns for the massage therapist to consider.

This chapter covers medical treatments that are frequently mentioned in the preceding chapters. In this chapter, common analgesics (pain relievers) are discussed in detail: the nonsteroidal anti-inflammatory drugs (NSAIDs), corticosteroids, and prescription opioid analgesics (narcotics). Surgery is discussed in detail, as well as organ and tissue transplant.

The chapter concludes with an alphabetical list of common side effects of medications and procedures. Corresponding massage therapy guidelines are described for each side effect (see Table 21-1).

General Principles

Two principles from Chapter 3 are central to this chapter: the Medication Principle and the Procedure Principle. These principles are nearly identical, but the second principle concerns surgery, diagnostic tests, and other procedures. These principles suggest a massage plan should adapt to the condition for which the medication (or procedure) is being used as well as to the medication (or procedure) itself.

These principles can be applied to any drug or treatment that might be encountered in massage therapy practice, and they can be adapted to a continuum of client presentations. In general, a strong treatment with strong side effects reflects a more serious condition and a gentle massage. A client who is taking a strong pain reliever usually has severe pain. The pain may emanate from an area that is unstable, malignant, or especially vulnerable to massage elements like pressure and movement. Avoid aggravating the underlying condition causing the pain. Moreover, strong treatment can alter the tissue and overall physiology significantly; in this situation, the client doesn't need massage to impose *another* strong change. Massage should support the body, not challenge it further. Massage helps the body integrate the changes it is already coping with, rather than add more.

In keeping with the Medication (or Procedure) Principle, the Four Medication Questions, introduced in Chapter 4, are repeated throughout this text, and used throughout this chapter. Here are the four questions a therapist should ask about any medication or medical procedure:

1. How do you spell it? (For looking it up in a reference or on the Internet.)
2. What is it for? (To adapt massage to the presenting condition.)
3. Is it effective? (To determine whether the presenting condition is still in force, requiring massage adjustments, or it has resolved.)
4. How does it affect you? Are there any side effects or complications of this medication or procedure? (To highlight any negative effects to adapt to in the massage session.)

Older adults are likely to be taking more than one medication, and massage therapists are in a good position to ask whether multiple treating physicians know about all the medications a patient is taking. Therapist's Journal 21-1 relates how a therapist did some digging about a client's medications, with surprising results.

Unintended Effects of Treatments

A side effect is any unintended action or effect of a drug or procedure that is outside the focus of treatment. It tends to be an undesirable symptom, such as nausea or stomach cramps. A complication of treatment, often used interchangeably with a side effect, usually refers to the development of more serious symptoms or conditions following a drug or procedure. Ulceration, bleeding, infection, and DVT are examples of complications. For simplicity, the term side effect is used here to mean

either a true side effect or a complication. (An *adverse effect* of a treatment is often used in the medical literature to describe an allergic reaction to a drug, but it, too, is used interchangeably with the other terms.).

Allergic reactions can vary from a mild case of hives to an acute case of anaphylaxis, or *anaphylactic shock*—a drop in blood pressure accompanied by breathing difficulty, requiring emergency medical attention. Virtually any medication

THERAPIST'S JOURNAL 21-1 *Catching Drug Interaction Precautions*

I have always been interested in medicine and health, and how drugs work. In massage school, my pathology teacher taught me to pay attention to any medications my clients were on, note how they affected the body, and so on.

But I had never had as complex a client as this one. She was assigned to me in a training clinic during a continuing education course. The night before the practice clinic I studied her health history, and she was taking a staggering list of medications—at least 10 or 12. Some were for cancer, some were for hypertension control, some for bone and joint conditions, and there were several psychotropic drugs. My eyes widened. In order to feel prepared for this client, I did some online research on each one to learn its indications, side effects, and contraindications.

In the process, I learned that some of her medications were used to treat side effects of other drugs. I also learned that some of them were not supposed to be taken together—there were clear drug interaction precautions. And some were not supposed to be taken by someone with high blood pressure. It was possible that this was already closely tracked by her physician. It also could be that she had several physicians: an oncologist, a primary care physician, and a psychopharmacologist or psychiatrist, and there was a lapse in communication. I made notes on each medication and the concerns.

When clinic time came the next day, my client wasn't there. I was almost relieved she might not come and I wouldn't have to use my carefully rehearsed speech. After everyone else's client was on the table, she finally arrived, rushing and apologetic. For a moment, I felt pressured to hurry the interview and get her on the table, too, but then I slowed myself down and gave time to the interview.

I didn't bring up the medications right away but waited until we went through some of the rest of the intake together. I asked her how her meds affected her, and what they were for. At that point, it seemed like there was enough of a rapport for me to say, "I hope you don't mind, but I looked up each medication because I didn't know what they were, and I wanted to learn about them." She seemed grateful that I had. I continued, "I'm not a doctor, but it looked to me like a couple of your medications (I listed them) shouldn't be taken together. Have you talked with your doctor about them?" She hadn't. I strongly encouraged her to talk with her primary care physician about them and the blood pressure issue. Then we went forward with the session, with several adaptations to medications and to her various conditions.

She seemed happy with the session. Afterward, she thanked me again for raising the issue of medications, and told me she would talk to her doctor about it. For my part, I was glad I said something. I never found out whether she actually followed up, but since then, this issue has come up a couple of other times in my practice. I think since massage therapists have a lot of time to spend with clients, this can come up from time to time. I'm glad that now I have a way to raise the issue that is well within my scope of practice and also encourages a client to stay on top of her own health care.

Michelle Zale
Milford, MA

can cause an allergic reaction. For an allergic response to any medication, the massage therapy guideline is the same: a physician referral. If severe allergy (anaphylaxis) is occurring, the situation is a medical emergency.

Throughout this text, whenever a medication is mentioned, some of its most common side effects are also addressed. A quick look at a drug product information sheet, available for each drug on the market, may reveal a staggering array of possible side effects. In general, prescription drugs tend to be stronger, with more unwanted effects than **over-the-counter (OTC)** medications, available for purchase without a prescription. Data about side effects are derived from drug studies, and pharmaceutical companies are required to list all potential side effects, not just the common ones. Decision Trees and discussions in this text focus on the most frequent side effects, and those with clear massage guidelines. Not all drugs or side effects are listed under each condition.

Routes of Administration

In pharmacology, a **route of administration** is the path by which a medication is brought into contact with the body. A **topical medication** is applied to the skin or mucous membrane, usually right where it is needed, for example, directly on a rash a mouth sore. Such a drug is designed to have a *local* effect, at the site. In contrast, in a **systemic medication**, the desired effect of the drug is throughout the body.

Medications with systemic effects include **oral medications** (taken by mouth) and **inhaled medications** (as in an asthma inhaler). Systemic effects can also come from **intravenous (IV)** delivery (directly into a vein), as in chemotherapy. Insulin is delivered by **subcutaneous injection** (under the skin), and fertility drugs are often administered by **intramuscular injection** (into a muscle). In a **transdermal patch**, a concentrated amount of medication is contained within an adhesive patch, through the skin, into the bloodstream. This can target the local tissues, as in the use of capsaicin for relief of neuropathic pain; it can also deliver systemic medication, as in a fentanyl patch for pain relief.

Medication delivery can also be intrathecal, in which medication is delivered into the spinal canal, as in the control of spasticity (see "Cerebral Palsy," online at http://thePoint. lww.com/Walton).

There are times when the route of administration figures into the massage therapy plan. With injected medications, find out how fast they are absorbed from the skin or muscle before using circulatory intent or friction at the site. This may be an hour, several hours, or longer, depending on the drug. If the absorption rate is not known, then 24 hours is a safe length of time to wait before using circulatory intent and focus at the site.

With a transdermal patch, take care not to dislodge the patch with too much focus, and avoid circulatory intent at the site. Most transdermal medications are carefully time-released, and there may be situations in which the doctor or nurse asks you to avoid the area entirely. The skin might be slightly irritated at the site of the patch, so avoid irritating it further.

Intravenous or intrathecal administration calls for an awareness of medical devices: a port or other vascular access device in the case of IV chemotherapy, or a pump placed in the abdomen for baclofen therapy (see "Cerebral Palsy," online). Here, position or pressure might need to be adjusted to avoid disturbing the device.

Most oral and IV medications do not require any other massage adjustments unless the medications are particularly strong in effect: corticosteroids, opioids, chemotherapy, and biologic therapy are examples of strong medications. Any time these types of medication are in use, it is a good idea to avoid general circulatory intent, and provide a gentle session overall. Typically, if strong medication is in use, a significant, complex, or unstable medical condition is present, and the stability of the tissues may be precarious. Strong medication is placing additional demand on the body's internal environment, especially the filtering organs. Against this backdrop, plan a gentle massage, one that is not expected to accelerate circulation or change the internal environment. Instead, provide a session that supports the body's rest and deepest healing.

Analgesics

Analgesia means pain relief, and an analgesic medication or procedure relieves pain. There are several classes of analgesic drugs. Three of them—the NSAIDs, corticosteroids, and opioid analgesics—are discussed here. Other medications used in pain relief, such as antiseizure medications and muscle relaxants, are covered in Chapter 10.

● NONSTEROIDAL ANTI-INFLAMMATORY DRUGS

Medications in this very large drug class are used as analgesics. These analgesics work as anti-inflammatories, because inflammation, which is common in injured or diseased tissues, causes nerve irritation and the experience of pain. The "nonsteroidal" designation distinguishes this class of drugs from corticosteroids, which also have an anti-inflammatory effect, but a different action and significantly more complex side effects. Hence, a nonsteroidal anti-inflammatory drug (NSAID) reduces the inflammation and uncomfortable symptoms along with it.

Background

Some NSAIDs are available OTC, and others require a prescription. This class of medications includes aspirin, ibuprofen (Advil, Motrin); naproxen (Anaprox, Naprosyn, Aleve); ketoprofen (Orudis); and celecoxib (Celebrex). Acetaminophen (Tylenol, Panadol) is sometimes classified as an NSAID, although its anti-inflammatory properties are quite weak, and it primarily acts as a fever reducer and pain reliever.

INDICATIONS

An indication is a condition which makes a certain treatment advisable. NSAIDs are indicated for mild to moderate pain, inflammation, and fever. Common indications for NSAIDs are:

• Arthritis (rheumatoid and osteoarthritis)
• Menstrual cramps
• Tendinitis

• Bursitis
• Minor injuries
• Common cold symptoms
• Back pain
• Headache
• Toothache

NSAIDs inhibit the synthesis of prostaglandins, substances produced in high concentrations by cells in an area of injury or trauma, contributing to pain, inflammation, and fever. Prostaglandins also support platelets in blood clotting, and they protect the stomach lining from damage by stomach acid. (Looking at these prostaglandin functions, you can guess what the side effects might be when their functions are inhibited.)

Aspirin is the oldest NSAID still in use, one of a class of salicylates. More recently developed NSAIDs work as cox inhibitors. They interfere with cox enzymes, which produce prostaglandins. Cox-1 is more active in protecting the lining of the GI tract, and cox-2 is more present and active at sites of inflammation.

NSAIDs are often used to relieve headaches, menstrual cramps, and the pain from injuries. They may be combined with other drugs to ease the symptoms of colds and allergies. Salicylates are used to thin the blood slightly and thus help prevent heart attack and stroke.

SIDE EFFECTS

The side effects and complications of NSAIDs arise from their effects on prostaglandins. For example, when platelets do not have the support of prostaglandins in clotting the blood, easy bruising and bleeding result. When the lining of the stomach is compromised, ulcers can develop and bleed. Since prostaglandins also regulate salt and therefore fluid balance in the body, fluid retention can occur.

An NSAID that blocks cox-1 also tends to cause ulcers and bleeding, and older adults are at increased risk of this side effect. A drug that selectively blocks cox-2 does not cause bleeding and ulcers the same way that cox-1 inhibitors do,

Nonsteroidal Anti-inflammatory Drugs (NSAIDs)

Medical Information

Massage Therapy Guidelines

Essentials

- Pain reliever used for mild to moderate pain; work by inhibiting cox-1 and cox-2 enzymes that enable prostaglandin synthesis

- Used to reduce inflammation, pain and fever; also used to prevent blood clots (aspirin); commonly used in arthritis, dysmenorrhea, minor injuries, back pain, common cold, headache

- Examples: aspirin, ibuprofen (Advil, Motrin), naproxen (Aleve), ketoprofen (Orudis), celecoxib (Celebrex)

- Ask about source of pain (see Chapter 4, follow-up pain questions) and adapt massage to source (see relevant chapter); work gently at affected site, if at all

- Be alert for self-medicating (continued use > 2 weeks medically discouraged); encourage client to report problem to physician

- If aspirin used to prevent blood clots, inquire about cardiovascular conditions, other cardiovascular medications (see Chapter 11)

- Determine which medication(s) client is taking; not all have same side effects

Side Effects and Complications

- Abdominal pain

- Nausea, vomiting

- Constipation

- Diarrhea

- Headache

- Drowsiness, dizziness

- Easy bruising and bleeding

- Fluid retention, edema

- Aggravation of hypertension; increased risk of heart attack, stroke

- Ulcers

- Kidney or liver failure (rare)

- Position for comfort, especially when prone; side-lying position may be welcome

- Position for comfort, gentle session overall; pressure to tolerance, slow speeds; no uneven rhythms or strong joint movement

- Gentle pressure at abdomen (level 2 max); medical referral if client has not had a bowel movement for several days

- Easy bathroom access; gentle session overall; avoid contact or pressure at abdomen that could aggravate.

- If headache severe or throbbing, see aggravation of hypertension, below; otherwise, position for comfort, especially prone; consider inclined table or propping; gentle session overall; pressure to tolerance; slow speed and even rhythm; general circulatory intent may be poorly tolerated

- Reposition gently, slow speed and even rhythm, slow rise from table, gentle transition at end of session

- Slight pressure modification (usually levels 2-3 are safe; physician input advised before increasing pressure to level 4)

- Urgent medical referral if client's doctor uninformed; otherwise, avoid general circulatory intent, avoid circulatory intent at site

- Urgent medical referral if client has not informed physician of NSAID use; emergency medical referral if signs/symptoms of spike in blood pressure (severe, throbbing headache) or stroke (see Chapter 10); follow-up on any cardiovascular conditions (see Chapter 11)

- Medical referral if client has not informed physician of gastrointestinal symptoms (see Peptic Ulcer Disease, Chapter 15)

- See Acute kidney failure, Chapter 18; Liver Failure, Chapter 16

FIGURE 21-1. A Decision Tree for NSAIDs. Not all side effects of all drugs are listed. Not all drugs cause all side effects.

and it targets sites of inflammation, where cox-2 is active. An example of a cox-2 inhibitor is celecoxib (Celebrex).

Common side effects of NSAIDs involve the GI tract: abdominal pain, nausea, vomiting, constipation, diarrhea, and reduced appetite. Headache, drowsiness, dizziness, insomnia, and rash are other common side effects. In some individuals, NSAIDs cause fluid retention and edema; in others, aggravation of hypertension. Rarer complications are kidney or liver failure, ulcers, and prolonged bleeding in the event of an injury or surgery. Prescription drugs such as Celebrex may contribute to heart attack or stroke in vulnerable individuals. These more serious complications tend to occur after chronic use. For this reason, they are stopped for a time before a surgical procedure. Acetaminophen has few side effects unless taken in large doses.

Because lower doses of these medications tend to be available OTC, individuals may self-medicate, continuing to take

them for pain management long after they would be medically recommended. NSAIDs are not meant for long-term use, and physicians discourage use for more than 2 weeks without ongoing monitoring.

MANAGEMENT OF SIDE EFFECTS

One of the most prevalent side effects of NSAIDs is stomach discomfort, so many people stop self-medicating (or their doctors stop prescribing) in the event of stomach pain. However, in an attempt to reduce the gastric side effects of NSAIDs, patients may take drugs that reduce the production of stomach acid. These include the famous "purple pill" (Nexium), or other common OTC drugs: Prevacid and Prilosec. If an NSAID causes a strong side effect, usually it's stopped and another medication is tried.

● INTERVIEW QUESTIONS

1. What is the name of the medication you are taking?
2. For what condition are you taking it?
3. Has the condition been seen by a doctor?
4. How long have you taken the medication?
5. How does it affect you?

Massage Therapy Guidelines

The answer to Question 1, especially when accompanied by the correct spelling of the medication, makes it possible to look up the medication. It is an easy thing to search for a medication and identify any potential massage therapy issues. You can use textbooks about pharmacology, written specifically for massage therapists (Persad, 2001; Wible, 2005, 2009). Useful Web sites such as www.medicinenet.com and www.drugs.com summarize each medication's use and adverse effects. Searching for "NSAIDs" or the specific name of the medication, you can begin to identify possible side effects or complications and ask the client about them in case they are not raised in Question 5.

Question 2 may return a specific medical condition, such as arthritis, but a likely response is simply pain, rather than a diagnosed condition. If the client does mention a diagnosed condition, do not assume the drug has resolved it; NSAIDs are designed to treat symptoms, not eradicate disease. The condition itself is often still present and may require some massage adjustments; refer to the appropriate chapter (see "Soft Tissue Injuries [Strain, Sprain, Tendinopathy, Tenosynovitis]," "Bursitis," Chapter 8; "Osteoarthritis," Chapter 9, "Dysmenorrhea," Chapter 19). If the client is taking aspirin as a mild blood thinner, then the physician has probably recommended it because of other cardiovascular issues (see Chapter 11). There may be additional massage therapy guidelines based on the condition, not just the medication.

Remember that NSAIDs affect inflammation and pain, but they do not treat the cause of it. Although the client's sensation and perception are still intact after taking an NSAID, the pain is not likely to be felt as strongly as it normally would. In this case, the client might call for more pressure than is advisable, or a longer, stronger stretch. Do not assume, because the symptoms and signs are milder, that you can work more deeply or apply an intense stretch to the area. Circulatory intent at the site might aggravate inflammation, and a strong stretch, or pressure that is too deep, might worsen the condition. Work gently at the site, and respect the healing process.

Be gentle when asking Question 3, because a client might feel defensive if he or she hasn't brought the condition to the attention of his or her doctor or has no doctor or no medical insurance. Asking this question may require some finesse and rapport, and the point of asking it is to determine whether a medical referral is advisable or even urgent. Many people self-medicate with NSAIDs because most of them are available OTC in some form. They may also self-diagnose. Short-term NSAID use for an occasional headache, sports injury, menstrual cramps, or muscle ache is not usually an issue, but chronic or repeated use can be a problem. It could mask the pain of a condition that needs medical attention.

Question 4 gives a good gauge of how long-standing the condition is and the medication use. Most physicians do not recommend NSAID use for more than a couple of weeks. Strongly urge the client to report the condition and medication use to his or her doctor, especially if side effects are apparent.

Question 5 should bring up any side effects to be considered in the massage plan. The massage therapy guidelines for side effects such as abdominal pain, constipation, and headache are described in the Decision Tree (Figure 21-1).

If signs or symptoms of more serious complications are present, a medical referral is typically urgent or immediate, and usually the medication is stopped or the dose is decreased. A slight increase in bruising or bleeding calls for slight adjustment in overall pressure, usually in the level 2–3 range. If the doctor agrees, a level 4 pressure may be possible. Any time fluid retention and edema are present, it's a good idea to avoid massage therapy with general circulatory intent; this is the Fluid Balance Principle (see Chapter 18). When systemic fluid balance is disturbed, avoid imposing the additional challenge of general circulatory massage. If the client also has cardiovascular issues, the client should certainly inform his or her doctor about the medication use. Some NSAIDs can aggravate hypertension and increase risk of heart attack or stroke, and the doctor needs to know about it to manage both conditions. Pay attention if the client reports a severe, throbbing headache, as it can be a sign of aggravated hypertension (see Chapter 11), and be alert for signs of stroke (see Chapter 10).

If your client reports having developed a rare complication of NSAID use, such as ulcers, or liver or kidney failure, see the appropriate chapter in this book for further massage guidelines (see "Peptic Ulcer Disease," Chapter 15; "Liver Failure," Chapter 16; "Acute Kidney Failure," Chapter 18).

Massage Research

As of this writing, there are no randomized, controlled trials (RCTs), published in the English language, on NSAIDs and massage indexed in PubMed or the Massage Therapy Foundation Research Database. The NIH RePORTER tool lists no active, federally funded research projects on this topic in the United States. No active projects are listed on the clinicaltrials.gov database (see Chapter 6).

Several review articles comment on the poor quality or lack of evidence for massage and other complementary therapies in the treatment of pain, injury, and muscle soreness, all conditions that are now treated with NSAIDs (Borenstein, 2007; Howatson and Someren, 2008; Neufeld and Cerrato, 2008). Future research comparing pharmacological (including NSAIDs) and nonpharmacological (including massage therapy) treatments of pain will be useful. In one study of cancer patients in chemotherapy, massage therapy was associated with less pain and NSAID use than controls (Post-White et al., 2003). More research is needed to answer this important question—whether massage therapy leads to reduced NSAID use in people with pain—before firm conclusions can be drawn.

Possible Massage Benefits

There is no specific massage therapy benefit related to NSAIDs. Focus on massage that addresses the *reason* for taking the medication—the mild to moderate pain. Massage therapy is likely to support someone in pain, whether chronic or acute. It may even provide significant pain relief. Sometimes just the full, firm, and simple contact of the hands—the "laying on of hands"—is just what an individual needs. Hands placed on the head or neck may ease a headache, and hands placed on a low back can relieve soreness. Sometimes hand placement elsewhere is just right, even though it might be poorly tolerated directly on the painful area. Be willing to rest your hands on a painful area, even if it's a sore stomach from an NSAID. At the very least, massage can soften the isolation of living alone with chronic pain.

Where appropriate, massage and joint movement on or near the site of pain can address the portion of pain due to muscle tension. Once this can be addressed, the pain-spasm-pain cycle is broken and the client can get even deeper relief of pain in the area (see "General Principles," Chapter 8). Sometimes this form of pain relief is necessary for an individual to realize how much of the pain was due to muscle tension.

● CORTICOSTEROIDS

Corticosteroids, also called *steroidal anti-inflammatories* or simply *steroids*, include cortisone, prednisone, and prednisolone. These are similar to the glucocorticoids produced by the adrenal cortex (see Chapter 17).

Background

Corticosteroids have two principal properties—anti-inflammatory and immunosuppressive—that make them effective in the treatment of a wide variety of conditions, including inflammatory conditions and autoimmune diseases.

INDICATIONS

Corticosteroids are used in autoimmune conditions such as systemic lupus erythematosus and Crohn disease. They are inhaled to treat allergies and asthma, to calm inflammation of the bronchial tubes. They effectively treat skin conditions involving dermatitis. In an organ or tissue transplant, corticosteroids serve as antirejection medications, by dampening the immune response.

Corticosteroids can aid cancer treatment in a number of ways. They can enhance the effectiveness of chemotherapy against certain types of cancer, diminish an adverse response to chemotherapy, increase appetite and help to avert weight loss, and promote positive mood. They might help relieve nausea and vomiting. By lessening swelling around a tumor, as in a brain tumor, corticosteroid treatment reduces pressure and pain. A single steroid medication, such as dexamethasone (Decadron), may have multiple effects in a cancer treatment regimen.

Corticosteroid medication may be used in small doses to replace missing cortisol in treating hypocortisolism (see Chapter 17). Such a small replacement dose is called a **physiological dose**, and it does not usually produce the same side effects as a much higher **pharmacological dose**. In most cases, a pharmacological dose is necessary for reducing inflammation or suppressing immunity. Steroids may be administered topically, as in dermatitis; orally, as in arthritis and lupus; through an inhaler, as in asthma; and by injection, such as directly into an area of tendinitis. The medication may also be delivered through an IV along with anticancer drugs. For the most part, corticosteroids are available only by prescription. An exception is mild topical steroid cream.

SIDE EFFECTS

Some side effects of corticosteroids depend on the dose and route of administration. Topical corticosteroids have two main side effects at the site: thinning the skin and causing acne, especially with chronic use. (With prolonged use of topical steroids over a significant area of the body, more serious complications can occur, such as bone loss.)

Short-term systemic (oral or IV) corticosteroid therapy causes fluid retention, often seen as swelling in the lower legs; hypertension, GI upset, stomach ulcers, mood changes, and insomnia. With long-term (longer than 3 weeks) therapy, corticosteroids can cause cataracts, glaucoma, hyperglycemia (see "Diabetes Mellitus," Chapter 17), decreased immunity, muscle weakness, and weight gain, with deposits of fat in the face, back of the neck ("buffalo hump"), and abdomen. Excess facial hair may appear. Thinned skin and easy bruising are common, and osteoporosis might result in pathologic fracture, especially in the spine (see "Osteoporosis," Chapter 9). Oral and IV steroid administration tends to cause the most severe side effects because of the systemic action. Other methods of administration deliver the drug more directly to the inflamed area.

High doses of steroids may be used in children with muscular dystrophy, in a controversial therapy to slow disease progression and preserve the ability to walk. High doses may also be used to treat a flare-up of multiple sclerosis, or other autoimmune disease. Sleep disturbances are common in both of these cases.

Inhaled corticosteroids sometimes stay in the mouth and throat instead of going the distance to the lungs. Side effects are sore throat, coughing, hoarseness, and dry mouth. Patients may develop **thrush**, a fungal infection of the mouth and throat, and they are thus urged to rinse the mouth after taking an inhaled steroid. As the immune system weakens with high doses, thrush is more likely.

Injected corticosteroids can cause pain near the injection site, infection, and shrinking of the soft tissue. For this reason, their use in a single area is limited.

MANAGEMENT OF SIDE EFFECTS

In general, the strong side effects and complications of steroids limit their use, and patients are closely monitored with prolonged use. Where possible, alternative medications are used, or drugs are rotated. With the host of side effects of corticosteroids, patients may be taking additional medications to control them. Antibiotics and antifungal agents are given in the event of infection. Osteoporosis is treated with bisphosphonates (see Chapter 9). Stomach irritation and ulcers are treated with appropriate medications (see "Peptic Ulcer Disease," Chapter 15).

● INTERVIEW QUESTIONS

1. What is the name of the medication you are taking? How do you take it (oral, inhaler, applied to the skin, injected, or IV)?
2. For what condition are you taking it?
3. What is the goal of the corticosteroid in your case? To reduce inflammation? To suppress immunity? To assist another treatment?
4. Is the medication working as intended?
5. How long have you taken this medication? In the past, have you had to take corticosteroids regularly, for long periods of time?
6. How does it affect you?

Corticosteroids

Medical Information	Massage Therapy Guidelines

Essentials

- Medications with antiinflammatory and immunosuppressive properties; most available only by prescription (some topical preparations OTC); used in inflammatory conditions including autoimmune conditions (lupus, Crohn disease), asthma, dermatitis, tendinitis, arthritis

- Used as antirejection medication in tissue and organ transplant; suppress host and donor immune activity

- Dexamethasone (Decadron) used in cancer treatment to enhance treatment, limit adverse effects of chemotherapy, improve mood, improve appetite, and reduce nausea and vomiting

→

- If systemic (oral, IV, or topical over large area) in pharmacological dose, avoid general circulatory intent
- If topical, avoid contact at site until medication absorbed, avoid aggravating condition
- If used for pain management, ask about source of pain (see follow-up questions for pain, Chapter 4) and adapt massage to source (see relevant chapter)
- If used for inflammatory condition, follow inflammation principle

→

- See Organ and Tissue Transplant section

→

- If used in cancer treatment, see Chapter 20

Side Effects and Complications

- Acne

- Thinned skin

- Thinning of bones (osteoporosis)

- Thinning and shrinking of soft tissue (at site of injected steroids)

- Fluid retention, edema (often in lower legs)

- Hypertension

- Gastrointestinal upset; stomach ulcers

- Mood swings

- Insomnia

- Cataracts

- Glaucoma

- Hyperglycemia (can aggravate diabetes)

- Decreased immunity, opportunisitc infections

- Muscle weakness

- Weight gain
- Adipose tissue at abdomen, face, base of neck
- Excess facial hair

- Easy bruising

- Sore throat, coughing, hoarseness, thrush (with inhaled steroids)

→

- Do not aggravate inflammation (see Acne vulgaris, Chapter 7)
- Gentle pressure at sites of thinned skin (if topical preparation); gentle pressure overall if systemic; use level 1-3 max, depending on physician consultation
- See Osteoporosis, Chapter 9
- Use gentle pressure at injection site (level 2-3 max in most cases); often a site of injury such as tendinitis
- Avoid general circulatory intent; follow Fluid Balance Principle (see Chapter 18)
- See Chapter 11
- Adjust position for client comfort, possibly avoiding flat prone position; avoid pressure in upper abdomen; see Peptic Ulcer Disease, Chapter 15
- Be sensitive to fluctuations in mood, and urge client to report to physician
- When appropriate, use sedative intent at end of day, activating/invigorating intent at beginning
- No massage adjustments
- No massage adjustments; client may prefer to avoid flat prone position
- See Diabetes, Chapter 17
- Follow standard precautions plus any additional infection control measures recommended by physician or requested by client
- If infection present, avoid general circulatory intent until it resolves; gentle pressure overall (2 or 3 max) depending on tolerance
- Gentle joint movement
- No massage adjustments

- Gentle pressure overall (level 2 or 3 max, depending on tissue stability)
- No general circulatory intent if thrush

FIGURE 21-2. A Decision Tree for corticosteroids. Not all side effects of all drugs are listed. Not all drugs cause all side effects.

Massage Therapy Guidelines

Outside of a simple, low-strength topical preparation for skin irritation, most corticosteroids require a prescription. For this reason, there may be a significant, if not serious, condition for your client to tell you about in order for you to prepare your massage plan. Because of the range of conditions that corticosteroids might treat, it's good to be prepared for anything—from severe eczema to hypercortisolism to a kidney transplant. Adapt accordingly. If inflammation is involved, avoid aggravating it.

With the answer to Question 1, you can look up information about the medication on the Internet or in other resources. The route of administration is relevant because of specific massage adjustments at the site of topical applications or injected medications. As always, avoid direct contact with a topical application until it has been absorbed. And be careful with pressure at an injection site, for example, at the site of an injured, inflamed tendon.

Most other routes of administration are considered systemic, with systemic effects. In most cases, avoid general circulatory intent. Side effects are not as strong with inhaled steroids as they are with oral and IV drugs, unless high doses are inhaled. Be mindful of an increased risk of cataracts, glaucoma, and osteoporosis in an elderly client and adjust accordingly.

Questions 2–4 should yield a clear picture of the reasons for the corticosteroid medication, its role in the treatment, and how problematic the indicating condition is. For example, if asthma is the issue, the massage adjustments are fairly straightforward (see Chapter 14), and a chronic, moderate form of eczema may require only adjustments at the site of the problem (see Chapter 7). On the other hand, a client in cancer treatment, or with a transplant history, may require a host of other massage adjustments. A client with an autoimmune condition, such as rheumatoid arthritis (see Chapter 9) or lupus (see Chapter 13), may well be taking other medications, and you will need to follow massage guidelines for those as well as for problems caused by the indicating disease.

Question 5 has particular relevance, because prolonged use of corticosteroids tends to thin the skin and bones. The skin becomes easily bruised and fragile, and your pressure should be adjusted at the site of a topical application, or overall for a systemic drug. Osteoporosis develops, and those who must take steroid medication regularly may have a heightened risk of fracture (see "Osteoporosis," Chapter 9). Prolonged steroid use is decreasing because modern drugs offer more alternatives to steroids for controlling chronic inflammation, but they are still the best choice for some people. It may be that pressure level 2 is the maximum appropriate; find out about the tissue stability and err on the cautious side.

> **The Unstable Tissue Principle.** *If a tissue is unstable, do not challenge it with too much pressure or joint movement in the area.*

Question 6 may highlight weakened bones and skin again, or a range of other effects. Refer to the side effects listed in the Decision Tree (see Figure 21-2) for an extensive list of guidelines. Note that additional medications may be taken to counter the side effects of corticosteroids; be sure to incorporate these into the massage plan, as well.

As you review the Decision Tree, keep in mind two side effects of systemic steroids for consideration in the massage plan: a shift in fluid balance and suppression of the immune system. If fluid retention has occurred, usually visible as swelling in the lower extremities, avoid general circulatory intent.

> **The Fluid Balance Principle.** *If fluid balance is off, causing either systemic swelling or dehydration, massage with general circulatory intent is contraindicated.*

If the client is vulnerable to infection, follow any specific hygienic precautions recommended by the nurse or doctor as well as your usual standard precautions. If concern about immunity is heightened, this could mean scheduling at certain low-volume times of day, or rescheduling if you have cold symptoms, such as a scratchy throat (see Neutropenia, Chapter 12).

Finally, the effects of corticosteroids on blood sugar and blood pressure, while well monitored, are important to bear in mind. Review "Diabetes Mellitus," Chapter 17, and any other cardiovascular conditions (see Chapter 11), as appropriate.

Massage Research

As of this writing, there are no RCTs, published in the English language, on corticosteroids and massage indexed in PubMed or the Massage Therapy Foundation Research Database. The NIH RePORTER tool lists no active, federally funded research projects on this topic in the United States. No active projects are listed on the clinicaltrials.gov database (see Chapter 6).

Possible Massage Benefits

Systemic corticosteroid medication comes with extensive, uncomfortable side effects, and the indications for steroid use are often serious. While there is no specific benefit of massage for someone on corticosteroids, well-placed massage or simple laying on of hands could ease discomfort. If the person is immunosuppressed, he or she may feel extremely isolated by the restrictions on activity. Companionship in the form of skilled touch can mean the world to someone who might literally be uncomfortable in his or her own skin.

● OPIOID ANALGESICS

Opioid analgesics, also called *narcotics,* are pain medications used for moderate to severe pain.

Background

The most familiar opioid is morphine, and other common ones are codeine, hydrocodone, and pethidine. These drugs act on the opiate receptors in the central nervous system (CNS) and peripheral nerves, and thereby interfere with pain transmission and perception. In these actions, they are similar to the natural pain-relieving substances of the body, *endorphins* and *enkephalins,* which moderate pain perception as well as the emotional response to pain. Opioids also depress respiration, act against the cough reflex, slow motility in the GI tract, and produce sleep.

INDICATIONS

Opioids have traditionally been used in the management of acute pain and cancer pain. More recently, they have been applied to chronic pain such as back pain, neuropathy, and pain due to shingles.

Long-acting opioids have been developed, making potent medications such as morphine, oxycodone, and fentanyl available in controlled release preparations for more successful pain management. Fentanyl is often delivered transdermally, through a *fentanyl patch.* Morphine is used to relieve shortness of breath in patients with pulmonary edema, congestive heart failure, and end-stage pulmonary disease.

Concerns about dependence on opioid medications have limited their use in the management of acute and chronic pain. In general, physiological and psychological dependence is uncommon; when it does occur, patients usually have a prior history of substance abuse. Drugs have been developed to minimize the potential for dependence. **Mixed narcotic agonist-antagonists** are designed to relieve pain with fewer toxic complications and less dependence. Examples are OxyContin, Darvon, Stadol, and Nubain. These might be used during childbirth or to reduce anxiety and pain before surgery.

Combination narcotic analgesics provide pain relief by combining an opioid analgesic with another drug, such as acetaminophen, aspirin, or another NSAID. Examples are Tylenol # 1, which includes acetaminophen and codeine. Oxycodone and aspirin are combined as Percodan. Oxycodone and acetaminophen are combined as Percocet.

SIDE EFFECTS

Although different people may react very differently to opioids, they are uniformly strong drugs with strong effects. Opioid analgesics can cause nausea and vomiting, and constipation is common. Itching is a side effect that may be mild or severe.

Opioids can also produce drowsiness and sleep; dizziness; and orthostatic hypotension. In some individuals at certain doses, confusion and delirium can occur. The respiration rate slows with opioids, and it must be reversed quickly if it slows enough to be life threatening. Heart palpitations may also be life threatening.

MANAGEMENT OF SIDE EFFECTS

Constipation is managed with diet, stool softeners, and laxatives. When opioids are used to treat chronic pain, nausea usually fades over time. If high doses of opioids are needed, and nausea persists, patients are given antiemetics.

Drowsiness and sedation also tend to ease over time when an opioid is used for chronic pain. Chronic, slowed respiration tends to fade with ongoing opioid use, but if it becomes acute, it may be reversed using medication.

Opioid-induced itching can be difficult to treat, as antihistamines and other traditional approaches are usually ineffective. Heavy emollients on the skin, and avoiding hot and drying baths, may be helpful. A switch in medication may be tried, in the hope that a different opioid produces less itching. In stubborn cases, a narcotic antagonist such as Naloxone or Ondansetron may be used.

● INTERVIEW QUESTIONS

1. What is the name of the medication you are taking?
2. How often do you take it, and how recently did you last take it?
3. For what condition are you taking it? Is this for acute or chronic pain?
4. Is the medication working as intended?
5. How does the medication affect you?

Massage Therapy Guidelines

An overarching guideline is to work gently with someone taking opioids because his perception might be diminished. Follow the Sensation Principle. At the same time, someone needing such a strong analgesic is usually in significant pain and discomfort. The condition itself calls for gentleness in massage, regardless of the medication.

Questions 1 and 2 are especially important to ask when a person is taking opioid analgesics. If possible, look up the medication to learn more about it. Asking about how recently and how often the client takes the medication, you can think about the timing and strength of the massage session. If the client has recently dosed, perception of pain will be diminished, calling for more caution; however, at that point, the pain relief may be at its best level, making comfortable positioning easier. The massage may be well tolerated if this is the case. On the other hand, if the dose was a while ago, take additional care in your pressure and positioning, to avoid aggravating the pain.

Adapt the massage to the painful condition and how stable it is. If a client has low-back pain that is highly unstable, avoid any joint movement or pressure in that area that could aggravate it. If the client has neuropathic pain or back pain that is easily activated, be sure to avoid any stimuli that precipitate or worsen it.

Ask Question 3 about the condition itself in order to determine whether it requires any massage adjustments. Most often, someone taking opioid medication is in rough shape. He or she may be coping with acute pain and perhaps pain that is unmanageable. He or she might have recently undergone a medical procedure such as an operation, or he or she may be at the end of life, managing multiple symptoms. In other, more chronic cases, opioid relief might allow an individual a reasonably high level of function, for example, in someone with neuropathic or back pain. These two ends of the spectrum obviously call for very different massage sessions. A gentle session is in order for a client who is quite compromised. A stronger session is likely to be well tolerated by a person who is more physically functional. The client's activity level is the key to determining how strong the overall massage can be, although even if the client is high functioning, it is a good idea to begin conservatively at the first session and monitor the dynamic between pain, medication, and massage over time before going more deeply.

Question 4 about the medication's effectiveness may be very important to ask. Obviously if it's not quite effective, you will work more carefully in the painful areas. But you can also serve as a gentle advocate for a client who needs more help. If the client states that he or she is still in pain, encourage the client to bring it to his or her doctor's or nurse's attention. Sometimes people need a gentle nudge to encourage them to complain. Not wanting to be labeled a complainer or malingerer, a person might tolerate unnecessary pain. Let your client know that he or she does not have to "wait out" the pain. Pain management, especially at the end of life, continues to improve, and there are more options available to manage pain well. If pain is unreported, encourage the person to report it.

Question 5 about the effects of the medication could uncover many undesirable side effects, or very few. Most of the common opioid side effects are listed on the Decision Tree, along with straightforward massage therapy guidelines (see Figure 21-3). Approaches to side effects such as nausea and itching are similar to those described in other chapters.

GI problems like constipation are common with opioids and may indicate abdominal massage strokes to facilitate elimination, but be certain there is no pressure contraindication at that site, for example, as in colorectal cancer. Massage adjustments for nausea and vomiting are in the Decision Tree.

There are three symptoms—drowsiness, dizziness, and orthostatic hypotension—that dictate a slow rise from the

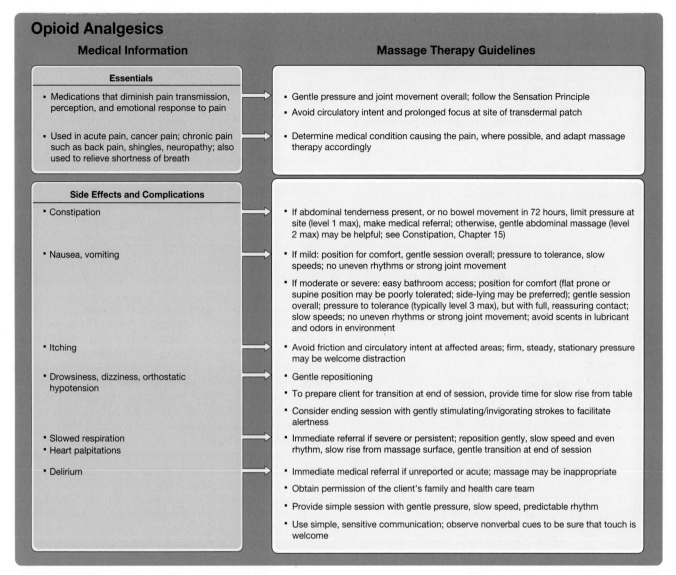

FIGURE 21-3. A Decision Tree for opioid analgesics (narcotic analgesics). Not all side effects of all drugs are listed. Not all drugs cause all side effects.

massage surface at the end of the session. If the setting permits it, it may be desirable to let the client relax and sleep at the end of the session.

Itchiness due to opioids can be severe—sometimes so intolerable that the drug is stopped. Massage therapy strokes and lubricant that might aggravate itching are obvious things to avoid. It may be that stationary, firm pressure provides a welcome distraction from the itching.

Slowed respiration and heart palpitations are potentially life-threatening complications of opioids. If they haven't been reported already, an immediate or emergency medical referral is in order. If the doctor is not concerned, then work gently and predictably, with a gentle transition at the end of the session.

A client who seems confused or agitated may be suffering from delirium associated with opioid toxicity or with the underlying condition. This might occur after a stressful event such as surgery or a hospital admission, or at the end of life. Urge the client's caregivers to report these signs to the client's doctor or nurse. Massage therapy may not be appropriate at this

time, but in the right situation, touch from a massage therapist can be reorienting and grounding. It is difficult to establish consent for massage with someone who is delirious, although the confusion might be punctuated by lucid moments. If touch is performed, it should be done with the permission of the client's family and health care team, and it should be simple and predictable in nature. Observe nonverbal cues to be sure that the touch is welcome.

Massage Research

As of this writing, there are no RCTs, published in the English language, on opioid analgesics and massage indexed in PubMed or the Massage Therapy Foundation Research Database.

The NIH RePORTER tool lists a federally funded pilot RCT, investigating the effects of a 40-minute massage on cerebrospinal fluid neurochemistry. The investigators are looking at several hormones and neurotransmitters over 6 hours following a massage and a control intervention. Shifts in these neurochemicals may provide mechanisms for massage effects on pain and other variables, and whether natural pain relief can substitute for pharmacological measures in some people. This will be the first known research to collect this specific data. Otherwise, no related projects are listed on the clinical-trials.gov database (see Chapter 6).

A large survey of complementary and alternative medicine (CAM) therapy use was performed on a sample of 908 individuals who were using opioids for chronic pain. Forty-four percent of them reported using one or more CAM therapies in the preceding 12 months, and of those, 27% used massage therapy (Fleming et al., 2007). These and other authors commented that further study is needed to know whether CAM therapies can reduce opioid use. See the Surgery section for further study on this question.

Possible Massage Benefits

Opioid analgesics are generally prescribed for the management of chronic, severe pain. Clinical observations suggest massage therapy can contribute to pain relief and help ease suffering. It may also ease some of the side effects of opioids, such as nausea or constipation.

If an individual is in such pain that opioid relief is needed, others around him or her might be reluctant to provide touch, for fear of hurting the person. A caring and careful massage therapist can, by example, provide a model of touch that encourages family and friends to touch, as well. By quietly modeling touch with the person, thereby offering permission for others to touch him, a massage therapist makes healing available to friends and family, as well as the client.

Surgery

Anytime a surgeon cuts, abrades, sutures, or applies laser treatment to a tissue it is called surgery. Most surgical procedures aim to repair, replace, sample, or remove a tissue or organ that is diseased or injured.

● BACKGROUND

Surgery is often classified into three categories, based on how pressing the situation is. Emergency surgery is performed within minutes of a hospital visit, usually an emergency room admission. It frequently is used when it's necessary to stop rapid internal bleeding, to avert a life-threatening event, or to save a limb. Urgent surgery has to be performed within hours of an acute event and includes the removal of an inflamed appendix or treatment of a colon that may perforate, as in acute diverticulitis. At the other end of the spectrum is elective surgery, which can be delayed and scheduled for a time when an individual may best recover from the operation. An example is a hip or knee replacement.

Surgeries are also classified according to invasiveness. In major surgery, general anesthesia is used. A team of surgeons is required, and the surgery is performed in an operating room. This procedure typically involves opening one of the major body cavities, such as the skull (*craniotomy*), the chest (*thoracotomy*), or the abdomen (*laparotomy*). Any time the surgeon has direct access to the tissues or organs involved, this is known as *open surgery*.

Minor surgery might also involve general anesthesia, but it often can be done with local or regional anesthesia. It does not require opening the major body cavities, and it can be performed by a single physician. Also called *outpatient surgery* or *day surgery*, the procedure can be done in a doctor's office, an ambulatory surgical center, or in an emergency room.

Less invasive surgical techniques are also used. A procedure can be done by making a small incision through which a surgical scope with lights and a viewing device is inserted. Compared to open surgery, small incisions result in less pain and fewer complications, such as bleeding. Shorter hospital stays mean patients can return to normal functioning more quickly. Abdominal surgery using a scope is *laparoscopic surgery*. Joint surgery using a scope is called *arthroscopic surgery*. Chest surgery using a scope is called *thoracoscopic surgery*.

There are four main categories of anesthesia. Local anesthesia occurs when an anesthetic is injected in a small area of the body, numbing only that area. It is often used to stitch up a wound or take a skin biopsy. With regional anesthesia, nerves are injected to numb the area of the body supplied by those nerves. In these two procedures, the patient remains awake. Spinal and epidural anesthesia are examples of regional anesthesia. The patient may receive anti-anxiety drugs to ease the experience. Regional anesthesia is also used for pelvic and lower extremity surgery.

In conscious sedation, also called *IV sedation*, pain medication is administered intravenously and a mild sedative is included in the IV infusion. It may be combined with regional anesthesia. The patient remains awake enough to swallow or cough, and to respond to questions from the surgical team. This type of anesthesia may be used for unpleasant or difficult procedures, such as a colonoscopy. The sedation may cause the person to forget the procedure.

In general anesthesia, the patient is unconscious, resulting from a medication that circulates in the blood, administered by inhalation or IV. Breathing is slowed, and in longer operations, *intubation*, the insertion of a breathing tube in the trachea, might be needed. Because general anesthesia affects the function of vital organs, the patient's heart rate and rhythm, blood pressure, breathing, and temperature must be monitored until the anesthesia wears off. While general anesthesia is not as safe as local or regional anesthesia, close monitoring means that complications are rare.

A surgical drain may be placed at the incision site (Figure 21-4). A tube leads to a collection bulb for excess fluid and blood from the area, to minimize the possibility of infection.

Drains are usually in place for a few days. The collection bulb volume is logged to determine the progress of the drainage. A dressing covers the insertion site.

Indications

The reasons to have surgery are many and varied, but diagnosis and treatment of conditions are always in mind. An example of diagnostic surgery is a needle biopsy of the liver, in which a sample of tissue is removed to check for liver disease. In cancer surgery, the removal of a tumor and lymph node may serve

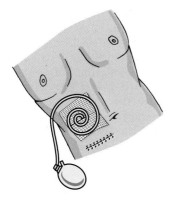

FIGURE 21-4. A surgical drain.

both diagnostic and therapeutic purposes at once, because the tissues are analyzed once they are removed from the body.

Most operations performed as part of treatment involve the removal or repair of an organ or tissue. The suffix *-ectomy* means the surgical removal of that part, as in an appendectomy, thyroidectomy, or splenectomy. Some of the reasons for tissue or organ removal are:

- Infection threatens rupture of the tissue and spread of the infection (as in an appendectomy)
- A gland is malfunctioning, causing excessive production of a substance (as in thyroidectomy)
- The organ is injured, and highly vascular, so that blood loss could be life threatening (as in splenectomy)
- The tissue or organ contains cancer cells (as in lumpectomy of the breast, prostatectomy, orchiectomy)

In other surgeries, tissues or organs such as the bladder, colon, or breast are repaired or reconstructed. In a transplant, an organ, such as the kidney, is replaced with a donor organ. Surgery may also involve the placement of a medical device or hardware to deliver a drug (as in the placement of a port for chemotherapy), or it can stabilize a tissue (as in the internal fixation of a fracture).

Side Effects

The side effects and complications of surgery are diverse. Immediate effects of surgery and anesthesia are nausea and vomiting. Patients may feel cold and groggy for some time. Spinal and epidural anesthesia may cause headaches. Postsurgical pain at the incision site is common, and drainage from the site continues for some time. Anesthesia and analgesics cause constipation.

The two most serious complications of surgery in the days afterward are infection and blood clots. Patients are monitored closely, with prophylactic care. Respiratory infection is a concern with longer hospital stays, regardless of the location of the surgery. For this reason, pulmonary function is carefully monitored. One "side effect" of managed care in the United States is shorter hospital stays, and a benefit is that fewer respiratory infections are contracted in the hospital. Another potential site of infection is the incision or drainage site. Antibiotics are administered, usually by IV, and aftercare literature instructs patients to watch for signs of infection.

Thrombosis is a concern after surgery, because an incision sets off platelet activity and a cascade of clotting events. Rogue clots can appear in the lower extremities, iliac veins, and in

other veins in the body. Preventive measures, aimed at getting blood moving through the veins, are the following: encouraging the patient to walk as soon as possible after surgery, and applying compression devices to the legs to keep blood from pooling there.

A surgical procedure can result in a temporary loss of function, depending on how much tissue was removed, replaced, reconstructed, or repaired, and how deep the affected tissues are. The area of the surgery dictates any functional impairment. If damage to motor nerves was unavoidable, for example, in an effort to remove a large tumor, function might be lost in the corresponding organs. Lingering scar tissue may restrict movement indefinitely.

Numbness or other sensation changes may occur if nerve pathways were injured during the surgery. For example, a common experience after breast cancer surgery is a strange numbness under the arm, noted when applying deodorant.

Medical devices that may be in use after surgery include a breathing tube in the throat, a tube in the nose or mouth, an IV, a catheter in the bladder, and adhesive pads on the chest to monitor heartbeat. Drainage tubes may be present, attached to collecting bulbs and inserted near or at the incision site.

Fatigue is a consequence of surgery and may linger for weeks. Although a standard recovery time is 6 weeks, many people are surprised by how tired they are during the weeks and months postsurgery.

Body image may suffer after surgery. With disfigurement comes anxiety and depression. Depending on how significantly the surgery changes the individual's appearance, and depending on the person's own unique emotional response to the surgery, self-esteem and body image can be greatly compromised.

Management of Side Effects

Standard treatments following surgery are antiemetics for nausea, stool softeners, and laxatives for constipation. Postoperative pain is managed with opioid analgesics, mixed narcotic agonist-antagonists, or combination narcotic analgesics. Pain medication is provided by IV, orally, through intramuscular injection, or via a transdermal patch.

Antibiotics are given to prevent or treat infection. Anticoagulants (and sometimes thrombolytics) are administered if DVT occurs, although the blood-thinning properties of anticoagulants must be balanced with the clotting the body needs to respond the surgical incision.

● INTERVIEW QUESTIONS

1. When was the surgery?
2. What was it for? Where? Was it effective?
3. Was it major or minor surgery?
4. How have you felt, and how do you feel now, since the surgery? Has your body recovered from the operation and the anesthesia?
5. Were there any problems or complications following the surgery?
6. Is there any pain resulting from the surgery? Where?
7. Is there any loss of sensation or function resulting from the surgery? Where?
8. What is your activity level since the surgery? Are there any medical restrictions on your activities?
9. Are you taking any medications related to the surgery? How do they affect you?

● MASSAGE THERAPY GUIDELINES

Approaches to massage therapy for clients who have recently undergone surgery are quite uniform across different types of procedures. The Decision Tree (Figure 21-5) lists the common side effects and massage guidelines.

Questions 1–3 about the surgery history are usually asked about procedures in the recent past, within the preceding 12 months. But in some cases, lingering effects of surgeries performed years ago are still relevant to the massage plan. Examples are the removal of lymph nodes during cancer surgery and the lifelong risk of lymphedema (see Chapter 20), or a neck injury that has been stabilized with plates or pins.

Incision sites must be handled delicately, especially if the surgery was done in the last few days or weeks. If fluids are still draining from the site, avoid contact with them, steering clear of the dressing. Gloves are necessary if fluid might come into contact with your hands. Also, avoid contact and lubricant at the site. Note that there may be more than one incision site—

several incisions for scopes and more for surgical drains—and ask the client to point to all of them.

Question 2, about the original reason for surgery and the effectiveness, is relevant if the initial problem still persists, as in a back injury that is still troublesome despite surgery. Be cautious in the affected area at first, monitoring the results of massage over time. If a condition is only partly resolved or is still healing, question the client about the condition, referring to appropriate chapters in this book. Examples of such conditions are a heart condition after bypass surgery (see Chapter 11), or cancer that has recurred after removal of the primary tumor (see Chapter 20).

Question 3 is most relevant for surgery in the past few months. If the client underwent major surgery in the last 12 weeks, then follow the DVT Risk Principles (see Chapter 11). Consider following it for longer if there are other DVT risk factors, if major surgery was performed on the lower extremities or hip, or a fracture was involved. For minor surgeries such as skin biopsies or other surface work, check with the

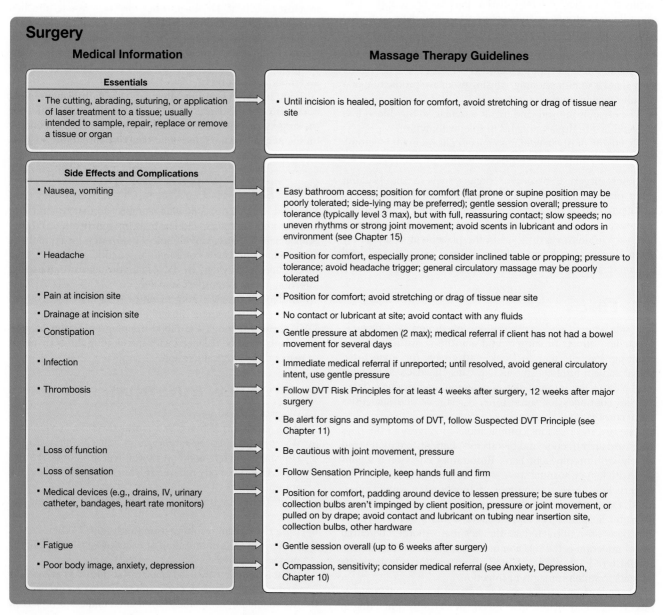

FIGURE 21-5. A Decision Tree for surgery.

patient's doctor and nurse to see whether it's necessary to be so careful; chances are that 4 weeks of DVT Risk Principles are more than sufficient.

Questions 4–7 address any lingering effects of surgery. The answers might reveal side effects such as fatigue, headache, nausea and vomiting, constipation, or pain at the incision site. There might have been surgery complications. If side effects or complications were a long time ago, they may not present an issue for massage therapy. If surgery was recent, the client may still be recovering. See the Decision Tree for massage adjustments in this case.

If there are lingering effects of anesthesia that reduce pain perception, or any analgesics that mask sensation, gentle work overall is indicated—especially in the areas of joint movement and pressure. This is true, too, for fatigue.

If the client has a headache, avoid massage with general circulatory intent. A gentle overall session is in order. These guidelines are advised, also, for anyone taking strong medications that reduce perception.

If the client is experiencing constipation, see Chapter 15 to know how to help. If the client has not had a bowel movement for several days, the client should contact his or her doctor. Avoid pressure above level 2 in the abdomen.

For pain at the incision site, have the client point to all incision sites. Adjust the client's position so that there is no pressure or drag at the site. Adjust pressure near the site to avoid any pull on the area, and if it is really sensitive, then be cautious with the drape, as well. Especially be alert to the drape pulling on the area as the client turns or repositions.

Question 5 about surgery complications points to two main issues: infection and DVT. Stay especially alert to the possibility of postoperative complications in the days after surgery. This is when the risks of DVT and infection are the highest. Signs of DVT (see Chapter 11) and signs of infection—fever plus the four signs of inflammation—should be brought to the client's attention and, if not reported to the doctor, strongly encourage an immediate or urgent referral. If infection is present, massage therapy with circulatory intent should be avoided until it has resolved. Use gentle techniques overall, including gentle pressure (maximum about 2 or 3, depending on tolerance).

If there has been loss in sensation, then follow the Sensation Principle in the affected area. Ask the client to point to the area and use gentle pressure—in the 1–3 range.

> *The Sensation Principle. In an area of impaired or absent sensation, use caution with pressure and joint movement.*

If there has been loss of function, ask more: Does it involve muscle weakness, movement restriction, or problems with organ function? Answers can be many and varied. If there is muscle weakness, avoid vigorous stretching at the involved joint in any direction. Massage pressure should be conservative on the muscle and any agonists and antagonists, unless you are working closely with a client's physical therapist or other rehabilitation staff. If there is simply restricted movement, massage therapy to free the area may be indicated, but scar work to free adhesions should be undertaken only with specialized training. If organ function is compromised, ask which organ and refer to the appropriate chapter for massage therapy guidelines.

Work around any surgical drains, ostomy sites, catheters, or IVs. Consider the tubing that connects to these areas to be part of the person—another appendage to avoid. On entering a patient's hospital or rehab room, take a visual survey of equipment to avoid stumbling or catching any lines. Position the client comfortably, avoiding impingement and taking care to avoid catching the drape on equipment as the client repositions. Avoid touching the tubing with lubricant at the insertion sites or any collection bulbs or other receptacles.

It can take a while to recover from major surgery, and if the client is still recovering, the overall massage should be gentle at first. Question 8 will help illuminate how well the client has recovered; a return to full activity, especially exercise, suggests that the person's tolerance of massage is strong, as well. Six weeks is a common surgery recovery time, although many people are surprised when it takes that long or longer. Even though a surgery seems remote and long ago after a few weeks, feelings of exhaustion may persist. This is why the activity level is such a good index for massage tolerance.

The second part of Question 8 can also help you plan the session. After surgery, a client is given a list of aftercare instructions. Infection is a real concern—either infection through an incision site or a drain or a respiratory infection from being vulnerable in the hospital. A client may be advised to avoid immersion in a bath or wetting the incision area in a shower. The client might be told to be alert for signs of infection or DVT and to contact his or her treating physician if any occur. The client might be told to limit lifting or movement in an area. You can "borrow the medical concern," keeping alert for signs of infection and DVT, and refer the client to his or her doctor for immediate care if any materialize. Apply any movement limitations to massage plan, and avoid aggravating the area with pressure near the site until it's healed.

The client's response to Question 9 could turn up a host of medications, depending on the nature of the surgery. Pain relievers are common and are addressed in this chapter. Review this section, and follow the Medication (or Procedure) Principle.

The main massage issues after surgery are summarized in Figure 21-6. Exceptions to these guidelines are only for very minor surgeries at the surface, such as the removal of small skin lesions. For a sense of the restrictions on activities and things patients must monitor after surgery, search the Internet for aftercare instructions for a given surgery. These are often placed on hospital Web sites in the "for patients" education section.

● MASSAGE RESEARCH

One of the largest clinical trials of massage therapy was funded by the U.S. Department of Veterans Affairs and carried out at two VA Medical Centers (Mitchinson et al., 2007). This study followed a sample of 605 veterans, average age 64 years, for the first 5 postoperative days in the hospital after major surgery. The subjects were randomized to three groups: usual care; usual care plus 20 minutes daily of individualized attention without touch; usual care plus 20 minutes of effleurage to the back each day.

The central outcome of interest was pain control. In all three groups, the pain intensity dropped to the same level by day 5 postsurgery, but pain intensity and unpleasantness declined significantly *faster* in the massage group than in the

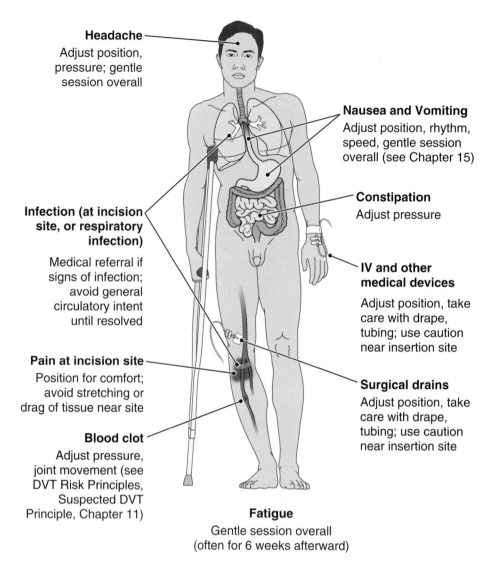

Headache
Adjust position,
pressure; gentle
session overall

Nausea and Vomiting
Adjust position, rhythm,
speed, gentle session
overall (see Chapter 15)

Constipation
Adjust pressure

**Infection (at incision
site, or respiratory
infection)**

Medical referral if
signs of infection;
avoid general
circulatory intent
until resolved

**IV and other
medical devices**

Adjust position, take
care with drape,
tubing; use caution
near insertion site

Pain at incision site
Position for comfort;
avoid stretching or
drag of tissue near site

Surgical drains
Adjust position, take
care with drape,
tubing; use caution
near insertion site

Blood clot
Adjust pressure,
joint movement (see
DVT Risk Principles,
Suspected DVT
Principle, Chapter 11)

Fatigue
Gentle session overall
(often for 6 weeks afterward)

FIGURE 21-6. Surgery: common side effects, complications, and massage therapy guidelines to consider. Specific instructions and additional massage therapy guidelines are in Decision Tree and text.

other groups. The strongest massage effects were seen on the 1st day postsurgery, typically a time of significant patient distress, analgesic use, and respiratory complications from opioid analgesics. Postoperative pain tends to develop right after surgery, and it can increase rapidly. Any pain relief during the acute postoperative period is extremely welcome, as anyone who has had major surgery can attest.

Of interest is the observation that there was no reduction in opioid use in the massage group compared to the others. The authors pointed out that massage was provided on a schedule (nightly), not as needed, the way pain medications are. They raised the question of whether opioid use could decrease if massage were delivered as needed. If pain relief can come to patients in nonpharmacologic ways, this could reduce patient distress, the need for opioids, and dangerous complications from their use. Moreover, the investigators reported no adverse effects related to the massage in the 200 patients who received it, suggesting that massage could be delivered on a large scale, safely, in a hospital setting. For anyone organizing a hospital massage program, this is important safety data.

An RCT of massage therapy in 605 patients is an achievement in the massage profession. It suggests expanding interest in massage therapy and greater dedication of research funds to massage. In and of itself, this is a promising sign.

● POSSIBLE MASSAGE BENEFITS

When a person is preparing for surgery, massage can help relieve anxiety. A relaxation massage the night before a procedure, or early the morning of the procedure, can be beneficial. After surgery, massage may help relieve pain, nausea, constipation, and fatigue. Judiciously applied, relaxing strokes could facilitate sleep and therefore healing.

Massage therapy may also help considerably with a client's body image after surgery. Surgery can be experienced as a traumatic event and, in some cases, brings about obvious changes in the body. Surgical scars and missing limbs or other tissue can be emotionally traumatic and difficult to accept. A therapist's acceptance of the changed body, and his or her compassion, may help cultivate the client's own acceptance and compassion for him- or herself.

Organ and Tissue Transplant

Advances in modern medicine have made it possible for tissue and whole organs to be transplanted from one individual to another, a phenomenon that would have been hard to dream of a few decades ago. In an **organ transplant**, also called a *solid organ transplant*, an intact organ such as a kidney or heart is transferred from one individual to another. In a **tissue transplant**, a smaller amount of tissue is transferred, as in fetal tissue or stem cells from the blood.

● BACKGROUND

Transplantation can be a complicated process, requiring thoughtful preparatory matching of the **graft**, the tissue or organ to be transplanted, and the recipient, or **host**. When the graft comes from a donor other than the patient, it is called an *allograft*. Transplantation with an allograft may involve enormous measures to prevent rejection, and careful monitoring. It is one of the strongest treatments available in medicine, with multiple, layered side effects and complications. A massage therapist working with transplant patients takes on a number of challenging tasks. Keeping track of the procedures and medications, as they may change, is one of them.

Indications

A transplanted heart, lung, kidney, or liver may make survival possible in the face of organ failure. When a vital organ starts to fail, essential functions are compromised. It is only a matter of time before homeostasis is lost, resulting in dysfunction in multiple body systems. In certain cases, a *solid organ transplant* can be lifesaving.

Depending on the type of transplant, the donor might be living or deceased. Examples of transplants with living donors are kidney, liver tissue, and stem cell. A heart transplant obviously requires an organ from a deceased donor. In most cases, a critical issue is the timely availability of a matching donor, that is, one whose tissue is compatible with that of the recipient, or host. The closer the match, the more likely the transplant will "take"—a process known as **engraftment**. Other types of transplants provide new organ tissue to the recipient. Tissue from the pancreas may be transplanted. A tendon from a cadaver might serve as a ligament in a recipient's knee. Even bone tissue can be transplanted.

A **stem cell transplant (SCT)** is the transplantation of stem cells into the blood of a patient. **Stem cells** are used from the blood or bone marrow because they are unspecialized cells, capable of differentiating into all blood cell types and generating new, healthy cells. They are extracted from the bloodstream in a SCT, or harvested directly from the bone marrow in a *bone marrow transplant (BMT)*. Even though the source of stem cells differs in the two procedures, the terms SCT and BMT are often used interchangeably. SCT is used in certain blood diseases, including hematologic cancers such as leukemia (see Chapter 12). The procedure is explained in Chapter 20.

In an **allogeneic** transplant, stem cells are used from a donor, with careful monitoring for the first 100 days, and a recovery time of around 1 year. In an **autologous** transplant, the patient's own cells are used and carefully treated before reintroduction, and the procedure often can be completed in a 3-week hospital stay with follow-up. In either case, additional medical procedures, monitoring, and medications are required to support a successful SCT.

Side Effects

In any transplant, complications occur when the donor tissue is different enough from the host's tissue that one is rejected by the other. The immune system, which recognizes and destroys tissue considered "other," may interfere with the desired outcome in this way. Strong immunosuppressive drugs are needed to manage the transition. In many cases, the need for these drugs is lifelong.

Because of the need for strong antirejection drugs, many side effects and complications occur during organ and tissue transplantation. At the outset of the treatment, most patients are unwell by definition, with some measure of tissue or organ failure. Not all patients have the same transplant experience; some sail through with fewer complications than others. Of all the types of transplants, allogeneic stem cell transplantation, in which high-dose chemotherapy and possible total body irradiation (TBI) are added to the procedure, is known for some of the strongest side effects in medicine (see Chapter 20).

Depending on the type of transplant, patients may experience the following problems:

- Low blood cell counts, and immunosuppression (from antirejection drugs, and additionally from high-dose chemotherapy in the case of a SCT)
- Organ or tissue rejection
- Organ or tissue failure (either the transplanted organ, or other organ affected by the procedure, such as liver, kidney)
- Graft-vs.- host disease (GVHD)
- GI effects (mouth sores, nausea, vomiting, heartburn, stomach pain, stomach ulcer, bloating, constipation, diarrhea)
- Tissue breakdown (thinned skin, slow wound healing, osteoporosis)
- Fluid balance changes (swelling of feet, face, hands; hypertension)
- Pain (in joints, muscles, stomach and abdominal pain, headache)
- General effects (fatigue, fever, dizziness, drowsiness, hypotension, weakness, violent shaking [*rigors*], tremor, seizures, insomnia, mood changes)

Of these complications, two warrant a closer look: antirejection drugs and GVHD.

Antirejection drugs include mycophenolate mofetil (CellCept), corticosteroids (Deltasone, Methylprednisolone), monoclonal antibodies (Zenapax, Orthoclone OKT3), cyclosporine A (Sandimmune, Neoral), tacrolimus (Prograf, Protopic), sirolimus (Rapamycin, Rapamune), and mitotic inhibitors (Cytoxan, Imuran). These drugs cause a host of side effects, including nausea, GI upset, constipation, diarrhea, mouth sores, fever, headache, seizures, tremor, *rigors* (shaking), edema, and hair loss.

At antirejection doses, corticosteroids can cause dramatic changes in physical appearance: acne, stretch marks, puffy face, obesity in the trunk, and weight gain due to increased appetite. The typical side effects of corticosteroids are aggravated at these doses: hypertension and hyperglycemia, osteoporosis, easy bruising, and mood swings can be problematic.

It is a dance: keeping antirejection in force but managing the side effects and complications of antirejection drugs at the same time. Some of the problems caused by antirejection drugs are temporary and tend to fade with continued use, and others, such as osteoporosis, worsen with continued use. For this reason, dosages are reduced as soon as possible to the minimum needed to prevent rejection. Yet immunosuppressants may be required indefinitely. In a kidney transplant, the risk of rejection is highest in the first 4 months, but it can occur at any time.

Antirejection drugs help prevent the patient's immune system from rejecting a donated organ or tissue, but rejection can go both ways, so these drugs also prevent the *donated tissue* from rejecting its new *host*. Throughout many types of transplants, patients are monitored carefully for **graft-vs.- host disease (GVHD)**, in which the donor immune cells (the graft) mount an immune response against the host's (patient's) tissues, perceived as foreign (see "Stem Cell Transplant," Chapter 20). GVHD can even occur when solid organs or other tissues are transplanted, because donor immune cells travel in those tissues, then react to the host environment.

Acute GVHD occurs soon after a transplant; chronic GVHD often develops after successful engraftment, and it can be lifelong. Unless they are working in a transplant unit, massage therapists are more likely to encounter the chronic form of GVHD.

Both acute and chronic GVHD range from mild to severe and reflect widespread inflammation of the skin, liver, and GI tract. In GVHD, scattered skin lesions typically appear at first in a painful or itchy rash. The disease is considered more severe when more of the body surface is involved. Eyes are dry, irritated, and light sensitive. GI disturbances are common. Obstructive lung disease might occur with respiratory distress, and neuropathic pain may set in. Muscle cramps and muscle weakness are typical. Serious cases of GVHD include fever, intense, generalized reddening of the skin, and peeling or shedding of the skin. Severe GVHD can be life threatening.

Other complications of transplant include infertility, cataracts, and injury to the heart and lungs. In the long term, the toxic effects of transplant medications can also lead to the development of cancer.

Management of Side Effects

People having transplants may be taking a whole array of medications to manage side effects. In general, these come under the following groups:

1. *Drugs to prevent or treat infection.* These include antivirals (Zovirax, Cytovene), antibiotics (Bactrim, Septra), and antifungal drugs (Mycostatin, Nilstat). Side effects include nausea, vomiting, diarrhea, GI upset, dizziness, confusion, nervousness, tremor, swelling, orthostatic hypotension, fatigue.

2. *Drugs for symptom management.* These include antiulcer medications (Propulsid, Pepcid, Prilosec), antihypertensives (Procardia XL, Florinef, Lasix), antihyperglycemics (various forms of insulin), antiemetics (see Chapter 20), and analgesics (this chapter). Standard drugs for diarrhea and constipation are used. IV nutrition may be needed, as well as transfusions of red blood cells (RBCs) and platelets.

● INTERVIEW QUESTIONS

1. When was the transplant?
2. What kind of transplant did you have? What was involved in the procedure?
3. How are you feeling now? What is your activity level? Are there any medical restrictions on your activities?
4. Are you taking any antirejection medications? Which ones?
5. What is your level of infection risk at this point?
6. Are you taking any medications to prevent or treat infection? Which ones?
7. Are you taking any other medications? Which medications, and for what purpose?
8. How do your medications affect you? Of the medications you are taking, what are the side effects that you experience?
9. How are your blood counts?
10. How are your skin, muscles, and bones? Are any of your doctors concerned about their stability? Does your skin bruise easily, or is there any osteoporosis?
11. Have you had any occurrences of GVHD?

● MASSAGE THERAPY GUIDELINES

Question 1 is pivotal to the massage plan. For a recent transplant (within the last year), the client may be weakened by the procedure and the strong medications needed to keep the transplant intact. During the interview, be sensitive to the possibility that repeating the whole story could be exhausting. This is especially true for fatigued and ill clients. Whenever possible, read up on the client's type of transplant beforehand. Some therapists, working within a facility, may have access to the patient's chart and can bypass the need to ask the patient so many questions.

Question 2 about the type of transplant is standard. A short summary of the steps involved in the transplant will help you understand the extent of the procedures. See the Decision Tree for guidelines. Much less detail is needed if the transplant took place years ago, was successful, and the person returned to a high level of function. For more recent procedures, a more extensive list of medications is likely. Ask about organ function, and adapt your massage plan to the current level of function.

Question 3 provides a picture of the client's current health and activity level. The client's activity tolerance will inform the massage therapy tolerance. A client who is still recovering from a transplant a few months later may be significantly curtailed in his or her activity by fatigue, weight gain, and other side effects of medications. On the other hand, a client who is years beyond the transplant may be fully functioning: taking care of children, moderately physically active, and so on. A massage therapy session would need to be significantly gentler for the first client than the second. Likewise, if activity restrictions are in place, they reflect the physician's level of concern for the client's overall health, and perhaps the health of individual organs. Vigorous activity is ill-advised (and the client rarely feels like it) until a transplant has fully "taken" and assumed a normal level of function. Massage accordingly.

Use Questions 3–6 to determine any infection control precautions. You can mirror any precautions that nurses or friends and family are following for the client. Where possible, ask the client ahead of time where he or she was treated, and go to the hospital's Web site for aftercare information. Hospitals

Organ and Tissue Transplant

Medical Information

Essentials

- The transfer of tissue or organs (graft) from one individual to another (host); used to replace diseased host tissue; requires careful matching of compatible tissues to prevent rejection between graft and host

Side Effects and Complications

- Immunosuppression

- Thrombocytopenia, easy bruising, bleeding

- Anemia

- Organ failure (liver, kidney)

- Vital Organ transplant

- Graft vs. host disease

- Nausea, vomiting, heartburn, stomach pain, stomach ulcer, bloating, constipation, diarrhea

- Mouth sores

- Thinned skin, slow wound healing

- Osteoporosis

- Swelling of feet, face, hands

- Hypertension

- Pain in joints and muscles

- Headache

- Fatigue

- Fever

- Dizziness, drowsiness, orthostatic hypotension

- Weakness

- Shaking (rigors)

- Tremor

- Seizures

- Insomnia

- Mood changes

Massage Therapy Guidelines

- Ask whether graft is fully functioning; if not, adapt massage plan to current level of function

- Be cautious if transplant recent (in last year)

- Adjust massage to activity level and activity tolerance, any medical restrictions on activities

- Follow hygeinic precautions (standard precautions, neutropenic precautions, or isolation precautions as recommended by health care team); no general circulatory intent; gentle pressure (level 1-3 max depending on tolerance, medical consultation); reschedule if you are ill or symptomatic

- Limit pressure depending on tissue stability; generally level 1-2 max; do not advance to level 3 without physician consultation; see Thrombocytopenia, Chapter 12

- Gentle session overall; reposition gently, slow speed and even rhythm, slow rise from table, gente transition at end of session; adjust ambient temperature; drape for warmth (see Anemia, Chapter 12)

- Follow Vital Organ Principle; see Chronic or Acute Kidney Failure, Chapter 18; see Liver Failure, Chapter 16

- Follow Vital Organ Principle unless/until organ is fully functioning

- No friction, lubricant, over affected skin; avoid general circulatory intent unless physician consulted; massage during acute GVHD may be inappropriate; use gentle holding with soft hands (pressure level 1 or 2)

- See Table 21-1; see Nausea, Peptic Ulcer Disease, Constipation, Diarrhea, Chapter 15

- Limit pressure at face; use alternative to face cradle if necessary

- Limit overall pressure (level 2-3 max for most)

- See Osteoporosis, Chapter 9

- Avoid general circulatory intent

- See Hypertension, Chapter 11

- No pressure or joint movement that might aggravate pain; monitor results

- Position for comfort, especially prone; consider inclined table or propping; gentle session overall; pressure to tolerance; slow speed and even rhythm; general circulatory intent may be poorly tolerated (see Headache, Chapter 10)

- Gentle session overall

- No general circulatory intent; gentle pressure (level 2-3 max, depending on tolerance)

- Reposition gently

- To prepare client for transition at end of session, provide time for slow rise from table

- Slow rise from table; reposition gently, limit joint movement

- Massage therapy with moving strokes not appropriate, but firm, steady, stationary pressure may be welcome

- No significant massage adjustments; see Parkinson Disease, Chapter 10

- See Seizures; Seizure Disorders, Chapter 10

- When appropriate, use sedative intent at end of day, activiting/invigorating intent at beginning

- Sensitivity to sudden mood changes; urge client to report to physician if unreported

FIGURE 21-7. A Decision Tree for organ and tissue transplant. Numerous side effects and complications listed here include effects of antirejection drugs, as well as effects of antivirals, antibiotics, antifungals, and additional drugs used to manage side effects.

specializing in organ and tissue transplants generally have excellent patient education materials, and many are easy to find on the Internet.

There may be few infection control precautions, or many. Your client may be confined to home and will require home visits, with everyone in contact required to mask and glove. It may be that the client is able to go out but must avoid crowded areas, the salad bar at restaurants, or even rooms with potted plants or pets, because of mold spores and other pathogens. Adapt your massage and massage setting, where applicable to these requirements.

Monitor your own health: be alert for signs of respiratory, GI, or skin infection. For example, if you have a scratchy throat or sniffles, inform your immunosuppressed client (and possibly the health care team). Even if you think your symptoms are caused by allergies rather than a cold, you will probably be prohibited from contact with the client, depending on where the client is in the recovery process. In Therapist's Journal 21-2, a massage therapist describes these measures, in the 1st year of her life as a transplant patient.

In general, if your client is vulnerable to infection, the infection control measures will be clear, and there is little guesswork. General circulatory intent is not recommended—it is too strong for someone whose body is still gaining strength.

Questions 7 and 8 should capture any medications for other conditions, such as hypertension, diabetes, ulcers, or other side effects. Space limits full discussion of every side effect here, but the principal side effects and complications, such as dizziness, insomnia, mood changes, and swelling, are listed in the Decision Tree, along with brief massage therapy guidelines (see Figure 21-7). Most related conditions, such as hypertension, osteoporosis, and peptic ulcer disease, are also addressed in preceding chapters. Be mindful of the Medication (or Procedure) Principle when learning about each of the client's medications.

> *The Medication Principle. Adapt massage to the condition for which the medication is taken or prescribed, and to any side effects.*

Question 9 about blood counts should be asked at each visit as long as the client is taking medication for the transplant. Blood counts can change over a period of days. In a SCT, white blood cells (WBCs) tend to return to function first after the transplant, followed by platelets and RBCs. Questions 4–6 probably caught any WBC issues, but if the answer to this question raises any problem in RBC or platelet counts, refer to Chapter 12 on blood conditions and Chapter 20 on cancer therapies for guidance. Easy bruising will limit your pressure to level 2, and possibly level 3 as the client improves.

Question 10 is a catchall question that directs you regarding pressure and joint movement. Because many antirejection drugs affect the skin, thinned skin and easy bruising dictate gentle pressure, probably in the level 1–3 range for most clients. If the client's skin or bones are particularly fragile, with high-dose or long-term corticosteroid use, then the lighter range might even be in order. The client's doctor or nurse can provide good guidance.

Question 11 about GVHD should be followed with more questions if the answer is yes. Ask how serious it was or is, which tissues were affected, and any symptoms. Your client might have mild, chronic GVHD on his or her chest, which

is easy to work around. Be cautious around any skin lesions; contact through a drape might be okay, but not lubricant, stroking, or friction. Limit your stationary pressure to level 1 or 2. Check with the physician about whether general circulatory intent is advised.

● MASSAGE RESEARCH

At the time of this writing, there are a few small studies of massage and transplant, all of them focused on SCT patients. One study reported that massage therapy was associated with improved comfort and fewer CNS complications in adult patients (Smith et al., 2003). Another suggested effects of massage on distress, fatigue, nausea, and anxiety at different time points in the SCT procedure (Ahles et al., 1999). Another group, looking at massage in caregivers of SCT patients, found significant declines in anxiety, depression, and fatigue in the massage group (Rexilius et al., 2002). And a report to the journal *Bone Marrow Transplantation* describes the use of a massage service in a BMT unit of children and adult patients (Davies et al., 2008)

At the time of this writing, a multi-site team is investigating the effects of massage therapy and humor therapy in children undergoing SCT (Phipps et al.). Led by a researcher at St. Jude Children's Research Hospital in Memphis, Tennessee, they are also testing massage therapy and relaxation training in the parents of these patients.

This researcher had already carried out a small pilot study of massage and other interventions in this population. In that study, massage seemed to have little effect on well-being or symptoms in patients but was associated with shorter engraftment time and earlier discharge from the hospital (Phipps et al., 2005). Investigators were careful not to overstate these surprising results; instead, they devoted themselves to this follow-up study to see if these outcomes are true effects of massage. A similar study is in progress at the University of California-San Francisco, where investigators are also adding massage training for the resident parents to use with their children (Mehling et al.,). The small studies in print so far do not provide conclusive evidence of massage benefit. However, they have raised some interesting questions for follow-up research, and it will be interesting to see what comes from these ongoing studies.

● POSSIBLE MASSAGE BENEFITS

Having a transplant can be a very isolating experience—literally as well as emotionally. The medical restrictions on activities interfere with many levels of normal life, especially in the realm of contact with others. With antirejection therapy and the profound immunosuppression that can result, patients are cautioned about sharing breathing space and touch with everyone they love and need. There can be an additional emotional overlay from perceiving others—one's children, partner, friends, and everyone on the street—as a potential source of germs. The level of fear that is engendered to keep the patient safe during this tender, important time is significant, in keeping with the life-threatening consequences.

Sometimes transplants do not work, and the potential for, or reality of, rejection can be frightening. Side effects and complications make it one of the most grueling medical procedures known. Coupled with the possibility that the therapy could be unsuccessful, the strength it takes to survive can make a marathon event into a terrifying one as well.

THERAPIST'S JOURNAL 21-2 *My Stem Cell Transplant*

In November of 2004, I had a routine colonoscopy. At the time my doctor asked to draw blood because my skin color was gray. But I didn't wear makeup, and I was busy with three small children, so I hadn't thought anything of it.

Shortly after returning home from the colonoscopy, the hospital called and asked me to return to the ER as soon as possible. Once there an ER doctor told me that my blood work showed leukemia. I was in disbelief. An oncologist was called in to do a bone marrow test and reassure me they would do all they could to treat my cancer. Results were positive for AML, and without immediate treatment, things did not look good. With that news, my whole life changed.

I knew I had limited options, and I didn't question the doctors' recommendations. I was admitted at once, and the following morning chemotherapy was started. After 3½ weeks I finally went into remission and was able to go home for a quick Christmas with my family. The following January, I was admitted to a cancer center for a SCT. It was an allogeneic transplant, and my brother was the donor. It was also my only option for survival.

For another 3½ weeks I lived in isolation, in a glassed-in, positive pressurized room. My IV pole was outside the room so that the nurses could service it without coming in. It was linked by a 50-ft clear tube to the port in my chest. I was under isolation precautions. Every magazine, every CD, everything was checked and wiped down before it was allowed in. When people came in, which was rarely, they wore gloves, gowns, and masks.

To wipe out my problematic white cells, I underwent several days of TBI. I lay on what looked like a stovetop for a few minutes each day. The side effects were terrible: Pain, bone pain, fatigue, and horrible mouth sores that made it hard to eat, drink, and swallow. I lost 75 pounds through the whole experience.

After that, in a move that turned out to be anticlimactic after all of the buildup, I received a bag of blood from my brother through an IV. He had been stuck about 150 times in an effort to get the needed supply of bone marrow out. He couldn't walk for 2 weeks! But they let him see me before he left. I visited my family via webcam and webphone. I missed them terribly.

Each day I would walk the sanitized hallway and see other patients on the transplant unit who were too sick to move. I thought, I'm doing okay, but I wished they were, too. A team of seven doctors would see me every morning and I tried hard to sit up, look at them, and look well so that they would think well of my prognosis.

I was released from the hospital with instructions to remain in my home for the next year. Everyone around me, including my kids, had to glove, mask, and sanitize. I used a separate bathroom, drank only bottled water, and followed strict food sanitation. For the most part, I followed instructions except to sneak out—bald, masked, and gloved—and watch my kids' plays at school. I think I terrified the other children! And I always came clean to my doctors: "I snuck out." They were reproachful. But I had to feel like a human when it came to my kids.

My medications during that year cost $4,000 a day. I had about 12 prescriptions and took 20 different pills daily. There was a time lag before insurance kicked in, so the pharmacy would do what they could, dispensing a $600 pill while they waited for insurance to approve it.

After a year, I could go out again, and several years later, I am well. My skin is very soft—my hair grew in curly and shiny, a function of the radiation. I am rosy-cheeked. I get colds a fair amount. I get a little jittery when I get sick, what are the implications? Will I be okay? I returned to my massage practice feeling weak but glad to be back. It took me 2 years to regain my strength so that I now have to ask whether my pressure is too deep! I volunteer for the "Soft Touch Program" at my local hospital, giving hand and foot massage to patients, and I always request the cancer unit. One very ill patient couldn't believe it would help him. He resisted but his wife urged him to try it. He was awestruck that it helped him relax and sleep! Now he calls me his "angel." I have welcomed the chance to give back.

Ann Mantzaris
Wallingford, CT

Touch that is skilled, compassionate, and unafraid can be especially welcome during this time, and massage therapists who work with inpatients or outpatients can help ease the isolation of the experience. Symptom relief from pain, nausea, fatigue, anxiety, and depression is possible, along with an experience of deep relaxation that can promote sleep, hope, and coping resources. At the very least, massage can provide a brief respite from the realities of a transplant experience. Massage therapists have many gifts to bring to the transplant recipient: simple gifts they hold in their own hands.

Massage Therapy, Medical Treatments, and Side Effects

Over a lifetime of massage practice, a therapist will encounter hundreds, and perhaps thousands of medications. Medications in common use will become familiar, as they appear repeatedly on the client health history form, or come up again and again in conversation.

The Medication Principle. Adapt massage to the condition for which the medication is taken or prescribed, and to any side effects.

Many medications, procedures, and side effects have appeared in this book, along with corresponding massage therapy guidelines, but space limits a full discussion of all of them. As specified in the Medication Principle (see Chapter 3), it is not necessary to have specific guidelines for each drug listed under every condition. Instead, once your client tells you about a medication, you can use several tools to reason your way to a massage plan:

1. The Four Medication Questions (see Chapter 4)
2. Drug texts and references for massage therapists (Wible, 2005, 2009; Persad, 2001)
3. Internet databases of medications and side effects, for example, at www.drugs.com or at the National Library of Medicine at www.nlm.nih.gov/medlineplus/druginformation.html

Used alone or in combination, these three tools can help you adjust your massage plan for most situations. A fourth tool appears in Table 21-1: an alphabetical list of common side effects, complications, and massage therapy guidelines. The information in this table is compiled for use with any medical condition, any drug or procedure, and many side effects. Locate a side effect and the corresponding massage therapy adjustments needed to work safely. If you are still not sure whether you have complete information, involve the client's doctor or nurse in the massage plan. If they are not available, work conservatively for the first session, and explain your reasoning to your client.

Massage therapists are increasingly called to work with vulnerable populations, multiple conditions, and complex treatments. As clients age, this trend will continue, and these factors can limit the massage plan at times. Within these limits, however, there are many rich and creative possibilities for touch.

TABLE 21-1.	MASSAGE THERAPY GUIDELINES FOR COMMON SIDE EFFECTS OF MEDICATIONS AND PROCEDURES

Abdominal Discomfort, Bloating, Gas

- Adjust for discomfort in lower abdomen (padding above and below for prone position, or use side-lying).

Anemia

- Gentle session overall; reposition gently, slow speed and even rhythm, slow rise from table, gentle transition at end of session.
- Adjust ambient temperature; drape for warmth (see "Anemia," Chapter 12).

Anxiety

- Encourage medical referral if unreported; inquire about anxiety triggers and avoid (see Anxiety, Chapter 10).

Arrhythmia

- Immediate/emergency medical referral if acute, if client has not reported to his/her doctor.

Bleeding

- Follow DVT Risk Principles (see Chapter 11).
- Use gentle pressure overall.
- Avoid contact with site.

Bone Pain

- Avoid strong joint movement; use gentle pressure; holding with still, soft hands may ease pain.

Bone Thinning

- Gentle overall pressure, gentle joint movement (see 'Osteoporosis," Chapter 9).

Bowel Urgency; Bowel Incontinence

- Easy bathroom access; gentle session overall; avoid contact or pressure at abdomen that could aggravate condition.

Breast Enlargement

- Position for comfort; pad above and below breasts in prone position if needed.

Bruising; Easy Bruising or Bleeding

- In general, use gentle pressure overall.
- If caused by low platelets, see "Thrombocytopenia," Chapter 12.
- If caused by antiplatelet drugs: Slight pressure modification overall (usually level 1–3, possibly 4); see Chapter 11.
- If caused by anticoagulants: Adjust pressure to stability of tissues; gentle pressure overall (level 1–2 maximum); with physician approval, can use pressure level 3 overall; see Chapter 11.
- If caused by thrombolytics: Adjust pressure to stability of tissues; overall pressure maximum level 1; work in close communication with client's doctor; see Chapter 11.

(continued)

TABLE 21-1.	MASSAGE THERAPY GUIDELINES FOR COMMON SIDE EFFECTS OF MEDICATIONS AND PROCEDURES (Continued)

Cardiotoxicity (Heart Muscle Damage)

- Rare, serious complication; heart function is usually well monitored if cardiotoxicity is anticipated; treatment typically stopped or reduced if it occurs.
- If client reports shortness of breath, dizziness, leg swelling, fatigue, rapid heartbeat, cough with bloody sputum, and has not reported symptoms to physician, emergency medical referral.
- If diagnosed condition, avoid general circulatory intent; immediate medical referral if symptoms worsening (see Congestive Heart Failure, Chapter 11).

Confusion

- Obtain permission of the client's family and health care team
- Provide simple session with gentle pressure, slow speed, predictable rhythm.
- Use simple, sensitive communication; observe nonverbal cues to be sure that the touch is welcome.

Constipation

- If abdominal tenderness present, or no bowel movement in 72 hours, limit pressure at site (level 1 max), make medical referral; otherwise, gentle abdominal massage (level 2 max) may be helpful; see "Constipation," Chapter 15.

Dehydration

- If symptoms/signs of mild dehydration (increased thirst; dry mouth; dark yellow urine; reduced urine output), gentle overall session (gentle pressure overall, slow speeds, even rhythm, avoid general circulatory intent); have drinking water available.
- If symptoms/signs of moderate dehydration (strong thirst; dark amber/brown urine; urine output down by half in past 24 hours; lightheadedness relieved by lying down; irritability; restlessness; muscle cramps; rapid heartbeat; arms/legs cool to touch), urgent medical referral; encourage hydration; if providing massage, gentle overall session, avoid general circulatory intent.
- If symptoms/signs of severe dehydration (rapid respiration rate; rapid heart rate; weak pulse; faintness not relieved by lying down; lightheadedness that persists after 2 minutes standing; behavior changes; confusion; sleepiness; anxiety; cold/clammy skin or hot/dry skin; little or no urination in last 12 hours), emergency medical referral.

Depression

- Compassion, sensitivity.
- Encourage medical referral if undiagnosed or untreated; be alert for complications (see "Depression," Chapter 10).

Diarrhea

- Easy bathroom access; gentle session overall; avoid contact or pressure at abdomen that could aggravate condition; be alert for signs of dehydration (see above). See "Diarrhea," Chapter 15.

Dizziness

- Medical referral if severe or persistent; reposition gently, slow speed and even rhythm, slow rise from table, gentle transition at end of session.

Drowsiness

- To prepare client for transition at end of session, provide time for slow rise from table.
- Consider ending session with gently stimulating/invigorating strokes to facilitate alertness (Wible, 2009)

Fatigue

- Gentle session overall; massage should offer support rather than further challenge; follow the Compromised Client Principle (see Chapter 3).

Fever

- No general circulatory intent; gentle pressure (level 2–3 maximum) overall; firm, nonmoving contact may be welcome; urge client to report this side effect to the doctor.

Flu-like Symptoms

- Use gentle pressure overall (level 2 max), avoid general circulatory intent; use even rhythms, slow speeds, limited joint movement; drape for comfort; consider shorter session. Stationary touch may be more welcome than moving touch.

(continued)

TABLE 21-1.	MASSAGE THERAPY GUIDELINES FOR COMMON SIDE EFFECTS OF MEDICATIONS AND PROCEDURES (Continued)

Gastrointestinal Upset

- Adjust position for comfort (consider inclined table for reflux/heartburn); pad to reduce pressure on area, or use side-lying position with hips flexed/legs drawn up).
- Consider scheduling massage at better times of day, away from peak side effect.
- See Abdominal discomfort, above; see "Nausea," "Diarrhea," "Constipation," Chapter 15.

Hair Loss

- Ask, "Would you like me to include massage of your head in the session? If so, how would you like me to work with that area?"
- Limit pressure, drag, or contact at head, to client preference.
- Avoid lubricant on wig or head scarf.

Hallucinations; Delusions

- Sensitive, caring communication; possible medical referral; communicate closely with caregivers.

Headache

- Position for comfort, especially prone; consider inclined table or propping; gentle session overall; pressure to tolerance; slow speed and even rhythm; general circulatory intent may be poorly tolerated (see Headache, Chapter 10).
- Urgent medical referral if headache moderate; if headache is severe, immediate medical referral is advised unless cause of headache is certain; in this case, massage is inadvisable, or stationary holds may be all that are tolerable.

Hot Flashes

- Adjust room temperature, drape; avoid hot pads, heat treatments, confining spa wraps.

Hypertension

- Usually BP is monitored closely if a drug elevates blood pressure, especially if the individual's BP is already high.
- If client reports severe, throbbing headache (possible spike in BP), emergency medical referral, especially if baseline BP (without medications) is high.

Hypotension; Orthostatic Hypotension

- Reposition gently.
- To prepare client for transition at end of session, provide time for slow rise from table.
- Consider ending session with gently stimulating/invigorating strokes (Wible, 2009).

Immunosuppression; Poor Immunity

- Always use standard precautions; follow any additional infection control precautions if recommended by client's doctor or nurse (see "Neutropenia," Chapter 12).
- Monitor your own health; if you have signs/symptoms of an infection such as a cold, offer client opportunity to reschedule, or follow client's preferences in this regard.

Infection

- If infection present, avoid general circulatory intent until resolved; use gentle pressure overall (level 2–3 maximum, depending on tolerance and severity of illness.
- For increased infection risk, be alert for signs/symptoms (fever, chills, signs of inflammation); urge medical referral if signs/symptoms of infection have not been reported to physician; urge immediate referral if signs appear at a surgical site.

Injection Site; Injection Site Reaction

- Avoid circulatory intent at injection site until drug is absorbed (24 hours is usually safe if absorption rate unknown); no circulatory intent or friction at site until reaction is resolved.

Insomnia

- When appropriate, use sedative intent at end of day, activating/invigorating intent at beginning.

Itching

- Avoid friction and circulatory intent at affected areas; firm, steady, stationary pressure may be welcome distraction.

Jitteriness, Restlessness

- Use even rhythms, firm, moderate pressure; position for comfort; adapt to need to move, shift, change positions.

(continued)

TABLE 21-1.	MASSAGE THERAPY GUIDELINES FOR COMMON SIDE EFFECTS OF MEDICATIONS AND PROCEDURES (Continued)

Liver Toxicity

- Rare, serious complication; liver function is usually well monitored if liver toxicity is anticipated; treatment typically stopped or reduced if it occurs.
- Be alert for signs (jaundice, nausea, vomiting, dark urine) and make urgent/immediate medical referral if symptoms are worsening or haven't been reported to physician.
- Avoid general circulatory intent; follow Filter and Pump Principle (see "Liver Failure," Chapter 16).

Low Platelets (Thrombocytopenia)

- Gentle overall pressure depending on platelet levels, tissue stability, and physician input; at moderately low levels (50–100K), pressure = level 2–3 maximum depending on ease of bruising; 20–50K, pressure = level 2 max; below 20K, pressure = level 1 max; see "Thrombocytopenia," Chapter 12.

Low Red Blood Cells

- See Anemia, above

Low White Blood Cells (Leukopenia; Neutropenia)

- Strict infection control; ask about neutropenic precautions and follow; monitor your own health; if you have signs/symptoms of any possible communicable disease (cold, flu, GI or skin condition), offer client opportunity to reschedule; see Neutropenia, Chapter 12.

Lymphedema

- If lymphedema is present, or client has a history of it, observe Quadrant Principle for Lymphedema History (see Chapter 13); refer to lymphedema therapist.
- If elevated risk of lymphedema but no history of it, observe Quadrant Principle for Lymphedema Risk (see Chapter 20).

Medical Devices

- Position for comfort, padding around device to lessen pressure; be sure tubes or collection bulbs aren't impinged by client position; pressure or joint movement, or pulled on by drape
- Avoid contact and lubricant on tubing near insertion site, collection bulbs, other hardware.

Mood Changes; Mood Swings

- No specific massage adjustments; patience, compassion.

Mouth Sores

- Limit pressure at face; use alternative to face cradle if necessary.

Muscle Weakness

- Avoid strong joint movement or stretches if joints are less stable.

Nausea, Vomiting

- If mild: position for comfort, gentle session overall; pressure to tolerance, slow speeds; no uneven rhythms or strong joint movement.
- If moderate or severe: easy bathroom access; position for comfort (flat prone or supine position may be poorly tolerated; side-lying may be preferred); gentle session overall; pressure to tolerance (typically level 3 max), but with full, reassuring contact; slow speeds; no uneven rhythms or strong joint movement; avoid scents in lubricant and odors in environment (see Chapter 15).

Nervousness, Trembling

- Use even rhythms, firm, moderate pressure; position for comfort; adapt to need to move, shift, change positions.
- Allow longer for relaxation effect of massage to occur.

Neuropathy; Peripheral Neuropathy

- If numbness, follow Sensation Principle, Sensation Loss, Injury Prone Principle (see Chapter 3).
- If pain, burning, discomfort, position for comfort, use pressure to tolerance.
- See "Peripheral Neuropathy," Chapter 10.

Numbness

- Follow Sensation Principle, Sensation Loss, Injury Prone Principle (see Chapter 3).

(continued)

TABLE 21-1.	**MASSAGE THERAPY GUIDELINES FOR COMMON SIDE EFFECTS OF MEDICATIONS AND PROCEDURES (Continued)**

Pain

- Adjust position for comfort, using bolsters, soft padding, pillows.
- Holding affected area with soft hands, no movement may ease pain.
- Urge medical referral if pain is worsening or persisting.

Rash

- Avoid lubricant, friction, and circulatory intent at site; limit stretching and friction of adjacent tissues to avoid drag at site.
- Inspect skin before each session; avoid contact if open lesions, or if cause unclear.
- Urge medical referral if client has not reported this side effect to doctor.
- See "General Principles," Chapter 7.

Renal Toxicity; Renal Failure

- Rare, serious complication; renal function is usually well monitored if renal toxicity is possible; treatment typically stopped or reduced if it occurs.
- Be alert for signs/symptoms (low urine volume, swelling in lower extremities, drowsiness, confusion, breathing difficulty, fatigue) and make immediate medical referral if symptoms have not been reported to physician.
- If renal toxicity is recent, avoid general circulatory intent; follow Filter and Pump Principle (see Acute Kidney Failure, Chapter 18).

Sedation

- Overall, extremely gentle pressure (level 1–2 maximum) and limited joint movement.
- Reposition gently, slow speed and even rhythm, gentle transition at end of session.

Seizures

- See Seizures, Seizure disorders, Chapter 10.

Sensation Loss

- See Numbness, Neuropathy, above

Sinus Congestion

- Limit flat prone and flat supine position; consider inclined table, seated, side-lying positions.

Skin Thinning

- Limit stretching and friction of tissues; limit pressure at affected areas (level 1–2 or 2–3 maximum for most, depending on tissue stability).

Stomach Ulcers

- See "Peptic Ulcer Disease," Chapter 15.

Swelling (Edema)

- Avoid general circulatory intent if systemic (e.g., face, hands, feet).
- Avoid circulatory intent at site without specialized training, identified cause of swelling (physician consultation is strongly advised)
- If swelling in lower extremities, consider DVT Risk Principles (see Chapter 11)

Tender Breasts

- Possible position changes for comfort; bolster with padding above and below breasts for prone position.

Thrombosis

- If signs and symptoms present (such as swelling, warmth, redness, palpable thrombus, discoloration, superficial venous dilation, pain, tenderness to touch), then follow Suspected DVT Principle see "Deep Vein Thrombosis," Chapter 11).
- If single strong risk factor present, or multiple risk factors, follow DVT Risk Principles (see "Deep Vein Thrombosis," Chapter 11).

Transdermal Patch

- Avoid dislodging transdermal patch; avoid focused pressure and circulatory intent at site of patch; consult physician or nurse if any question about advisability of massage around patch.

Urinary Frequency, Urgency, Incontinence

- Easy bathroom access; advise medical referral if symptoms are worsening or persisting.

(continued)

TABLE 21-1.	MASSAGE THERAPY GUIDELINES FOR COMMON SIDE EFFECTS OF MEDICATIONS AND PROCEDURES (Continued)

Weight Gain

- No massage adjustments (except positioning if necessary).

Weight Loss (Cachexia)

- Gentle session overall; extremely gentle session overall if client is cachexic; limit joint movement if loss of muscle mass makes joints unstable.
- Use extra care around vulnerable vascular and nerve endangerment sites.

SELF TEST

1. Describe the differences between a side effect, complication, and adverse effect.
2. What are the Four Medication Questions and why are they important?
3. Describe how NSAIDs work, and give two examples of massage adjustments for a client taking an NSAID.
4. What are the primary functions of corticosteroids?
5. What are common effects of corticosteroids on bone and skin, and what adjustments to massage might be necessary due to these side effects?
6. Explain the effect of corticosteroid medication on fluid balance and the corresponding massage therapy guideline.
7. Describe the differences between opioid analgesics, mixed narcotic agonist-antagonists, and combination narcotic analgesics.
8. How is the Sensation Principle relevant in working with a client who is taking an opioid medication? For a client after surgery?
9. In the case of a client who has had surgery, what are the two main complications that are monitored carefully after surgery by medical staff? How does each influence the massage plan?

10. According to research, how might massage therapy benefit a postoperative patient?
11. How is a client's activity level after surgery or transplant helpful in planning a massage session?
12. Describe how to adjust massage to any medical devices that might be in place after surgery.
13. What is the purpose of antirejection medications in a tissue or organ transplant? How would you adjust to these medications?
14. According to research, how might massage therapy benefit a client during a SCT?
15. Using Table 21-1, compare the massage guidelines and side effects for the following:
    - Mild vs. severe dehydration
    - Mild vs. moderate nausea
    - Hypertension vs. hypotension
    - Easy bruising caused by antiplatelet drugs vs. bruising caused by anticoagulants

 For answers to these questions and to see a bibliography for this chapter, visit http://thePoint.lww.com/Walton.

Index

Note: Page numbers followed by *b* indicate boxes; those followed by *t* indicate table. Page numbers in italics indicate figures.